AF710826

The Handbook of Health Behavior Change

Second Edition

SALLY A. SHUMAKER, PHD, is Professor of Public Health Sciences and Internal Medicine, and Head of the Section on Social Sciences and Health Policy at The Wake Forest University School of Medicine. In addition, she is director of the Women's Center of Excellence. She holds a doctorate in Social Psychology from The University of Michigan with post-doctoral training in environment and health from the University of California (Irvine and Los Angeles). Dr. Shumaker's primary areas of research interest include women's health, psychosocial factors in primary and secondary prevention of chronic disease, health behavior change and adherence, aging, and health-related quality of life (HRQL).

ELEANOR B. SCHRON, MS, RN, is a Senior Research Nurse with the Clinical Trials Scientific Research Group, of The National Heart, Lung, and Blood Institute. Previously she was a Health Science Analyst with the Office of Health Research, Statistics and Technology, Office of the Assistant Secretary for Health, and Nurse Consultant with the Division of Peer Review of the Office of Professional Standards Review Organizations, Health Care Financing Administration, both within the Department of Health and Human Services. Ms. Schron received her Master's degree in Psychiatric/Mental Health Nursing from the University of Maryland. Her clinical experience includes work in public health, psychiatric/mental health services, and intensive and coronary care areas. Her professional interests include quality-of-life evaluation, adherence in clinical trials and practice, informed consent, clinical trials methodology and administration, women's health, and dissemination of research findings.

JUDITH K. OCKENE, PHD, is Professor of Medicine and Director of the Division of Preventive and Behavioral Medicine at the University of Massachusetts Medical School. Her Ph.D. is in Counseling Psychology from Boston College, and she has a Master's in Science Education. Dr. Ockene's major research has been in the investigation of factors which affect lifestyle behavior change, factors which affect healthcare providers' practice behaviors, women's health, and the relationship of lifestyle behaviors to disease. Her clinical work has involved interventions for cigarette smoking, nutritional behavior, exercise, stress, coping with disease, and the management of other disease-related behaviors.

WENDY L. McBEE, MA, is a Research Associate in Public Health Sciences, Section on Social Sciences and Health Policy, at The Wake Forest University School of Medicine. Ms. McBee received her Master's degree in Psychology from Wake Forest University. Her primary areas of interest include women's health, dementia, health behavior change, disease management, and psychosocial measurement. Currently, Ms. McBee is a project manager for a large, multicenter, randomized clinical trial examining the effects of hormone replacement therapy on the incidence and progression of dementia in older women, the Women's Health Initiative-Memory Study.

The Handbook of Health Behavior Change

Second Edition

Sally A. Shumaker, PhD
Eleanor B. Schron, RN, MS
Judith K. Ockene, PhD
Wendy L. McBee, MA
Editors

Springer Publishing Company

Copyright © 1998 by Springer Publishing Company, Inc.

All rights reserved

No part of this publication may be reproduced, stored in a retrieval system, or transmitted in any form or by any means, electronic, mechanical, photocopying, recording, or otherwise, without the prior permission of Springer Publishing Company, Inc.

Springer Publishing Company, Inc.
11 West 42nd Street
New York, NY 10036

Cover design by Janet Joachim
Acquisitions Editor: Bill Tucker
Production Editor: Jeanne Libby

Library of Congress Cataloging-in-Publication Data

The handbook of health behavior change / edited by Sally A. Shumaker . . . [et al.
— 2nd ed.
p. cm.
Includes bibliographical references and index.
ISBN 0-8261-6782-9
1. Health behavior. 2. Health attitudes. 3. Self-care, Health. 4. Behavior modification. I. Shumaker, Sally A.
RA776.9.H36 1998
613—dc21 98-25632
CIP

Printed in the United States of America

Contents

Contributors

David B. Abrams, Ph.D.
The Miriam Hospital/Brown University School of Medicine
Division of Behavioral & Preventive Medicine
Providence, RI

David G. Altman, Ph.D.
Department of Public Health Sciences
Section on Social Sciences & Health Policy
The Wake Forest University School of Medicine
Winston-Salem, NC

Catherine J. Atkins, Ph.D.
Department of Psychology
San Diego State University
San Diego, CA

Marshall H. Becker, Ph.D., M.P.H.
Deceased

Beth C. Bock
Division of Behavioral & Preventive Medicine
Miriam Hospital/Brown University School of Medicine
Providence, RI

Belinda Borrelli, Ph.D.
The Miriam Hospital/Brown University School of Medicine
Division of Behavioral & Preventive Medicine
Providence, RI

Viktor E. Bovbjerg, M.P.H., Ph.D.
Williamson Institute for Health Studies
Medical College of Virginia
Richmond, VA

Lora E. Burke, M.S.N., R.N.
University of Pittsburgh
School of Nursing
Center for Nursing Research
Pittsburgh, PA

David F. Cella, Ph.D.
Director, Center on Outcomes, Research & Education (CORE)
Evanston, IL

Margaret A. Chesney, Ph.D.
Department of Epidemiology & Biostatistics
School of Medicine
University of California, San Francisco
San Francisco, CA

Matthew M. Clark
Division of Behavioral & Preventive Medicine
Miriam Hospital/Brown University School of Medicine
Providence, RI

Noreen M. Clark, Ph.D.
Dean
University of Michigan
School of Public Health
Ann Arbor, MI

Michael A. Rapoff, Ph.D.
Chief, Behavioral Sciences
Department of Pediatrics
University of Kansas Medical Center
Kansas City, KS

Kurt M. Ribisl, Ph.D.
Stanford Center for Research in Disease Prevention
Stanford University School of Medicine
Palo Alto, CA

Andrew L. Ries, M.D.
Division of Pulmonary & Critical Care Medicine
Northwest Lipid Research Clinic & Dept. of Medicine
University of California, San Diego
La Jolla, CA

Paul G. Salmon, Ph.D.
Department of Psychology
University of Louisville
Louisville, KY

Saki F. Santorelli, Ed.D.
Divsion of Preventive and Behavioral Medicine
Center for Mindfulness in Medicine, Health Care, and Society
University of Massachusetts Medical Center
Worcester, MA

Elizabeth A. Schlenk, Ph.D., R.N.
University of Pittsburgh
School of Nursing
Center for Nursing Research
Pittsburgh, PA

William G. Shadel, Ph.D.
The Miriam Hospital/Brown University School of Medicine
Division of Behavioral & Preventive Medicine
Providence, RI

Ashley W. Smith, B.A.
University of Pittsburgh Cancer Institute
Behavioral Medicine and Oncology
Pittsburgh, PA

Michelle Toshima
Dept. of Rehabilitation Medicine
School of Medicine
University of Washington
Seattle, WA

Kathleen Weeks, M.S.
The Johns Hopkins Asthma & Allergy Center
Baltimore, MD

SECTION I

Behavior Change and Maintenance: Theory and Measurement

Judith K. Ockene, Editor

This book represents a detailed review of selected theoretical and empirical literature on the individual, interpersonal, social, and cultural factors that inhibit or promote individual behavior change and the application of the findings to clinical practice. Chapters in Section I review several theories and models of behavior change addressing factors which have an effect at the level of the individual.

Theories and models provide a basis for predicting behavior change and maintenance, developing interventions to achieve changes in health-promoting and disease-preventing behaviors, and evaluating the outcomes of the interventions. The variety of theories and models available provide insights into the different factors affecting health-promoting behaviors, with no single model being all-encompassing.

In order to address behavior change at all levels, it is necessary for the practitioner and the researcher to integrate theories and models into a framework of constructs that interact across the theories at each level of change, as well as between levels of change. As Lawrence Green noted in the preface to Section I in the first edition of this book:

> Each (theory or model) is an approximation of a different slice of reality, or a different perspective on the same slice . . . The framework should emerge inductively from personal experience in practice (and research). Theories and their variables can then be attached to the practitioner's (researcher's) personal framework deductively by asking of each theory how it fits, what it adds, or what it explains among the cause-effect relationships one presumes to be operating in one's practice (research).

The first chapter in Section I, written by Clark and Becker, reviews several models and theories of adherence and disease management directed at health promotion and preventive behavior, illness behavior, and sick-role behavior. These include, among others, the Health Belief Model, Theory of Planned Action, Theory of Planned Behavior, Behavioral-Cognitive Theory, Self-Regulation Model, and a model of Disease Self-Management. There is also a discussion of how to apply these models and theories to enhance adherence. Other chapters present the Relapse Prevention Model, the Transtheoretical Model of Behavior Change, and a Model of Provider-Patient Interaction and its application to health behavior change. Methodological problems and measurement issues in adherence behaviors are described in the last chapter of this section.

Even though there are many theories and models available, there is still much we have not been able to explain or "prove" about why and how people make changes. To fill in the black box of behavior change, we must be able to move "outside the dots" and not be limited by theories. Theory can be used to guide us, but should not constrain our creativity. We must be open to integrating, expanding, and testing our theories in order to expand our base of knowledge.

Measurement, which is addressed in chapter 5, allows us to test the key theoretical constructs in order to build on the theories and eventually support or dismiss them. Standardized, well-validated measures are needed to evaluate the major constructs. While measurement is important for testing and building on theories, as Lawrence Green noted in the first edition of this book,

> The problem with measurement and controlled experimental testing of theories as criteria of their relative worth is that these criteria bias the

> selection toward the more simplistic or mechanistic slices of reality, the more concrete and observable variables, and the theories for which measurement instruments with known psychometric or sociometric properties are at hand. Reductionism becomes rampant; empiricism becomes empirical; technology becomes technocracy. (p. 2)

We must constantly be open to finding creative ways of designing and implementing interventions and measuring outcomes and be ever mindful to not get caught "inside the dots" with limited vision of how to broaden our perspectives.

1

Theoretical Models and Strategies for Improving Adherence and Disease Management

Noreen M. Clark and Marshall H. Becker

It is apparent that the ultimate success of efficacious preventive and curative regimens is usually dependent upon individuals' willingness to undertake and maintain the required behaviors. Unfortunately, data indicate that poor adherence to professional advice often occurs wherever some form of discretionary action or self-administration is involved. Estimates are that, on average, only one-third of patients correctly follow physicians' directions. Sackett (1976) points out that scheduled appointments for treatment are missed 20 to 50% of the time; about 50% of patients do not take prescribed medications in accordance with instructions; and recommended changes in habitual behaviors are even less frequently adhered to (e.g., smoking cessation programs are considered to be unusually effective if more than one-third of the entrants have stopped smoking by the end of 6 months; dietary restrictions are often not observed; and large percentages drop out of weight-control programs).

Given the extensive documentation of suboptimal public participation in screening, immunization, and other preventive health efforts, as well as low levels of individual adherence to prescribed medical therapies (c.f., Col,

---

This chapter is revised by Dr. Clark based on Dr. Becker's original work and is dedicated to his memory.

Fanale, & Kronholm, 1990; Fotheringham & Sawyer, 1995; Sackett & Snow, 1979), it is not surprising that behavioral scientists devote extensive conceptual and empirical effort toward the explanation and prediction of individuals' health-related decisions. This chapter reviews theoretical frameworks that have been advanced to elucidate the nonadherence phenomenon. In large part, these have been used to address the behavior of medicine-taking. In the last two decades, discussions of the concept of compliance or adherence to clinical recommendations have been expanded to include the wider range of activities patients must undertake to manage their health problems more effectively. Therefore, conceptual frameworks for patient self-management also are included in this review. Finally, major approaches and techniques are identified that have been advanced for health professionals to use to ameliorate problems in adherence and effective patient management of disease.

MODELS OF ADHERENCE AND DISEASE MANAGEMENT

The reasons individuals voluntarily elect to engage in health-directed activities were categorized years ago (Kasl & Cobb, 1966) into three major classes:

1. to prevent illness or to detect it at an asymptomatic stage ("health behavior");
2. in the presence of symptoms, to obtain diagnosis and to discover suitable treatment ("illness behavior"); and
3. in the presence of defined illness, to undertake/receive treatment aimed at restoration of health or at halting disease progression ("sick-role behavior").

More recently, the first category (health behavior) has also been discussed as "health promotion and preventive behavior" (Glanz, Lewis, & Rimer, 1990). Illness and sick-role behavior are often referred to as "disease management" (Lorig, Laurin, & Holman, 1984).

Family Use of Health Services

From a mainly sociological perspective, Andersen (1968, 1995) developed a behavioral model to identify determinants of family utilization of health services. In this framework, behavior is seen as dependent upon (1) the predisposition of the family to use services; (2) their ability to secure services; and (3) their need for such services.

The "predisposing" component of the model includes family characteristics existing prior to the onset of illness that result in differences in propensity to use health services, including demographic variables; social structure variables; and health beliefs and attitudes about medical care, physicians, and disease. These predisposing variables are not seen as directly responsible for use of health services, but rather as determinants of variation in "inclination" toward use; thus, Andersen suggests that patterns of utilization are affected by individuals in various age groups having different types and amounts of illness, by families with different social structural characteristics having different lifestyles (in terms of physical and social environment and behavior patterns), and by variations of belief in the efficacy of medical care.

The second model component refers to conditions that permit the use of health services, or that make these services available. "Enabling" conditions include both family resources (e.g., family income and savings, health insurance, or other source of third-party coverage) and community resources (e.g., availability of health services and health personnel).

When appropriate predisposing and enabling conditions are present, variations in perception of illness (or the probability of its occurrence) and the manner of response to illness (or potential illness) will determine the use of health services. The first subcomponent, perceived "need," is measured by (1) subjective perceptions of illness (including reported disability days, number of symptoms experienced, and self-reported general state of health) and (2) clinical evaluation of illness (usually based on the weighing of reported symptoms for probability of need for care by age group) (Andersen & Newman, 1973). Finally, reaction to illness is measured by the pattern of seeing a doctor for symptoms (on a continuum from "doctor not seen for any symptoms" to "doctor seen for all symptoms") and by receipt of regular physical examinations.

In specifying hypotheses generated by the model, Andersen (1968) stated that "the amount of health services used by a family will be a function of the predisposing and enabling characteristics of the family and its need for medical care" (p.19). The components of the model are hypothesized to contribute independently to the understanding of differential utilization of health services—and need, which represents factors most directly related to use, is expected to be more important than either predisposing or enabling components.

This model has been employed with varying degrees of explanatory success in several early studies using surveys of large national samples (c.f., Andersen, 1968; Andersen & Anderson, 1979; Andersen, Kravits, & Anderson, 1975; Dutton, 1978). More recently, Wolinsky and colleagues (1995) and Stump, Johnson, and Wolinsky (1995) showed constructs from Anderson's model to be associated with hospital and physician use by older adults. Potvin, Camirand, and Beland (1995) used the model to predict mammography use, and Berkanovic and Hurwicz (1995) assessed physcian visits by patients with arthritis. Evans and Stoddart (1990) have shown that personal health practices such as diet and exercise interact with formal health services to influence outcome.

Health Belief Model

The Health Belief Model (HBM) was developed in the early 1950s by a group of social psychologists at the U.S. Public Health Service (Rosenstock, 1974) in an attempt to understand "the widespread failure of people to accept disease preventives or screening tests for the early detection of asymptomatic disease" (p. 328); it was later applied to patients' responses to symptoms (Kirscht, 1974) and to following prescribed medical regimens (Becker, 1974).

The basic components of the HBM are derived from a well-established body of psychological and behavioral theory whose various models hypothesize that behavior depends mainly upon two variables: (1) the value placed by an individual on a particular goal and (2) the individual's estimate of the likelihood that a given action will achieve that goal (Maiman & Becker, 1974). When these variables were conceptualized in the context of health-related behavior, the correspondences were: (1) the desire to avoid illness (or if ill, to get well) and (2) the belief that a specific health action will prevent (or ameliorate) illness (i.e., the individual's estimate of the threat of illness and of the likelihood of being able, through personal action, to reduce that threat).

Specifically, the HBM consists of the following dimensions (Figure 1.1): *Perceived Susceptibility*, or one's subjective perception of the risk of contracting a condition; *Perceived Severity*, or feelings concerning the seriousness of contracting an illness (or of leaving it untreated); While low perceptions of seriousness might provide insufficient motivation for behavior, very high perceived severity might inhibit action; *Perceived Benefits*, or beliefs regarding the effectiveness of the various actions available to reduce the disease threat; *Perceived Barriers*, or the potential negative aspects of a particular health action that may act as impediments to undertaking the recommended behavior; and *Cues to Action*, or stimuli to trigger the decision-making process.

In the HBM context, it is understood that diverse demographic, personal, structural, and social factors are capable of influencing health behaviors. However, these variables are believed to work through their effects on the individual's health motivations and subjective perceptions, rather than functioning as direct causes of health action (Becker et al., 1977).

Of all the existing models of health-related behaviors, the HBM has received the most extensive research attention. A large body of evidence has

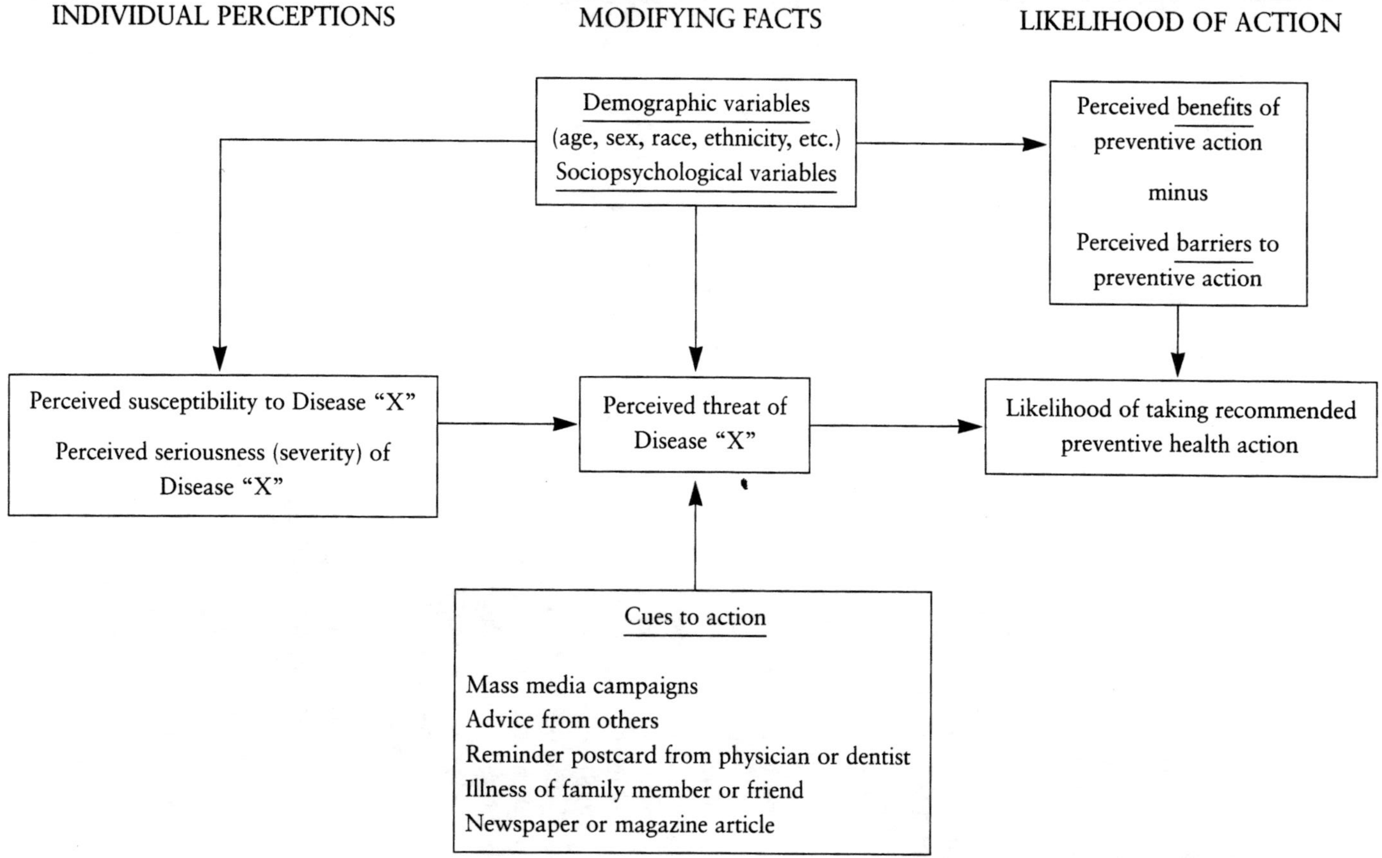

Figure 1.1 The health belief model.

From M.H. Becker, R.H. Drachman, & J.P. Kirscht (1974). A field experiment to evaluate various outcomes of continuity of physician care. *American Journal of Public Health, 64,* 1062–1070. Reprinted with permission.

accumulated in support of the HBM's ability to account for the undertaking of preventive health actions, seeking diagnoses, and following prescribed medical advice (i.e., adherence to regimens). A review (Janz & Becker, 1984) summarized findings from 46 HBM-related investigations (18 prospective, 28 retrospective). Twenty-four studies examined preventive health behaviors (PHB); 19 explored sick-role behaviors (SRB); and 3 addressed clinic utilization. A "significance ratio" was constructed that divides the number of positive, statistically significant findings for an HBM dimension by the total number of studies reporting significance levels for that dimension.

In the preponderance of cases, each HBM dimension was found to be significantly associated with the health-related behaviors under study; overall, the significance ratio orderings (in descending order) were "barriers" (89%); "susceptibility" (81%); "benefits" (78%); and "severity" (65%). Findings from prospective studies were at least as favorable as those obtained from retrospective research. Also, the model has been shown to be associated with preventive behavior, for example, cancer screening (Aiken, West, Woodward, & Reno, 1994; Clasen, Vernon, Mullen, & Jackson, 1994) and dental behavior (Barker, 1994). It has also predicted disease management, including diabetes (Pham, Fortin, & Thibaudeau, 1996), and HIV disease (Catt, Stygall, & Catalan, 1995; Muma, Ross, Parcel, & Pollard, 1995).

Investigators have considered combining HBM constructs and others from social cognitive theory, specifically self-efficacy, that is, the confidence people have in their ability to undertake given behaviors. Clark and colleagues (1988) added self-efficacy to dimensions of the health belief model and found that the variance explained in the management of asthma by school-aged children did not increase significantly.

Despite the body of findings ranking HBM dimensions to health actions, Janz and Becker (1984) note that the HBM is a psychosocial model; as such, it is limited to accounting for as much of the variance in individuals' health-related behaviors as can be explained by their attitudes and beliefs. It is clear that other forces influence health actions as well; for example: (1) some behaviors (e.g., cigarette smoking, tooth brushing) have a substantial habitual component obviating any ongoing psychosocial decisionmaking process; (2) many health-related behaviors are undertaken for what are ostensibly non-health related reasons (e.g., dieting to appear more attractive; stopping smoking or jogging to attain social approval); and (3) economic or environmental factors may prevent the individual from undertaking a preferred course of action (e.g., a worker in a hazardous environment; a resident in a city with high levels of air pollution). Furthermore, the model is based on the premise that "health" is a highly valued concern or goal for most individuals, and also that "cues to action" are widely prevalent; where these conditions are not satisfied, the model is not likely to be useful in, or relevant to, explaining behavior.

Theory of Reasoned Action

In the approach taken by Ajzen and Fishbein (1980), intention to perform a behavior can be accounted for by a combination of attitudes about an action and perceptions of likely normative reactions to that action. More specifically, the Theory of Reasoned Action focuses on the individual's attitude toward the behavior (i.e., the person's beliefs that the behavior leads to certain outcomes) and their evaluations of these outcomes and of the subjective norm (i.e., the person's beliefs that certain individuals or groups think he or she should or should not undertake the behavior, weighted by the person's desire to comply with their wishes). As with the HBM, sociodemographic factors operate only through their influences on the determinants of behavioral intention. Intention will result in behavior if there is an opportunity to act. This model also emphasizes normative influences that might affect intention for any reason, health-related or otherwise, thus adding a strong cultural component to the prediction of behavior.

This model has been successfully applied in the areas of smoking (Jaccard, 1975) and intentions to engage in family planning (Fishbein & Jaccard, 1973) and obtain Pap tests for cervical cancer (Seibold & Roper, 1979). However, much of this research used college students as subjects, and less data are available related to other adult populations.

Theory of Planned Behavior

The Theory of Planned Behavior is an extension of Ajzen and Fishbein's Theory of Reasoned Action and is appropriate for both volitional and nonvolitional behaviors. Here, performance of a behavior is a function of the strength of a person's attempt to perform a behavior and the degree of control the person has over that behavior. Control includes both personal and external factors that influence the behavior, such as having a workable plan, skills, knowledge, time, money, willpower, and opportunity.

Intention to try to perform the behavior is the immediate determinant of an attempt to perform the behavior. Intention is seen as a function of an individual's attitude toward trying and their subjective norm with regard to trying. Consistent with the Theory of Reasoned Action, the relative influence of attitude and subjective norm on intention is dependent on the behavioral goal. For some behaviors, the attitudinal component will be the major determinant of intention, while for others, the importance of social pressure will be the primary influence. In general, the more favorable an individual's attitude toward attempting a behavior, and the more the individual believes that significant others are in favor of his or her trying, the stronger will be his or her intention to try.

The Theory of Planned Behavior goes beyond the Theory of Reasoned Action in identifying determinants of attitude toward trying to perform a behavior. The person's overall attitude toward trying a behavior is weighted by the person's subjective estimate of the likelihood of success or failure of performance and depends on the behavioral goal. Subjective estimate of likelihood of success or failure is a function of beliefs about the presence or absence of personal and external factors that may facilitate or inhibit performance. Attitudes toward trying and succeeding or failing are a function of the individual's beliefs about the consequences of successful or unsuccessful attempts and their evaluation of these consequences.

Subjective norm, the second major determinant of intention to try, is defined as the person's beliefs regarding what significant others think they should or should not do. Subjective norm concerning a behavioral goal is viewed as a recommendation by significant others that is based on their approval of the behavior and their belief that the attempt is likely to succeed.

Other attempts to expand the Theory of Reasoned Action are incorporated in Ajzen's description of the Theory of Planned Behavior. The author stresses the distinction between the intention to try and what an individual really expects to do ("behavioral expectations"). According to Ajzen (1985), behavioral expectation is seen as a "person's estimate of the likelihood that he actually will perform a certain behavior" (p.33). Behavioral expectation is viewed as a function of intention to try and the individual's belief in his or her ability to control a behavior. Factors influential in perception of behavioral control include past experience, confidence in subjective judgement of control, availability of a detailed plan of action, and general self-knowledge.

In summary, the Theory of Planned Behavior states that variables important in determining an attempt to perform a behavior "include beliefs about the likely consequences of success and failure, the perceived probabilities of success and failure, normative beliefs regarding important referents, and motivation to comply with these referents" (p. 36). In general, individuals will try to perform a behavior if they believe that the benefits of success are outweighed by the benefits of failure, and if they feel that significant others (with whom they want to comply) believe they should attempt to perform the behavior. Successful performance of the behavior will be the end result if individuals have sufficient control over internal and external factors that influence such performance.

The Theory of Reasoned Action is described as a "special case" of the Theory of Planned Behavior. "The two theories are identical when the subjective probability of success and the degree of control over internal and external factors reach their maximal values" (p. 36). When this occurs, the behavior is purely volitional and the Theory of Reasoned Action can be applied. The Theory of Planned Behavior is more appropriate when the probability of success and actual control over performance of a behavior are less than perfect.

In a recent review of the range of studies examining the theory (Godkin

& Kok, 1996), it was shown to perform quite well across several types of behavior in predicting *intention* to behave. For predicting *actual* behavior, however, the models' efficacies were found to vary. For example, correlations were quite low for clinical and screening behaviors, but much higher for addictive and HIV/AID-related behavior. The reviewers suggest that the addition of other variables, including role beliefs and "moral norms," would make the models more robust.

Health Decision Model

Proposed as "a third generation model of patient behavior that focused more specifically on health decisions" (Eraker, Kirscht, & Becker, 1984, p. 260), the Health Decision Model attempted to combine decision analysis, behavioral decision theory, and health beliefs to yield a unifying model of health decisions and resultant behavior. The model included contributions from the "patient preferences" literature (Eraker & Politser, 1982). Decision analysis provided a quantitative means for patients to express their preferences about critical trade-offs between benefits and risk—and at times, between quantity and quality of life (McNeil, Keeler, & Adelstein, 1975; Weinstein & Fineberg, 1980). Behavioral decision theory extends this quantitative emphasis by identifying a number of general inferential rules that patients use to reduce difficult mental tasks to simpler ones (Eraker & Sox, Jr., 1981; Tversky & Kahneman, 1974).

The relationships among health beliefs, decision analysis, and behavioral decision theory were demonstrated in a study on patient preferences of variations in the way information is presented to patients. McNeil, Pauker, Sox, and Tversky (1982) examined the results of surgery and radiation treatment for lung cancer and found that preferences for alternative therapies shifted when the outcomes were framed in terms of probability of living or the probability of dying. The investigators also found that people relied more on preexisting beliefs regarding the treatments than on statistical data presented to them. These preexisting beliefs may help to explain why some patients, based on decision-analysis criteria, are treated in a manner not reflecting their underlying preferences.

The Health Decision Model also recognizes the importance of other factors affecting health decisions and behavior, such as knowledge, experience, and social and demographic variables. The bidirectional arrows and feedback loops reflect the notion that adherence behavior can change health beliefs. The model also includes concepts related to the efficacy of the prescribed regimen, motivational variables involving the person's assessment of the importance of good health, and "cues to action" that refer specifically to the patient-physician interaction (Eraker, Becker, Strecher, & Kirscht, 1985).

Model of Illness Behavior

A decision-theoretic, anthropological approach to understanding illness behavior, which focuses on "the information that a person might be expected to process during an occurrence of illness," provided the framework for Fabrega's (1973, p. 473) model. ("Illness" refers to the culturally defined state that forms the basis of decisions about medical treatment; thus, the model has cross-cultural application.) This model tries to order and categorize the stages an individual passes through in recognizing and responding to illness by concentrating on (1) the information to be evaluated and acted upon; (2) the time-ordering of events in the decision process; and (3) reducing variation in processes and events of the health illness-medical treatment cycle by providing constant and repetitive structure for channeling and processing medically relevant information.

Fabrega (1973) posited that the individual has four systems that provide "coding units . . . [or] norms or experienced levels of variations" (p. 473), which permit continuous monitoring of health-related happenings and processes. Put another way, the four systems are involved in information processing: coding, classifying, and ordering events related to symptoms and to feelings of illness. The systems are both open and interjoined, each contributing to illness behavior: (1) the biological system, which focuses on chemical and physiologic processes; (2) the social system, which executes relationships with other individuals, groups, and institutions; (3) the phenomenologic system, which is concerned with the individual's state of awareness and self-definition; and (4) the memory system, which includes earlier illness occurrences and accompanying medical attitudes and beliefs and which serves as a continual influence on the other three systems.

The model provides an abstract definition of illness behavior outlined in nine stages describing the sequence of decisions people make during illness. In order for this model of illness behavior to operate, Fabrega specified three assumptions. First, illness must be recognized as undesirable; that is, the model is not applicable to individuals who favor or who deny disease states and thus would not be motivated to undertake remedial action. Second, illness must be perceived as a discrete occurrence, rather than as an undifferentiated and constant state managed by habitual behaviors (which do not require decisions of illness definition and treatment selection). Finally, individuals must make their illness decisions based on rational evaluations of optimal treatment actions (rather than on random or irrational bases).

In summary, Fabrega (1974) developed a behavioral framework to study how social and cultural behavior influences the individual's processing of information about illness and decisions about medical treatment; he suggests that the model be used in cross-cultural comparisons of the disvalues or costs of illness. Although difficulties in operationalizing the variables contained in the model are acknowledged, it is proposed that it be used as a rubric for empirical studies that would yield an "estimate" of the key variables (c.f., Fabrega, 1977; Fabrega & Zucker, 1977).

Self-Regulation Model

Leventhal, Meyer, and Gutmann (1980) view self-regulation as a solution to dealing with the basic problem of locus of control in adherence theory. The fundamental notion is that

> the individual functions as a feedback system. He or she establishes behavioral goals, generates plans and responses to reach these goals, and establishes criteria for monitoring the effects of his/her responses on movement toward or away from the goal. This information is then used to alter coping techniques, set new criteria for evaluating response outputs, and revise goals. The individual is, therefore, an information processing system that regulates his/her relationship to the environment. (p. 34)

The analogy provided is one of the person as scientist—formulating hypotheses about physiology and the effects of illness and creating a mental picture of ability to take actions to prevent or cure illness.

Leventhal's self-regulation model contains components that depict a process not unlike Fabrega's approach: (1) extracting information from the environment; (2) generating a representation of the illness danger to oneself; and (3) planning and acting, which involves imagining response alternatives to deal with the problem and emotions it generates, then taking selected actions to achieve specific effects. Here the feedback loop is achieved by the last step: (4) monitoring or appraising how one's coping reactions affected the environmental problem and oneself. "Each component is a set of processes, each operates within its own set of rules, each has its own potentials" (p. 35).

Data from Cameron, Leventhal, and Leventhal (1995) illustrate that in this model individuals use self-regulation to adapt to perceived health threats, for example, symptoms. In a study of 366 men and women using clinics of a University Hospital, they found that care-seeking was a function of the characteristics of the symptoms patients identified as distinctive signs of illness, and not of the level of life stresses they experience. Leventhal, Hansell, Diefenbach, Leventhal, and Glass (1996) have shown mood state to be related to physical symptoms patients report. In this self-regulation model, therefore, patients' adherence to a regimen is thought to be influenced by their perceptions and evaluations of the presence or absence of symptoms. Also, this model relies to a fair degree on Bandura's formulations regarding reciprocal determinism and self-regulation, and both this work and Bandura's (1986) social cognitive theory arise from a common theoretical heritage that strongly suggests the importance of the approach to understanding adherence behaviors.

Social Cognitive Theory

Bandura's (1986) discussion of social learning attempts to explain and predict behavior using several key concepts: incentives, outcome expectations, and efficacy expectations. Bandura (1977) outlined the roles of these concepts in the paradigm of a person engaging in a behavior that will have a consequent outcome; here, behavior change and maintenance are a function of (1) expectations about the outcomes that will result from engaging in a behavior and (2) expectations about one's ability to engage in or execute the behavior. Thus, "outcome expectations" consist of beliefs about whether a given behavior will lead to given outcomes, whereas "efficacy expectations" consist of beliefs about how capable one is of performing the behavior that leads to those outcomes. The two have been shown to be linked in predicting, for example, adoption and maintenance of exercise (D. O. Clark, Patrick, Grembowski, & Durham, 1995), and self-management of epilepsy (DiIorio, Hennessy, & Manteuffel, 1996). It should be emphasized that both outcome and efficacy expectations reflect a person's beliefs about capabilities and the connections between behavior and outcome. Thus it is these perceptions, and not necessarily "true" capabilities, that influence behavior. In addition, it is important to understand that the concept of self-efficacy relates to beliefs about capabilities of performing specific behaviors in particular situations (Schunk & Carbonari, 1984); self-efficacy does not refer to a personality characteristic or to a global trait that operates independently of contextual factors (Bandura, 1986). This means that individuals' efficacy expectations will vary greatly depending on the particular task and context that confronts them.

Bandura argued that perceived self-efficacy influences all aspects of behavior, including the acquisition of new behaviors (e.g., a sexually active young adult learning how to use a particular contraceptive device), inhibition of existing behaviors (e.g., decreasing or stopping cigarette smoking), and disinhibition of behaviors (e.g., resuming sexual activity after a myocardial infarction). Self-efficacy also affects people's choices of behavioral settings, the amount of effort they will expend on a task, and the length of time they will persist in the face of obstacles. Finally, self-efficacy affects people's emotional reactions, such as anxiety and distress and thought patterns. Thus, individuals with low self-efficacy about a particular task may ruminate about their personal deficiencies, rather than thinking about accomplishing or attending to the task at hand; this, in turn, impedes successful performance of the task.

According to Bandura, efficacy expectations vary along dimensions of magnitude, strength, and generality. "Magnitude" refers to the ordering of tasks by difficulty level. Persons having low-magnitude expectations feel capable of performing only the simpler of a graded series of tasks, while those with high-magnitude expectations feel capable of performing even the most difficult tasks in the series. "Strength" refers to a probabilistic judgment of how certain one is of one's ability to perform a specific task (Bandura, 1984). "Generality" concerns the extent to which efficacy expectations about a particular situation or experience generalize to other situations. For example, the beliefs of post-myocardial infarction patients about their endurance capabilities generated during supervised exercise testing may or may not generalize to unsupervised exercising at home.

Efficacy expectations are learned from four major sources (Bandura, 1977, 1986). The first, termed "performance accomplishments," refers to learning through personal experience where one achieves mastery over a difficult or previously feared task and thereby enjoys an increase in self-efficacy. Performance accomplishments attained through personal experience are the most potent source of efficacy expectations.

The second source is "vicarious experience," which includes learning that occurs through observation of events or other people. These events or people are referred to as "models" when they display a set of behaviors or stimulus array that illustrates a certain principle, rule, or response. In order for modeling to affect an observer's self-efficacy positively, however, it is important that the model can be viewed as overcoming difficulties through determined effort rather than with ease, and that the model be similar to the observer with regard to other characteristics (e.g., age, gender). Additionally, modeled behaviors presented with clear rewarding outcomes are more effective than modeling with unclear or unrewarded outcomes.

"Verbal persuasion" constitutes the third source of efficacy expectations. This method is quite familiar to all health workers who have exhorted patients to persevere in their efforts to change behavior.

Finally, one's "physiological state" provides information that can influence efficacy expectations. Bandura noted that because high physiological arousal usually impairs performance, people are more likely to expect failure when they are very tense and viscerally agitated. For example, people who experience extremely sweaty palms, a racing heartbeat, and trembling knees prior to giving a talk find that their self-efficacy plummets; to someone just beginning an exercise program, fatigue and mild aches and pains may be mistakenly interpreted as a sign of physical inefficacy. Self-efficacy has been shown to predict HIV risk behavior among low-income women (Sikkema et al., 1995), survival of patients with

COPD (Kaplan, Ries, Prewitt, & Eakin, 1994), and frequency of breast self-examination (Friedman, Nelson, Webb, Hoffman, & Baer, 1994) among other outcomes.

While this presentation of social cognitive theory emphasizes cognitive-perceptual dimensions, it should be noted that Bandura (1986) recognized the influence of the social environment. Although the cognitive-motivational aspects of the theory have recently received the most attention, situational determinants are essential to the theory as well. It is important to distinguish self-efficacy from a number of other concepts with which it is sometimes linked and frequently confused. This confusion occurs in part because the personality traits, states, and processes that these concepts represent can influence efficacy expectations or be influenced by them.

"Health locus of control" refers to a generalized expectation about whether one's health is controlled by one's own behavior or by forces external to oneself (Wallston & Wallston, 1984) and has been a focus of many studies (see for example, Chen, 1995; Furnham & Steele, 1993; Ziff, Conrad, & Lachman, 1995). Health is an outcome, while self-efficacy focuses on beliefs about the capacity to undertake behavior(s) that may not lead to desired outcomes (such as health). Bandura (1986) illustrated the importance of the distinction between locus of control and self-efficacy by noting that the conviction that outcomes (e.g., good health) are determined by one's own action can have any number of effects on self-efficacy and behavior. For example, people who view their health as personally determined, but who believe they lack the skills needed to carry out the behaviors that would result in good health, would experience low self-efficacy and approach those activities with a sense of futility.

"Self-esteem" refers to liking and respect for oneself that has some realistic basis (Crandall, 1978) and is a construct that has received considerable attention in the health literature (see for example, Fisher, Schneider, Pegler, & Napolitano, 1991; Ireys, Gross, Werthamer-Larsson, & Kolodner, 1994; Torres, Fernandez, & Maceira, 1995). Thus self-esteem is concerned with an evaluation of self-worth, while self-efficacy relates to an evaluation of specific capabilities in specific situations. Bandura (1984) highlighted the distinction between the two concepts by pointing out that people can have high self-efficacy for a task from which they derive no self-pride (e.g., being able to brush one's teeth well) or have low self-efficacy for a task but have no loss of self-worth (e.g., not being able to ride a unicycle). However, he observes that people often try to develop self-efficacy in activities that give them a sense of self-worth, so that the two concepts are frequently intertwined.

"Coping," according to Lazarus and Folkman's (1984) conceptualization, is viewed as a process; like Bandura, they downplayed notions of coping that emphasize generalized dispositional concepts such as self-esteem. Coping style has been shown to be associated with hardiness and health (McCracken, Semenchuk, & Goetsch, 1995; Williams, Wiebe & Smith,

1992). "Secondary appraisal" is defined as an individual's evaluation of what might and can be done in the face of a threat or challenge. During this complex process, a person takes into account (either consciously or unconsciously) (1) which coping strategies are available; (2) the likelihood that some strategy will accomplish the expected outcome; and (3) whether one can apply that strategy or strategies effectively. Clearly the second part of this process is similar to the notion of outcome expectation, while the third is equivalent to self-efficacy. Thus, within Lazarus and Folkman's framework, efficacy expectations are part of secondary appraisal.

"Learned helplessness" (see for example, Koestner & Zuckerman, 1994; Lindroth, Strombeck, Brossner, Gullberg, & Wollheim, 1994) refers to cognitive, affective, and motivational deficits that result from exposure to uncontrollable events. The attributional reformulation of learned helplessness suggests that there are two types of helplessness: personal and universal. Personal helplessness occurs when an individual lacks the requisite controlling response in a situation, but believes this response is available to others; that is, the individual believes that although he or she cannot control the outcome, others in the same situation could. In the case of universal helplessness, the individual still lacks the requisite response but believes that the outcome is independent of any response he or she or others could make. Abramson, Garber, and Seligman (1980) view this distinction between personal and universal helplessness as consistent with Bandura's distinction between efficacy and outcome expectancies. Low efficacy and high outcome expectations characterize universal helplessness.

A Model Of Disease Self-Management

Drawing from social cognitive theory, and especially the construct of self-regulation, N. M. Clark (1977); N. M. Clark & Starr (1994); N. M. Clark and colleagues (1988) propose a framework for conceptualizing disease management by patients with acute or chronic conditions. In this model (see Figure 1.2) self-regulation is viewed as a means by which patients determine what is effective and what isn't, given their specific goals. They make these determinations influenced by their social context and according to the resources they have available. The model is based on three assumptions. First, several factors predispose one to manage a disease. Second, patient management is the conscious use of strategies to manipulate situations to reduce the impact of disease on daily life. One learns which strategies do or do not work through processes of self-regulation. Third, illness management is not an end in itself but the means to other ends. These ends include: improved physiologic status; reduction of symptoms and other clinical manifestations of disease; improved functioning; reduced side effects; appropriate health care use; and, perhaps most important, better quality of life as perceived by the patient.

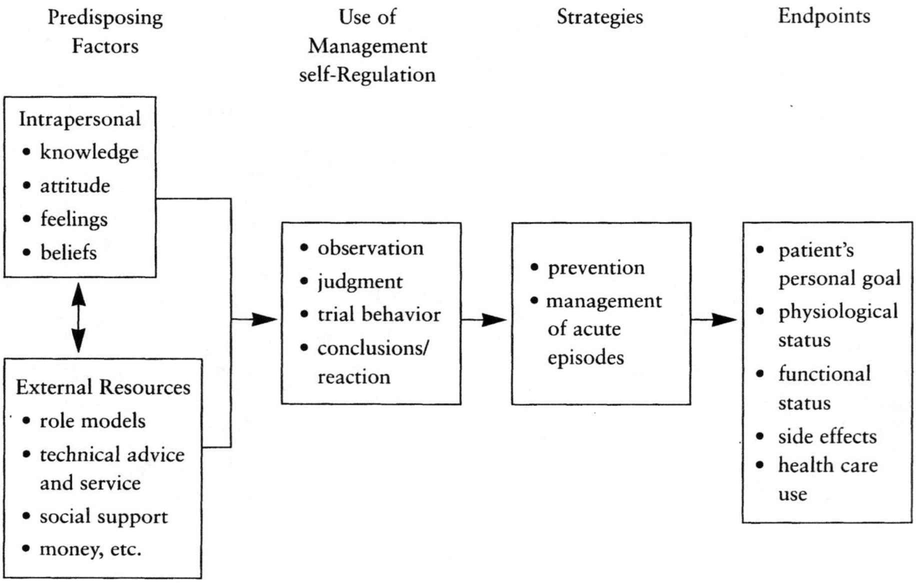

Figure 1.2 A model of disease self-management. Self-regulation is in part a function of predisposing intrapersonal and external factors. Self-regulating individuals, influenced by the factors, employ management strategies to achieve a personal goal or endpoint. Other endpoints of concern to clinicians and other health care professionals result from these effects (N. M. Clark, N. S. Starr, 1994, p.555).

Articles in the literature have proposed that individuals draw from a base of knowledge and by virtue of their attitudes, beliefs, and feelings make decisions and take actions (N. M. Clark & Zimmerman, 1990). Important external factors that enhance or enable disease management also have been proposed. These include role models from whom management strategies can be learned, technical professional advice and service, social support, and money to obtain care and maintain an adequate physical environment. It also must be noted that while knowledge, attitudes, and feelings are the basis for action, these can also change as a result of behavior (Bandura, 1986).

An individual uses his or her intrapersonal and external resources and through processes of self-regulation tries to reach a personal goal. An example would be a child who wants to play full-court basketball who believes he is susceptible to respiratory problems, thinks medicines will help and so uses them preventively, works out a procedure for taking a breather when active, seeks moral support from his or her friends and coaches, and uses other strategies that enable him or her to reach the personal goal. The child learns which strategies are effective through self-regulation. Self-regulation may be particularly important in diseases where there is no sure-fire formula an individual can use to control symptoms or deal with crucial interpersonal relationships. In these illnesses, patients (and families) must exercise a high level of decisionmaking in the absence of health professionals. The self-regulatory processes in which they engage entail observing situations where the disease contributes to problems in reaching their goals; judging what types of actions might ameliorate the situation; using management strategies, that is, trying out new behaviors; and drawing conclusions or reacting to the effects of the behavior. Two important reactions are that the behavior resulted in the desired effect and that one can effectively carry out the behavior, i.e., self-efficacy (as defined by Bandura, 1986). Using strategies to prevent symptoms, manage them effectively, and manage the interpersonal relationships needed to control the effects of the disease should lead to important outcomes. These likely include a better quality of life for the patient, including reaching a personal goal, as well as improved health status as determined by the clinician, more appropriate use of health services, and so on. Elements of the model have been shown to be related to disease self-management (c.f., N. M. Clark, Evans, Zimmerman, Levison & Mellins, 1994).

Behavior Modification

Finally, an approach to understanding and influencing adherence behaviors that is substantially different from the cognitive themes emphasized in the previously described models and frameworks is represented by behavior modification. This emphasizes the roles played by habit and skill in attempts to modify undesirable personal (or "lifestyle") behaviors and brings to bear a wide variety of techniques (e.g., contingency contracting, self-monitoring, counter-conditioning, covert sensitization, relaxation, environmental engineering) (Matarazzo, Weiss, Herd, Miller, & Weiss, 1984; Melamed & Siegel, 1980). It is not reasonable to suggest a single "model" for behavior modification, although the concepts of behavioral consequences and stimulus control are fairly common in these approaches. The general plan that this approach frequently follows is this: identify the problem and describe it in behavioral terms; select a target behavior that is measurable; identify the antecedents and consequences of the behavior, set behavioral objectives; devise and implement a behavior-change program; and evaluate the program. Since cognitive and behavioral models and approaches both have much to offer, it seems reasonable to assume that our best bets for effective interventions to improve adherence will be strategies that combine these elements.

HEALTH PROVIDER STRATEGIES FOR IMPROVING PATIENTS' ADHERENCE AND DISEASE MANAGEMENT

Much research has been devoted to identifying the "determinants" of self-management and adherence to professional recommendations (Becker, 1990), and a smaller number of investigations has attempted to evaluate the efficacies of different strategies aimed at increasing the level of patient management and acceptance of suggested and prescribed therapies (N. M. Clark et al., 1995). While no all-purpose solution to these problems has been discovered, sufficient practical knowledge and techniques have evolved to provide a foundation for efforts to address them. Listed below are some of the more commonly employed (and promising) approaches to enhancing adherence and effective management of disease by patients, with an emphasis on feasible interventions implemented by different members of the healthcare team.

Providing Information

Investigations of the usefulness of providing various kinds of information have revealed a number of important considerations that influence the likelihood of patient adherence (Maiman & Becker, 1980). Unfortunately, data regarding knowledge and adherence are, in the aggregate, neither consistent nor clear-cut; some studies have found no relationship between levels of patient information and adherence to therapy. One interpretation of the studies in this area is that regimen-related knowledge is necessary in compliance, but more general disease-related knowledge may predict adherence.

A number of studies conducted by Ley and colleagues (1972, 1976; Ley, Bradshaw, Eaves, & Walker, 1973) in the 1970s identified factors associated with failure to follow therapeutic recommendations. These factors, which seem valid in clinical experience, included poor recall (after 5 minutes patients forget one-half of the clinicians' instructions), recall according to the timing of messages (material presented in the first third of the discussion is best remembered), selective recall (patients recall diagnosis better than therapy recommendations), recall through labeling and categorizing messages (simple reorganization of a list of fifteen medical statements into labeled categories enhanced recall by 50%), recall through repetition (well-organized messages repeated several times in a simple leaflet significantly improved adherence to a weight-loss plan).

In the 1960s, Korsch and colleagues (Korsch, Gozzi, & Francis, 1988; Korsch & Negrets, 1972) found patients' understanding of information is diminished by language common in the clinical setting (e.g., "follow-up", "incubation period", "work-up"), and that by modifying messages delivered to the patient, improvements in communication could be achieved in as few as 5 minutes of clinician time.

Modifying Regimen Characteristics and Assessing Patients' Skills

Rates of adherence tend to be lower when the therapeutic regimen is complex, of long duration, dependent on alteration of the patients' lifestyle, inconvenient, or expensive (cf., Becker & Maiman, 1981). The regimen can be made less complex by reducing the number of different medications required. This can be accomplished by avoiding the routine prescription of nonessential medicine and by avoiding unnecessary doses or variations in scheduling. Complexity can also be modified by emphasizing the necessity of adherence to particularly critical aspects of the treatment ("prioritizing" the regimen); by breaking the treatment plan into less complex stages that can be implemented sequentially ("graduated regimen implementation"); and by minimizing both inconvenience and forgetfulness by matching the regimen schedule to the patient's regular daily activities ("tailoring" the regimen) (Sackett et al., 1978).

Frequency of dosing is also a consideration, and newer, longer-lasting drugs are helping to simplify and enhance drug regimens. The ability to adhere to medical recommendations has been shown to be associated with the level of patient skill in administering a drug. For example, Larsen, Hahn, Ekholm, and Wick (1994) found low skill levels among patients using metered dose inhalers (MDIs). Also, patients' skills deteriorate over time. One group of investigators (Kesten, Elias, Cartier, & Chapman, 1994) found that 2 weeks after patients rehearsed and demonstrated medicine use to nurses in the clinic, their skills significantly decreased. Data suggest (c.f., Wasilewski et al., 1996) that even when a regimen has been reduced in its complexity, patients must be taught how to use medicines and demonstrate their proficiency in every encounter with the clinician in order to correct deteriorating skills. Further, patients must know how to determine if the medical regimen is working and be able to identify signs of an emergency situation, should it occur.

Modifying Health Beliefs

Considerable attention has been given to conceptualizing patient nonadherence as a problem in health-related decisionmaking, wherein the individual is guided by attitudes and beliefs that may operate independently of levels of information, objective features of the condition and the regimen, and so forth (Cummings, Becker, & Maile, 1980). Beliefs that have been found most consistently to produce significant relationships with adherence to health and medical care recommendations have been the components of the Health Belief Model (Janz & Becker, 1984), social-normative variables (Ajzen, 1985), and self-efficacy (Strecher, DeVellis, Becker, & Rosenstock, 1986). It is therefore recommended that more attention be paid to both monitoring and motivating the patient along these belief dimensions. Such an adherence-oriented history can be viewed as a critical extension of the usual medical history and be made a routine part of the examination process.

Reinforcing Elements of the Treatment Experience

One way to alter the treatment experience is the contingency contract, wherein both parties set forth a treatment goal, the specific obligations of each party in attempting to accomplish that goal, and a time limit for its achievement. Data support the provider-client contract as a tool for improving patient adherence (Janz, Becker, & Hartman, 1984). Contracts offer a written outline of expected behavior, the involvement of the patient in the decisionmaking process concerning the regimen and the opportunity to discuss potential problems and solutions with the health care provider, a formal commitment to the program from the patient, and rewards, such as additional time spent with the provider or lottery tickets, that create incentives for achieving compliance goals.

Enlisting Family and Social Support

Evidence suggests that social support (particularly support provided by the patient's family) plays an important role in influencing adherence and self-management (see for example, Higgins, Budney, Bickel, & Badger, 1994; Kulik & Mahler, 1993; LaGreca et al., 1995). The family can enhance supervision of the patient, as well as provide assistance and encouragement. Social support seems to be especially important in long-term treatment plans that require continuous action on the part of the patient. A family's own health beliefs and its evaluation of the patient's illness and treatment plan may influence adherence. Success is greatest when the family's normal roles and patterns are compatible with the illness of the patient or when the family members are willing to make accommodating changes in their lives and in the family environment.

Enhancing the Provider-Patient Relationship

A partnership between provider and patient is essential to managing disease (see, for example, Bartholomew, Parcel, Swank & Czyzewski, 1993; Conway, Pond, Hamnett, & Watson, 1995; Lorenc & Branthwaite, 1993). Barriers to effective communication have been identified in studies of physician-patient interaction. Becker described five specific patient responses (Becker, 1990). Patients often: 1) feel they are wasting the physician's valuable time; (2) omit details they deem unimportant; (3) are embarrassed to mention things they think will place them in an unfavorable light; (4) do not understand medical terms; and (5) may believe the physician has not really listened and therefore does not have the information needed to make a good treatment decision. Obviously, both diagnosis and therapy decisions are affected when patients do not fully inform physicians.

Desired outcomes, such as improved communication, the patient's greater satisfaction with the visit, and the patient's willingness to follow the therapeutic plan are more likely when the provider's behavior reflects principles of good communication and regimen management. These principles have been identified in studies of the general population of adults (Becker, 1990). They may not always apply to cultural subgroups, but they serve as useful guides for clinicians. Communication is improved when the professional:

1. is attentive to the patient;
2. elicits the patient's underlying concerns about the condition;
3. constructs reassuring messages that alleviate fears;
4. addresses immediate concerns the family expresses;
5. engages the patient in interactive conversation through use of open-ended questions, simple language, and analogies to teach important concepts;
6. tailors the regimen by eliciting and addressing potential problems in the timing, dosage, or side effects of the medicines recommended;
7. uses appropriate nonverbal encouragement and verbal praise when the patient reports using correct disease management strategies;
8. elicits the patient's immediate objective related to control of the disease and reaches an agreement with the patient and the family on a short-term goal;
9. reviews the long-term plan for the patient's treatment so the patient knows what to expect over time, knows the situations under which the physician will modify treatment, and knows the criteria for judging the success of the treatment plan; and
10. helps the patient plan in advance for decisionmaking about the condition.

These ten factors were examined in a survey of 149 physicians and have been shown to cluster into three categories of behavior (N. M. Clark et al., 1997): focus on the treatment plan; congenial demeanor; and reassuring communication.

As would be expected, health professionals who believe these strategies to be valuable have been shown to use them more frequently in interactions with patients. Further, these behaviors on the part of providers appear to be associated with self-management of disease by their patients.

SUMMARY

Lack of effective disease self-management by the patient and adherence to clinical recommendations remains a substantial threat to the efficacy of preventive and therapeutic regimens. This chapter has summarized and depicted the major elements of a number of well-known and widely employed psychological, sociological, and anthropological models of health-related decisionmaking and action and has summarized some of the major strategies advanced in the empirical literature for increasing adherence and self-management. While further theoretical conceptualization and empirical investigation regarding determinants of (and strategies for influencing) patient adherence are certainly still needed, the variables identified and suggestions offered in this chapter provide the foundation for a rational program that can be implemented by health care providers and public health planners wishing to improve levels of patient cooperation with health-related recommendations.

REFERENCES

Abramson, L. Y., Garber, J., & Seligman, M. E. P. (1980). Learned helplessness in humans: An attributional analysis. In J. Garber & M. E. P. Seligman (Eds.), *Human helplessness: Theory and applications* (pp. 49–74). New York: Academic Press.

Aiken, L. S., West, S. G., Woodward, C. K., & Reno, R. R. (1994). Health beliefs and compliance with mammography-screening recommendations in asymptomatic women. *Health Psychology, 13*, 122–129.

Ajzen, I. (1985). From intentions to actions: A theory of planned behavior. In J. Kuhl & J. Beckman (Eds.), *Action control: From cognition to behavior* (pp. 11–39). New York: Springer Verlag.

Ajzen, I., & Fishbein, M. (1980). *Understanding attitudes and predicting social behavior*. Englewood Cliffs, NJ: Prentice-Hall.

Andersen, R. (1968). *A behavioral model of families' use of health services*. Chicago: University of Chicago, Center for Health Administration Studies.

Andersen, R. (1995). Revisiting the behavioral model and access to medical care: Does it matter? *Journal of Health and Social Behavior, 36*, 1–10.

Andersen, R., & Anderson, O. W. (1979). Trends in the use of health services. In H. E. Freeman, S. Levine, & L. G. Reeder (Eds.), *Handbook of medical sociology* (pp. 371–91). Englewood Cliffs, NJ: Prentice-Hall.

Andersen, R., Kravits, J., & Anderson, O. W. (Eds.). (1975). *Equity in health services: Empirical analyses in social policy*. Cambridge, MA: M.A. Ballinger.

Andersen, R., & Newman, J. F. (1973). Societal and individual determinants of medical care utilization in the United States. *Milbank Memorial Fund Quarterly/Health and Society, 51*, 95–124.

Bandura, A. (1977). Self-efficacy: Toward a unifying theory of behavioral change. *Psychological Review, 84*, 191–215.

Bandura, A. (1984). Recycling misconceptions of perceived self-efficacy. *Cognitive Therapy and Research, 8*, 231–255.

Bandura, A. (1986). *Social learning theory*. Englewood Cliffs, NJ: Prentice-Hall.

Barker, T. (1994). Role of health beliefs in patient compliance with preventive dental advice. *Community Dentistry and Oral Epidemiology, 22*, 327–30.

Bartholomew, L. K., Parcel, G. S., Swank, P. R., & Czyzewski, D. I., Measuring self-efficacy expectations for the self-management of cystic fibrosis. *Chest*, 103(5), 1524–1530.

Becker, M. H. (1974). The health belief model and sick role behavior. *Health Education Monographs, 2*, 409–419.

Becker, M. H. (1990). Theoretical models of adherence and strategies for improving adherence. In S. A. Shumaker, E. Schron, & J. Ockene (Eds.), *The handbook of health behavior change* (pp. 5–43). New York: Springer Publishing.

Becker, M. H., Haefner, D. P., Kasl, S. U., Kirscht, J. P., Maiman, L. A., & Rosenstock, I. M. (1977). Selected psychosocial models and correlates of individual health-related behaviors. *Medical Care, 15* (Suppl), 27–46.

Becker, M. H., & Maiman, L. A. (1981). Patient compliance. In K. L. Melmon (Ed.), *Drug therapeutics: Concepts for physicians* (pp. 65–79). New York: Elsevier.

Berkanovic, E., & Hurwicz, M. L. (1995). Physician visits by rheumatoid arthritis patients: A prospective analysis. *Arthritis Care and Research, 8*, 73–79.

Cameron, L., Leventhal, E. A., & Leventhal, H. (1995). Seeking medical care in response to symptoms and life stress. *Psychosomatic Medicine, 57*, 37–47.

Catt, S., Stygall, J., & Catalan, J. (1995). Acceptance of zidovudine (AZT) in early HIV disease: The role of health beliefs. *AIDS Care, 7*, 225–229.

Chen, W. W. (1995). Enhancement of health locus of control through biofeedback training. *Perceptual and Motor Skills, 80*, 395–398.

Clark, D. O., Patrick, D. L., Grembowski, D., & Durham, M. L. (1995). Socioeconomic status and exercise self-efficacy in late life. *Journal of Behavioral Medicine, 18*, 355–376.

Clark, N. M. (1997). Self-regulation of heart disease and hypertension. In D. S. Gochman (Ed), *Handbook of health behavior research*. New York: Plenum.

Clark, N. M., Evans, D., Zimmerman, B. J., Levison, M. J., & Mellins, R. B. (1994). Patient and family management of asthma: Theory-based techniques for the clinician. *Journal of Asthma, 31*, 427–435.

Clark, N. M., Gong, M., Schork, M. A., Maiman, L. A., Evans, D., Hurwitz, M. E., Roloff, D., & Mellins, R. B. (1997). A scale for assessing health care providers' teaching and communication behavior regarding asthma. *Health Education and Behavior, 24*, 245–256.

Clark, N. M., Nothwehr, F., Gong, M., Evans, D., Maiman L. A., Hurwitz, M. E., Roloff, D., & Mellins, R. B. (1995). Physician-patient partnership in managing chronic illness. *Academic Medicine, 11*, 957–959.

Clark, N. M., Rosenstock, I., Hassan, H., Wasilewski, Y., Evans, D., Feldman, C., & Mellins, R. (1988). The effect of health beliefs and feelings of self-efficacy on self-management behavior of children with a chronic disease. *Patient Counseling and Education, 11*, 131–139.

Clark, N. M., & Starr, N. S. (1994). Management of asthma by patients and families. *American Journal of Respiratory and Critical Care Medicine, 149*, S54–S66.

Clark, N. M., & Zimmerman, B. J. (1990). A social cognitive view of self-regulated learning about health. *Health Education Research, 5*, 371–379.

Clasen, C. M., Vernon, S. W., Mullen, P. D., & Jackson, G. L. (1994). A survey of physician beliefs and self-reported practices concerning screening for early detection of cancer. *Social Science Medicine, 39*, 841–849.

Col, N., Fanale, J. E., & Kronholm, P. (1990). The role of medication noncompliance and adverse drug reactions in hospitalizations of the elderly. *Archives of Internal Medicine, 150*, 841–845.

Conway, S. P., Pond, M. N., Hamnett, T., & Watson, A. (1996). Compliance with treatment in adult patients with cystic fibrosis. *Thorax, 51* (1), 29–33.

Crandall, R. (1978). The measurement of self-esteem and related constructs. In J. P. Robinson & P. R. Shaver (Eds.), *Measures of social psychological attitudes* (pp. 87–94). Ann Arbor, MI: Institute of Social Research, University of Michigan.

Cummings, K. M., Becker, M. H., & Maile, M. C. (1980). Bringing the models together: An empirical approach to combining variables used to explain health actions. *Journal of Behavioral Medicine, 3*, 123–145.

DiIorio, C., Hennessy, M., & Manteuffel, B. (1996). Epilepsy self-management: A test of a theorectical model. *Nursing Research, 45*, 211–217.

Dutton, D. B. (1978). Explaining low use of health services by the poor: Costs, attitudes or delivery systems? *American Sociological Review, 43*, 348–368.

Eraker, S. A., Becker, M. H., Strecher, V. J., & Kirscht, J. P. (1985). Smoking behavior, cessation techniques, and the health decision model. *American Journal of Medicine, 78*, 817–825.

Eraker, S. A., Kirscht, J. P., & Becker, M. H. (1984). Understanding and improving patient compliance. *Annals of Internal Medicine, 100*, 258–268.

Eraker, S. A., & Politser, P. (1982), How decisions are reached: Physician and patient. *Annals of Internal Medicine, 97*, 262–268.

Eraker, S. A., & Sox, H. C., Jr. (1981). Assessment of patients' preferences for therapeutic outcomes. *Medical Decision Making, 1*, 29–39.

Evans, R. G., & Stoddart, G. L. (1990). Producing health, consuming health care. *Social Science and Medicine, 31*, 1347–1363.

Fabrega, H., Jr. (1973). Toward a model of illness behavior. *Medical Care, 11*, 470–484.

Fabrega, H., Jr. (1974). *Disease and social behavior: An interdisciplinary perspective.* Cambridge, MA: Massachusetts Institute of Technology Press.

Fabrega, H., Jr. (1977). Perceived illness and its treatment: A naturalistic study in social medicine. *British Journal of Preventive and Social Medicine, 31*, 213–219.

Fabrega, H., Jr., & Zucker, M. (1977). Comparison of illness episodes in a pluralistic setting. *Psychosomatic Medicine, 39*, 325–343.

Fishbein, M., & Jaccard, J. (1973). Theoretical and methodological considerations in the prediction of family planning intentions and behavior. *Representative Research in Social Psychology, 4*, 37–51.

Fisher, M., Schneider, M., Pegler, C., & Napolitano, B. (1991). Eating attitudes, health-risk behaviors, self-esteem, and anxiety among adolescent females in a suburban high school. *Journal of Adolescent Health, 12*, 377–384.

Fotheringham, M. J., & Sawyer, M. G. (1995). Adherence to recommended medical regimens in childhood and adolescence. *Journal of Pediatric Child Health, 31*, 72–78.

Friedman, L. C., Nelson, D. V., Webb, J. A., Hoffman, L. P., & Baer, P. E. (1994). Dispositional optimism, self-efficacy and health beliefs as predictors of breast self-examination. *American Journal of Preventive Medicine, 10*, 130–135.

Furnham, A., & Steele, H. (1993). Measuring locus of control: A critique of general, children's, health- and work-related locus of control questionnaires. *British Journal of Psychology, 84*, 443–479.

Glanz, K., Lewis, F. M., & Rimer, B. K. (Eds.). (1990). The scope of health education: Parameters of a maturing field. In, *Health behavior and health education: Theory, research and practice* (pp. 3–16). San Francisco: Jossey-Bass.

Godkin, G., & Kok, G. (1996). Theory of P.B.: A review of its application to health related behaviors. *American Journal of Health Promotion, 11*, 87–96.

Higgins, S. T., Budney, A. J., Bickel, W. K., & Badger, G. J. (1994). Participation of significant others in outpatient behavioral treatment predicts greater cocaine abstinence. *American Journal of Alcohol Abuse, 20*, 47–56.

Ireys, H. T., Gross, S. S., Werthamer-Larsson, L. A., & Kolodner, K. B. (1994). Self-esteem of young adults with chronic health conditions: Appraising the effects of perceived impact. *Developmental and Behavioral Pediatrics, 15*, 409–415.

Jaccard, J. (1975). A theoretical analysis of selected factors important to health education strategies. *Health Education Monographs, 3*, 152–167.

Janz, N. K., & Becker, M. H. (1984). The health belief model: A decade later. *Health Education Quarterly, 11*, 1–47.

Janz, N. K., Becker, M. H., & Hartman, P. E. (1984). Contingency contracting to enhance patient compliance: A review. *Patient Education and Counseling, 5*, 165–178.

Kaplan, R. M., Ries, A. L., Prewitt, L. M., & Eakin, E. (1994). Self-efficacy expectations predict survival for patients with chronic obstructive pulmonary disease. *Health Psychology, 13*, 366–368.

Kasl, S. V., & Cobb, S. (1966). Health behavior, illness behavior, and sick role behavior: I. Health and illness behavior. *Archives of Environmental Health, 12*, 246–266.

Kesten, S., Elias, M., Cartier, A., & Chapman, K. R. (1994). Patient handling of a multidose dry power inhalation device for albuterol. *Chest, 105*, 1077–1081.

Kirscht, J. P. (1974). The health belief model and illness behavior. *Health Education Monographs, 2*, 387–408.

Koestner, R., & Zuckerman, M. (1994). Causality orientations, failure, and achievement. *Journal of Personality, 62*, 321–346.

Korsch, B. M., Gozzi, E. K, & Francis, V. (1968). Gaps in doctor-patient communication. I. Doctor-patient interaction and patient satisfaction. *Pediatrics, 42*, 855–871.

Korsch, B. M., & Negrete, V. F. (1972). Doctor-patient communication. *Scientific American, 227*, 66–74.

Kulik, J. A., & Mahler, H. I. M. (1993). Emotional support as a moderator of adjustment and compliance after coronary artery bypass surgery: A longitudinal study. *Journal of Behavioral Medicine, 16*, 45–63.

LaGreca, A. M., Auslander, W. F., Greco, P., Spetter, D., Fisher, E. B., & Santiago, J. V. (1995). I get by with a little help from my family and friends: Adolescents' support for diabetes care. *Journal of Pediatric Psychology, 20*, 449–476.

Larsen, J. S., Hahn, M., Ekholm, B., & Wick, K. A. (1994). Evaluation of conventional press-and-breathe metered-dose inhaler techniques in 501 patients. *Journal of Asthma, 31*, 193–199.

Lazarus, R. S., & Folkman, S. (1984). *Stress, appraisal and coping*. New York: Springer Publishing.

Leventhal, E. A., Hansell, S., Diefenbach, M., Leventhal, H., & Glass, D. C. (1996). Negative affect and self-report of physical symptoms: Two longitudinal studies of older adults. *Health Psychology, 15*, 193–199.

Leventhal, H., Meyer, D., & Gutmann, M. (1980). The role of theory in the study of compliance to high blood pressure regimens. In R. B. Haynes, M. E. Mattson, & T. O. Engebretson, Jr. (Eds.), *Patient compliance to prescribed antihypertensive medication regimens: A report to the National Heart, Lung, and Blood Institute* (NIH Publication No. 81–2102). (pp. 1–58) Washington, DC: U.S. Department of Health and Human Services.

Ley, P. (1972). Primacy, rated importance, and the recall of medical statements. *Journal of Health and Social Behavior, 13*, 311–317.

Ley, P. (1976). Towards better doctor-patient communications. In A. E. Bennett (Ed.), *Communications between doctors and patients* (pp. 77–98). London: Oxford University Press.

Ley, P., Bradshaw, P. W., Eaves, D., & Walker, C. M. (1973). A method for increasing patients' recall of information presented by doctors. *Psychological Medicine, 3*, 217–220.

Lindroth, Y., Strombeck, B., Brossner, M., Gullberg, B., & Wollheim, F. A. (1994). Learned helplessness and its correlation to impairment, pain, anxiety and depression in rheumatoid arthritis. *Scandanavian Journal Rheumatology, 23*, 299–304.

Lorenc, L., & Branthwaite, A. (1993). Are older adults less compliant with prescribed medication than younger adults? *British Journal of Clinical Psychology, 32* (Part 4), 485–492.

Lorig, K., Laurin, J., & Holman, H. R. (1984). Arthritis self-management: A study of the effectiveness of patient education for the elderly. *The Gerontologist, 24*, 455–457.

Maiman, L. A., & Becker, M. H. (1974). The health belief model: Origins and correlates in psychological theory. *Health Education Monographs, 2*, 336–353.
Maiman, L. A., & Becker, M. H. (1980). The clinician's role in patient compliance. *Trends in Pharmacological Sciences, 1*, 457–459.
Matarazzo, J. D., Weiss, S. M., Herd, J. A., Miller, N. E., & Weiss, S. M. (Eds.). (1984). *Behavioral health: A handbook of health enhancement and disease prevention*. New York: Wiley.
McCracken, L. M., Semenchuk, E. M., & Goetsch, V. L. (1995). Cross-sectional and longitudinal analyses of coping responses and health status in persons with systemic lupus erythematosus. *Behavioral Medicine, 20*, 179–187.
McNeil, B. J., Keeler, E., & Adelstein, S. J. (1975). Primer on certain elements of medical decision making. *New England Journal of Medicine, 293*, 211 –215.
McNeil, B. J., Pauker, S. G., Sox, H. C., Jr., & Tversky, A. (1982). On the elicitation of preferences for alternative therapies. *New England Journal of Medicine, 306*, 1259–1262.
Melamed, B. G., & Siegel, L. J. (1980). *Behavioral medicine: Practical applications in health care*. New York: Springer Publishing.
Muma, R. D., Ross, M. W., Parcel, G. S., & Pollard, R. B. (1995). Zidovudine adherence among individuals with HIV infection. *AIDS Care, 7*, 439–447.
Pham, D. T., Fortin, F., & Thibaudeau, M. F. (1996). The role of the health belief model in amputees' self-care adherence to diabetes self-care behaviors. *The Diabetes Educator, 22*, 126–132.
Potvin, L., Camirand, J., & Beland, F. (1995). Patterns of health services utilization and mammography use among women aged 50 to 59 years in the Quebec Medicare system. *Medical Care, 33*, 515–530.
Rosenstock, I. M. (1974). Historical origins of the health belief model. *Health Education Monographs, 2*, 328–335.
Sackett, D. L. (1976). The magnitude of compliance and noncompliance. In D. L. Sackett & R. B. Haynes (Eds.), *Compliance with therapeutic regimens* (pp. 9–25). Baltimore: Johns Hopkins University Press.
Sackett, D. L., Haynes, R. B., Gibson, E. S., Taylor, D. W., Roberts, R. S., & Johnson, A. L. (1978). Patient compliance with antihypertensive regimens. *Patient Counselling and Health Education, 1*, 18–21.
Sackett, D. L., & Snow, J. C. (1979). The magnitude of compliance and noncompliance. In R. B. Haynes, D. W. Taylor, & D. L. Sackett (Eds.), *Compliance in health care* (pp. 11–22). Baltimore, MD: Johns Hopkins University Press.
Schunk, D. H., & Carbonari, J. P. (1984). Self-efficacy models. In J. D. Matarazzo, S. M. Weiss, J. A. Herd, N. E. Miller, & S. M. Weiss (Eds.), *Behavioral health: A handbook of health enhancement and disease prevention* (pp. 230–247). New York: Wiley.
Seibold, D., & Roper, R. (1979). Psychosocial determinants of health care intentions: Test of the Triandis and Fishbein models. In D. Nimmo (Ed.), *Communication yearbook 3* (pp. 111–123). New Brunswick, NJ: Transaction Books.
Sikkema, K. J., Koob, J. J., Cargill, V. C., Kelly, J. A., Desiderato, L. L., Roffman, R. A., Norman, A. D., Shaboazz, M., Copeland, C., Winett, R. A., Steiner, S., & Lemke, A. L. (1995). Levels and predictors of HIV risk behavior among women in low-income public housing developments. *Public Health Reports, 110* (6), 707–713.

Strecher, V. J., DeVellis, B. McE., Becker, M. H., & Rosenstock, I. M. (1986). The role of self-efficacy in achieving health behavior change. *Health Education Quarterly, 13*, 73–92.

Stump, T. E., Johnson, R. J., & Wolinsky, F. D. (1995). Changes in physician utilization over time among older adults. *Journal of Gerontology: Social Sciences, 50B*(1), S45–S58.

Torres, R., Fernandez, F., & Maceira, D. (1995). Self-esteem and value of health as correlates of adolescent health behavior. *Adolescence, 30*, 403–412.

Tversky, A., & Kahneman, D. (1974). Judgment under uncertainty: Heuristics and biases. *Science, 185*, 1124–1131.

Wallston, B. S., & Wallston, K. A. (1984). Social psychological models of health behavior: An examination and integration. In A. Baum, S. Taylor, & J. E. Singer (Eds.), *Handbook of psychology and health* (Vol. IV) (pp. 215–222). Hillsdale, NJ: Erlbaum.

Wasilewski, Y., Clark, N. M., Evans, D., Levison, M. J., Levin, B., & Mellins, R. B. (1996). Factors associated with emergency department visits by children with asthma and implications for health education. *American Journal of Public Health, 86*, 1410–1415.

Weinstein, M. C., & Fineberg, H. V. (Eds.). (1980). *Clinical decision analysis*. Philadelphia: W. B. Saunders.

Williams, P. G. Wiebe, D. J., & Smith, T. W. (1992). Coping processes as mediators of the relationship between hardiness and health. *Journal of Behavioral Medicine, 15*, 237–255.

Wolinsky, F. D., Johnson, R. L., & Stump, T. E. (1995). The risk of mortality among older adults over an eight-year period. *The Gerontologist, 35*, 150–161.

Ziff, M. A., Conrad, P., & Lachman M. E. (1995). The relative effects of perceived personal control and responsibility on health and health-related behaviors in young and middle-aged adults. *Health Education Quarterly, 22*, 127–142.

2

Relapse Prevention and the Maintenance of Optimal Health

G. Alan Marlatt and William H. George

WHAT IS RELAPSE PREVENTION?

Relapse Prevention (RP) is a self-control program designed to help individuals to anticipate and cope with the problem of relapse in the habit-change process. *Relapse* refers to a breakdown or failure in a person's attempt to change or modify a particular habit pattern, such as stopping "bad habits" or developing new, optimal health behaviors. Based on the principle of social-learning theory (Bandura, 1986), RP combines behavioral skill-training procedures, cognitive therapy, and lifestyle rebalancing. Because the RP model combines behavioral and cognitive components, it is similar to other cognitive-behavioral approaches that have been developed in recent years as an outgrowth and extension of more traditional behavior therapy programs.

The RP model initially developed as a behavioral maintenance program for use in the treatment of addictive behaviors (Marlatt & Gordon, 1980, 1985). Goals of addiction treatment are either to refrain totally from performing a target behavior (e.g., to abstain from drug use) or to impose regulatory limits or controls over the occurrence of a behavior (e.g., to diet as a means of controlling food intake).

Relapse prevention can be applied either as a maintenance strategy to prevent relapse or as a more general approach to lifestyle change. The aim of maintenance strategies is to prevent or intervene in the relapse process after the initiation of behavior change (e.g., to prevent a recent ex-smoker from returning to habitual smoking). As such, RP procedures are designed to enhance the maintenance of behavior change, and may be applied regardless of the theoretical orientation or intervention methods applied during the initial treatment phase. Once an alcoholic has stopped drinking, for example, RP methods can be applied toward the effective maintenance of abstinence, regardless of the methods used to initiate abstinence (e.g., attending AA meetings, pharmacotherapy, voluntary cessation).

The second application of the RP model is a more general one: to facilitate changes in personal habits to reduce the risk of physical disease or psychological stress. A balanced lifestyle is characterized by enhanced awareness and a harmonious balance between "want" and "should" activities. The development of "positive addictions" (Glasser, 1974) such as physical exercise and meditation is recommended as part of the lifestyle rebalancing program.

TREATMENT VERSUS MAINTENANCE: SEPARATE PROCESSES?

To illustrate the distinction between treatment and maintenance as separate processes or stages in the modification of addictive behaviors, consider the example of an alcoholic or problem drinker who is motivated to change. A wide variety of procedures and techniques is available that may be effective in getting an alcoholic to stop drinking; examples include comprehensive inpatient programs, pharmacotherapy, dietary management, marital or family counseling, group therapy, occupational therapy, behavior modification, religious conversions, Alcoholics Anonymous, and so forth. Some techniques are directed more toward initially getting the person to stop drinking (i.e., oriented toward the initial cessation of the problem behavior), whereas others are directed more toward the long-term maintenance of this change.

A typical response to the high relapse rate in addiction treatment has been to increase the number of initial treatment techniques, and to build a more comprehensive broad-spectrum or multimodal treatment package designed to facilitate cessation of the target behavior (Marlatt & Gordon, 1985). The underlying assumption here seems to be that if sufficient components are added to the initial treatment program, the effects on treatment outcome will somehow last longer. There are two major drawbacks to the multimodal approach to treatment. First, recent evidence suggests that the more techniques and procedures that are applied during treatment, the more difficult it becomes for the client to maintain compliance with the program requirements (e.g., S. Hall, 1980). Second, many, if not all, of the intervention techniques are directed primarily toward initial behavior change only, and not toward the long-term maintenance of this change. Frequently treatment techniques are geared primarily toward cessation of the target behavior, whether it be smoking, alcohol consumption, overeating, or the performance of other problem behaviors (e.g., sexual exhibitionism). What is often overlooked in this focus on initial cessation is that the maintenance of change, once induced, may be governed by entirely different principles than those associated with initial cessation.

One important difference between initial treatment procedures and those designed to enhance maintenance effects over time is that the former techniques are often externally administered to the client by the therapist (e.g., pharmacotherapy, assertive training, and contingency contracting), whereas maintenance procedures are often left to the client to "self-administer". An exception to this distinction is the use of externally applied "booster" sessions, in which a technique such as pharmacotherapy is readministered to the client at various intervals following treatment in an attempt to bolster and reinforce the effects of the initial treatment program. The goal of teaching the client self-administered maintenance techniques, on the other hand, is to train the client to become his or her own therapist, and to carry on the thrust of the intervention program after the termination of the formal therapeutic relationship. Instead of relying on willpower during the maintenance phase, a successful graduate of this type of program would be well-grounded in self-monitoring and self-management skills. This self-control orientation is characteristic of the RP approach.

RELAPSE: TWO OPPOSING DEFINITIONS

At a recent workshop for alcoholism and drug counselors, members of the audience were asked to share their subjective associations to the term *relapse*. Here are some of their replies: "treatment failure", "return to illness", "falling back into addiction", "failure and guilt", and "breakdown." These associations are reflected in one definition of "relapse" given in *Webster's New Collegiate Dictionary*: "A recurrence of symptoms of a disease after a period of improvement". This definition corresponds with the dichotomous view of treatment outcome fostered by the disease model: one is either "cured" (or the symptoms are in remission) or one has relapsed (recidivism). It has been standard practice in the addictions field to view any use of drugs following an abstinence-oriented treatment program as indicative of relapse. Relapse is thus seen as an end state—the end of the road, a dead end.

There are a number of problems with this rather pessimistic approach to relapse. If the black/white dichotomy of abstinence/relapse is assimilated by the individual while in treatment, this may set up an expectation leading to a self-fulfilling prophecy, in which any violation of abstinence will send the pendulum to the other extreme of relapse.

Another problem with the traditional definition of relapse is its association with the return of the disease state. The cause of the relapse is usually attributed to internal biological factors associated with the disease condition (Brickman et al., 1982). Behaviors associated with relapse come to be equated with the emergence of symptoms signaling the reactivation of the underlying disease, much as the experience of fever and chills serves as a signal of relapse in malaria. This emphasis on internal causation carries the implicit message that there is nothing much one can do about the outbreak of symptoms—how does one prevent a fever from breaking out? This outlook tends to ignore the influence of situational and psychological factors as potential determinants in the relapse process. It also reinforces the notion that the individual who experiences a relapse is a helpless victim of circumstances beyond his or her control.

An alternative approach to the issue of relapse is reflected in Webster's second definition of relapse: "Relapse is the *act* or *instance* of backsliding, worsening, or subsiding". Italics are added here to emphasize that a relapse can be viewed as a *single act* of falling back: a single mistake, an error, a slip. A more appropriate word to refer to the singular occurrence of the behavior in question (e.g., the first drink or cigarette following a period of abstinence) would be *lapse* (as in a "lapse" of attention). The same dictionary defines 'lapse" as "a slight error or slip . . . a temporary fall esp. from a higher to a lower state". One thinks here of a skater in competition who trips and falls on the ice: whether the skater gets up again and continues to perform depends to a large extent on whether the fall is seen as a 'lapse" or a "relapse"—as a single slip (mistake) or as an indication of total failure.

In the RP approach, relapse is viewed as a transitional process, a series of events that may or may not be followed by a return to pretreatment baseline levels of the target behavior. It is possible to view the alcoholic who takes a single drink after a period of abstinence as someone who has made a slight excursion over the border between abstinence and relapse. Whether this first lapse is followed by a return to abstinence depends considerably on the personal expectations of the individual involved. The RP approach attempts to provide the individual with the necessary skills and cognitive strategies to prevent the single occurrence of a lapse from snowballing into a total relapse. Rather than pessimistically looking upon a relapse as a dead end, the RP approach views it as a fork in the road, with one path returning to the former problem behavior and the other continuing in the direction of positive change.

Different questions arise when one adopts this alternative perspective of relapse (Brownell, Marlatt, Lichtenstein, & Wilson, 1986). Are there any specific situational events that serve as precipitating triggers for relapse? Are the determinants of the first lapse the same as those assumed to govern a total relapse? Is it possible for an individual to covertly "plan" a relapse by setting up a situation in which it is virtually impossible to resist temptation? At which points in the relapse process is it possible to intervene and alter the course of events and thus prevent a return to the former habit pattern? How does the individual react to and conceptualize the events preceding and following a relapse, and how do these reactions affect the person's subsequent behavior? Is it possible to prepare persons in treatment to anticipate the likelihood of a relapse so that they may engage in preventive alternative behaviors? To borrow a term from the medical model, can we develop prevention procedures that would "inoculate" the individual against the inevitability of relapse?

To answer these and other questions, it is necessary to engage in a detailed microanalysis of the relapse process itself. This fine-grained approach focuses upon the various determinants of relapse, including the immediate precipitating circumstances and the longer chain of events that may or may not precede the relapse episode. In addition, the role of such cognitive factors as expectation and attribution is examined in detail, particularly those related to the individual's reactions to the relapse. A microanalysis of the relapse process is justified by the old maxim that we can learn much from our mistakes. Rather than being seen as an indication of failure, a relapse can be viewed more optimistically as a challenge, an opportunity for new learning to occur.

OVERVIEW OF THE RELAPSE MODEL

In the following overview, only the highlights of the RP model are presented. Background research and theory leading to the development of this model can be found in Cummings, Gordon, and Marlatt (1980), Marlatt (1978, 1982, 1996a, b), Marlatt and Gordon (1980, 1985), and Shiffman and Wills (1985). The following overview draws extensively from these previously published accounts of the model. It represents an updated version of the RP overview presented by Marlatt and George (1984, 1990) and previously updated in George (1989), Marlatt and Barrett (1994). The present update critiques recent validation studies of the relapse taxonomy, summarizes recent outcome findings, and considers the extended range of problems for which RP has been applied.

High-Risk Situations: The Relapse Taxonomy

The relapse taxonomy provides a structure for classifying relapse circumstances (Marlatt, 1996a). The taxonomy evolved from empirical scrutiny of relapse episodes (Marlatt, 1978).

A base assumption of the taxonomy is that the individual experiences a sense of perceived control while maintaining abstinence (or complying with other rules governing the target behavior). The behavior is under control so long as it does not occur during this period; the longer the period of successful abstinence (or compliance), the greater the individual's perception of self-control. This perceived control will continue until the person encounters a high-risk situation. A high-risk situation is defined broadly as any situation (including emotional reactions to the situation) that poses a threat to the individual's sense of control and increases the risk of potential relapse.

Classification of the circumstances associated with reinitiation of addictive behaviors led to a taxonomy of relapse episodes. In an analysis of 311 initial relapse episodes obtained from clients with a variety of problem behaviors (problem drinking, smoking, heroin addiction, compulsive gambling, and overeating), we identified three primary high-risk situations that were associated with almost three quarters of all the relapses reported (see Cummings et al., 1980, for a description of other high-risk situations). A brief description of the three categories associated with the highest relapse rates follows.

1. Negative emotional states (35% of all relapses in the sample)

These are situations in which the individual is experiencing a negative (or unpleasant) emotional state, mood, or feeling such as frustration, anger, anxiety, depression, boredom, and so forth, prior to or at the same time that the first lapse occurs. For example, a smoker in the sample gave the following description of a relapse episode

> It had been raining continually all week. Saturday I walked down to the basement to do laundry and I found the basement filled with a good three inches of water. To make things worse, as I went to turn on the light to see the extent of the damage, I got shocked from the light switch. Later that same day I was feeling real low and knew I had to have a cigarette after my neighbor, who is a contractor, assessed the damage at over $4,000. I went to the store and bought a pack.

2. Interpersonal conflict (16% of the relapses)

These are situations involving an ongoing or relatively recent conflict associated with any interpersonal relationship, such as marriage, friendship, family members, or employer-employee relations. Arguments and interpersonal confrontations occur frequently in this category. A gambler who had been abstaining from betting on the horses described his relapse in the following terms

> I came home late from a horrible day on the road and I hadn't stepped in the house 5 minutes before my wife started accusing me of gambling on the horses. Racetrack, hell! I told her if she didn't believe me, I'd give her a real reason to file for divorce. That night I spent $450 on the Longacres track.

3. Social pressure (20% of the sample)

These are situations in which the individual is responding to the influence of another person or group of people who exert pressure on the individual to engage in the taboo behavior. Social pressure may either be direct (direct interpersonal contact with verbal persuasion) or indirect (e.g., being in the presence of others who are engaging in the same target behavior, even though no direct pressure is involved). Here is an example of direct social pressure given by a formerly abstinent problem drinker in our sample

> I went to my boss's house for a surprise birthday dinner for him. I got there late and as I came into the living room everyone had a drink in hand. I froze when the boss's wife asked me what I was drinking. Without thinking, I said, 'J&B on the rock's".

In these early analyses of relapse episodes, we found more similarities than differences in relapse categories across the various addictive behaviors. These same three high-risk situations are frequently found to he associated with relapse, regardless of the particular problem involved (problem drinking, smoking, gambling, heroin use, or overeating). This pattern of findings lends support to our hypothesis that there is a common mechanism underlying the relapse process across different addictive behaviors.

The above classification structure emerged as prominent among taxonomic systems emphasizing psychological precipitants of relapse (Connors, Maisto, & Donovan, 1996). The relapse taxonomy has stimulated considerable clinical innovation (e.g., Annis, Schober, & Kelly, 1996) and empirical research (e.g., Vuchinich & Tucker, 1996). In an extensive multi-site project investigating the taxonomy, investigators reported data replicating, extending, and qualifying various aspects of the taxonomy (Lowman, Allen, Stout, & the Alcohol Relapse Group, 1996).

Microanalysis of Proximal Relapse Determinants

We postulated that if an individual can cope effectively with the high-risk situation (e.g., is assertive in counteracting social pressures), the probability of relapse decreases significantly. The individual who copes successfully with the situation is likely to experience a sense of mastery or perception of control. Successful mastery of one problematic situation is often associated with an expectation of being able to cope successfully with the next challenging event. The expectancy of being able to cope with successive high-risk situations as they develop is closely associated with Bandura's notion of self-efficacy (Bandura, 1977, 1986), defined as the individual's expectation concerning the capacity to cope with an impending situation or task. A feeling of confidence in one's abilities to cope effectively with a high-risk situation is associated with an increased perception of self-efficacy, a kind of "I know I can handle it" feeling. As the duration of the abstinence (or period of controlled use) increases, and the individual is able to cope effectively with more and more high-risk situations, perception of control increases in a cumulative fashion. The probability of relapse decreases accordingly.

What happens if an individual does not cope successfully with a high-risk situation? The person may never have acquired the coping skills involved, or the appropriate response may be inhibited by fear or anxiety. Perhaps the individual fails to recognize and respond to the risk involved before it is too late. Motivational deficits may also undermine acquired coping strategies. Whatever the reason, as self-efficacy decreases in the precipitating high-risk situation, one's expectations for coping successfully with subsequent problem situations also begin to decrease. If the situation also involves the temptation to engage in the prohibited behavior as a means of attempting to cope with the stress involved, the stage is set for a probable relapse. The probability of relapse is enhanced if the individual holds positive expectancies about the effects of the activity or substance involved. Often the person will anticipate the immediate positive effects of the activity, an anticipation based on past experience, while ignoring or not attending to the delayed negative consequences involved. The lure of immediate gratification becomes the dominant figure in the perceptual field as the reality of the full consequences of the act recedes into the background. For many persons, smoking a cigarette or taking a drink has long been associated with coping with stress. "A drink would sure help me get through this" or "If only I could have a smoke, I would feel more relaxed" are common beliefs of this type. Positive outcome expectancies are a primary determinant of alcohol use/abuse and other forms of substance abuse (e.g., Brown, 1993; Brandon, Wetter, & Baker, 1996). Expectancies figure prominently as determinants of relapse in the RP model (Marlatt, 1987; Marlatt & Rohsenow, 1980).

Coping skills play an important role in relapse (e.g., Connors, Maisto, & Zwiak, 1996; Miller, Westerberg, Harris, & Tonigan, 1996). The inability to cope effectively in a high-risk situation, coupled with positive outcome expectancies for the effects of the habitual coping behavior, greatly increases the probability that an initial lapse will occur. On the one hand, the individual is faced with a high-risk situation with no coping response available;

self-efficacy decreases as the person feels less able to exert control. On the other hand, there is the lure of the old coping response, the drink, the drug, or other substance. At this point, unless a last-minute coping response or a sudden change of circumstance occurs, the individual may cross over the border from abstinence (or controlled use) to relapse. Whether or not this first excursion over the line, the first lapse, is followed by a total relapse depends to a large extent on the individual's perceptions of the "cause" of the lapse and the reactions associated with its occurrence.

The requirement of abstinence is an absolute dictum. Once someone has crossed over the line, there is no going back. From this all-or-none perspective, a single drink or cigarette is sufficient to violate the rule of abstinence: once committed, the deed cannot be undone. After a lapse experience, the person is likely to experience a decrease in self-efficacy, frequently coupled with a sense of helplessness and a tendency to passively give in to the situation. "It's no use, I can't handle this" is a common reaction. To account for this reaction to the transgression of an absolute rule, we have postulated a mechanism called the *Abstinence Violation Effect* or AVE (Curry, Gordon, & Marlatt, 1987; Marlatt & Gordon, 1985). The AVE is postulated to occur under the following conditions: Prior to the first lapse, the individual is personally committed to an extended or indefinite period of abstinence. The intensity of the AVE will vary as a function of several factors, including the degree of prior commitment or effort expended to maintain abstinence, the duration of the abstinence period (the longer the period, the greater the effect), and the subjective value or importance of the prohibited behavior to the individual. We hypothesize that the AVE is characterized by two key cognitive-affective elements: cognitive dissonance (conflict and guilt), and a personal attribution effect (blaming the self as the cause of the relapse). Subsequent work has extended and elaborated conceptual and methodological indicators of the AVE (e.g. Miller et al., 1996; Shiffman, et al. 1996).

Covert Antecedents and Relapse Set-Ups

In the foregoing discussion of the immediate determinants and reactions to relapse, the high-risk situation is viewed as the precipitating or triggering situation associated with the initial lapse or first "slip" following a period of abstinence or controlled use. In many of the relapse episodes we have studied in our research program, the first lapse is precipitated in a high-risk situation that the individual unexpectedly encounters. In many cases, the person is not expecting the high-risk situation to occur, and/or is generally insufficiently prepared to cope effectively with the circumstances as they arise. Quite often, individuals will suddenly find themselves in a rapidly escalating situation that cannot be dealt with effectively.

For example, one of our clients who had a serious drinking problem experienced her first lapse after several weeks of abstinence when she treated a new friend to lunch. A last-minute change of plans led them to eat at a restaurant that served alcoholic beverages. Just moments after their arrival, a cocktail waitress approached their table and asked for drink orders. Our client's friend ordered a cocktail first, and then the waitress turned to the client saying, "And you?" She too ordered a drink, the first of a series of events that culminated in a full-blown relapse. As the client said later, "I didn't plan it and I wasn't prepared for it." Suddenly confronted with a high-risk situation (a social pressure situation, in which the client was influenced both by her friend's ordering a drink and by the waitress asking her for an order), she was unable to cope effectively.

In other relapse episodes, however, the high-risk situation appears to be the last link in a chain of events preceding the first lapse. In another case study, for example, the client was a compulsive gambler who came to us for help in controlling his habit, which had caused him numerous marital and financial problems. Although he had abstained from all gambling for about 6 months, he had had a relapse and was unable to regain abstinence. We asked the client, a resident of Seattle, to describe this last relapse episode. "There's nothing much to talk about," he began. "I was in Reno and I started gambling again." Reno, Nevada is clearly a high-risk city for any gambler trying to maintain abstinence. We then asked him to describe the events preceding his arrival in Reno (Reno is 1,000 miles from Seattle). A close analysis of this chain of events led us to the conclusion that this client had covertly set up or "planned" the relapse. Although our client strongly denied his responsibility in this covert planning process, it was clear to us that there were a number of choice points (forks in the road) preceding the relapse where the client "chose" an alternative that led him closer to the brink of relapse. He finally ended up in a downtown Reno casino where he succumbed to a slot machine, an event that triggered a weekend-long binge of costly gambling. It was as if he had placed himself in a situation that was so risky only a moral Superman could have resisted the temptation to resume gambling.

Why do some clients appear to set up their own relapse? From a cost-benefit perspective, a relapse can be seen as a very rational choice or decision for many individuals. The benefit is swift in coming: the payoff of immediate gratification (and the chance of hitting the jackpot). For many, the reward of instant gratification far outweighs the cost of potential negative effects that may or may not occur sometime in the distant future (especially if one is a gambler at heart). Why not take the chance—this time it might be different, and perhaps it could be done with impunity? Cognitive distortions such as denial and rationalization make it much easier to set up one's own relapse episode: One may deny both the intent to relapse and the importance of long-range negative consequences. There are also many excuses to rationalize the act of indulgence.

One of the most tempting rationalizations is that the desire to indulge is justified. This justification is exemplified in the title of a book describing the drinking lifestyles of derelict alcoholics: *You Owe Yourself a Drunk* (Spradley, 1970). Our research findings and clinical experience in working with a variety of addictive behavior problems suggest that the degree of balance in a person's daily life has a significant impact on the desire for indulgence or immediate gratification. Here we are defining "balance" as the degree of equilibrium that exists in one's daily life between those activities perceived as external demands (or "shoulds") and those perceived as activities the person engages in for pleasure or self-fulfillment (the "wants"). Paying household bills and performing routine chores or menial tasks at work would count highly as "shoulds" for many individuals. At the other end of the scale are the "wants"—the activities the person likes to perform and gains some immediate gratification from engaging in (e.g., going fishing, taking time off for lunch with a friend, or engaging in a creative work task). Other activities represent a mixture of "wants" and "shoulds". We find that a lifestyle encumbered with a preponderance of perceived "shoulds" is often associated with an increased perception of self-deprivation and a corresponding desire for indulgence and gratification. It is as if the person who spends his or her entire day engaged in activities that are high in external demand (often perceived as "hassling" events) attempts to balance this disequilibrium by engaging in an excessive "want" as a means of justifying self-indulgence at the end of the day (e.g., drinking to excess in the evening).

Assessment and Intervention Strategies

In this section, we present highlights of the RP assessment and intervention strategies. We first discuss strategies that are designed to teach the client how to anticipate and cope with the possibility of relapse, how to recognize and cope with high-risk situations that may precipitate a lapse, and how to modify their cognitions and other reactions and thus prevent a single lapse from developing into a full-blown relapse. Because these procedures are explicitly focused on the immediate precipitants of the relapse process, we refer to them collectively as specific intervention strategies. Second, we present strategies designed to rebalance the client's lifestyle and to identify and cope with covert determinants of relapse. We refer to these procedures as global self-control strategies.

Both specific and global RP strategies can be placed in three main categories: skill training, cognitive reframing, and lifestyle rebalancing. Skill-training strategies include both behavioral and cognitive responses to cope with high-risk situations. Cognitive reframing procedures are designed to provide the client with alternative cognitions concerning the nature of the habit-change process (i.e., to view it as a learning process), to introduce coping imagery to deal with urges and early warning signals, and to reframe reactions to the initial lapse (restructuring of the AVE). Finally, lifestyle rebalancing strategies (e.g., relaxation and exercise) are designed to strengthen the client's overall coping capacity and to reduce the frequency and intensity of urges and craving that are often the product of an unbalanced lifestyle.

Which of the various intervention techniques should be applied with a particular client? It is possible to combine techniques into a standardized "package," with each subject receiving identical components, if the purpose is to evaluate the effectiveness of a package program. Most readers, however, will be applying the RP model with clients in an applied clinical setting. In contrast to the demands of treatment outcome research, clinicians typically prefer to develop an individualized program of techniques for each client. The individualized approach is the one we recommend for most clients. Specific techniques should be selected based on a carefully conducted assessment program (Donovan & Marlatt, 1988). Therapists are encouraged to select intervention techniques based on their initial evaluation and assessment of the client's problem and general lifestyle pattern. The overall goal of the specific intervention procedures is to teach the client to anticipate and cope with the possibility of relapse: to recognize and cope with high-risk situations that may precipitate a slip, and to modify cognitions and other reactions so as to prevent a single lapse from developing into a full-blown relapse.

The first step in the prevention of relapse is to teach the client to recognize high-risk situations that may precipitate or trigger a relapse. Here, the sooner one becomes aware that one is involved in a chain of events that increases the probability of a slip or lapse, the sooner one can intervene by performing an appropriate coping skill and/or recognize and respond to the discriminative stimuli associated with entering a high-risk situation, using these cues both as warning signals and as reminders to engage in alternative or remedial action.

In a metaphor we often use, the client in a self-control program is likened to a driver setting out on a highway journey. The trip itinerary (i.e., moving from excessive drug use to abstinence) includes both "easy" and "hard" stretches of road. From this metaphorical perspective, the high-risk situations are equivalent to those dangerous parts of the trip requiring extra caution and skill to prevent a mishap. The discriminative stimuli that signal a high-risk situation can be thought of as highway signs providing the driver with information about upcoming dangers and risks on the road (e.g., "Icy patches ahead: SLOW to 25"). The responsible, alert driver is trained to keep an eye out for these signs and to take appropriate action. Similarly, the person attempting to refrain from engaging in a particular target behavior (e.g., smoking or drinking) must be on the lookout for cues that signal the proximity of potentially troublesome situations. These cues are early warning signals; the sooner they are noticed, the easier it is to anticipate what lies around the next bend and to take appropriate steps for effectively dealing with the situation.

An essential aspect of teaching clients to handle high-risk situations more effectively is to first enable them to identify and anticipate these situations. Earlier we discussed prototypic kinds of high-risk situations. However, the identification of high-risk situations is ultimately an individualized question requiring idiographic assessment procedures. Whenever it is possible to have clients keep a record of their addictive behaviors for a baseline period prior to treatment, self-monitoring procedures offer an effective method for assessing high-risk situations. As little as 2 weeks of self-monitoring data can often highlight the situational influences and skill deficits that underlie an addictive behavior pattern.

In the assessment of self-efficacy, the client is presented with a list of potential relapse situations. For each situation, the client uses a rating scale to estimate his or her subjective expectation of successful coping. Ratings across a wide range of situations enable the individual to identify both problematic situations and skill deficits in need of remedial training. Results from these types of assessment can later dictate the focus of skill-training procedures. Self-efficacy scales have been developed for addictive behavior problems such as smoking (Condiotte & Lichtenstein, 1981) and alcoholism (Annis, 1986).

Determining the adequacy of preexisting coping abilities is a critical assessment target. In a treatment outcome investigation aimed at teaching alcoholics to handle situational temptations, Chaney, O'Leary, and Marlatt (1978) devised the Situational Competency Test to measure coping ability. In this technique, the client is presented with a series of written or audiotaped descriptions of potential relapse situations. Each description ends with a prompt for the client to respond. Later, the client's responses to the scenes are scored on a number of dimensions, including response duration and latency, degree of compliance, and specification of alternative behaviors.

Carefully executed assessment procedures will enable the individual to identify many high-risk situations. The client must then learn an alternative approach for responding to these situations. A first step in this new approach is to recognize that high-risk situations are best perceived as discriminative stimuli, signaling the need for behavior change in the same way that road signs signal the need for alternative action. When viewed in this way, these situations can be seen as junctures where choices are made, rather than as inevitable and uncontrollable challenges that must be endured. In this light, the choice to simply avoid or take a detour around risky situations becomes more available to the individual. However, routine avoidance of particular high-risk situations is unrealistic. Therefore, clients must acquire coping skills that enable them to cope with these situations.

Remedial skill training necessitated by identification of coping skill deficits is the cornerstone of the RP treatment program. When the individual lacks coping skills, a variety of remedial skills can be taught. The content of the skill-training program is variable and will depend on the needs of the individual. Possible content areas include assertiveness, stress management, relaxation training, anger management, communication skills, and general social and/or dating skills. In addition to these specific content areas, the RP approach routinely includes training in more general problem-solving skills (Goldfried & Davison, 1976). The advantage of this latter feature is that it provides the client with a set of highly flexible skills that are generalizable across situations and problem areas. Equipping the client with general problem-solving skills obviates the need for overreliance on rote memorization and execution of the relatively mechanized behavioral prescriptions that often typify content-focused skill-training programs. In skill training, the actual teaching procedures are based on the work of McFall (1976) and other investigators. The range of methods includes behavior rehearsal, instruction, coaching, evaluative feedback, modeling, and role playing. In addition, Meichenbaum's (1977) work on cognitive self-instruction has proven especially valuable for teaching clients constructive self-statements. For troubleshooting and consolidating the newly acquired skills, regular homework assignments are an essential ingredient in skill training.

To reiterate, implementation of a specific skill-training program will be dictated by the client's unique profile of high-risk situations. If the individual typically drinks or overdrinks after arguments with a spouse or significant other, then communication or anger-management skills are indicated. If risky encounters revolve around contact with the opposite sex, then dating and social skills may be recommended. The person's high-risk situations determine the skill training requirements.

In some instances, it will be impractical to rehearse the new coping skills in real-life situations. This problem can be surmounted through relapse rehearsal. In this procedure, the client is instructed to imagine being in actual high-risk situations, but performing more adaptive behaviors and thinking more adaptive thoughts. The emphasis here is on coping rather than mastery imagery. That is, the individual is encouraged to visualize that he or she is successfully handling the difficult situation through some effortful struggle, rather than through easy mastery. To emphasize self-efficacy enhancement, the client may be instructed to imagine that the rehearsed experience is accompanied by mounting feelings of competence and confidence. As a consequence, the person experiences heightened expectations of successful coping in future real-life situations, thereby reducing the probability of relapse.

We have found that the relapse rehearsal procedure can be readily carried out as an intersession homework assignment.

That the client may fail to effectively employ these coping strategies and experience a slip must be anticipated. The client's postslip reaction is a pivotal intervention point in the RP model, because it determines the degree of escalation from a single isolated slip to a full-blown relapse. The first step in anticipating and dealing with this reaction is to devise an explicit therapeutic contract to limit the extent of substance use if a slip occurs. The contract specifications should be worked out individually with the client. However, the fundamental method of intervention after a slip is to use cognitive restructuring to counter the cognitive and affective components of the AVE. The main objective here is to enable the client to construe the slip as a unique occurrence—a mistake. If instead the client views the slip as an irreversible failure and succumbs to the conflict, guilt, and personal attribution that characterize the AVE, then a full-blown relapse is more likely to occur. A highly useful technique here is to have the client carry a wallet-sized reminder card with instructions to read and follow in the event of a slip. The text of this card should include the name and phone number of a therapist or treatment center to be called, as well as a cognitive reframing antidote to the AVE.

The final thrust in the RP self-management program is the global intervention procedure of lifestyle rebalancing. It is insufficient to teach clients mechanistic skills for handling high-risk situations and regulating consumption. A comprehensive self-management program also must improve the client's overall lifestyle and thus increase his or her capacity to cope with more pervasive stress factors, antecedents to the occurrence of high-risk situations. To accomplish this training, a number of treatment strategies have been devised to short-circuit the covert antecedents to relapse and promote mental and physical wellness.

In an unbalanced lifestyle, a persistent and continuing disequilibrium between "shoulds" and "wants" can pave the way for relapse by producing a chronic sense of deprivation. To reiterate: when the individual perceives his or her lifestyle as predominated by duties and obligations and as lacking commensurate indulgence in gratifying activities, then a sense of deprivation begins to accrue. As these feelings mount, the person may experience a growing desire to treat himself or herself to an immediately gratifying indulgence. For most clients, drug use is a source of immediate gratification and a method for restoring balance to an "unfairly" lopsided equation. This desire for indulgence translates into urges, cravings, and cognitive distortions that lead clients "unintentionally" closer to the brink of relapse.

An effective method to induce clients to view the disequilibrium of "wants" and "shoulds" as a precursor of relapse is to have them self-monitor the number of "wants" and "shoulds" that prevail in their lives. By keeping a daily record of duties and obligations on one hand and indulgences on the other, clients can soon become acutely aware of the discrepancy between "shoulds" and "wants." Next, the client should be encouraged to seek a restoration of balance by making time each day to engage in worthwhile indulgences, including more positive addictions. Glasser (1974) described negative addictions (e.g., excessive drinking) as activities that initially feel good but produce long-term harm. Conversely, positive addictions (e.g., running) produce short-term discomfort while yielding long-range benefits. After short-range disincentives have been surmounted, a positive addiction acquires a great deal of attraction value for the individual and comes to be perceived as a want. At this point, the person feels deprived if prevented from engaging in the activity. Furthermore, positive addictions contribute toward the person's long-term health and well-being, while also providing an adaptive coping response for life stressors and relapse-risk situations. As long-range health benefits accrue, the person begins to develop more self-confidence and self-efficacy.

Activities having potential for positive addiction include aerobic exercise, meditation and other relaxation techniques (Marlatt & Marques, 1977). Such activities offer an easily learnable and readily available method for achieving a constructive "high" experience. We have found that regular aerobic exercise (running) is associated with a significant reduction in drinking behavior among heavy drinkers (Murphy, Pagano, & Marlatt, 1986).

Despite the efficacy of these techniques for counteracting feelings of deprivation that would otherwise predispose the individual toward relapse, occasional urges and cravings may still surface from time to time. For this reason, various urge-control procedures are recommended. Sometimes urges and cravings are directly triggered by external cues, such as the sight of one's favorite beer mug or wine goblet in the kitchen cabinet, or meeting an old friend who is a heavy smoker. The frequency of these externally triggered urges can be substantially reduced by employing simple stimulus control techniques aimed at minimizing exposure to these cues. In some instances, avoidance strategies offer the most effective way of reducing the frequency of externally triggered urges. Certain events or situations, such as the biweekly poker games or the wine section of the local grocery, may just have to be avoided temporarily while the individual develops more coping skills. Generally, avoidance strategies can often come in handy for dealing with unexpected high-risk situations that emerge. A selection of viable avoidance strategies can enhance the individual's sense of choice when confronted with dangerous situations.

In teaching clients to cope with urge and craving experiences, it is important to emphasize that the discomfort associated with these internal events is natural. Often the person undergoing cravings has a tendency to feel as though the discomfort will continue to mount precipitously until resistance collapses under the overwhelming weight of a ballooning urge. In working with this concern, we stress that urges and cravings are often triggered by environmental cues; they rise in intensity, reach a peak, and then subside. In this respect, urges can be likened to waves in the sea: they rise, crest, and fall. Using this metaphor, we encourage the client to wait out the urge, to look forward to the downside, and to endure that time when the urge discomfort is peaking.

Recall that urges and cravings may not always operate at a conscious level, but may become masked by cognitive distortions and defense mechanisms. As such, they can still exert a potent influence by allowing for "apparently irrelevant decisions" that inch the person closer to relapse. To counter this, we train the client to see through these self-deceptions by recognizing their true meanings. Explicit self-talk can help in making apparently irrelevant decisions seem more relevant. By acknowledging to oneself that certain "minidecisions" (e.g., keeping wine at home in case friends drop over) actually represent urges and cravings, one becomes able to use these experiences as early warning signals. An important objective in these urge-control techniques is to enable the individual to externalize urges and cravings and to view them with detachment. Another way to achieve this detachment is to encourage the client to deliberately label the urge as soon as it registers into consciousness. Urges should be viewed as natural occurrences that happen in response to environmental and lifestyle forces, rather than as signs of being a failure and indicators of future relapse.

EMPIRICAL SUPPORT AND FUTURE DIRECTIONS

The empirical underpinnings of the RP model discussed in this chapter have been reviewed by Marlatt and Gordon (1985). Early outcome studies, along with research on the role of expectancies (self-efficacy and outcome expectancies) and coping skills in the habit-change process, have provided general support for the model (Abrams, Niaura, Carey, Monti, & Binkoff, 1986; Brownell et al., 1986; Shiffman & Wills, 1985). The model is now beyond its formative stages of development. Several aspects of the model have been subjected to empirical investigation in recent years.

The Relapse Taxonomy: Current Status

A potential limitation of our original relapse taxonomy is its reliance on retrospective self-reports of individuals, who may have been attributionally biased by having experienced a relapse. However, recent research using a prospective design replicated the initial findings. As we had observed earlier

(Marlatt & Gordon, 1980), Hodgins, el-Guebaly, and Armstrong (1995) found that negative emotional states emerged as the most frequent relapse trigger; social pressure and interpersonal events were also influential relapse determinants. In another recent article, negative emotional states were a primary determinant of drinking for both individuals in treatment for alcohol problems and for heavy drinkers in the general population (Cunningham, Sobell, Sobell, Gavin, & Annis, 1995).

Recent efforts to evaluate the construct validity (Maisto, Connors, & Zywiak, 1996), and predictive validity (Stout, Longabaugh, & Rubin, 1996) of our taxonomy failed to generate supportive data. However, these investigations suffered serious conceptual flaws. In these studies, investigators hypothesized that pretreatment relapse triggers would determine posttreatment relapse. According to this hypothesis, the circumstances of a previous "baseline" relapse assessed retrospectively should predict the circumstances of later relapse episodes. This conceptualization contradicts the logic of the RP model, where a lapse results from a dynamic interplay among proximal situational conditions, coping skills, self-efficacy, and expectancies. Instead, these investigators assumed static linkages between exposure to specific stimulus conditions and the occurrence of relapse drinking. Their conceptualization of relapse also failed to consider the RP logic that relapse is best predicted from an idiographic profile of high-risk situations rather than from a singular situation. Furthermore, the investigators defined relapse in a way that violates a crucial assumption of the RP model: The individual has to have made a voluntary choice or decision to change a target behavior. Because of these conceptual problems, as well as methodological problems concerning long periods of retrospective recall and nonconsideration of interloping treatment effects, these studies failed to constitute sound tests of the RP taxonomy. Nevertheless, these studies and others have usefully identified important limitations and qualifications of RP taxonomy (e.g. Longabaugh, Rubin, Stout, Zwiak, & Lowman, 1996; Rubin, Stout, & Longabaugh, 1996). Furthermore, these recent studies have generated valuable suggestions for improving the precision of the taxonomy (Donovan, 1996; Kadden, 1996).

RP Related Constructs

Because of the developmental and interactive nature of the RP model, efforts to predict relapse solely from exposure to high-risk situations are inherently limited. For instance, we have found that assessment of the patient's actual coping abilities (Chaney et al., 1978) or ratings of self-efficacy have been the most reliable proximal determinants of posttreatment relapse (Marlatt, Baer, & Quigley, 1995). After finding that high-risk situations (operationalized as negative life events) did not predict posttreatment alcoholic relapse but that other RP constructs did predict relapse, Miller et al., (1996) concluded: "This suggests that it is not the mere occurrence of potentially stressful events, but the client's resources for coping with them that predict whether or not the client will relapse to drinking" (p. S169).

In the above prospective study, Miller and his colleagues specifically tested the predictive power of five RP constructs (Miller et al., 1996). Four constructs predicted alcoholic relapse: coping responses, self-efficacy, positive expectancies, and belief in the disease model of alcoholism (a proxy for the Abstinence Violation Effect). When these constructs were examined jointly, two emerged as optimally predictive: lack of coping responses and disease model beliefs. Thus, in analyses approximating a comprehensive test of the RP model and its constituent elements, the model was generally supported.

RP Related Treatments

Most research has been conducted in the areas of alcohol dependency and smoking, although work is underway applying the RP model to other addictive behaviors. In the alcohol field, the pioneering work of G. K. Litman and her colleagues at the Addiction Research Unit at the Maudsley Hospital has provided valuable insight into the role of coping with high-risk situations as a factor that discriminates between alcoholics who relapse after treatment and those who "survive" or show a good treatment outcome. Litman and her co-workers have provided extensive documentation of relapse situations and associated coping responses related to treatment outcome (Litman, 1980; Litman, Eiser, Rawson, & Oppenheim, 1977, 1979; Litman, Eiser, & Taylor, 1979).

Similar research on the role of coping as a factor reducing relapse risk among ex-smokers has been described by Shiffman and his colleagues (e.g., Shiffman, 1982, 1984, 1989, 1993; Shiffman, Read, Maltese, Rapkin, & Jarvik, 1985). Related studies in the smoking area have shown that self-efficacy ratings are valid predictors of subsequent treatment outcome (Baer & Lichtenstein, 1988; Condiotte & Lichtenstein, 1981; DiClemente, 1981). Recent studies continue to attest to the importance of self-efficacy as a predictor of smoking outcomes (e.g., Carey, Kalra, Carey, Halperin, & Richards, 1993; Gulliver, Hughes, Solomon, & Dey, 1995).

Skill-training approaches also have received some attention in the treatment outcome literature. To take a specific example from our own skill-training research with alcoholic clients (Chaney et al., 1978), the client's responses to the Situational Competency Test are first considered in planning the specific skill-training program. For one particular client, the problem may involve an inability to resist social pressure to indulge; for another, the problem may involve a deficit in coping with feelings of loneliness or depression. In the skill-training program described in the study by Chaney and colleagues, alcoholics in treatment met together in a small group for a series of treatment sessions. Each group was led by two therapists, who began by describing a particular high-risk situation. The group members then discussed the situation and generated various ways of responding to it. The therapists then modeled an appropriate coping response and practiced it in front of the group. During this procedure, each client received individualized feedback from group members and specific coaching and instructions from the therapists. The client was then required to repeat the coping response until it matched the therapists' criteria for adequacy. This particular skill-training program was evaluated in a year-long follow-up study in comparison with two control groups: a group that spent an equivalent amount of time discussing their emotional reactions to the same high-risk situations (as in psychodynamic group therapy), and a no-treatment control condition (regular hospital program only). The skill-training condition proved to be more successful than either control group, showing a significant improvement at the one-year follow-up period for such variables as amount of post-treatment drinking, duration of time spent drinking before regaining abstinence, and frequency of periods of intoxication. Positive results for skill training with alcoholics have been reported elsewhere as well (e.g. Jones & Lanyon; 1981; O'Farrell, Choquette, Cutter, Brown, & McCourt, 1993; Oei & Jackson, 1982).

Numerous outcome studies have now appeared in the literature evaluating the efficacy of treatments based on the RP model. In a review of 24 such studies of various substance abusers, Carroll (1996) found consistent support for RP's superiority to no treatment, inconsistent support for its superiority over discussion control conditions, and consistent support for RP being as effective as other active treatments. Though not generally superior to other treatments, Carroll concluded that RP holds particular promise in three areas: reducing severity of relapses when they occur, enhancing durability of effects following cessation, and matching patient to treatment, particularly for patients at higher levels of impairment. Moreover, in some studies, RP demonstrated delayed emergent effects, suggesting superior effects to other treatments during the maintenance stage of habit change.

Range of Treatment Applications

A final question concerns the range of application of the RP model. Expanding the range of RP from initial work on alcoholism to encompass other addictions is shaped by two basic considerations. First, RP focuses on psychological determinants of substance-use behavior. Therefore, explanatory principles essential to the model are not constrained by the pharmacological or physiological properties of alcohol or other substances. Second, model building has kept pace with mainstream work in psychology stressing causal explanations that have generality across all behaviors. Thus, RP's wide scope readily encompasses habit change problems traditionally thought of as addictive behaviors in the usual sense of the term: excessive use of alcohol, tobacco, or other drugs, gambling, and eating disorders. The primary focus has been on the application of RP principles to the modification of such problems.

Outside of addictions, one area of application that has received considerable attention is sexuality. In the treatment of the sexual aggressor (e.g., pedophiles and rapists), the overall goal is the same as it often is in the treatment of addiction: to abstain from engaging in the taboo behavior (George & Marlatt, 1989). Projects by Laws (Laws, 1989), Pithers (e.g. Pithers, Marques, Gibat, & Marlatt, 1983), Marques (e.g., Marques, 1988) and others (e.g., G. C. N. Hall, 1995; Neidigh, 1991) have explored the application of the RP model in the treatment of sexual aggression. Preliminary results indicate that RP has promising effects as an adjunctive element to sexual offender treatment (G. C. N. Hall, 1995; Miner, Marques, Day, & Nelson, 1990). In addition, the RP model has been applied to treatment of sexual dysfunction for promoting retention of postreatment improvements (e.g., McCarthy, 1993; Rosen, Leiblum, & Spector, 1994). Another aspect of sexuality where RP has been applied is in reduction of AIDS-related sexual risk-taking behaviors (e.g., Wexler, Magura, Beardsley, Josepher, 1994).

We stated, at the outset, that RP was designed to help individuals anticipate and cope with lapse/relapse in the habit-change process. This broad aim subsumes two basic goals: to prevent occurrence of a lapse/relapse, and to promote a healthy lifestyle resistant to relapse-prone forces. Consequently, RP can potentially be applied to almost any problem where there is a need to establish and maintain long-term behavior change. In the mental health domain, examples include the application of RP to treatment of obsessive compulsive disorder (Hiss, Foa, & Kozak, 1994), to treatment of excessive interpersonal dependency (Overholser & Fine, 1994), and to prevention of depression relapse in seriously mentally ill patients (Clare & Singh, 1994). In the physical health domain, examples include the application of RP to compliance with oral health care treatment (McCaul, Bakdash, Geboy, & Gerbert, et al., 1990; Tedesco, 1987) and compliance with exercise regimens (Simkin & Gross, 1994). RP has been applied even to maintenance problems that bear little or no resemblance to addictions or health care, such as the "transfer of training" problem in retention of business managerial training (Marx, 1982). Given that pursuits aimed at improving health and other lifestyle practices typically involve the initiation and maintenance of habit change, the range of applications of the RP model is likely to grow

The RP model enjoys emerging empirical support. Though many of the model's basic tenets have received support, further work is needed to establish the solidity, and to clarify the limitations, of these principles. In light of recent findings on the relapse taxonomy, investigators should remain mindful that their research operationalizations are faithful to the underlying assumptions, component postulates, and dynamic gestalt of the RP model. Research on the effectiveness of the RP approach for treating various addictive behaviors and other pertinent disorders has generally been supportive. Overall, these developments encourage confidence in the RP model; however, more research is needed. Based on future research, refinement of the basic assumptions and clinical applications of the relapse prevention model will undoubtedly occur.

REFERENCES

Abrams, D. B., Niaura, R. S., Carey, K. B., Monti, P. M., & Binkoff, J. A. (1986). Understanding relapse and recovery in alcohol abuse. *Annals of Behavioral Medicine, 8*, 27–32.

Annis, H. M. (1986). A relapse prevention model for treatment of alcoholics. In W. R. Miller & N. Heather (Eds.), *Treating addictive behaviors* (pp. 407–421). New York: Plenum.

Annis, H. M., Schober, R., & Kelly, E. (1996). Matching addiction outpatient counseling to client readiness for change: The role of structured relapse prevention and counseling. *Experimental and Clinical Psychopharmacology, 4*, 37–45.

Baer, J. S., & Lichtenstein, E. (1988). Classification and prediction of smoking relapse episodes: An exploration of individual differences. *Journal of Consulting and Clinical Psychology, 56*, 104–110.

Bandura, A. (1977). *Social learning theory*. Englewood Cliffs, NJ: Prentice-Hall.

Bandura, A. (1986). *Social foundations of thought and action: A social cognitive theory*. Englewood Cliffs, NJ: Prentice-Hall.

Brandon, T. H., Wetter, D. W., & Baker, T. B. (1996). Affect, expectancies, urges, and smoking: Do they conform to models of drug motivation and relapse? *Experimental and Clinical Psychopharmacology, 4*, 29–36.

Brickman, P., Rabinowitz, V. C., Karuza, J., Coates, D., Cohn, E., & Kidder, L. (1982). Models of helping and coping. *American Psychologist, 37*, 368–384.

Brown, S. A. (1993). Drug effect expectancies and addictive behavior change. *Experimental & Clinical Psychopharmacology, 1*, 55–67.

Brownell, K. D., Marlatt, G. A., Lichtenstein, E., & Wilson, G. T. (1986). Understanding and preventing relapse. *American Psychologist, 41*, 765–782.

Carey, M. P., Kalra, D. L., Carey, K. B., Halperin, S., & Richards, C. S. (1993). Stress and unaided smoking cessation: A prospective investigation. *Journal of Consulting & Clinical Psychology, 61*, 831–838.

Carroll, K. M. (1996). Relapse prevention as a psychosocial treatment: A review of controlled clinical trials. *Experimental and Clinical Psychopharmacology, 4*, 46–54.

Chaney, E. F., O'Leary, M. R., & Marlatt, G. A. (1978). Skill training with alcoholics. *Journal of Consulting and Clinical Psychology, 46*, 1092–1104.

Clare, L., & Singh, K. (1994). Preventing relapse in psychotic illness: A psychological approach to early intervention. *Journal of Mental Health, 3*, 541–550.

Condiotte, M. M., & Lichtenstein, E. (1981). Self-efficacy and relapse in smoking cessation programs. *Journal of Consulting and Clinical Psychology, 49*, 648–658.

Connors, G. J., Maisto, S. A., & Donovan, D. M. (1996). Conceptualizations of relapse: A summary of psychological and psychobiological models. *Addiction, 91*: Supplement, S5–S13.

Connors, G. J., Maisto, S. A., & Zwiak, W. H. (1996). Understanding relapse in the broader context of post-treatment functioning. *Addiction, 91*: Supplement, S173–S189.

Cummings, C., Gordon, J. R., & Marlatt, G. A (1980). Relapse: Strategies of prevention and prediction. In W. R. Miller (Ed), *The addictive behaviors: Treatment of alcoholism, drug abuse, smoking, and obesity* (pp. 291–321). Oxford: Pergamon.

Cunningham, J. A., Sobell, M. B., Sobell, L. C., Gavin, D. R., & Annis, H. M. (1995). Heavy drinking and negative affect situations in a general population and a treatment sample: Alternative explanations. *Psychology of Addictive Behaviors, 9*, 123–127.

Curry, S. G., Gordon, J. R., & Marlatt, G. A (1987). Abstinence violation effect: Validation of an attributional construct with smoking cessation. *Journal of Consulting and Clinical Psychology, 55*, 145–149.

DiClemente, C. C. (1981). Self-efficacy and smoking cessation maintenance. *Cognitive Research and Therapy, 5*, 175–187.

Donovan, D. M. (1996). Marlatt's classification of relapse precipitants: Is the emperor still wearing clothes? *Addiction, 91*: Supplement, S131–S137.

Donovan, D. M., & Marlatt, G. A. (1988). *Assessment of addictive behaviors: Behavioral, cognitive, and physiological processes*. New York: Guilford.

George, W. H. (1989). Marlatt and Gordon's Relapse Prevention model: A cognitive-behavioral approach to understanding and preventing relapse. *Journal of Chemical Dependency Treatment, 2*, 125–152.

George, W. H., & Marlatt, G. A. (1989). Relapse prevention as a treatment for addictive disorders: Application to sex offenders. In D. R. Laws (Ed.), *Relapse prevention with sex offenders* (1–31). New York: Guilford.

Glasser, W. (1974). *Positive addiction*. New York: Harper & Row.

Goldfried, M. R., & Davison, G. C. (1976). *Clinical behavior therapy*. New York: Holt, Rinehart & Winston.

Gulliver, S. B., Hughes, J. R., Solomon, L. J., & Dey, A. N. (1995). An investigation of self-efficacy, partner support and daily stresses as predictors of relapse to smoking in self-quitters. *Addiction, 90*, 767–772.

Hall, G. C. N. (1995). The preliminary development of theory-based community treatment of sexual offenders. *Professional psychology: Research & practice, 26*, 478–483.

Hall, S. (1980). Self-management and therapeutic maintenance: Theory and research. In P. Karoly & J. J. Steffen (Eds.), *Toward a psychology of therapeutic maintenance: Widening perspectives* (pp. 263–300). New York: Gardner.

Hiss, H., Foa, E. B., & Kozak, M. J. (1994). Relapse prevention program for treatment of obsessive compulsive disorder. *Journal of Consulting and Clinical Psychology, 62*, 801–808.

Hodgins, D. C. , el-Guebaly, N., & Armstrong, S. (1995). Prospective and retrospective reports of mood state before relapse to substance use. *Journal of Consulting and Clinical Psychology, 63*, 400–407.

Jones, S. L., & Lanyon. R. I. (1981). Relationship between adaptive skills and sustained improvement following alcoholism treatment. *Journal of Studies on Alcohol, 42*, 521–525.

Kadden, R. M. (1996). Is Marlatt's relapse taxonomy reliable or valid? *Addiction, 91*: Supplement, S139–S145.

Laws, D. R. (1989). *Relapse prevention with sex offenders*. New York: Guilford Press.

Litman, A. (1980). Relapse in alcoholism: Traditional and current approaches. In G. Edwards & M. Grant (Eds.), *Alcoholism treatment in transition* (pp. 294–303). Baltimore: University Park Press.

Litman, G. K., Eiser, J. R., Rawson, N. S B., & Oppenheim, A. N. (1977). Towards a typology of relapse: A preliminary report. *Drug and Alcohol Dependence, 2*, 157–162.

Litman, G. K., Eiser, J. R., Rawson, N. S. B., & Oppenheim, A. N. (1979). Differences in relapse precipitants and coping behaviours between alcoholic relapsers and survivors. *Behaviour Research and Therapy, 17*, 89–94.

Litman, G. K., Eiser, J. R., & Taylor, C. (1979). Dependence, relapse and extinction: A theoretical critique and behavioral examination. *Journal of Clinical Psychology, 35*, 192–199

Longabaugh, R., Rubin, A., Stout, R. L., Zwiak, W. H., & Lowman, C. (1996). The reliability of Marlatt's taxonomy for classifying relapses. *Addiction, 91*: Supplement, S73–S88.

Lowman, C., Allen, J., Stout, R. L., & The Alcohol Relapse Group (1996). Replication and extension of Marlatt's taxonomy of relapse precipitants: Overview of procedures and results. *Addiction, 91*: Supplement, S51–S71.

Maisto, S. A., Connors, G. J., & Zywiak, W. H. (1996). Construct validation analyses on the Marlatt typology of relapse precipitants. *Addiction, 91*: Supplement, S89–S97.

Marlatt, G. A. (1978). Craving for alcohol, loss of control, and relapse: A cognitive-behavioral analysis. In P. E. Nathan, G. A. Marlatt, & T. Loberg (Eds.), *Alcoholism: New directions in behavioral research and treatment* (pp. 271–314). New York: Plenum.

Marlatt, G. A. (1982). Relapse prevention: A self-control program for the treatment of addictive behaviors. In R. B. Stuart (Ed.), *Adherence, compliance, and generalization in behavioral medicine* (pp. 329–378). New York: Brunner/Mazel.

Marlatt, G. A. (1987). Alcohol, the magic elixir: Stress, expectancy, and the transformation of emotional states. In E. Gottheil, K. A. Druly, S. Pashko, & S. P. Weinstein (Eds.), *Stress and addiction* (pp. 302–322). New York: Brunner/Mazel.

Marlatt, G. A. (1996a). Taxonomy of high-risk situations for alcohol relapse: Evolution and development of a cognitive-behavioral model of relapse. *Addiction, 91*: Supplement, S37–S50.

Marlatt, G. A. (1996b). Lest taxonomy become taxidermy: A comment on the relapse replication and extension project. *Addiction, 91*: Supplement, S37–S50.

Marlatt, G. A., Baer, J. S., & Quigley, L. A. (1995). Self-efficacy and addictive behavior. In A. Bandura (Ed.), *Self-efficacy in changing societies* (pp. 289–315). New York: Cambridge University Press.

Marlatt, G. A. & Barrett, K. (1994). Relapse prevention. In M. Galanter & D. Kleber (Eds.), *The textbook of substance abuse treatment* (pp. 285–299). New York: American Psychiatric Press.

Marlatt, G. A., & George, W. H. (1984). Relapse prevention: Introduction and overview of the model. *British Journal of Addiction, 79*, 261–273.

Marlatt, G. A., & George, W. H. (1990). Relapse prevention and the maintenance of optimal health. In S. Shumaker, E. Schron, & J. K. Ockene (Eds.), *The handbook of health behavior change* (pp. 44–63). New York: Springer Publishing Co.

Marlatt, G. A., & Gordon, J. R. (1980). Determinants of relapse: Implications for the maintenance of behavior change. In P. O. Davidson & S. M. Davidson (Eds.), *Behavioral medicine: Changing health lifestyles* (pp. 410–452). New York: Brunner/Mazel.

Marlatt, G A., & Gordon, J. R. (Eds). (1985). *Relapse prevention: Maintenance strategies in the treatment of addictive behaviors*. New York: Guilford.

Marlatt, G. A., & Marques, J. K. (1977). Meditation, self-control, and alcohol use. In R. B. Stuart (Ed.), *Behavioral self-management: Strategies, techniques, and outcomes* (pp. 117–153). New York: Brunner/Mazel.

Marlatt, G. A., & Rohsenow, D. R. (1980). Cognitive processes in alcohol use: Expectancy and the balanced placebo design. In N. K. Mello (Ed.), *Advances in substance abuse* (Vol. 1, pp. 159–199). Greenwich, CT: JAI Press.

Marques, J. K. (1988). The sex offender treatment and evaluation project: California's new outcome study. *Annals of the New York Academy of Sciences, 528*, 235–243.

Marx, R. D. (1982). Relapse prevention for managerial training: A model for maintenance of behavior change. *Academy of Management Review, 7*, 433–441.

McCarthy, B. W. (1993). Relapse prevention strategies and techniques in sex therapy. *Journal of Sex and Marital Therapy, 19*, 142–146.

McCaul, K. D., Bakdash, M. B., Geboy, M.J., Gerbert, B., et al. (1990). Promoting self-portective health behaviors in dentistry. *Annals of Behavioral Medicine, 12*, 156–160.

McFall, R. M. (1976). *Behavioral training: A skill-acquisition approach to clinical problems*. Morristown, NJ: General Learning Press.

Meichenbaum, D. (1977). *Cognitive-behavior modification*. New York: Plenum.

Miller, W. R., Westerberg, V. S., Harris, R. J., & Tonigan, J. S. (1996). What predicts relapse? Prospective testing of antecedent models. *Addiction, 91*: Supplement, S155–S171.

Miner, M. H., Marques, J. K., Day, D. M. & Nelson, C. (1990). Impact of relapse prevention in treating sex offenders. *Annals of Sex Research, 3*, 165–185.

Murphy, T. J., Pagano, R. R., & Marlatt, G. A. (1986). Lifestyle modification with heavy alcohol drinkers: Effects of aerobic exercise and meditation. *Addictive Behaviors, 11*, 175–186.

Neidigh, L. (1991). Implications of a relapse prevention model for treatment of sexual offenders. *Journal of Addictions & Offender Counseling, 11*, 42–50.

Oei, T. P. S., & Jackson, P. R. (1982). Social skills and cognitive behavioral approaches to the treatment of problem drinking. *Journal of Studies in Alcohol, 43*, 532–547.

O'Farrell, T. J., Choquette, K. A. Cutter, H. S. G., Brown, E. D., & McCourt, W. F. (1993). Behavioral marital therapy with and without additional couples relapse prevention sessions for alcoholics and their wives. *Journal of Studies in Alcohol, 54*, 652–666.

Overholser, J. C., & Fine, M. A., (1994). Cognitive-behavioral treatment of excessive interpersonal dependency: A four-stage psychotherapy model. *Journal of Cognitive Psychotherapy, 8*, 55–70.

Pithers, W. D., Marques, J. K., Gibat, C. C., & Marlatt, G. A. (1983). Relapse prevention with sexual aggressives: A self-control model of treatment and maintenance of change. In J. G. Greer & I. R. Stuart (Eds.), *The sexual aggressor: Current perspectives on treatment* (pp. 214–239). New York: Van Nostrand Reinhold.

Rosen, R. C., Leiblum, S. R., & Spector, I. P. (1994). Psychologically based treatment of male erectile disorder: A cognitive-interpersonal model. *Journal of Sex & Marital Therapy, 20*, 67–85.

Rubin, A., Stout, R. L., & Longabaugh, R. (1996). Gender differences in relapse situations. *Addiction, 91*: Supplement, S111–S120.

Shiffman, S. (1982). Relapse following smoking cessation: A situational analysis. *Journal of Consulting and Clinical Psychology, 50*, 71–86.

Shiffman, S. (1984). Coping with temptations to smoke. *Journal of Consulting and Clinical Psychology, 52*, 261–267.

Shiffman, S. (1989). Trans-situational consistency in smoking relapse. *Health Psychology, 8*, 471–481.

Shiffman, S. (1993). Smoking cessation treatment: Any progress? *Journal of Consulting & Clinical Psychology, 61*, 718–722.

Shiffman, S., Hickcox, M., Paty, J. A., Gnys, M., Kassel, J, D., & Richards, T. J. (1996) Progression from a smoking lapse to relapse: Prediction from abstinence violation effects, nicotine dependence, and lapse characteristics. *Journal of Consulting & Clinical Psychology, 64*, 993–1002.

Shiffman, S., Read, L., Maltese, J., Rapkin, D., & Jarvik, M. E. (1985). Preventing relapse in ex-smokers: A self-management approach. In G. A. Marlatt & J. R. Gordon (Eds.), *Relapse prevention: Maintenance strategies in the treatment or addictive behaviors* (pp. 472–520). New York: Guilford.

Shiffman, S., & Wills, T. A. (Eds.) (1985). *Coping and substance use*. New York: Academic Press.

Simkin, L. R., & Gross, A. M. (1994). Assessment of coping with high-risk situations for exercise relapse among healthy women. *Health Psychology, 13*, 274–277.

Spradley, J. P. (1970). *You owe yourself a drunk*. Boston: Little, Brown.

Stout, R. L., Longabaugh, R., & Rubin, A. (1996). Predictive validity of Marlatt's relapse taxonomy versus a more general relapse code. *Addiction, 91*: Supplement, S99–S100.

Tedesco, L. (1987). *Cognitive-behavioral enhancment of oral health status*. Unpublished manuscript, State University of New York at Buffalo.

Vuchinich, R. E., & Tucker, J. A. (1996). Alcoholic relapse, life events, and behavioral theories of choice: A prospective analysis. *Experimental and Clinical Psychopharmacology, 4*, 19–28.

Wexler, H. K., Magura, S., Beardsley, M. M., & Josepher, H. (1994). ARRIVE: An AIDS education/relapse prevention model for high-risk parolees. *International Journal of the Addictions, 29*, 361–386.

3

The Transtheoretical Model of Behavior Change

James O. Prochaska, Sara Johnson, and Patricia Lee

The Transtheoretical Model is an integrative framework for understanding how individuals and populations progress toward adopting and maintaining health behavior change for optimal health. The Transtheoretical Model uses stages of change to integrate processes and principles of change from across major theories of intervention, hence the name "Transtheoretical." This model emerged from a comparative analysis of leading theories of psychotherapy and behavior change. The search was for a systematic integration of a field that had fragmented into more than 300 theories of psychotherapy (Prochaska, 1979). The comparative analysis identified only ten processes of change, such as consciousness-raising from the Freudian tradition, contingency management from the Skinnerian tradition, and helping relationships from the Rogerian tradition.

In an empirical analysis of self-changers compared to smokers in professional treatments, we assessed how frequently each group used each of the ten processes (Prochaska & DiClemente, 1982). Our research participants kept saying that they used different processes at different times in their struggles with smoking. These naive subjects were teaching us about a phenomenon that was not included in any of the multitude of therapy theories. They were revealing to us that behavior change unfolds through a series of stages (Prochaska & DiClemente, 1983).

From the initial studies of smoking, the stage model rapidly expanded in scope to include investigations and applications with a broad range of health and mental health behaviors. These include alcohol and substance abuse, anxiety and panic disorders, delinquency, eating disorders and obesity, high-fat diets, HIV/AIDS prevention, mammography screening, medication compliance, unplanned pregnancy prevention, pregnancy and smoking, radon testing, sedentary lifestyles, sun exposure, and physicians practicing preventive medicine. Over time these studies have expanded, validated, applied, and challenged the core constructs of the Transtheoretical Model.

CORE CONSTRUCTS

The Transtheoretical Model has concentrated on five stages of change; ten processes of change; the pros and cons of changing; self-efficacy; and temptation as core constructs. The Transtheoretical Model is also based on critical assumptions about the nature of behavior change and interventions that can best facilitate such change. These core constructs and critical assumptions will be discussed in this section. Each core construct has been subjected to a wide variety of studies across a broad range of behaviors and populations. These also will be presented here.

Stages of Change

The stage construct is important in part because it represents a temporal dimension. Change implies phenomena occurring over time, but, surprisingly, none of the leading theories of therapy contained a core construct representing time. Behavior change was often construed as an event, such as quitting smoking, drinking, or overeating. The Transtheoretical Model construes change as a process involving progress through a series of six stages.

Precontemplation is the stage in which people are not intending to take action in the foreseeable future, a time frame usually measured as the next 6 months. People may be in this stage because they are uninformed or underinformed about the consequences of their behavior. Alternatively, they may have tried to change a number of times and become demoralized about their abilities to change. Both groups tend to avoid reading, talking, or thinking about their high-risk behaviors. They are often characterized in other theories as “resistant” or “unmotivated” clients, or as “not ready” for therapy or health promotion programs. The fact is that traditional health promotion programs were not ready for such individuals, and were not motivated to match their needs.

Contemplation is the stage in which people are intending to change in the next 6 months. They are now aware of the pros of changing, but are also acutely aware of the cons. This balance between the costs and benefits of changing can produce profound ambivalence that can keep people stuck in this stage for long periods of time. We often characterize this phenomenon as chronic contemplation or behavioral procrastination. These folks are also not ready for traditional action-oriented programs.

Preparation is the stage in which people are intending to take action in the immediate future, usually measured as during the next month. They have typically taken some significant action in the past year. These individuals have a plan of action, such as joining a health education class, consulting a counselor, talking to their physician, buying a self-help book, or relying on a self-change approach. These are the people we should recruit for such action-oriented programs as smoking cessation, weight loss, or exercise.

Action is the stage in which people have made specific overt modifications in their lifestyles within the past 6 months. Since action is observable, behavior change often has been equated with action. In the Transtheoretical Model, however, action is only one of six stages. Not all modifications of behavior count as action in this model. People must attain a criterion that scientists and professionals agree is sufficient to reduce risks for disease. In smoking, for example, the field used to count reduction in the number of cigarettes as action, or switching to low-tar and low-nicotine cigarettes. Now the consensus is clear: only total abstinence counts. In the diet area, there is a consensus that less than 30% of calories should be consumed from fat; but there are those who believe that this guideline needs to be lowered to 25% or even 20%.

Maintenance is the stage in which people are working to prevent relapse, but do not apply change processes as frequently as do people in action. They are less tempted to relapse and increasingly more confident that they can continue their changes. Based on temptation and self-efficacy data, we estimated that maintenance lasts from 6 months to about 5 years. While this estimate may seem somewhat pessimistic, longitudinal data in the 1990 Surgeon General's report gave some support to this temporal estimate (U.S. Department of Health and Human Services (USDHHS), 1990). After 12 months of continuous abstinence, the percentage of individuals who returned to regular smoking was 43%. It was not until 5 years of continuous abstinence that the risk for relapse dropped to 7%.

Termination is the stage in which individuals have zero temptation and 100% self-efficacy. No matter whether they are depressed, anxious, bored, lonely, angry or stressed, they are sure they will not return to their old unhealthy habit as a way of coping. It is as if they never acquired the habit in the first place. In a study of former smokers and alcoholics we found that less than 20% of each group had reached the criteria of zero temptation and total self-efficacy (Snow, Prochaska, & Rossi, 1992). These criteria may be too strict, or it may be that this stage is an ideal goal for the majority of people. In other areas, like exercise, consistent condom use, and weight control, the realistic goal may be a lifetime of maintenance. Since termination may not be a practical reality for a majority of people, this stage has not been given as much emphasis in our research.

Processes of Change

These are the covert and overt activities that people use to progress through the stages. Processes of change provide important guides for intervention programs, since these processes are like the independent variables that people need to apply to move from stage to stage. Ten processes have received the most empirical support in our research to date.

Consciousness-raising involves increased awareness about the causes, consequences and cures for a particular problem behavior. Interventions that can increase awareness include feedback, education, confrontation, interpretation, bibliotherapy, and media campaigns.

Dramatic relief initially produces increased emotional experiences, followed by reduced affect if appropriate action can be taken. Psychodrama, role-playing, grieving, personal testimonies, and media campaigns are examples of techniques that can move people emotionally.

Self-reevaluation combines both cognitive and affective assessments of one's self-image with and without a particular unhealthy habit; for example, one's image as a couch potato and an active person. Value clarification, healthy role models, and imagery are techniques that can move people evaluatively.

Environmental reevaluation combines both affective and cognitive assessments of how the presence or absence of a personal habit affects one's social environment, for example, the effect of smoking on others. It can also include the awareness that one can serve as a positive or negative role model for others. Empathy training, documentaries, and family interventions can lead to such re-assessments.

As an example, here is a brief television spot from California's anti-tobacco campaign, designed to help smokers in precontemplation to progress. A middle-aged man clearly in grief says, "I always worried that my smoking would cause lung cancer. I was always afraid that my smoking would lead to an early death. But I never imagined that it would happen to my wife." Then on the screen is flashed the message, "50,000 deaths per year due to passive smoking—California Department of Health."

There are no action directives in this intervention, but there is (1) consciousness-raising—"50,000 deaths per year"; (2) dramatic relief—around the grief, guilt and fear that can be reduced if appropriate action is taken; (3) self-reevaluation—examination of how individuals think and feels about themselves as smokers; and (4) environmental reevaluation—how the individual feels and thinks about the effects of their smoking on their environment.

Self-liberation is both the belief that one can change and the commitment and recommitment to act on that belief. New Year's resolutions, public testimonies, and multiple, rather than single, choices can enhance what the public calls "willpower." Motivative research indicates that people with two choices have greater commitment than people with one choice; those with three choices have even greater commitment; but four choices doesn't enhance willpower (Miller & Bernab, 1983). So with smokers, for example, three excellent action choices are cold turkey, nicotine fading, and nicotine replacement.

Social liberation requires an increase in social opportunities or alternatives, especially for people who are relatively deprived or oppressed. Advocacy, empowerment procedures, and appropriate policies can produce increased opportunities for minority health promotion, gay health promotion, and health promotion for impoverished people. These same procedures can also be used to help all people change, for example, through the use of smoke-free zones or salad bars in school cafeterias, and provision of easy access to condoms and other contraceptives.

Counterconditioning requires the learning of healthier behaviors that can substitute for problem behaviors. Relaxation can counter stress; assertion can counter peer pressure; nicotine replacement can substitute for cigarettes, and fat-free foods can be safer substitutes.

Stimulus control removes cues for unhealthy habits and adds prompts for healthier alternatives. Avoidance, environmental reengineering, and self-help groups can provide stimuli that support change and reduce risks for relapse. Planning parking lots with a 2 minute walk to the office and putting art displays in stairwells are examples of reengineering that can encourage more exercise.

Contingency management provides consequences for taking steps in a particular direction. While contingency management can include the use of punishments, we found that self-changers rely on rewards much more than on punishments. Consequently, reinforcements are emphasized, since a philosophy of the stage model is to work in harmony with how people change naturally. Contingency contracts, overt and covert reinforcements, positive self-statements, and group recognition are procedures for increasing reinforcement and the probability that healthier responses will be repeated.

Helping relationships combine caring, trust, openness, and acceptance as well as support for the healthy behavior change. Rapport-building, a therapeutic alliance, counselor calls, and buddy systems can be sources of social support.

Decisional Balance

This core construct reflects the individual's relative weighing of the pros and cons of changing. Originally, we relied on Janis and Mann's (1977) model of decisionmaking that included four categories of pros (instrumental gains for self and others, and approval for self and others). The four categories of cons were instrumental costs to self and others, and disapproval from self and others. In a long series of studies attempting to produce this structure of eight factors, we always found a much simpler structure—just the pros and cons of changing.

Self-Efficacy

This is the situation-specific confidence that people have when they can cope with high-risk situations without relapsing to their unhealthy or high-risk habit. This construct was integrated from Bandura's (1977, 1982) self-efficacy theory.

Temptation

This core construct reflects the intensity of urges to engage in a specific habit when in the midst of difficult situations. In our research, we typically find three factors reflecting the most common types of tempting situations: negative affect or emotional distress, positive social situations, and craving.

CRITICAL ASSUMPTIONS

The following are a set of assumptions that drive our theory, research, and practice.

1. No single theory can account for all of the complexities of behavior change. Therefore, a more comprehensive model will most likely emerge from an integration across major theories.
2. Behavior change is a process that unfolds over time through a sequence of stages.
3. Stages are both stable and open to change, just as chronic behavioral risk factors are both stable and open to change.
4. Without planned interventions, populations will remain stuck in the early stages. There is no inherent motivation to progress through the stages of intentional change as there seems to be in stages of physical and psychological development.
5. The majority of at-risk populations are not prepared for action and will not be served by traditional action-oriented prevention programs. Health promotion can have much greater impacts if it shifts from an action paradigm to a stage paradigm.
6. Specific processes and principles of change need to be applied at specific

stages if progress through the stages is to occur. In the stages of change, paradigm intervention programs must be matched to each individual's stage of change.

7. Chronic behavior patterns usually are under some combination of biological, social, and self-control. Stage-matched interventions have been primarily designed to enhance self-controls.

EMPIRICAL SUPPORT: BASIC RESEARCH

Stage Distribution

If we are to match the needs of entire populations, we need to know the stage distributions of specific high-risk behaviors. Table 3.1 presents results from a series of studies on smoking that have clearly demonstrated that less than 20% of smokers are in the preparation stage in most populations (e.g., Velicer et al., 1995). Approximately 40% of smokers are in the contemplation stage and another 40% are in precontemplation. These results show that action-oriented cessation programs will not match the needs of the vast majority of smokers.

With a sample of 20,000 members of an HMO, the stage distribution was assessed for 15 health behaviors (Rossi, 1992b). While there are variations in the distributions, for these high-risk behaviors, the results support a general rule of thumb: 40% of the population is in precontemplation, 40% in contemplation, and 20% in preparation.

Pros and Cons Structure Across 12 Behaviors

As indicated earlier, the pros and cons of decisional balance have a much simpler structure than Janis and Mann's (1977) theory suggests. Across studies of 12 different behaviors (smoking cessation, quitting cocaine, weight control, dietary fat reduction, safer sex, condom use, exercise acquisition, sunscreen use, radon testing, delinquency reduction, mammography screening, and physicians practicing preventive medicine), the two-factor structure was remarkably stable.

Integration of Pros and Cons and Stages of Change Across 12 Health Behaviors

Stage is not a theory; it is a variable. A theory requires systematic relationships between a set of variables, ideally culminating in mathematical relationships. Figure 3.1 presents systematic relationships between stages and pros and cons of changing for 12 health behaviors.

TABLE 3.1 Distribution of Smokers by Stage* Across Four Different Samples

Sample	Precon-templation	Contemplation	Preparation	Sample Size
Random Digit Dial	42.1%	40.3%	17.6%	4,144
4 USA Worksites	41.1%	38.7%	20.1%	4,785
California	37.3%	46.7%	16.0%	9,534
RI High Schools	43.8%	38.0%	18.3%	208

* These studies assess current smokers; therefore, no respondents are in action or maintenance.

In all 12 studies, the cons of changing are higher than the pros for people in precontemplation (Prochaska et al., 1994). In all 12 studies, the pros increase between precontemplation and contemplation. There are no systematic differences in the cons between precontemplation and contemplation. However, from contemplation to action for all 12 behaviors, the cons of changing are lower in action than in contemplation. In 11 of the 12 studies, the pros of changing are higher than the cons for people in action.

These basic findings suggest principles for progressing through the stages (Prochaska, 1994b). To progress from precontemplation to contemplation, the pros of changing must increase. To progress from contemplation to action, the cons of changing must decrease. So with people in precontemplation, we would target the pros for intervention and save the cons until after they progress to contemplation. Before progressing to action, we would want to see the pros and cons crossing over, taking a state where the pros are higher than the cons as a sign of being well prepared for action. Having the pros high enough and the cons low enough are part of what it takes to be well-prepared to progress to maintenance without relapsing.

Strong and Weak Principles of Progress

Across these same 12 studies, mathematical relationships were found between the pros and cons of changing and progress across the stages. The Strong Principle is:

$$\text{PC} -> \text{A} \cong 1 \text{ S.D.} \uparrow \text{PROS}$$

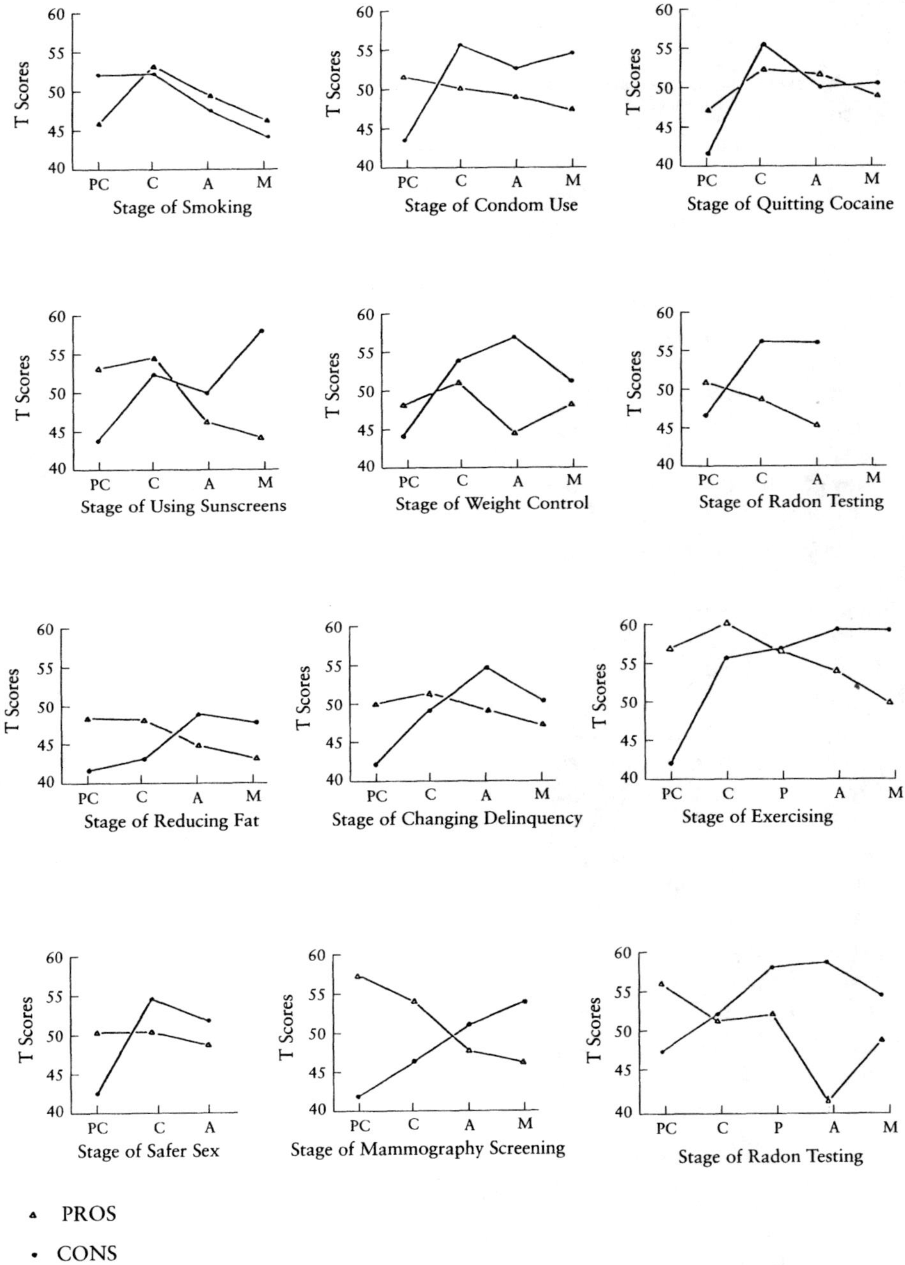

Figure 3.1 The pros and cons (in T scores) by stages of change for each of 12 problem behaviors (PC = precontemplation; C = contemplation; P = preparation; A = action; M = maintenance).

Progress from contemplation to action involves approximately one standard deviation (S.D.) increase in the pros of changing. On intelligence tests, a one S.D. increase would be 15 points, which is a substantial increase.

The Weak Principle is:
$$PC -> A \cong .5 \text{ S.D.} \downarrow \text{CONS}$$

Progress from precontemplation to action involves approximately .5 S.D. decrease in the cons of changing.

One practical implication of these principles is that the pros of changing must increase twice as much as the cons must decrease. Perhaps twice as much emphasis should be placed on raising the benefits as on reducing the costs or barriers. For example, if couch potatoes in precontemplation can only list 5 pros of exercise, then being too busy will be a big barrier to change. But if program participants come to appreciate that there can be more than 50 benefits for 60 minutes of exercise a week, being too busy becomes a relatively smaller barrier.

Processes of Change Across Behaviors

One of the assumptions of the transtheoretical model is that there is a common set of change processes that people can apply across a broad range of behaviors. The higher-order structure of the processes (experiential and behavioral) has been replicated across problem behaviors better than specific processes have (Rossi, 1992a). Typically we have found support for our standard set of 10 processes across such behaviors as smoking, diet, cocaine use, exercise, condom use, and sun exposure. However, the structure of the processes across studies has not been as consistent as the structure of the stages and the pros and cons of changing. In some studies, we find fewer processes, occasionally we find evidence for one or two more. It is also very possible that with some behaviors, fewer change processes may be used. With an infrequent behavior such as a yearly mammogram, for example, fewer processes may be required to progress to long-term maintenance (Rakowski, Dube, & Goldstein, in press; Rakowski, Ehrich, et al., in press).

Relationship Between Stages and Processes of Change

One of our earliest empirical integrations was the discovery of systematic relationships between the stage people were in and the processes they were applying. This discovery allowed us to integrate processes from theories that were typically seen as incompatible and in conflict. For example, Freudian theory, that relied almost entirely on consciousness-raising for producing change, was viewed as incompatible with Skinnerian theory, that relied entirely on contingency management for modifying behavior. The self-changers themselves did not know that these processes were theoretically incompatible, and they taught us that processes from very different theories needed to be emphasized at different stages of change. Table 3.2 presents our current empirical integration (Prochaska, DiClemente & Norcross, 1992). This integration suggests that in early stages people apply cognitive, affective, and evaluative processes to progress through the stages. In later stages, people rely more on commitments, conditioning, contingencies, environmental controls, and support for progressing toward termination.

Table 3.2 has important practical implications. To help people progress from precontemplation to contemplation we need to apply such processes as consciousness-raising and dramatic relief. Applying processes like contingency management, counterconditioning, and stimulus control to people in precontemplation would represent a theoretical, empirical, and practical mistake. But for people in action, such strategies would represent an optimal matching.

As with the structure of the processes, the integration of the processes and stages has not been as consistent as the integration of the stages and pros and cons of changing. While part of the problem may be due to the greater complexity of integrating 10 processes across five stages, the processes of change need more basic research.

APPLICATIONS OF THE TRANSTHEORETICAL MODEL: SMOKING CESSATION INTERVENTIONS AS EXAMPLES

Smoking is costly to individual smokers and to society. In the United States, approximately 47,000,000 Americans continue to smoke. Over 400,000 preventable deaths per year are attributable to smoking (USDHHS, 1990). Globally, the problem promises to be catastrophic. Of the people alive in the world today, 500,000,000 are expected to die from this single behavior, losing approximately 5 billion years of life to tobacco use (Peto & Lopez, 1990). If we can make even modest gains in our science and practice of smoking cessation, we could prevent millions of premature deaths and help preserve billions of years of life.

Currently, smoking cessation clinics have little impact. When offered for free by HMOs in the United States, such clinics recruit only about 1% of subscribers who smoke. Such behavior health services simply cannot make much difference if they treat such a small percentage of the problem (Orleans et al., 1988).

TABLE 3.2 Stages of Change in Which Change Processes Are Most Emphasized

	Stages of Change				
	Precontemplation	Contemplation	Preparation	Action	Maintenance
Processes	Consciousness raising				
	Dramatic relief				
	Environmental reevaluation				
		Self-reevaluation			
			Self-liberation		
				Contingency management	
				Helping relationship	
				Counterconditioning	
				Stimulus control	

Startled by such statistics, behavioral scientists took health promotion programs into communities and worksites. The results are now being reported, and in the largest trials ever attempted, the outcomes are discouraging. In the Minnesota Heart Health project, for example, 40 million was spent with 5 years of intervention in four communities totaling 400,000 people. There were no significant differences between treatment and control communities on smoking, diet, cholesterol, weight, blood pressure, and overall risks for cardiovascular disease (Luepker et al., 1994).

What went wrong? The investigators speculate that they may have diluted their programs by targeting multiple behaviors. But the COMMIT (1995) trial had no effects with its primary target of heavy smokers, and only a small effect with light smokers. The good news is that most of the effect occurred for the less educated segment of the population, with an 11 percentage point difference. Similarly, the largest worksite cessation programs produced no significant differences between intervention and comparison studies (Glasgow, Terborg, Hollis, 1995; Severson, & Boles, 1996). Part of the problem is that the control populations were improving, making it more difficult for the intervention groups to outperform them.

A closer look at participation rates may explain some of the disappointing results. In the Minnesota study, nearly 90% of smokers in both the treatment and control communities had processed media information about smoking in the past year, but only about 10% had been advised to quit by their physicians (Lando et al., 1995). Furthermore, only about 3% had participated in the most powerful behavioral programs, such as individualized and interactive clinics, classes and contests. In one of the Minnesota Heart Health studies, smokers were randomly assigned to one of three recruitment methods for home-based cessation programs (Schmidt, Jeffrey & Hellerstedt, 1989). These announcements generated 1 to 5% participation rates, with a personalized letter achieving the best results. We can not have much impact on the health of our communities if we only interact with a small percentage of populations at high risk for disease and early death.

One alternative is to shift from an action paradigm to a stage paradigm, in order to increase our reach and interact with a much higher percentage of populations at risk. Let us examine how the stage paradigm has been applied to five of the most important phases of planned interventions.

Recruitment

Recall that action-oriented cessation programs falter in this first phase of intervention and produce low participation rates. Table 3.1 reported results that can help explain such low rates. Across four different samples, 20% or less of smokers were in the preparation stage (Velicer et al., 1995). When we advertised or announced action-oriented programs, we were explicitly or implicitly targeting less than 20% of a population. The other 80% plus were left on their own.

In two home-based programs with approximately 5,000 smokers in each study, we reached out either by telephone alone or by personal letters, followed by telephone calls if needed, and recruited smokers to stage-matched interventions. For each of five stages, these interventions included self-help manuals, individualized computer feedback reports based on assessments of the pros and cons, processes, self-efficacy and temptations, and/or counselor protocols based on the computer reports. Using these proactive recruitment methods and stage-matched interventions, we were able to generate participation rates of 82 to 85%, respectively (Prochaska, Velicer, Fava & Laforge, 1996; Prochaska, Velicer, Fava & Rossi, 1996). Such quantum increases in participation rates provide the potential to generate unprecedented impacts with entire populations of smokers.

Population impact equals participation rate times the rate of efficacy or action. If a program produced 30% efficacy (such as long-term abstinence), it has historically been judged to be better than a program that produced 25% abstinence. However, a program that generates 30% efficacy but only 5% participation has an impact of only 1.5% (30% × 5%). A program that produces only 25% efficacy but 60% participation has an impact of 15%. With health promotion programs, this would be equal to 1000% greater impact on a high-risk population.

The stage paradigm would shift our outcomes from efficacy alone to impact. To achieve such high impact, we need to shift from reactive recruitment, where we advertise or announce our programs and react when people reach us, to proactive recruitments, where we reach out to interact with all potential participants.

Proactive recruitment alone will not work. In an intensive recruitment protocol, Lichtenstein & Hollis (1992) had physicians spend up to 5 minutes with each smoker simply to recruit the smoker for an action-oriented cessation clinic. If that didn't work, a nurse spent 10 minutes to persuade each smoker to sign up, followed by 12 minutes with a videotape, a health educator, and even a proactive counselor call if necessary. The base rate was 1% participation. This proactive protocol resulted in recruitment of 35% of smokers in precontemplation. Only 3% showed up for the clinic, and 2% finished the course. With a combination of smokers in the contemplation and preparation stages, 65% signed up, 15% showed up, and 11% finished up.

To optimize our impacts, we need to use proactive protocols to recruit participants to programs that match the stage they are in. Once we generate high recruitment rates, we then have to be concerned about high retention rates, lest we lose many of the initial participants in our health promotion programs.

Retention

One of the skeletons in the closet of psychotherapy and behavior change interventions is their relatively poor retention rates. Across 125 studies, the average retention rate was only about 50% (Wierzbicki & Pekarik, 1993). Furthermore, this meta-analysis found few consistent predictors of which participants would drop out prematurely and which would continue in therapy. In studies on smoking, weight control, substance abuse, and a mixture of DSM-III disorders, stage-of-change measures proved to be the best predictors of premature termination. Figure 3.2 presents the stage profile of three groups of therapy participants: the pretreatment stage profile of the entire 40% who dropped out prematurely (as judged by their therapists) was that of patients in precontemplation. The 20% who terminated quickly but appropriately had a profile of patients in action. Using pretreatment stage-related measures, we were able to correctly classify 93% of the three groups (Medeiros & Prochaska, 1996).

We simply cannot treat people with a precontemplation profile as if they were ready for action interventions and expect them to stay in treatment.

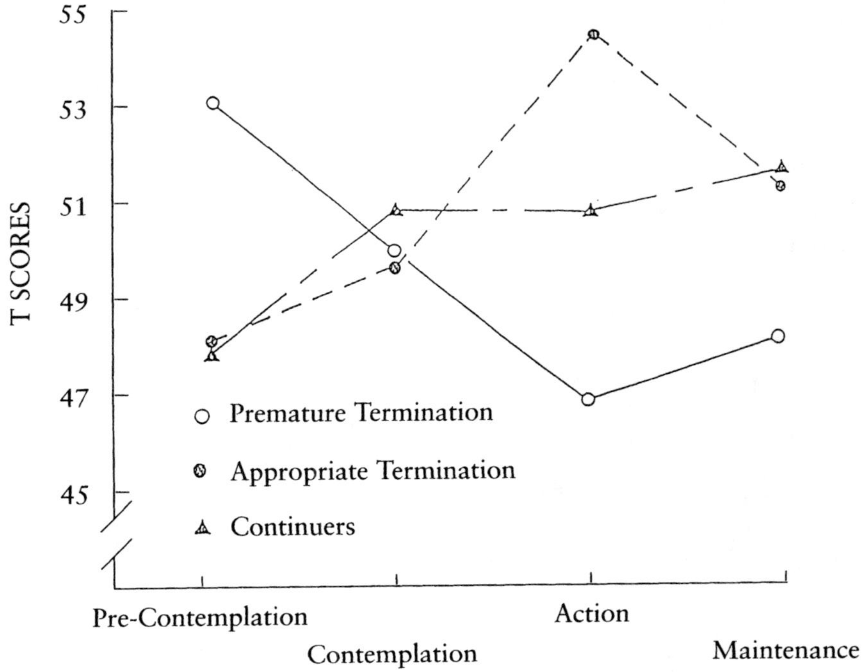

Figure 3.2 Pre-therapy stage profiles for premature terminators, appropriate terminators, and continuers.

Relapse prevention strategies would be indicated with smokers who are taking action, but those in precontemplation are more likely to need dropout prevention strategies.

The best strategy we have found to promote retention is matching our interventions to stage of change. In four smoking cessation studies using such matching strategies, we found we were able to retain smokers in the precontemplation stage at the same high levels as those who started in the preparation stage (Prochaska, 1994a).

Progress

The amount of progress participants make following health promotion programs is directly related to the stage they were in at the start of the interventions. This *stage effect* is illustrated in Figure 3.3, where smokers initially in precontemplation show the smallest amount of abstinence over 18 months and those in preparation progress the most (Prochaska et al., 1992). Across 66 different predictions of progress, we found that smokers starting in contemplation were about two-thirds more successful than those in precontemplation at 6-, 12- and 18-month follow-ups. Similarly, those in preparation were about two-thirds more successful then those in contemplation at the same follow-ups (Prochaska, Velicer, Fava, & Laforge, 1996; Prochaska, Velicer, Fava, & Rossi, 1996).

These results can be used clinically. A reasonable goal for each therapeutic intervention with smokers is to help them progress one stage. If over the course of brief therapy they progress two stages, they will be about 2.66 times more successful at longer-term follow-ups (Prochaska, Velicer, Fava, Ruggiero, et al., 1996).

This strategy has been taught to more that 3500 primary-care physicians, nurses, and physicians' assistants in Britain's National Health System. With stage-matched counseling, the strategic goal is to help each patient progress one stage following one brief intervention. One of the first reports is a marked improvement in the morale of such health promoters intervening with all patients who smoke, abuse substances, and have unhealthy diets (Mason, 1996). These professionals now have strategies that match the needs of all of their patients, not simply the minority prepared to take action. Furthermore, these professionals can assess progress across stages in the majority of these patients, where previously, when taking action was their only measure of movement they experienced mostly failure.

Process

To help populations progress through the stages, we need to understand the processes and principles of change. One of the fundamental principles for progress is that different processes of change need to be applied at different stages of change. Classic conditioning processes like counterconditioning, stimulus control, and contingency control can be highly successful for participants taking action, but can produce resistance with individuals in precontemplation. With these individuals, more experiential processes, such as consciousness-raising and dramatic relief, can move people cognitively and affectively, and help them shift to contemplation (Prochaska, Norcross et al., 1994).

After 15 years of research, we have identified 14 variables on which to intervene in order to accelerate progress across the first five stages of change

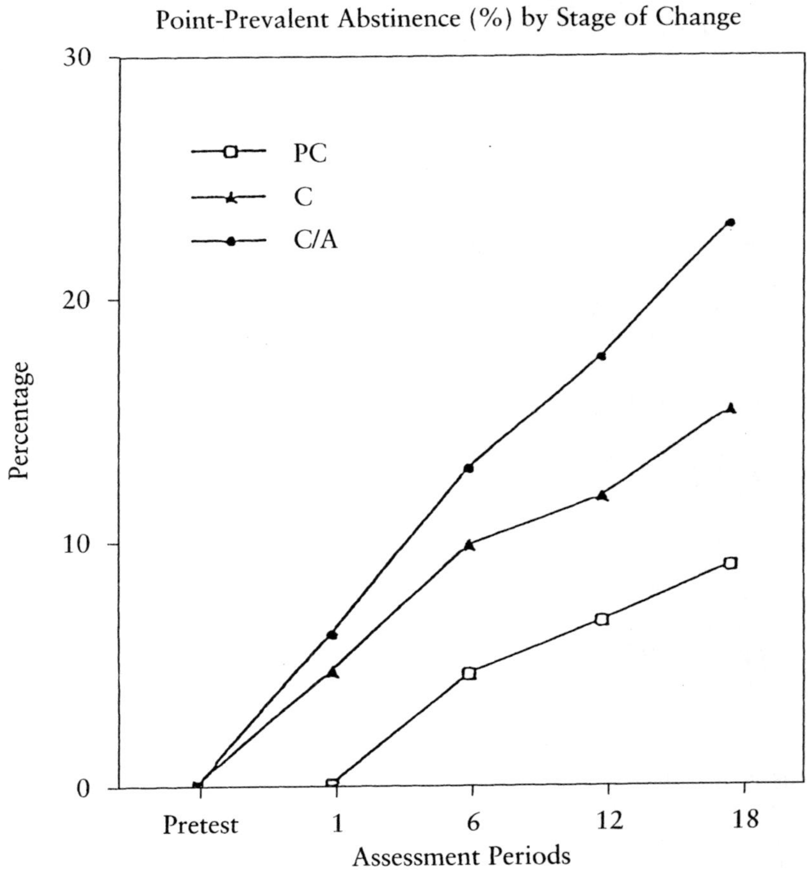

Figure 3.3 Percentage abstinent over 18 months for smokers in Precontemplation (PC), Contemplation (C), and Preparation (C/A) stages before treatment (N = 570).

(Prochaska et al., 1994). At any particular stage, we only need to intervene with a maximum of six variables. To help guide individuals at each stage of change, we have developed computer-based expert systems that can deliver individualized and interactive interventions to entire populations (Velicer et al., 1993). These computer programs can be used alone or in conjunction with counselors.

Outcomes

In our first large-scale clinical trial we compared four treatments: One of the best home-based action-oriented cessation programs (Standardized); stage-matched manuals (Individualized); expert system computer reports plus manuals (Interactive); and counselors plus computers and manuals (Personalized). We randomly assigned by stage 739 smokers to one of the four treatments (Prochaska, DiClemente, Velicer, & Rossi, 1993).

In the computer condition, participants completed by mail or telephone 40 questions. The answers were entered in our central computers and generated feedback reports. These reports informed participants about their stage of change, their pros and cons of changing, and their use of change processes appropriate to their stages. At baseline, participants were given positive feedback on what they were doing correctly and guidance on which principles and processes they needed to apply more in order to progress. In two progress reports delivered over the next 6 months, participants also received positive feedback on any improvement they made on any of the variables relevant to progressing. Thus, demoralized and defensive smokers could begin progressing without having to quit and without having to work too hard. Smokers in the contemplation stage could begin taking small steps, such as delaying their first morning cigarette for an extra 30 minutes. They could choose small steps that would increase their self-efficacy and help them become better prepared for quitting.

In the personalized condition, smokers received four proactive counselor calls over the 6 month intervention period. Three of the calls were based on the computer reports. Counselors reported much more difficulty in interacting with participants without any progress data. Without scientific assessments, it was much harder for both clients and counselors to tell whether any significant progress had occurred since their last interaction.

Figure 3.4 presents point prevalence abstinence rates for each of the four treatment groups over 18 months with treatment ending at 6 months (Prochaska, DiClemente et al., 1993). The two self-help manual conditions paralleled each other for 12 months. At 18 months, the stage-matched manuals moved ahead. This is an example of a delayed action effect, which we often observe with stage-matched programs specifically and others have observed with self-help programs generally (Glynn, Anderson, & Schwartz,

1992). It takes time for participants in early stages to progress all the way to action. Therefore, some treatment effects as measured by action will be observed only after considerable delay. However, it is encouraging to find treatments producing therapeutic effects months and even years after treatment ended.

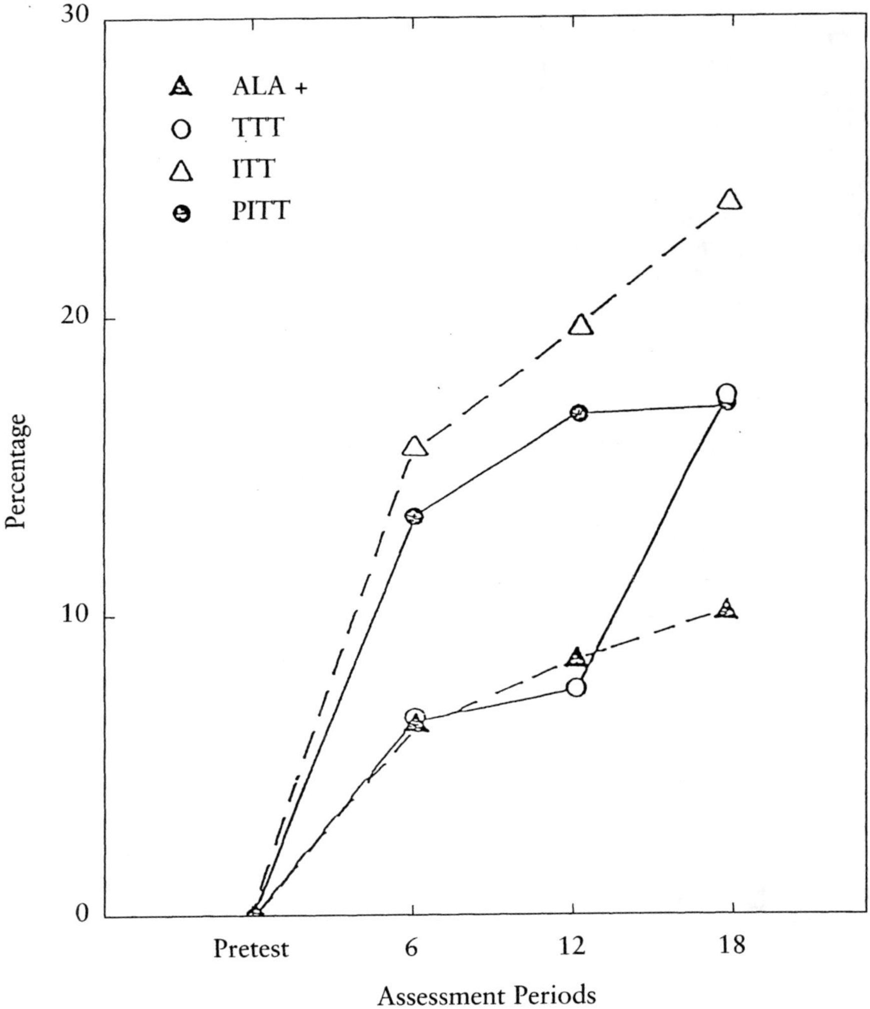

Figure 3.4 Point prevalence abstinence (%) for four treatment groups at pretest and at 6, 12, and 18 months. (ALA += standardized manuals; TTT = individualized stage-matched manuals; ITT = interactive computer reports; PITT = personalized counselor calls).

The computer-alone and computer-plus-counselor conditions paralleled each other for 12 months. Then, the effects of the counselor condition flattened out while the computer-condition effects continued to increase. We can only speculate as to the delayed differences between these two conditions. Participants in the personalized condition may have become somewhat dependent on the social support and social control of the counselor calling. The last call took place after the 6 months assessment, and benefits would be observed at 12 months. Termination of the counselors could result in no further progress because of the loss of social support and control. The classic pattern in smoking cessation clinics is rapid relapse beginning as soon as the treatment is terminated. Some of this rapid relapse could well be due to the sudden loss of social support or social control provided by the counselors and other participants in the clinic.

In this clinical trial, smokers were recruited reactively. They called us in response to advertisements, announcements, and articles. How would their results compare to the smokers proactively recruited to our programs? Most

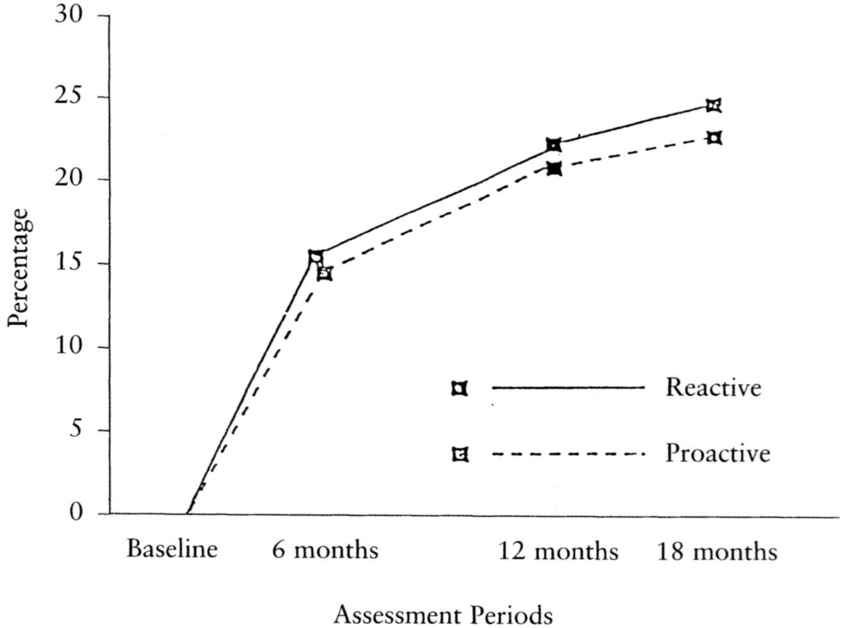

Figure 3.5 Point prevalence abstinence rates for smokers recruitment by Reactive vs. Proactive strategies and treated by stage-matched home-based expert system computer reports.

people would predict that smokers who call us for help would succeed more than smokers who we called to help.

Figure 3.5 shows the remarkable results of studies comparing smokers whom we called (reactive) (Prochaska, DiClemente, et al., 1993) to those whom we called (proactive) (Prochaska, Velicer, Fava, et al., 1996). Both groups received the same home-based expert system computer reports delivered over a 6-month period. While the reactively recruited subjects were slightly more successful at each follow-up, what is striking is how similar are the results.

If these results continue to be replicated, health promotion programs will be able to produce unprecedented impacts on entire populations. We believe that such unprecedented impacts require scientific and professional shifts:

1. from an action paradigm to a stage paradigm;
2. from reactive to proactive recruitment;
3. from expecting participants to match the needs of our programs to having our programs match their needs;
4. and from clinic-based to community-based behavioral health programs, still applying the field's most powerful individualized and interactive intervention strategies.

With these types of shifts in health promotion, we may be better prepared to respond to the huge unmet needs and the great opportunities related to the prevention of chronic diseases and premature death.

FUTURE RESEARCH

While expert system technology may be one of the waves of the future, adequate data sets are needed to develop the decision rules for each TTM variable, and computers are necessary to handle the complexity of stage-matching on these variables. One does not need a computer to generate stage-tailored health promotion materials. What does research demonstrate regarding the efficacy of stage-tailored interventions? There have been a series of studies across problem areas supporting the efficacy of stage-tailored health education materials when compared to action-oriented materials or no treatment (Campbell et al., 1994; Greene, Rossi, Reed, Willey, & Prochaska, 1994; Marcus, Banspach, Lefebvre, Rossi, & Carleton, 1992; Skinner, Strecher, & Hospers, 1994). In contrast, however, for smoking cessation, stage-tailored manuals did not outperform the "gold standard" ALA manuals, while the stage-matched expert system group clearly outperformed the action-oriented manuals (Prochaska, DiClemente, et al., 1993). In the most recent smoking cessation studies, the stage-matched expert system intervention was compared to stage-tailored manuals in different groups that received series of 1, 2, 3, or 6 doses. In this study, stage-matched expert systems clearly outperformed stage-tailored manuals (Prochaska, Velicer, Fava, & LaForge, 1996; Prochaska, Velicer, Fava, & Rossi, 1996; Prochaska, Velicer, Fava, Ruggiero, Rossi, & LaForge, 1996). Furthermore, the stage-tailored intervention group did not outperform the proactive-assessment-alone control group. We believe that proactive assessment alone does produce some active effect, which may have negated the difference between the stage-tailored and assessment-alone conditions. Further research is needed to determine the relative efficacy, impact, and cost-effectiveness of stage-matched interactive systems compared to non-interactive stage-tailored programs.

While we are encouraged by the research results to date, much still needs to be done to advance the Transtheoretical Model. Basic research needs to be done with other theoretical variables, such as perceived risk, subjective norms, and severity of the problem, to determine if such variables relate systematically to the stages and if they predict progress across particular stages. More research is needed on the structure of the processes and stages of change across a broad range of health behaviors. What modifications are most needed for specific types of behavior; for example, are fewer processes needed perhaps for infrequent behaviors, such as annual mammograms? What additional behaviors, such as stress, gambling, depression and social isolation, could be understood from a stage perspective? Does the model hold only for changing chronic behaviors, like smoking, or can it be useful with acute conditions, like acute depression?

Can the stage model be useful in describing, explaining, and predicting changes beyond the individual level, such as changes in couples, families, organizations, and communities? What happens when two or more people are trying to change together and they are in different stages? Can social policies be made more effective by matching policies to a community's stage of readiness to change? Are there particular types of public health campaigns, such as media campaigns, that can best produce progress in communities in early stages of change?

How do diverse populations respond to stage-matched interventions and to high-tech systems? How might this program best be tailored to meet the needs of diverse populations?

At the individual level, much more research needs to be done on the most cost-effective interventions for producing progress through the stages across a variety of health behaviors. What are the minimum interventions needed to accelerate progress at each stage?

The Transtheoretical Model is a dynamic theory of change and it must remain open to modification as more students, scientists, and practitioners apply the stage model to a growing number of theoretical and public health problems.

SUMMARY

Research to date supports the Transtheoretical perspective that the adoption and maintenance of health behavior change involves progress through a series of stages. Such progress can be accelerated and facilitated by matching particular processes and principles of change to populations and individuals at each stage of change. Proactively applying stage-matched interventions can greatly increase participation, retention, progress, and impact rates in entire populations at risk for chronic disease and premature death.

REFERENCES

Bandura, A. (1977). Self-efficacy: Toward a unifying theory of behavior change. *Psychological Review, 84*, 191–215.

Bandura, A. (1982). Self-efficacy mechanism in human agency. *American Psychologist, 37*, 122–147.

Campbell, M. K., DeVellis, B. M., Strecher, V. J., Ammerman, A. S., DeVellis, R. F., & Sandler, R. S. (1994). Improving dietary behavior: The effectiveness of tailored messages in primary care settings. *American Journal of Public Health, 84*, 783–787.

COMMIT Research Group. (1995). Community Intervention Trial for Smoking Cessation (COMMIT): I. Cohort results from a four-year community intervention. *American Journal of Public Health, 85*, 183–192.

Glasgow, R. E., Terborg, J. R., Hollis, J. F., Severson, H. H., & Boles, S. M. (1995). Take Heart: Results from the initial phase of a work-site wellness program. *American Journal of Public Health, 85*, 209–216.

Glynn, T. J., Anderson, D. M., & Schwarz, L. (1992). Tobacco use reduction among high risk youth: Recommendations of a National Cancer Institute Expert Advisory Panel. *Preventive Medicine, 24*, 354–362.

Greene, G. W., Rossi, S. R., Reed, G. R., Willey, C., & Prochaska, J. O. (1994). Stages of change for reducing dietary fat to 30% of energy or less. *Journal of the American Dietetic Association, 94*, 1105–1110.

Janis, I. L., & Mann, L. (1977). *Decision making: A psychological analysis of conflict, chance and commitment*. New York: Free Press.

Lando, H. A., Pechacek, T. F., Pirie, P. L., Murray, D. M., Mittelmark, M. B., Lichtenstein, E., Nothwehyr, F., & Gray, C. (1995). Changes in adult cigarette smoking in the Minnesota Heart Health Program. *American Journal of Public Health, 85*, 201–208.

Lichtenstein, E., & Hollis, J. (1992). Patient referral to smoking cessation programs: Who follows through? *Journal of Family Practice, 34*, 739–744.

Luepker, R. V., Murray, D. M., Jacobs, D. R., Mittelmark, M. B., Bracht, N., Carlaw, R., Crow, R., Elmer, P., Finnegan, J., Folsom, A. R., Grimm, P. J., Hannan, R., Jeffrey, R., Lando, H., McGovern, P., Mullis, R., Perry, L., Pechacek, P., Pirie, J. M., Sprafka, R., Wiesbrod, R., & Blackburn, H. (1994).

Community education for cardiovascular disease prevention: Risk factor changes in the Minnesota Heart Health Program. *American Journal of Public Health, 84*, 1383–1393.

Marcus, B. H., Banspach, S. W., Lefebvre, R. C., Rossi, J. S., & Carleton, R. A. (1992). Using the stages of change model to increase the adoption of physical activity among community participants. *American Journal of Health Promotion,* 6, 424–429.

Mason, P. (1996). *Helping people change: Train the trainers courses for health promotion in primary care.* Unpublished training manual. Birmingham, England.

Medeiros, M. E., & Prochaska, J. O. (1996). *Predicting termination and continuation status in psychotherapy using the Transtheoretical Model.* Manuscript under review.

Miller, R. C., & Berman, J. S. (1983). The efficacy of cognitive behavior therapies: A quantitative review of the research evidence. *Psychological Bulletin, 94*, 39–53.

Orleans, C. T., Schoenback, V. J., Salmon, M. A., Wagner, E. A., Pearson, D. C., Fiedler, J., Quade, D., Porter, C. Q., & Kaplan, B. A. (1988, November). Effectiveness of self-help quit smoking strategies. Paper presented in annual meeting of the Associatiòn for the Advancement of Behavior Therapy, New York, NY.

Peto, R., & Lopez, A. (1990). World-wide mortality from current smoking patterns. In B. Durstone & K. Jamrogik (Eds.), *The global war: Proceeding of the Seventh World Conference on Tobacco and Health* (pp. 62–68). East Perth, Western Australia: Organizing Committee of Seventh World Conference on Tobacco and Health.

Pinto, B. M., & Marcus, B. H. (1995). A stages of change approach to understanding college students physical activity. *Journal of American College Health, 44*, 27–31.

Prochaska, J. O. (1984). *Systems of psychotherapy: A transtheoretical analysis* (2nd ed.). Pacific Grove, CA: Brooks-Cole.

Prochaska, J. O. (1994a, April). Staging: A revolution in health promotion. Master science lecture at the annual meeting of the Society for Behavioral Medicine, Boston, Massachusetts.

Prochaska, J. O. (1994b). Strong and weak principles for progressing from Precontemplation to Action based on twelve problem behaviors. *Health Psychology, 13*, 47–51.

Prochaska, J. O., & DiClemente, C. C. (1982). Transtheoretical Therapy: Toward a more integrative model of change. *Psychotherapy: Theory, Research and Practice, 19*, 276–288.

Prochaska, J. O., & DiClemente, C. C. (1983). Stages and processes of self-change of smoking: Toward an integrative model of change. *Journal of Consulting and Clinical Psychology, 51*, 390–395.

Prochaska, J. O., DiClemente, C. C., & Norcross, J. C. (1992). In search of how people change: Applications to the addictive behaviors. *American Psychologist, 47*, 1102–1114.

Prochaska, J. O., DiClemente, C. C., Velicer, W. F., & Rossi, J. S. (1993). Standardized, individualized, interactive and personalized self-help programs for smoking cessation. *Health Psychology, 12*, 399–405.

Prochaska, J. O., Norcross, J. C., & DiClemente, C. C. (1994). *Changing for good.* New York: William Morrow.

Prochaska, J. O., Velicer, W. F., Fava, J., & Laforge, R. (1996). *Toward disease state management for smoking: Stage matched expert systems for a total managed care population of smokers.* Manuscript under review.

Prochaska, J. O., Velicer, W. F., Fava, J., & Rossi, J. (1996). *A stage matched expert system intervention with a total population of smokers.* Manuscript under review.

Prochaska, J. O., Velicer, W. F., Fava, J., Ruggiero, L., Rossi, J., & Laforge, R. (1996). *Stage, interactive, dose response, counseling and stimulus control computer effects in a total managed care population of smokers.* Manuscript under review.

Prochaska, J. O., Velicer, W. F., Rossi, J. S., Goldstein, M. G., Marcus, B. H., Rakowski, W., Fiore, C., Harlow, L., Redding, C. A., Rosenbloom, D., & Rossi, S. R. (1994). Stages of change and decisional balance for twelve problem behaviors. *Health Psychology, 13*, 39–46.

Rakowski, W., Dube, C. E., & Goldstein, M. G. (in press). Considerations for extending the transtheoretical model of behavior change to screening mammography. *Health Education Research.*

Rakowski, W., Ehrich, B., Dube, C. A., Pearlman, D. N., Goldstein, M. G., Rimer, B. K., Woolverton, H., & Peterson, K. K. (in press). Screening mammography and constructs from the Transtheoretical Model: Associations using two definitions of the stages-of-adoption. *Annals of Behavioral Medicine.*

Rossi, J. S. (1992b, April). *Stages of change for 15 health risk behaviors in an HMO population.* Paper presentation at 13th meeting of the Society for Behavioral Medicine, New York, NY.

Rossi, J. S. (1992a, August). *Common processes of change across nine problem behaviors.* Paper presentation at 100th meeting of American Psychological Association, Washington, DC.

Schmid, T. L., Jeffrey, R. W., & Hellerstedt, W. L. (1989). Direct mail recruitment to house-based smoking and weight control programs: A comparison of strengths. *Preventive Medicine, 18*, 503–517.

Skinner, C. S., Strecher, V. J., & Hospers, H. J. (1994). Physician recommendations for mammography: Do tailored messages make a difference? *American Journal of Public Health, 84*, 43–49.

Snow, M. G., Prochaska, J. O., & Rossi, J. S. (1992). Stages of change for smoking cessation among former problem drinkers: A cross-sectional analysis. *Journal of Substance Abuse, 4*, 107–116.

Sorensen, G., Thompson, B., Glantz, K., Feng, Z., Kinne, S., DiClemente, C. C., Emmons, K., Heimendinger, J., Probart, c., & Lichtenstein, E. (1996). Work site-based cancer prevention: Primary results from the working well trial. *American Journal of Public Health, 86*, 939–947.

U.S. Department of Health and Human Services. (1990). *The health benefits of smoking cessation: A report of the Surgeon General* (DHHS Publication No. CDC 90-8416). Washington, DC: U.S. Government Printing Office.

Velicer, W. F., Fava, J. L., Prochaska, J. O., Abrams, D. B., Emmons, K. M., &

Pierce, J. (1995). Distribution of smokers by stage in three representative samples. *Preventive Medicine, 24*, 401–411.

Velicer, W. F., Prochaska, J. O., Bellis, J. M., DiClemente, C. C., Rossi, J. S., Fava, J. L., & Steiger, J. H. (1993). An expert system intervention for smoking cessation. *Addictive Behaviors, 18*, 269–290.

Wierzbicki, M., & Pekarik, G. (1993). A meta-analysis of psychotherapy dropout. *Professional Psychology: Research and Practice, 29*, 190–195.

4

Models for Provider-Patient Interaction: Applications to Health Behavior Change

Michael G. Goldstein, Judith DePue, Alessandra Kazura, and Raymond Niaura

---

Physicians and other healthcare providers play an important role in providing patients with health information, educating patients about medical conditions and risk for disease, helping patients adhere to treatment plans, and motivating and assisting patients to alter unhealthy behaviors and adopt healthy behaviors. These activities will in turn improve risk factors, improve health outcomes, and reduce morbidity and mortality. Health care providers have ample opportunity, as approximately 76% of the U.S. population visit a physician in a year, with an average of 5.3 visits per year (National Center for Health Statistics, 1990). Moreover, patients view their physicians as having a great deal of influence over their health-related behaviors. For example, a physician's recommendation is a stronger predictor of screeening mannography than women's beliefs and perceptions (Lerman, Rimer, Trock, Balshem & Engstrom, 1990; National Cancer Institute Breast Cancer Screening Consortium, 1990). However, several population surveys have reported relatively low rates of such physician interventions. Studies of community-based primary care physicians' clinical cancer prevention activities found that, at baseline, only 34–49% of patients reported they received recommendations to reduce fat and increase fiber in their diet (Dietrich et al., 1992) and only 1–2% of patients' charts documented dietary counseling (McPhee, Bird, Fordham, Rodnick, & Osborn, 1991). Other surveys have shown 51–90% of physicians reported they advise most smokers to quit (Fortmann, Sallis, Magnus, & Farquhar, 1995; Goldstein et al., 1993; Lewis, Clancy, Leake, & Schwartz, 1991; Orleans, George, Houpt, & Brodie, 1985; Wells, Lewis, Leake, Schleiter, & Brook, 1986). While many physicians consider these practices important, there are clearly many remaining barriers to their consistent use.

In this chapter, we will first describe the barriers to delivery of behavior change interventions in health care settings. Then, we will describe several models which may be used to enhance provider-patient interaction to facilitate patient adherence and behavior change. We will review a Systems Model described by Walsh and McPhee (1992) and a Patient Path Model (Pommerenke & Dietrich, 1992a), both of which integrate patient and provider factors with the health care delivery system and organizational factors which impact the delivery of care and patient outcomes. We also discuss three models which focus in more detail on the provider-patient interaction: the Transtheoretical Model (Prochaska & DiClemente, 1986); Motivational Interviewing (Miller & Rolnick, 1991); and a Patient-Centered Patient Education model (Grueninger, Duffy, & Goldstein, 1995) The latter approach integrates features from the first two, and emphasizes the importance of tailoring interventions to the specific needs of patients and utilizing counseling skills to enhance the outome of the encounter. Examples of interventions are given to illustrate potential applications of these models.

BARRIERS TO PROVIDER INVOLVEMENT IN PATIENT ADHERENCE AND BEHAVIOR CHANGE INTERVENTIONS

Barriers to provider involvement in patient education and counseling can be categorized as deficits in knowledge, deficits in skill, attitudinal barriers, and organizational barriers (see Table 4.1). While most physicians recognize the importance of health promotion and risk-factor reduction, they have limited knowledge of behavior change principles and interventions, and they lack knowledge about patient education materials and other resources (Kottke, Battista, DeFriese, & Brekke, 1988; Orleans et al., 1985). Many physicians rely on simply providing advice because they have inadequate knowledge of effective patient education and counseling techniques, such as checking for understanding, addressing feelings about change, enhancing motivation, and negotiating a plan (Grueninger et al., 1995; Kottke et al., 1988; Lazare, Putnam, & Lipkin, 1995; Orleans et al., 1985; Ockene, 1988). Inadequate knowledge of methods leads to lack of success, which in turn, leads to reduced motivation to practice patient education (Grueninger et al., 1995).

TABLE 4.1 Barriers to Provider Involvement in Behavior Change Interventions

Physician Barriers

- Knowledge Deficit
  - Adherence and behavior change principles
  - Effectiveness of physician intervention
  - Intervention methods
  - Resources for patients: materials and referrals
- Skill Deficit
  - Interviewing/assessment/diagnostic skills
  - Patient education skills
  - Behavioral counseling skills
  - Maintenance/relapse prevention skills
- Beliefs and Attitudes
  - Patients don't want to change or can't change
  - Perceived ineffectiveness in helping patients adhere to treatment or change
  - Lack of confidence in helping patents adhere or change
  - Emphasis on final outcomes
  - Disease-oriented biomedical approach
  - Provider-centered, directive style
  - Moralistic view of behavior problems
- Poor personal health habits
- Dearth of role models practicing preventive care

Organizational Barriers

- Limited use of reminder systems, tracking logs
- Little or no reimbursement for patient education, counseling, or preventive services
- Poor coordination with self-help and behavioral treatment programs
- Limited involvement of office staff in patient education/health promotion activities

Note. From "Behavior medicine strategies for medical patients" In A. Stoudemire (Ed.), *Clinical psychiatry for medical students* (2nd ed., pp. 671–693) by M. G. Goldstein, L. Ruggiero, B. J. Guise, & D. B. Abrams, 1994, Philadelphia: J. B. Lippincott. Copyright 1994, 1990 by J. B. Lippincott Company. Adapted with permission.

A second important barrier is lack of skills, including interviewing and assessment skills to make an adequate diagnosis of the patient's educational needs, skills to motivate and to assist the patient with behavior change, and skills to help the patient maintain the new behaviors and adhere to the treatment plan. Medical education for physicians has neglected training in patient education and counseling skills, while nursing and other allied health disciplines have offered a somewhat greater emphasis on this. Because of lack of both knowledge and skills, physicians have reported lack of confidence for intervening on risk-factor change (Orleans et al., 1985). Lack of confidence is also a function of attitudes, such as perceived lack of effectiveness and a tendency to measure success by final outcomes, such as abstinence from smoking, rather than recognizing that lasting behavior change occurs only after multiple trials and through intermediate steps. This focus on final outcomes is unfortunate, because it is common for smokers to make many quit attempts before being successful, and the best 1-year abstinence rates reported from smoking cessation interventions in a primary care medical setting are only 10–20% (Fiore et al., 1996; Schwartz, 1992). Practitioners may not realize that this rate of "success" represents more than two times the rate that is achieved with no provider intervention (Fiore et al., 1996). The perceived lack of effectiveness also fuels the attitude that patients don't want to change or can't change. Provider attitudes are also shaped by the prevailing model in medicine, the biomedical model, which emphasizes a focus on diagnosis and treatment of disease and undervalues the role of behavior on health and disease. Traditional medical training has not yet adopted a systems-based biopsychosocial model which embraces the role of the patient, family, community, and other social forces in shaping health and illness (Engel, 1977).

Despite an increased emphasis in recent years on teaching prevention in health care training programs, very few role models are available to students that emphasize patient education and preventive care. This contributes to the belief of many physicians that health promotion activities are outside their role or they are uninteresting or unchallenging (Nutting, 1986). Providers may also harbor negative or moralistic attitudes towards patients who exhibit problematic behaviors such as drinking or smoking, or who don't follow their recommendations. These attitudes may interfere with providers' willingness or capacity to assist these patients to change. Finally, providers with negative personal health practices are less likely to counsel patients regarding prevention (Frank & Kunovich-Frieze, 1995; Lewis et al., 1991) and male physicians appear to be less likely than female physicians to offer mammography and Pap smears (Lurie et al., 1993; Frank & Kunovich-Frieze, 1995) and schedule general prevention visits (Osborn, Bird, McPhee, Rodnick, & Fordham, 1991).

Organizational barriers to provider involvement in adherence and behavior change counseling include limited reimbursement for counseling and preventive care services, lack of self-help or other patient education resources, poor coordination with behavioral treatment programs or other referral resources, and limited involvement of office staff in patient education and health promotion activities (Goldstein, Ruggiero, Guise, & Abrams, 1994; Kottke, Brekke, & Solberg, 1993; Mayer & Beardall, 1995; McPhee & Detmer, 1993; Pommerenke & Dietrich, 1992a). Many medical offices are not organized to provide patient education or preventive care services amidst the competing demands of an office full of sick patients. Providers need monitoring systems to alert them that a patient is due for her mammogram, reminder systems to prompt them to ask patients about smoking, and systems to reorder patient education materials when they are low. The effectiveness of reminders on the delivery of preventive services by physicians and other health care providers has been conclusively demonstrated in multiple studies (Goldstein et al., 1994; Kottke et al., 1993; Mayer & Beardall, 1995; McPhee & Detmer, 1993; I. S. Ockene et al., 1996; Pommerenke & Dietrich, 1992a). For example, a series of intervention trials sponsored by the National Cancer Institute showed that physician skills in smoking-cessation counseling could be improved and their frequency of counseling with patients increased; however, the overall quit rates among the population of smokers in the practice were most likely to be increased when physicians were also provided with prompts to remind them to bring up the topic with smokers (Manley, Epps, Husten, Glynn, & Shopland, 1991). Thus, organizational factors can undermine or enhance the positive efforts of individual providers.

A SYSTEMS MODEL OF CLINICAL PREVENTIVE CARE

Walsh and McPhee's Systems Model of Clinical Preventive Care (Walsh & McPhee, 1992) draws upon concepts from a variety of models, including the health belief model (Becker, Haefner, & Kasl, 1977), social learning theory (Bandura, 1977), the PRECEDE model (Green, Eriksen, & Schor, 1988), and the Diffusion and Adoption Model (Orlandi, 1987). However, the Walsh and McPhee model departs from these previous models, as it recognizes influences on both the patient and the clinician as contributors to the preventive behavior; each with predisposing, enabling, and reinforcing factors (see Figure 4.1). Predisposing factors are the cognitive, attitudinal, and perceptual factors that influence a patient's or a clinician's willingness to engage in health-behavior change (Green et al., 1988; Walsh & McPhee, 1992). Enabling factors are the skills and resources necessary to perform the behavior and reinforcing factors are those that support or reward the preventive activity (Green et al., 1988; Walsh & McPhee, 1992). Walsh and

McPhee further postulate that these factors influence the patient-provider interaction which determines the final outcome (e.g. physical activity by the patient or a screening test conducted by the provider). In addition, the model recognizes other factors which independently influence both the physician and the patient, including health care delivery/organizational factors, preventive activity fatctors, and situational factors/cues to action. Barriers may be present at any level in this model to interfere with accomplishment of preventive activity. Although Walsh and McPhee focussed only on the delivery of preventive care, their model may also be applied to other health-care targets, such as delivery of care for a chronic illness (e.g., management of diabetes, congestive heart failure, or hypertension). In the following section, we will delineate the factors that comprise the Systems Model of Clinical Preventive Care in more detail.

The patient and the provider both contribute predisposing factors which may influence their decisionmaking, including demographic factors (e.g., age, income, gender), beliefs, attitudes, self-efficacy, and prior experiences and expectations. For example, patients as well as providers who are ori-

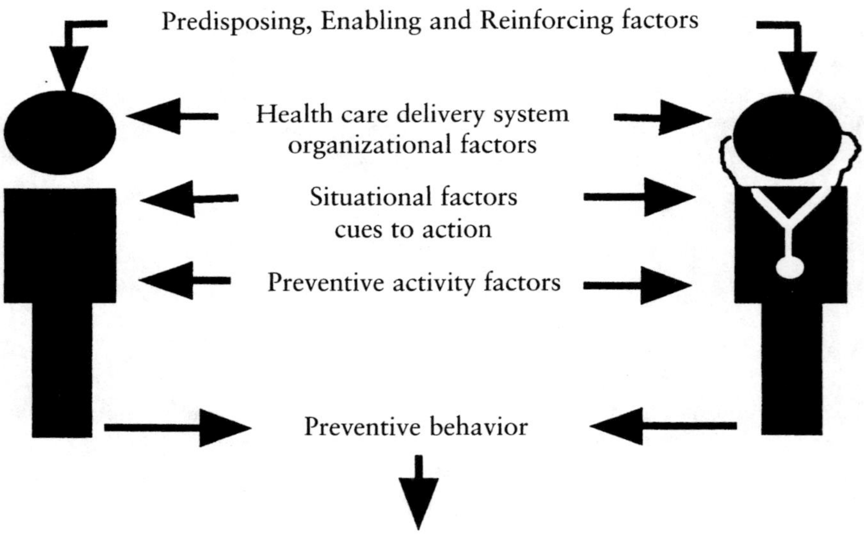

Figure 4.1 A Systems Model of Clinical Preventive Care.

From "A Systems Model of Preventive Care: An Analysis of Factors Influencing Patient and Physicians," by J.M. Walsh and S.J. McPhee, 1992, *Health Education Quarterly, 19,* p 159. Copyright 1992 by SOPHE, Published by John Wiley & Sons, Inc.

ented to curative medicine may be less receptive to delivery of preventive care during office visits. If either one holds this attitude, it can undermine accomplishment of desired outcomes. Similarly, patient's fear of having cancer coupled with the belief that the diagnosis is a death sentence may be a potent barrier to having a cancer-screening test. Conversely, patients who understand the benefits of screening, particularly if they know they are at increased risk, may be more likely to follow a provider's recommendation to undergo screening. As noted previously in this chapter, a provider's personal risk and behavior also may serve as predisposing factors and influence the delivery of counseling (Frank & Kunovich-Frieze, 1995; Lewis et al., 1991). For example, providers who smoke were less likely to deliver smoking cessation advice, and very physically active internists were more likely to counsel about exercise (Lewis et al., 1991). Enabling factors include knowledge, skills (e.g., ability to read, for patients; training in counseling, for physicians), resources (e.g., educational materials), and physiologic factors (e.g., low dependence on nicotine; for patients). For patients, higher education, higher income, and medical insurance also serve as enabling factors, while physician-enabling factors include knowledge of current recommendations and adequate time during the visit (Walsh, 1992). Reinforcing factors are often missing, at least immediately, for many preventive activities, or they may not be directly rewarding in themselves. Social support and approval by peers are reinforcing factors for both providers and patients, as is patient satisfaction for providers. Achievement of desired outcomes also may be reinforcing for both patients and providers. For providers, discovery of new, early-stage cancers is particularly reinforcing. On the other hand, past failures and disappointments on the part of either patients or providers may become a barrier to further efforts to promote change.

Healthcare delivery system/organizational factors affect both the physician and the patient to independently influence provision of preventive care. These factors include access to care, availability of technology and personnel, convenience of services to the patient, organizational priorities, structure of the office, reimbursement, and coordination with other community services. Organizational priorities usually determine the structure of the encounter, including the nature of the problems to be discussed and time allocated, and/or how fees are assigned. Preventive care is often assigned a lesser priority when time is restricted. Preventive activity factors refer to the characteristics of the screening test or preventive behavior itself which influence whether it is performed. For example, some screening tests have high false-positive rates, which discourages their use by physicians. Other tests may be very cost-effective, but involve discomfort (pelvic examination for Pap smear screening). Increasing physical activity may be an enjoyable preventive activity for some patients but uncomfortable or distasteful for others. Cost of a test or treatment is another important factor specific to the preventive activity. Situational factors/cues to action can influence performance of preventive activities either as internal factors (e.g., symptoms which cue a patient to make an office visit) or external (e.g., reminders to providers and/or patients; media coverage or advertising). Providers may utilize computer reminders to signal them that a patient is due for a routine test. Patients may use reminders to signal them to keep on their exercise schedule.

The Systems Model for Clinical Prevention offers a valuable means to recognize the many factors which influence the patient-physician intervention. Many of these factors may in fact be outside of the provider's control, such as availability of medical insurance or reimbursement. However, a key contribution of this model is the recognition of the influence of organizational and situational factors on the delivery of care and, specifically, the importance of office systems (e.g., reminders, convenient office hours) and a supportive office team who will reinforce the providers' messages. A weakness of this model is its static nature, as it does not describe a time course or pathway for receipt of a given patient education or preventive activity. Also, patient and provider factors are considered independently, with little attention paid to the interaction between provider and patient. The content of the interaction is not emphasized (except for the delivery of a message) and the process of the interaction (e.g., communication strategies and styles) is not considered.

THE PATIENT PATH MODEL

Pommerenke and Dietrich (Pommerenke & Dietrich, 1992a) offer the Patient Path Model (See Figure 4.2) as a conceptual framework to identify opportunities to enhance preventive care, taking into account practice characteristics, office systems, daily practice habits of physicians and their office staff, as well as patient factors. While the Patient Path Model incorporates many of the same factors as the Systems Model described above, albeit with different terminology, it offers the advantage of describing the intervention as a pathway through the medical encounter. Therefore, the framework to understand barriers and the opportunities to influence the encounter become more clear at logical junctures along the path. In this model, the path crosses four "spheres of influence":

1. The patient, including knowledge of the benefits of the target behavior, and money to pay for the medical visit or procedure;
2. the patient's environment, including support from family for screening;
3. the physician, including their skills, attitudes, and awareness of the patient's risk; and
4. the physician's environment, including office hours, office systems to prompt, track, and follow-up on screening and/or counseling interventions.

The patient's path is described through three different phases of the medical encounter: a) before the encounter; b) during the provider encounter; and c) after the encounter.

Before the Encounter

Many patient and patient environment factors serve as a starting point for the encounter. These include the patient's cultural background, language,

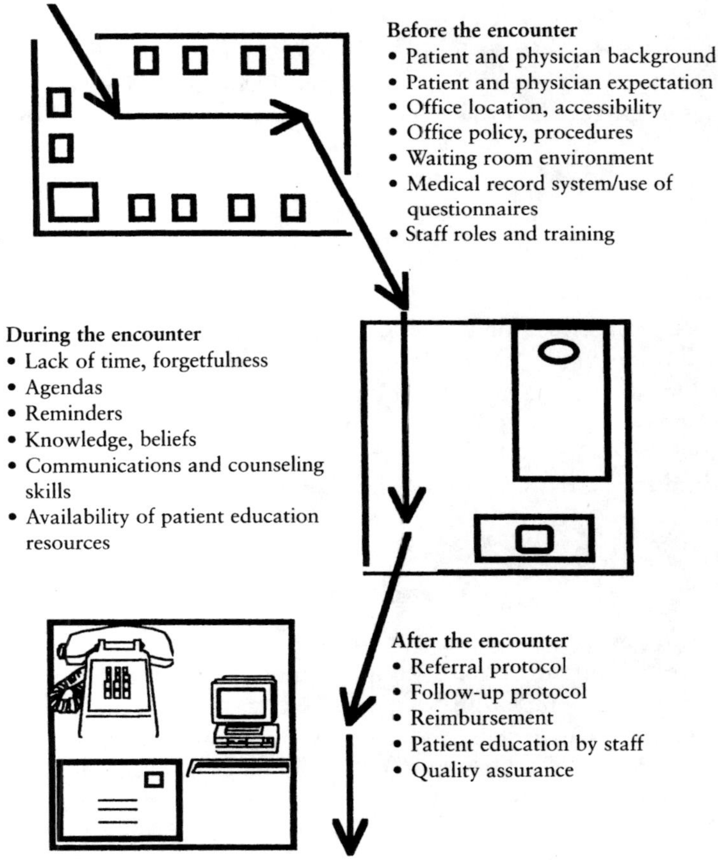

Figure 4.2 The patient path model.

From "Improving and Maintaining Preventive Services, Part 1: Applying the Patient Path Model," by F.A. Pommerenke and A. Dietrich, 1992a, *Journal of Family Practice, 34,* p. 87. Copyright 1992 Appleton & Lange.

socioeconomic status, and health behaviors. Physician factors also set the stage, such as insurance regulations, national politics, media influence, and their personal background. While some of these factors are outside the provider's control, the office can attempt to minimize such potential barriers, for example, by offering evening or weekend hours to accommodate people who work, or offering bilingual staff to accommodate language barriers. Efforts to insure courteous reception staff and to minimize waiting time also will influence the content of the encounter. The presence of posters, displays, and patient education materials in the waiting room may stimulate the patient to think about a behavioral or preventive issue and bring it up for discussion during the visit with the provider. The use of patient questionnaires or history forms prior to the visit (e.g., mail or in-office) facilitates assessment of patients' baseline behavior and provides a prompt for both the patient and provider. Technological advances now permit questionnaire data that is collected in the office to be rapidly analyzed and fed back to the provider and patient to aid tailoring of subsequent patient education and counseling interventions (Campbell et al., 1994).

During the Provider Encounter

The quality of the face-to-face interaction can be influenced by use of prompts, such as recording of smoking status among the vital signs noted at the visit (Fiore et al., 1995). Effective communication skills of the provider as well as other staff, can also ease discussion of sensitive behavioral topics or screening procedures. The physical layout of the office is important, for example, to insure availability of exam rooms, to accommodate patient privacy, and to insure that patient education materials are readily available to all providers.

After the Encounter

Practice organizational systems continue to influence patient compliance with recommendations. For example, follow-up protocols will offer reinforcement or assistance with a patient's commitment to quit smoking or will help insure the patient pursues a screening referral. Follow-up can take the form of office visits, telephone contacts, mailings or even on-line computer contact, and can be handled by a variety of office staff. The assignment of specific office staff to deliver follow-up contact can improve efficiency and increase the liklihood that follow-up will be provided.

Pommerenke and Dietrich recommend that the Patient Path Model can serve to help providers review their clinical practice procedures to identify problem areas and opportunities for improvement. Dietrich and colleagues utilized an earlier version of the Patient Path Model to test an intervention to increase the delivery of selected preventive services in primary care practices (Dietrich et al., 1992). Physicians in 98 practices were randomly assigned to receive: a day-long educational intervention aimed at enhancing physician knowledge, attitudes, and skills relevant to cancer prevention; an office system intervention based on the Patient Path Model that included three visits from a project facilitator over 3 month; both; or neither. The office system intervention was associated with a significant increase in six of ten preventive practices (mammography, clinical breast exam, recommendation for breast self-exam, stool occult blood, recommendation to reduce fat, and advice to smokers to quit) while the educational intervention was associated with an increase in only one practice (mammography) (Dietrich et al., 1992). As a result of their experience, Pommerenke and Dietrich have identified several principles for improving preventive services on an organizational level in primary care practices (Pommerenke & Dietrich, 1992b).

We have found the Patient Path Model model to be highly useful when assisting community-based primary care providers to enhance their pateint education, counseling, and preventive activites. We are currently employing the Patient Path Model as a component of an office-based intervention to increase the delivery of cancer preventive services in primary care practices. The project, "Promoting Cancer Prevention in Primary Care," is funded by the National Cancer Institute, and will test the impact of an office-based intervention on patient, provider, and office level outcomes. Because the Patient Path Model focuses on the opportunities for providing interventions to patients during their path through a typical office visit, the model is easily understood by clinicians participating in the trial. The office-based intervention includes an initial meeting with physicians, other clinicians, and office staff to revieiw their current cancer prevention activities and develop a plan to improve their practices in this area over a 2-year period. At this initial meeting, we utilize a story board which "follows the path" that a typical patient takes as she progresses through an office visit. In response to this stimulus, providers are able to identify opportunities for enhancing current activities in such areas as identification of patient risk (e.g., through the use of questionnaires while the patient is in the waiting room; assessment of risk when vital signs are taken or the patient is placed in an exam room), use of chart prompt to convey information about risk to the provider, face-to-face counseling by providers and other office staff, provision of patient education materials, delivery of screening tests, chart monitoring of delivered services, and arrangement of follow-up contact. The inclusion of all office staff in this process facilitates teamwork, as well as delegation of specific activities to staff best suited to these tasks (e.g, receptionists may hand out questionnaires; medical technologists may assess smoking status; an office manager orders patient education resources; a nurse provides follow-up phone counseling). In addition, providing multiple messages from multiple providers has been demonstrated to enhance patient behavior change, at least for smoking cessation (Kottke et al., 1988). Though the results of "Promoting Cancer Prevention in Primary Care" will not be available till 1999, the incorporation of the Patient Path Model into our office-based intervention has been quite useful in engaging participating providers in a process to promote change.

In summary, the Patient Path Model identifies opportunities before, during, and after a medical office visit for enhancing the delivery of preventive care. Like the Systems Model described above, the Patient Path Model emphasizes system and organizational factors which can facilitate the delivery of preventive services and identifies both patient and provider factors which influence the outcome of a clinical encounter. Also, like the Systems Model, the Patient Path Model can be applied to the provision of care for chronic medical conditions. An advantage of the Patient Path Model over the Systems Model is its focus on identifiable phases of the medical encounter and the easy application of the model to the analysis of actual office practice environments. It is easily understood by providers who might utilize the model to assess and improve their own behavior. Moreover, the Patient Path model emphasizes the important roles of multiple members of the office staff team in the delivery of interventions to enhance patient behavior change. However, the Patient Path model puts little emphasis on the actual content and process of the patient-provider interaction. Though provider communication and counseling skills are included as factors in the Patient Path Model, the elements of effective patient education and counseling are not featured. We will now review three models that focus on the content and process of provider-patient interaction: The Transtheoretical Model of Change (Prochaska & DiClemente, 1986); Motivational Interviewing (Miller & Rolnick, 1991), and finally a Patient-Centered Patient Education Model (Grueninger et al., 1995) that incorporates aspects of the other two.

MODELS TO ENHANCE PROVIDER-PATIENT INTERACTION

The Transtheoretical Model of Change (TTM)

Prochaska and DiClemente (Prochaska & DiClemente, 1986) found that individuals progress through a series of five stages when making lifestyle changes (see Figure 4.3): precontemplation (unaware of a problem and no plan to change in foreseeable future); contemplation (ambivalence about changing with no commitment to change); preparation (intends to take action within the next month and has made some changes in the past year); action (has made commitment to change and is actively attempting to make behavior change); and maintenance (has successfully made change, but still needs to monitor behavior to prevent slips and relapse). Prochaska and DiClemente (1986) found that individuals may take several years to progress through these stages, and they may also recycle through the stages repeatedly. Moreover, individuals at different stages utilize different behavioral change strategies, and respond best to interventions that are linked to these strategies (Prochaska, DiClemente & Norcross, 1992). For example, consciousness-raising strategies will more likely help a person in the contemplation stage, while stimulus-control strategies will more likely help the person ready for action. Conversely, it may not be useful to provide instructions or recommendations for action to persons in the precontemplation or contemplation stages who have not yet made a commitment to change. Thus, assessment of stage of change is very important to enable matching of appropriate patient education and counseling strategies to the individual (Prochaska & Goldstein, 1991). Strategies appropriate for counseling patients in the precontemplation and contemplation stages include: providing personalized information and feedback about the problem and its effect on patients' health status; helping patients express feelings about the problem and assess how they feel about themselves with respect to the problem; and offering to help with associated problems that are barriers to change. Action-oriented counseling strategies include assisting patients to develop and implement a plan; teaching skills; providing direct services (e.g., screening, pharmacotherapy for smoking cessation; an exercise prescription); and referring for further education, screening or treatement. (See Chapter 3 for more information on the Transtheoretical Model of Change and the section on the Patient-Centered Patient Education Model, below, for more specifics about how to incorporate the principles of the TTM into a counseling strategy.)

By recognizing how people change, providers may redefine success as moving patients along the continuum of stages of change, rather than defining success only as reaching desirable final outcomes, such as smoking cessation (Prochaska & Goldstein, 1991). Further, they can help patients view relapse as a common part of the process, and view it as a learning opportunity rather than as a failure. This orientation may help providers experience less frustration in facilitating behavior-change and thus reduce an important barrier to their engaging in behavior change interventions. Indeed, this was our experience with a population-based sample of 279 primary care physicians who participated in a controlled research trial, "Physicians Counseling Smokers" (Goldstein, MacDonald, Niaura & Dube´, 1993), which tested an academic detailing strategy (Soumerai & Avorn, 1990) for disseminating the National Cancer Institute (NCI) physician-delivered smoking cessation counseling protocol (Glynn & Manley, 1989). "Office staff consultants" (i.e., academic detailers) visited with physicians and office staff in their office up to 5 times over a 1-year intervention period. A central feature of our intervention was to inform physicians about the TTM and help them to utilize it within the framework of the NCI brief counseling approach. Preliminary results suggest that the physicians who received the intervention significantly increased the amount of time they spent counseling smokers (by self-report) and also reported a significant increase in self-efficacy for counseling smokers (Willey et al., 1996). These effects at the physician level also produced increased smoking cessation rates among the population of patients served by the physicians receiving the academic detailing intervention (Willey et al., 1996).

The TTM has also been applied to understanding physician behavior change by members of our research group (Goldstein et al., 1993); and others (Main, Cohen & DiClemente, 1995). Physician adoption of recommended practices or guidelines can be understood as occurring along the

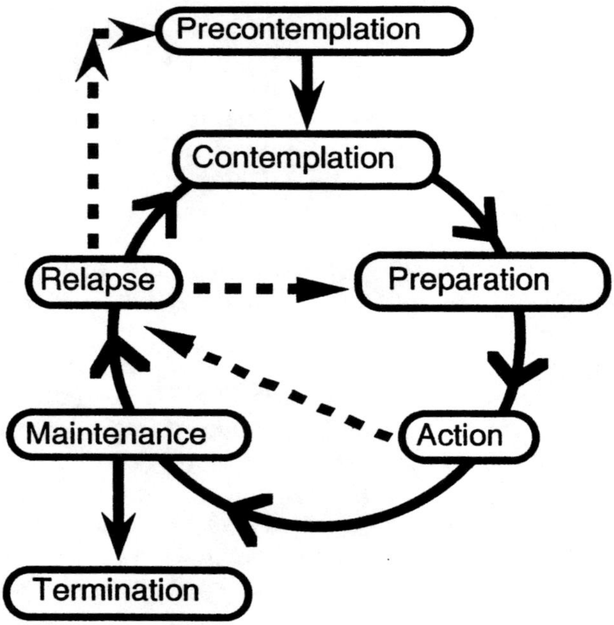

Figure 4.3 The stages of change.

From "Stages of Change in the Modification of Problem Behaviors," by J.O. Prochaska and C.C. DiClemente, 1992, *Pro Behav Modif, 28,* pp. 184–214.

continuum of stages of change, from precontemplation (not at all interested in adopting the guideline or behavior in the near future), to contemplation (ambivalent about adopting the behavior), to preparation (taking steps to adopt the behavior), to action and maintenance (consistently perfoming the behavior for a specified period of time). The "Physicians Counseling Smokers " project described above also utilized the TTM to develop a menu of intervention options that allowed the academic detailer to tailor interventions to the physician's stage of adoption of smoking cessation protocols (Goldstein et al., 1993). Cohen and colleagues (Cohen, Halvorson, & Gosselink, 1994) have also utilized the TTM to develop an intervention to enhance the delivery of a number of cancer-prevention activities in primary care. Though preliminary results from the Physicians Counseling Smokers project are positive (see above), the utility of applying the TTM to changing physician behavior is yet to be determined.

Motivational Interviewing

Motivational Interviewing (Miller & Rolnick, 1991) is a model or strategy of patient counseling which may be utilized to enhance patient behavioral change. This model incorporates theory from the Transtheoretical Model (Prochaska & DiClemente, 1986), Health Beliefs Model (Becker et al., 1977); Protection-Motivation Theory (Rippetoe & Rogers, 1987), and patient-centered approaches of Carl Rogers (Rogers, 1951; Rogers, 1959) and others (J. K. Ockene et al., 1988). It was developed primarily for treatment of alcohol addiction, but it is now increasingly being applied to other behaviors. It is especially helpful for patients who seem "stuck" in patterns of behavior that are harmful or potentially harmful by helping them resolve ambivalence and move along the path of change. Motivational Interviewing has been used effectively as a means of enhancing self-efficacy, increasing cognitive dissonance, and directing dissonance reduction toward behavior change.

Miller and Rolnick (1991) describe five general principles which underly this approach: (1) express empathy, (2) develop discrepancy; (3) avoid argumentation; (4) roll with resistance, and (5) support self-efficacy. Empathic warmth and reflective listening is employed throughout the movitational interviewing process. This style involves use of open-ended questions, legitimization of the patient's feelings, and validation of the patient's freedom to change or not change without judging. Respect for patients can be shown by accepting, while not necessarily condoning, their level of readiness to change, and by expressing support and willingness to help when they are ready to change. Ambivalence should be acknowledged as a normal part of the change process.

Developing discrepancy is done by raising patients' awareness of the consequences of their present behavior and highlighting the discrepancy between their present behavior and their own important personal goals. Wherever possible, patients are allowed to present their own reasons for change. The provider should avoid argumentation and labeling of the patient; arguments are counterproductive, and often lead to defensiveness. When the provider observes resistance by the patient, this should be a cue to change strategies. Rolling with resistance involves inviting the person to consider new information or perspectives and helping the patient to identify solutions, without imposing the provider's ideas. The provider can support self-efficacy by offering a range of alternative approaches and expressing encouragement that will help build on patients' past successes. The provider also should encourage patients to believe that they can change if they really want to, and that the decision to do so is up to them.

The menu of strategies for exploring concerns and options for change (Miller & Rolnick, 1991) are listed in assending order, with the more non-threatening strategies listed first. It is best to start with strategies close to the top of the list for persons less ready to change. These strategies have been adapted to accommodate other target behaviors beyond substance use, for which they were originally developed.

1. Ask about (target behavior) in detail, "Tell me about your (smoking)"; "How does your smoking affect you now?";
2. Ask about a typical day: "Describe your diet over the course of a typical day";
3. Ask about lifestyle and stresses: "What kind of stress are you under?" "How does (your use of alcohol) help you deal with your stress?";
4. Ask about health, then target behavior; a discussion about health concerns can lead to an open question, "I wonder where do you feel your typical diet fits in here?";
5. Ask about the good things, then the less good things: "What are the good things about your smoking?" "What are the not-so-good things?" While the goal is to explore concerns, it is important to recognize that less good things are not necessary concerns. However, the interviewer can use this discussion to lead to a question, "I wonder, how much does that bother you?";
6. Ask about target behavior in the past and now: "What's the difference between your (activity level) now and 10 years ago?" If the target behavior is substance use, this question can lead to a discussion about tolerance;
7. Provide information and ask, "What do you think?" "Would you like some information about what a low-fat diet would look like?" Then, after providing the information, ask, "What do you make of that?";
8. Ask about concerns directly. Only if the patient appears ready and

willing talk about this: "What concerns do you have about your (diabetes)?"; and

9. Ask about the next step. "I wonder where does this leave you now?" "It sounds like you're concerned about———. I wonder what is the next step?" Any negotiation is best done by eliciting possibilities from the patient.

Thus, Motivational Interviewing offers a specific approach for counseling the majority of patients who are in early stages of change and thus not ready to commit to specific treatment or behavioral change. A relative drawback of this approach, as originally outlined by Miller and Rollnick (1991), is the amount of time (45–120 minutes) and skill (several days of training) needed to provide the motivational intervention. A brief version of motivational interviewing that utilizes one or two of the nine strategies listed above has also been described (Rollnick, Heather, & Bell, 1992).

Patient-Centered Patient Education

The Patient-Centered Model of care has origins in the work of Rogers (Rogers, 1951) and Balint and colleagues (Balint, Hunt, Joyce, Marinker & Woodcock, 1970). Levenstein, Stewart, and colleagues (Levenstein, 1984; Levenstein, McCracken, McWhinney, Stewart & Brown, 1986; Stewart et al., 1995) have amplified the model and defined key components of a clinical method to be used by healthcare providers in communicating with patients. These are illustrated in an integrated model in Figure 4.4. Collaboration between doctor and patient is considered essential to defining healthcare problems and to choosing treatment options, including any behavioral changes to be made by the patient.

Related to the Patient-Centered Model are clinical and research paradigms on the medical interview (Cohen-Cole, 1991; Lipkin, Putnam & Lazare, 1995; Wissow, Roter, & Wilson, 1994); doctor-patient communications (Inui & Carter, 1995; Waitzkin, 1984); patient education (Green, 1984; Mullen & Green, 1990), and motivational interventions (Miller & Rolnick, 1991). All of these represent a movement away from a focus on physical explanations and solutions for suffering and dysfunction. They also share, either explicitly or implicitly, a value on an egalitarian process for developing the meaning of health experiences and prioritizing goals in medical encounters. Leopold and colleagues (Leopold, Cooper, & Clancy, 1996) use the term "sustained partnership" to emphasize those qualitative and structural aspects of the patient-centered doctor-patient relationship which distinguishes it from "continuity" or simply seeing the same provider across time. Although acknowledging that roles are unequal and that the responsibility for developing the relationship rests with the physician, the sustained

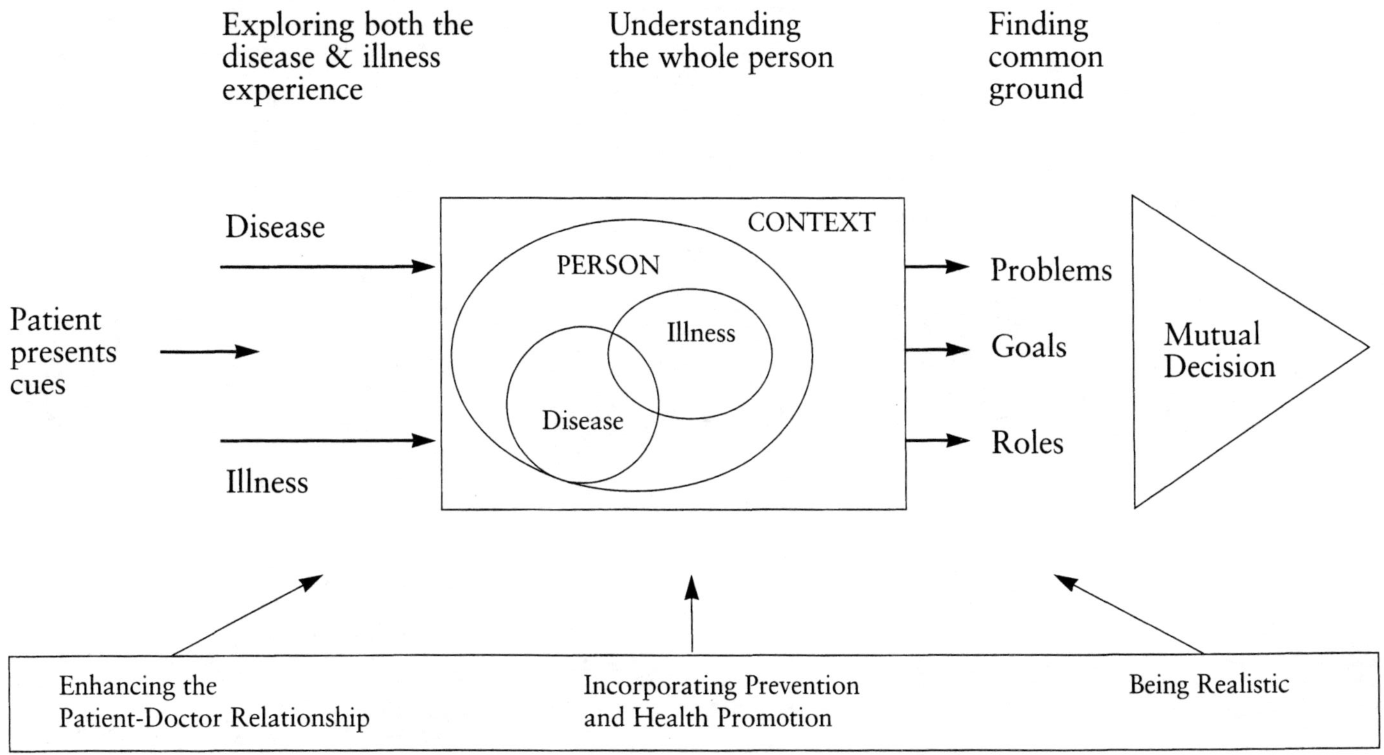

Figure 4.4 Patient-centered clinical model.

From *Patient-Centered Medicine: Transforming the Clinical Method*, p. 267, by M. Stewart, J. Brown, W. Weston, I. McWhinney, C. McWilliam, and T. Freeman, 1995, Thousand Oaks, CA. Sage, Copyright 1995 by Sage Publications, Inc.

partnership model describes a collaboration between doctor and patient in the control of communication and decisionmaking for health care. In this model, physician characteristics which are difficult to quantify, such as the ability to empathize, are viewed as critical to positive outcomes in patient satisfaction and health status.

Roter and Hall (1992), among others, have developed methods for studying physician behaviors which reflect the use of a collaborative care model. These tools include monitoring both content and nonverbal expressions in conversations between physicians and patients. Wissow, Roter, and Wilson (1994) have demonstrated that parents disclosed more psychosocial information when interviewed by pediatricians who used direct questions about psychosocial issues, statements of support, and statements indicating sympathetic and attentive listening than when interviewed by pediatricians who did not use these skills.

The Patient-Centered Patient Education Model (Grueninger et al., 1995) incorporates the principles of patient-centered care and applies them to the task of patient education and counseling, the "third function" of the medical interview (Cohen-Cole, 1991; Lazare et al., 1995). The first two functions are: (1) determining and monitoring the nature of the problem; and (2) developing, maintaining and concluding the therapeutic relationship (Cohen-Cole, 1991; Lazare et al., 1995). This model also is based on earlier work by Grueninger et al. 1989 and J. K. Ockene and colleagues (J. K. Ockene, 1987a; J. K. Ockene et al., 1988), and incorporates elements of the Transtheoretical Model of Prochaska and DiClemente (Prochaska & DiClemente, 1986) and Motivational Interviewing (Miller & Rolnick, 1991).

In the Patient-Centered Patient Education Model (see Figure 4.5), Grueninger and colleagues (Grueninger et al., 1995; Grueninger, Goldstein, & Duffy, 1989) defined five domains of assessment and intervention:

1. cognitive (knowledge and awareness about the problem, the targeted behavior, and benefits of change);
2. attitudinal (beliefs, intentions, readiness to change);
3. instrumental (instrumental skills needed to effect change, such as using an inhaler, performing blood glucose monitoring);
4. behavioral (coping skills needed to maintain change); and
5. social (social support and use of resources).

Assessment at each level involves gathering information about barriers and resources that may hinder or help change. Intervention involves correcting misunderstandings, providing information, solving problems, teaching skills, acknowledging feelings and beliefs, and offering support to overcome barriers and utilize resources. The process is continually interactive, involving dialogue and negotiation with the patient. By actively engaging the patient in the process of setting goals and making decisions regarding treatments, the provider encourages the patient's ownership of the problem and facilitates the patient's commitment to the care plan.

The Five A's: A Basic Approach to Behavioral Counseling

The National Cancer Institute and, more recently, the Agency for Health Care Policy and Research promote a brief, physician counseling strategy for smoking cessation known as the "Four A's": Ask (about smoking at every

Levels of Patient Education	**Doctor–Patient Interaction** (Assessment and Intervention)
1. Cognitive Level Information	Assess awareness, knowledge, concepts Explain facts, clarify, provide information
2. Attitudinal Level Beliefs Intentions Stage of change	Assess attitudes, beliefs, stage of change, to change Acknowledge feelings, build commitment
3. Instrumental Level Instrumental skills	Assess instrumental skills Instruct and practice necessary skills
4. Behavioral Level Coping behavior Coping skills	Assess behavioral cues, consequences and conditions; assess coping skills Find incentives, reinforcements and rewards; teach behavioral skills
4. Social Level Social support	Assess social support, resources Mobilize support, resources

Figure 4.5 Patient-centered education model.

From "Behavioral Medicine Strategies for Medical Patients," [p. 675], by M.G. Goldstein, L. Ruggicio, B.J. Guise, and D.B. Abrams; in A. Stoudemirc (Ed.), *Clinical Psychiatry for Medical Students* (2nd ed., pp. 671–693) 1993, Philadelphia: J.B. Lippincott. Copyright 1994, 1990 by J.B. Lippincott Company.

TABLE 4.2 A Patient-Centered Approach to Behavior Change Intervention: The Five A's

ADDRESS THE AGENDA
Attend to patient's agenda
Express desire to talk about target behavior
ASSESS
Assess knowledge, beliefs, concerns, feelings
Assess previous experience with change
Assess stage of change
ADVISE
Provide personalized information and advice
ASSIST
Provide support
Negotiate an intervention plan
Identify personal barriers and resources
ARRANGE FOLLOW-UP

Note. Adapted from (Glynn & Manley, 1989; Goldstein et al., 1994; Grueninger et al., 1995; Grueninger et al., 1989; Levenkron & Greenland, 1987; Ockene, 1987b).

opportunity), *A*dvise (all smokers to stop), *A*ssist (the patient in stopping), *A*rrange follow-up visits (Fiore et al., 1996; Glynn & Manley, 1989). This strategy was further adapted to conform to the Patient-Centered Patient Education Model by Goldstein and colleagues (Goldstein, DePue, & Niaura, 1993; Goldstein et al., 1994; Prochaska & Goldstein, 1991) to include five A's: *A*ddress the Agenda, *A*ssess, *A*dvise, *A*ssist, and *A*rrange follow-up (see Tables 4.2 and 4.3). Although originally developed as a strategy for brief smoking cessation counseling, the five A's can be applied to any generic patient education or counseling task.

At the beginning of a session, the provider first insures that the patient's agenda has been addressed, including the presenting problems for the visit and any other concerns the patient has raised. In addition, the provider brings up any issues which may relate to the patient's current medical problems or to preventive care needs (e.g., "I'd like to talk to you about . . ."). Next the provider assesses the patient's knowledge, beliefs, concerns, feelings,

TABLE 4.3 A Patient-Centered Approach to Behavior Change Intervention: The Five A's (Expanded)

Address the Agenda

  Attend to patient's agenda

  Express desire to talk about target behavior

    "I'd like to talk to you about ———"

  Define problem

    "You have ———"

    "This means ———"

Assess

  Assess and clarify patient's knowledge, beliefs, and concerns

    "What do you know about ———?"

  Assess and clarify patients's feelings about risk and change in behavior

    "How do you feel about ———?"

  Assess previous experience with change

    "What have you tried in the past?"

  Assess stage of change and clarify patient's goals

    "Are you willing to ——— (e.g. stop smoking, change your diet) now?"

    "Are you considering changing ——— in the next few weeks?"

  Assess pros and cons for change

    "What reasons do you have for wanting (and not wanting) to change?"

Advise

  Provide personalized information regarding risk and benefits of change

  Provide physiologic feedback when available

    "Your test results (physical findings, etc.) indicate that ——— is affecting your health."

  Tell patient that you strongly advise change

Assist

  Provide support, understanding, praise, and reinforcement

    "I can help you by ———"

    "It's often difficult to change ———"

    "It's great that you're considering ———"

  Describe intervention options

  Negotiate an intervention plan; match intervention to stage of change

  For Precontemplators and Contemplators:

TABLE 4.3 *(continued)*

Review patient's pros and cons for change; reinforce pros
Express willingness to help patient address cons
Provide more information, feedback
Address feelings
Encourage to consider change
For patients in Preparation and Action stages:
Negotiate selection among options
Solve problems with implementation
"What problems might arise with ——"
Provide resources (e.g., written materials)
Identify additional resources
"What (or who) might help you with ——"
Teach skills/recommend specific strategies
Consider a written contract/prescription
Refer, when appropriate
Arrange Follow-Up
Reaffirm plan
"Now, what are you going to do?"
Arrange follow-up appointment or call
"I'd like to see you again on ——"

Note. Adapted from (Glynn & Manley, 1989; Goldstein et al., 1994; Grueninger et al., 1995; Grueninger et al., 1989; Levenkron & Greenland, 1987; Ockene, 1987b).

and readiness to change (e.g., "What do you know about . . .?" "What do you feel about . . .?" "Are you considering changing . . . in the next few weeks?"). If the provider determines that the patient is not in the preparation or contemplation stage, he/she should try to help the patient develop awareness of the need for change and commitment. The "advice" step is gauged accordingly ("I understand you are not ready to move on this right now, but I strongly encourage you to think about it"). Providing personalized feedback about test results or other physiologic effects of the patient's lifestyle is also helpful to bolster the advice. The assist step for patients who are not ready for action involves helping the patient review their pros and cons for change, discuss feelings about past efforts to change, correct any misunderstandings, and/or provide additional information. Motivational interventions based on Motivational Interviewing (Miller & Rolnick, 1991) could be incorporated here. For the patient who is ready to change, the advice step would encourage a specific commitment ("It's great that you are ready to work on this. I would like you to make a plan that you will begin"). The assist step, for an individual ready for action, would include negotiating among options, solving anticipated problems, recommending specific strategies, identifying additional sources of support, and making referrals (see Table 4.3 for more detail). Finally, arranging follow-up reinforces the concern being expressed by the provider and encourages the patient to follow through on their commitment, whether it is to think about change or to proceed with an action plan. The follow-up could be accomplished through an appointment or a phone call ("I'd like to talk to you again about this on . . .").

This five-A strategy can be incorporated into a medical visit in as little as 3 minutes. For the motivated provider who is willing to spend more time on patient education and counseling, the five-A strategy can be utilized to provide a more substantial counseling intervention.

As noted previously, both the Systems Model and the Patient Path Model identify organizational and practice level factors which will affect the delivery and success of any office-based intervention that targets patient behavior change. Therefore, the five-A counseling approach must be considered within the context of multiple other opportunities within the practice setting for enhancing patient adherence to treatment and patient behavioral change. Several office-level interventions may enhance the effectiveness of the 5 A approach. For example, the use of patient risk factor assessment tools may help to streamline the assessment process. Use of printed informational and self-help booklets also may help the provider to deliver a tailored message. Patients who have experienced repeated problems with adherence or failures during previous change efforts, who have high levels of physical or psychological dependence on risk behavior, or who have poor social support may require more intensive interventions. In these circumstances, use of health educators or clinicians with specific training in patient education and counseling or referrals to other professionals who specialize in treatment of the targeted behavior may be helpful.

While lack of counseling skills is a barrier to providers' engaging in counseling about behavior change, there is evidence that such skills as these can be taught to physicians in residency programs and to physicians in practice (J. K. Ockene et al., 1995; J. K. Ockene et al., 1988; Strecher et al., 1991). Further, there is evidence that even minimal physician-delivered interventions are effective in improving rates of smoking cessation (Fiore et al., 1996; Willey et al., 1996).

REFERENCES

Balint, M., Hunt, J., Joyce, D., Marinker, M., & Woodcock, J. (1970). *Treatment or diagnosis: A study of repeat prescriptions in general practice.* Philadelphia: Lippincott.

Bandura, A. (1977). Self-efficacy: Toward a unifying theory of behavior change. *Psychological Review, 84*, 191–215.

Becker, M., Haefner, D., & Kasl, S. (1977). Selected psychosocial models and correlates of individual health-related beliefs. *Medical Care, 15*(5 Suppl), 27–46.

Campbell, M., DeVellis, B., Strecher, V., Ammerman, A., DeVellis, R., & Sandler, R. (1994). Improving dietary behavior: The effectiveness of tailored messages in primary care practice. *American Journal of Public Health, 84*, 783–787.

Cohen, S., Halvorson, H., & Gosselink, C. (1994). Changing physician behavior to improve disease prevention. *Preventive Medicine, 23*, 284–291.

Cohen-Cole, S. (1991). *The medical interview: The three function approach*. St. Louis: Mosby/Yearbook.

Dietrich, A. J., O'Connor, G. T., Keller, A., Carney, P. A., Levy, D., & Whaley, F. S. (1992). Cancer: improving early detection and prevention. A community practice randomised trial [see comments]. *BMJ, 304*(6828), 687–91.

Engel, G. (1977). The need for a new medical model: A challenge for biomedicine. *Science, 196*, 129–136.

Fiore, M., Bailey, W., Cohen, S., Dorfman, S., Goldstein, M., Gritz, E., Heyman, R., Hollbrook, J., Jaen, C., Kottke, T., Lando, H., Mecklenbrg, R., Mullen, P., Nett, L., Robinson, L., Stitzer, M., Tommasello, A., Villejo, L., & Wewers, M. (1996). *Smoking cessation: Clinical Practice Guideline No. 18* (AHCPR Publication No. 96-0692). Bethesda, MD: Agency for Health Care Policy and Research.

Fiore, M. C., Jorenby, D. E., Schensky, A. E., Smith, S. S., Bauer, R. R., & Baker, T. B. (1995). Smoking status as the new vital sign: Effect on assessment and intervention in patients who smoke [see comments]. *Mayo Clinic Procedures, 70*, 209–213.

Fortmann, S., Sallis, J., Magnus, P., & Farquhar, J. (1995). Attitudes and practices of physicians regarding hypertension and smoking: The Stanford Five City Project. *Preventive Medicine, 14*, 70–80.

Frank, E., & Kunovich-Frieze, T. (1995). Physicians' prevention counseling behaviors: Current status and future directions. *Preventive Medicine, 24*, 543–545.

Glynn, T. J., & Manley, M. W. (1989). *How to help your patients stop smoking: A National Cancer Institute manual for physicians* (Vol. NIH Publication 89-3064). Bethesda, MD: National Cancer Institute.

Goldstein, M., DePue, J., Eaton, R., Dube, C., Rakowski, W., & Willey-Lessne, C. (1993, March). *A population- based survey of physicians' smoking counseling behavior*. Paper presented at the Annual Meeting of the Society of Behavioral Medicine, San Francisco, CA.

Goldstein, M. G., DePue, J., & Niaura, R. (1993). The role of primary care physicians in smoking cessation. *Rhode Island Medicine, 76*, 515–22.

Goldstein, M. G., MacDonald, N. A., Niaura, R. S., & Dube, C. (1993). Dissemination of physician-based smoking cessation interventions. In S. Burns,

S. Cohen, E. Gritz, & T. Kottke (Eds.), *Tobacco and the clinician; Interventions for medical and dental practice* (pp. 342–355). Bethesda, MD: National Center Institute.

Goldstein, M. G., Ruggiero, L., Guise, B. J., & Abrams, D. B. (1994). Behavioral medicine strategies for medical patients. In A. Stoudemire (Ed.), *Clinical psychiatry for medical students* (2nd ed., pp. 671–693). Philadelphia: Lippincott.

Green, L. (1984). Health education models. In J. Matarazzo, S. Weiss, J. Herd, N. Miller, & S. Weiss (Eds.), *Behavioral health: A handbook for health enhancement* (pp. 181–198). New York: Wiley.

Green, L., Eriksen, M., & Schor, E. (1988). Preventive practices by physicians: Behavioral determinants and potential interventions. *American Journal of Preventive Medicine, 4*(4(Suppl), 101–107.

Grueninger, U., Duffy, F., & Goldstein, M. (1995). Patient education in the medical encounter: How to facilitate learning, behavior change and coping. In M. J. Lipkin, S. Putnam, & A. Lazare (Eds.), *The medical interview: Clinical care, education, research* (pp. 122–133). New York: Springer Verlag.

Grueninger, U. J., Goldstein, M. G., & Duffy, F. D. (1989). Patient education in hypertension: Five essential steps. *Journal of Hypertension, 7*, S93–S98.

Inui, T., & Carter, W. (1995). A guide to the research literature on doctor/patient communication. In M. J. Lipkin, S. Putnam, & A. Lazare (Eds.), *The medical interview: Clinical care, education, research* (pp. 482–488). New York: Springer Verlag.

Kottke, T. E., Battista, R. N., DeFriese, G. H., & Brekke, M. L. (1988). Attributes of successful smoking cessation interventions in medical practice: A meta-analysis of 39 controlled trials. *JAMA, 259*(19), 2883–9.

Kottke, T., Brekke, M., & Solberg, L. (1993). Making "time" for preventive services. *Mayo Clinic Procedures, 688*, 785–791.

Lazare, A., Putnam, S., & Lipkin, M. J. (1995). Three functions of the medical interview. In M. J. Lipkin, S. Putnam, & A. Lazare (Eds.), *The medical interview: Clinical care, education, research* (pp. 3–19). New York: Springer Verlag.

Leopold, N., Cooper, J., & Clancy, C. (1996). Sustained partnership in primary care. *Journal of Family Practice, 42*, 129–137.

Lerman, C., Rimer, B., Trock, B., Balshem, A., & Engstrom, P. F. (1990). Factors associated with repeat adherence to breast cancer screening. *Preventive Medicine, 19*, 1–12.

Levenkron, J. C., & Greenland, P. (1987). Validation of the University of Rochester Risk Factor Interview Scale. *American Journal of Preventive Medicine, 3*, 153–156.

Levenstein, J. (1984). The patient-centered general practice consultation. *South Africa Family Practice, 5*, 276–282.

Levenstein, J. H., McCracken, E. C., McWhinney, I. R., Stewart, M. A., & Brown, J. B. (1986). The patient-centered clinical method: I. A model for the doctor-patient interaction in family medicine. *Family Practice, 3*, 24–30.

Lewis, C. E., Clancy, C., Leake, B., & Schwartz, J. S. (1991). The counseling practices of internists. *Annals of Internal Medicine, 114*(1), 54–58.

Lipkin, M. J., Putnam, S., & Lazare, A. (Eds.). (1995). *The medical interview: Clinical care, education, research*. New York: Springer Verlag.

Lurie, N., Slater, J., McGovern, P., Ekstrum, J., Quam, L., & Margolis, K. (1993). Preventive care for women: Does the sex of the physician matter? *New England Journal of Medicine, 329*, 478–482.

Main, D., Cohen, S., & DiClemente, C. (1995). Measuring physician readiness to change cancer screening: Preliminary results. *American Journal of Preventive Medicine, 11*, 54–58.

Manley, M., Epps, R. P., Husten, C., Glynn, T., & Shopland, D. (1991). Clinical interventions in tobacco control: A National Cancer Institute training program for physicians. *JAMA, 266*, 3172–3173.

Mayer, W., & Beardall, R. (1995). Translating science into practice: Cancer prevention in primary care medicine. In P. Greenwald, B. S. Kramer, & D. Weed (Eds.), *Cancer prevention and control* (pp. 411–433). New York: Dekker.

McPhee, S. J., Bird, J. A., Fordham, D., Rodnick, J. E., & Osborn, E. H. (1991). Promoting cancer prevention activities by primary care physicians. Results of a randomized, controlled trial. *JAMA, 266*, 538–544.

McPhee, S. J., & Detmer, W. M. (1993). Office-based interventions to improve delivery of cancer prevention services by primary care physicians. *Cancer, 72*(3 Suppl), 1100–1112.

Miller, W. R., & Rolnick, S. (1991). *Motivational interviewing: Preparing people to change addictive behavior*. New York: Guilford.

Mullen, P., & Green, L. (1990). Educating and counseling for prevention: From theory and research to principles. In R. Goldbloom & L. RS (Eds.), *Preventing disease: Beyond the rhetoric* (pp. 474–479). New York: Springer Verlag.

National Cancer Institute Breast Cancer Screening Consortium. (1990). Screening mammograpy: A missed clinical opportunity? Results of the NCI Brease Cancer Screening Consortium and National Health Interview Survey Studies. *JAMA, 264*, 54–58.

National Center for Health Statistics. (1990). Health, United States, 1989 ((PHS90-1232): Washington, DC: U. S. Department of Health and Human Services.

Nutting, P. (1986). Health promotion in primary medical care: Problems and potential. *Preventive Medicine, 15*, 537–548.

Ockene, I. S, Hebert, J. R, Ockene, J. K, Merriam, P. A, Hurley, T. G., & Saperia, G. M. (1996). Effect of training and a structured office practice on physician-delivered nutrition counseling: The Worcester-Area Trial for Counseling in Hyperlipidemia (WATCH). *American Journal of Preventive Medicine, 12*, 252–258.

Ockene, J. K. (1987a). Physician-delivered interventions for smoking cessation: strategies for increasing effectiveness. *Preventive Medicine, 16*, 723–737.

Ockene, J. K. (1987b). Smoking intervention: the expanding role of the physician [editorial]. *American Journal of Public Health, 77*, 782–783.

Ockene, J. K, Ockene, I., Quirk, M., Hebert, J., Saperia, G., Luppold, R., PA, M., & Ellis, S. (1995). Physician training for patient-centered nutrition counseling in a lipid intervention trial. *Preventive Medicine, 24*, 563–570.

Ockene, J. K., Quirk, M. E., Goldberg, R. J., Kristeller, J. L., Donnelly, G., Kalan, K. L., Gould, B., Greene, H. L., Harrison, A. R., Pease, J., & et al. (1988). A residents' training program for the development of smoking intervention skills . *Archives of Internal Medicine, 148*, 1039–1045.

Orlandi, M. A. (1987). Promoting health and preventing disease in health care settings: An analysis of barriers. *Preventive Medicine, 16*, 119–130.

Orleans, C. T., George, L. K., Houpt, J. L., & Brodie, K. H. (1985). Health promotion in primary care. A survey of U.S. family practitioners. *Preventive Medicine, 14*, 636–647.

Osborn, E. H., Bird, J. A., McPhee, S. J., Rodnick, J. E., & Fordham, D. (1991). Cancer screening by primary care physicians: Can we explain the differences? [see comments]. *Journal of Family Practice, 32*, 465–471.

Pommerenke, F. A., & Dietrich, A. (1992b). Improving and maintaining preventive services, Part 2: Practical principles for primary care. *Journal of Family Practice, 34*, 92–97.

Pommerenke, F. A., & Dietrich, A. (1992a). Improving and maintaining preventive services. Part 1: Applying the patient path model. *Journal of Family Practice, 34*, 86–91.

Prochaska, J. O., & DiClemente, C. C. (1986). Towards a comprehensive model of change. In W. R. Miller & N. Heather (Eds.), *Treating addictive disorders: Processes of change* (pp. 3–27). New York: Plenum.

Prochaska, J. O., & DiClemente, C. C. (1992). Stages of change in the modification of problem behaviors. *Progress In Behavior Modification, 28*(183), 183–218.

Prochaska, J. O., DiClemente, C. C., & Norcross, J. C. (1992). In search of how people change. Applications to addictive behaviors. *American Psychologist, 47*, 1102–1114.

Prochaska, J. O., & Goldstein, M. G. (1991). Process of smoking cessation: Implications for clinicians. *Clinics In Chest Medicine, 12*, 727–735.

Rippetoe, P., & Rogers, R. (1987). Effects of components of protection-motivation theory on adaptive and maladaptive coping with a health threat. *Journal of Personality and Social Psychology, 52*, 596–604.

Rogers, C. (1951). *Client-oriented therapy: Its current practical implications and theory*. Cambridge, MA: Riverside.

Rogers, C. (1959). A theory of therapy, personality, and interpersonal relationships as developed in the client-centered framework. In E. Koch (Ed.), *Psychology, the study of a science: Formulations of the person and the social context* (Vol. 3, pp. 184–256). New York: McGraw-Hill.

Rollnick, S., Heather, N., & Bell, A. (1992). Negotiating behaviour change in medical settings: The development of brief motivational interviewing. *Journal of Mental Health, 1*, 25–37.

Roter, D., & Hall, J. (1992). *Doctors talking with patients/Patients talking with doctors: Improving communication in medical visits*. Westport, CT: Auburn.

Schwartz, J. L. (1992). Methods of smoking cessation. *Medical Clinics of North America, 76*, 451–476.

Soumerai, S. B., & Avorn, J. (1990). Principles of educational outreach ("academic detailing") to improve clinical decision making. *Journal of the American Medical Association, 263*, 549–556.

Stewart, M., Brown, J., Weston, W., McWhinney, I., McWilliam, C., & Freeman, T. (1995). *Patient-centered medicine: Transforming the clinical method*. Thousand Oaks, CA: Sage.

Strecher, V. J., O'Malley, M. S., Villagra, V. G., Campbell, E. E., Gonzalez, J. J.,

Irons, T. G., Kenney, R. D., Turner, R. C., Rogers, C. S., Lyles, M. F. (1991). Can residents be trained to counsel patients about quitting smoking? Results from a randomized trial. *Journal of General Internal Medicine, 6*, 9–17.

Waitzkin, H. (1984). Doctor-patient communication. *Journal of the American Medical Association, 252*, 2441–2446.

Walsh, J. M. (1992). Cancer screening in older adults [see comments]. *Western Journal of Medicine, 156*, 495–500.

Walsh, J. M., & McPhee, S. J. (1992). A systems model of clinical preventive care: An analysis of factors influencing patient and physician. *Health Education Quarterly, 19*, 157–175.

Wells, K. B., Lewis, C. E., Leake, B., Schleiter, M. K., & Brook, R. H. (1986). The practices of general and subspecialty internists in counseling about smoking and exercise. *American Journal of Public Health, 76*, 1009–1013.

Willey, C., Goldstein, M., Niaura, R., DePue, J., Velicer, W., & Prochaska, J. (1996 March). *Smoking cessation outcomes of a physician counseling and home-based expert system intervention.* Paper presented at the Annual Meeting of the Society of Behavioral Medicine, Washington, DC.

Wissow, L. S., Roter, D. L., & Wilson, M. E. (1994). Pediatrician interview style and mothers' disclosure of psychosocial issues. *Pediatrics, 93*, 289–295.

5

Measuring Adherence With Medication Regimens in Clinical Care and Research

Cynthia S. Rand and Kathleen Weeks

When patients' therapies don't work, clinicians often adjust dosages, order more diagnostic tests or switch to different, sometimes more risky treatments. When a clinical trial does not find a significant treatment effect for a promising investigative drug, that therapy may be judged inefficacious and abandoned as a possible treatment option. All too often, however, the cause of the ineffective therapy lies not with the drug or treatment, but rather with patient or provider behavior. Clinicians and researchers who do not measure patient adherence appropriately are at risk of misjudging the causes of treatment ineffectiveness.

Patient adherence is the necessary interface between efficacious therapies and treatment effectiveness. Studies which have measured patient adherence with medication regimens have repeatedly documented the magnitude of medication nonadherence across all diseases and therapies. Estimates are

Correspondence to:
Cynthia S. Rand, Ph.D.
The Johns Hopkins Asthma & Allergy Center
Division of Pulmonary & Critical Care Medicine
5501 Hopkins Bayview Circle
Baltimore, Maryland 21224

that 50–65% of all outpatients do not adhere appropriately to their medication regimens (Berg, Dischler, Wagner, Raia, & Palmer-Shevlin, 1993; Melnikow & Kiefe, 1994; Schaub, Steiner, & Vetter, 1993). Patient adherence with a physician's behavioral recommendations such as weight loss, exercise, and smoking cessation is even poorer (Brownell, Marlatt, Lichtenstein, & Wilson, 1986).

Nonadherence to prescribed treatment has implications for clinicians in several critical areas. Most obviously, a patient who does not adhere to a short- or long-term medical regimen may not get the complete therapeutic benefits. A physician can often be misled by patient nonadherence to conclude that the prescribed treatment is inadequate or inappropriate. This, in turn, can lead to costly diagnostic procedures, or even dangerous intensification of therapy, when the patient would have been served best by accurately following the originally prescribed regimen.

Another serious consequence of patient nonadherence is the compromise of clinical drug trials. A new treatment can easily be judged ineffective if subjects do not adhere adequately to the treatment protocol. So critical is the issue of adherence to the evaluation of drug efficacy that some researchers have suggested that clinical studies are of only limited value without the inclusion of valid measures of adherence (Besch, 1995; Melnikow & Kiefe, 1994).

DEFINING AND CLASSIFYING ADHERENCE

"Adherence" or "compliance" may be broadly defined as the degree to which patient behaviors coincide with the clinical recommendations of health care providers. Despite the fact that clinicians and researchers alike categorize patients as being either compliant or noncompliant, such adherence is not inherently a dichotomous variable. There is no gold standard for what defines "satisfactory' versus "poor" adherence across all health behaviors. Factors such as the dosage necessary for therapeutic effectiveness, the risks of nonadherence, and the clinical or research goals will all influence the criteria for good adherence. Appropriate adherence must be situationally defined, with parameters of good adherence explicitly delineated and appropriate to the medication regimen or health behavior under study. How one chooses to define good adherence is integrally related to the way in which adherence will best be measured. A broadly defined, flexible criterion of acceptable adherence may not need precise measurement methodology. In contrast, when detailed and exact adherence data are necessary, the measurement instruments should be comparably precise. Assessment of adherence in a clinical trial, for example, must be as rigorous as possible in order to ensure the fundamental integrity of the study's conclusions.

In both clinical care and research settings, measuring and classifying patients' patterns of medication uses is as necessary as assessing overall adherence level. Understanding patterns of medication use is important in the evaluation of treatment response and efficacy and in developing strategies to enhance adherence. The expected patient behavior is "appropriate adherence"—that is, using medications exactly as prescribed and consistently over time. The most obvious form of noncompliance is chronic "under use"—where a patient regularly uses less medication than is prescribed. Although underuse is most often considered a risk for poor disease control, for some patients, underuse may be an effective self-management or self-titration strategy when treatment has been overprescribed (Steiner, Fihn, Blair, & Inui, 1991). Patients also may have "erratic adherence," in which medication use alternates between adherent use (usually when symptomatic) and underuse or total nonuse (when asymptomatic). Patients with erratic adherence may present for treatment during symptom exacerbations with apparent complete adherence to their prescribed regimen. Erratic adherence may also reflect forgetfulness, stress, changed schedules, running out of medication, or other barriers to full adherence. The term "drug holiday" is sometimes used to describe multi-day lapses in medication use. Finally, some patients using pain or symptom-relieving drugs, such as inhaled beta-agonists, on an as-needed basis (i.e., PRN) , may be prone to "over-use" during exacerbations. This may cause a patient to delay seeking care or lead to complications associated with excessive medication use (Sears & Rea, 1987; Spitzer et al., 1992).

METHODS FOR MEASURING ADHERENCE

Several investigators have published excellent reviews of adherence measurement research, and the reader is referred to them for greater detail (Berg et al., 1993; Besch, 1995; Dunbar, 1980; Gordis, 1976; Masur, 1981; Melnikow & Kiefe, 1994). As these reviewers have noted, all of the most commonly used methods for assessing adherence have both strengths and weaknesses that must be considered in their use. Adherence measures can be divided into "indirect methods" (presumed used) and "direct methods" (confirmed use).

Indirect Measures

Clinician Judgment

In everyday clinical care, health care providers form thumbnail impressions of how well each of their patients is following their prescribed regimens. These judgments necessarily shape the patient-provider interaction, the selected therapy, and the follow-up plan. Several classic studies have shown, however, that physicians generally greatly overestimate the degree to which their patients comply with their directives (Davis, 1966; Kasl, 1975; Paulson, Krause, & Iber, 1977). A study by Mushlin and Appel (1977) found that when medical interns and residents attempted to make assessments of an individual patient's medication adherence, they were accurate only 25% of the time.

Physicians not only overestimate patient adherence, they are also poor predictors of which specific patients will be good or poor adherers. Steele, Jackson, and Gutmann (1990) used qualitative, sociolinguistic methodology to evaluate how primary care physicians assess patient adherence with antihypertensive therapies. They found that these physicians identified only 53% of the adherence problems in the 38 critical case encounters. Physicians who used indirect approaches to assessment (e.g., "Have you noticed any changes since you started taking your medicine?") were the least successful in identifying adherence problems (0/9 correct); simple, direct questioning (e.g., "You've been taking your medications?") was moderately successful (8/13 correct); and information-intensive strategies (open-ended queries about patterns of medication use) was the most successful approach (8/10 correct). The investigators conclude that a "nonaccusatory, open-ended, information-intensive approach can be a sensitive and productive tool for the diagnosis of patient's adherence status" (Steele et al., 1990, pp. 299). The lack of physician skill in identifying patients with adherence difficulties has been attributed to a medical education focus that neglects communication skills and attention to psychosocial issues. A study by Steiner and colleagues (1991), however, found that even nurse-practitioners (a profession that emphasizes patient education and communication) were poor judges of patient adherence. Nurse-practitioners in a V.A. clinic treating hypertensive patients correctly identified only 23.1% of the poorly adherent patients and misclassified 22.5% of the more adherent patients as partial compliers. Clinical judgments based on preconceived beliefs about the attributes of the "typical" compliant patient are destined to fail. Patient characteristics such as race, education, gender, SES, and personality have not been found to be reliable predictors of adherence. Physician interviewing skills and the qualities of the patient-provider interaction will be more important in both measuring and facilitating adherence than will stereotypical beliefs about adherence (Dimatteo et al., 1993; Dunbar-Jacob, 1993; Heszen-Klemens & Lapinska, 1984; Holloway, Rogers, & Gershenhorn, 1992; Sackett & Haynes, 1976).

Self-Report

Self-report of medication use is a common measure of adherence in both clinical trials and behavioral intervention studies. Patient self-reports may be collected by interview (De Geest et al., 1995), diaries (Rodewald & Pichichero, 1993) and questionnaires (Moriskey, Green, & Levine, 1986). No cross-disease, validated adherence-specific questionnaire is currently in common use, in part because most self-report questionnaires of adherence have been designed for specific diseases and studies, or because they are often embedded in more general disease self-management measures (Dolce et al., 1991; Rand & Wise, 1994). Self-report is an inexpensive, simple, measurement strategy that is applicable to different regimens, is generally brief, and has face validity. In addition, self-report (particularly in the clinical setting) is the best measure for collecting information about patient beliefs, attitudes, and experiences with medication regimens. For example, the patient who misunderstands a dosing regimen, or who has altered her regimen because of fear of side effects, will not be identified by objective adherence assessments (Britten, 1994; Donovan & Blake, 1992). Personal, financial, social, or physical barriers to adherence can only be revealed by thoughtful measurement of patient self-reports. Morgan interviewed patients using anti-hypertensive medications in inner London and found that traditional cultural beliefs among Afro-Caribbeans about the long-term harmful effects of these medications leads to reduced adherence with prescribed therapies and increased use of herbal remedies (Morgan, 1995). Pachter and Weller (1993) found that lower levels of acculturation among Puerto Rican asthmatics was associated with poorer medication adherence.

As a quantitative measure of medication use, self-report has been found to have a highly variable degree of accuracy (Coutts, Gibson, & Paton, 1992; Gonder-Frederick, Julian, Cox, Clark, & Carter, 1988; Mason, Matsuyama, & Jue, 1995; Sheiner, Rosenberg, Marathe, & Peck, 1974; Waterhouse, Calzone, Mele, & Brenner, 1993). A study by Spector and colleagues (1986) compared asthmatic patients' self-reports of inhaler usage with the objective adherence data collected by a medication monitoring device called a Nebulizer Chronolog (discussed below). They found that while all subjects self-reported using the inhaler on more than half of the study days, the measured medication usage indicated that only 52.6% of the subjects actually did so. Coutts and colleagues (1992) and Gibson and colleagues (Gibson, Ferguson, Aitchison, Paton, 1995) have used the Nebulizer Chronolog to examine metered dose inhaler compliance with anti-inflammatory therapies in children. Like Spector and colleagues, they found that patient self-reports of adherence recorded in asthma diaries significantly overestimated adherence.

Similar findings have been reported on the accuracy of patient self-reports for anti-hypertensive medications (Rudd et al., 1989), anti-epileptics (Cramer, Mattson, Prevey, Scheyer, & Oullette, 1989), and arthritis medications (Kraag, Gordon, Menard, Russell, & Kalish, 1994). Self-reports of adherence will be influenced by the demand characteristics on the setting in which the information is collected. The desire to please the physician or investigator can lead patients to exaggerate reports of medication use. Patients with memory impairment (related to illness, age, concurrent medications or stress) may not be able to accurately self-report their usage pattern of any one medication. Patients on long-term medication regimens may be able to correctly recall recent usage patterns, but may fail to report their adherence patterns 4 months prior to their physician visit. Physicians' and investigators' sensitivity and skill in eliciting patients' self-reports will certainly influence the reliability and usefulness of the information they receive.

While self-report may not be a sufficient measure of adherence in many settings (particularly in research), it is probably a necessary measure in all settings. For, when carefully collected, this information can provide invaluable insight into the nature of patients' problems with adherence. Additionally, because there is no evidence to suggest that adhering patients will misrepresent themselves as nonadherers (Gordis, 1976), this measurement technique will allow the simple identification of many candid nonadherers.

Medication Measurement

Medication measurement has frequently been used as a relatively simple, yet objective measure of adherence (Gordis, 1976; Hilbrands, Hoitsma, Koene, 1995; Koch, Giardina, Ryan, MacQueen, & Hilgartner, 1993). Counting pills, checking prescription refills, or weighing inhaler canisters or liquid medication are examples of measures which allow researchers to infer the degree of medication adherence. This method requires that the clinician or investigator know exactly how much medication the patient began the measurement period with and how much medication should have been used during this period.

Medication measurement has been used to provide objective data on the relationship between adherence with therapy and disease exacerbations. Hilbrands and colleagues (1995) used pill counts to evaluate adherence with immunosuppressive and antihypertensive drugs among adult patients who had received a renal transplant in the previous year. They found that overall adherence was generally good (87% to 64% of patients were fully adherent); however, there was considerable variability, both within patients for different drugs, and between patients. Patients who experienced a subsequent rejection episode had lower compliance with immunosuppressive drugs than did patients without a rejection episode, and compliance appeared to improve in these patients after the rejection month.

Du Bard, Goldenberg, Copper, and Hauth (1993) evaluated adherence with low-dose aspirin therapy for the prevention of pre-eclampsia. They compared pill-count estimations of adherence with a biochemical measure (serum thromboxane B_2) and found that women with a pill count greater than 100% had lower biochemical levels of the drug than did women with pill counts <95%, suggesting that pills may have been discarded. This phenomenon of medication "dumping" has been described by a number of investigators (Mawhinney et al., 1991; Rand et al., 1992; Urquhart, 1991) and appears to be a common occurrence when medication measurement is used in a clinical trial setting to confirm compliance.

In some settings, medication measurement can serve as both an adherence intervention tool and an outcome measure. Koch and colleagues (1993) contracted with 23 pediatric patients with thalassemia to improve adherence with desferrioxamine iron chelation therapy. Patients were asked to increase the number of days they used the subcutaneous pump delivery system, and the number of empty desferrioxamine vials served as a basis for reinforcement and adherence documentation. By the end of the 6-month program, patients' use of the pump had climbed from 4.5 to approximately 5.5 days per week. Koch and colleagues note that because of the need for parental supervision during therapy and the high cost of desferrioxamine, it was unlikely that patients would deceptively empty vials.

Medication measurement need not be confined to clinic visits. Cromer and colleagues (Cromer, Steinberg, Gardner, Thornton, & Shannon, 1989) studied adherence with therapy for iron deficiency among 71 adolescents using a home pill count (conducted by research staff), serum ferritin levels, and urinary assays for tracer riboflavin. Pill counts in this setting were found to be highly correlated with biochemical indices of compliance, suggesting that this measurement strategy is an accurate method for measuring adherence.

While these adherence data are both objective and reasonably simple to collect, they are limited by several factors. Medication measures can easily be influenced by a patient's efforts to deceive the investigator. As discussed, some patients may discard medication to appear adherent. Medications are often shared within households, particularly when family members are on the same medication (i.e., common antihypertensives), or for particular types of medications (i.e., tranquilizers, antibiotics, sleeping pills). Additionally, medication measures give no indication of the accuracy of dosages or the timing of medication (Christensen, 1978). However, in situations where patients are unthreatened by the consequences of reporting nonadherence, the pattern of medication use is not critical, and where the likelihood of medication-sharing is low, medication measurement is a useful, objective, and valid means of assessing adherence.

Automated Pharmacy Database-Review

As managed care has expanded and the technology for health care utilization data tracking and management has become more sophisticated, it has become increasingly feasible to monitor patients' medication adherence by examining pharmacy databases. Pharmacy databases can provide information on the exact regimen prescribed, the amount of medication dispensed, and the timing of refills. This data can be used to calculate roughly the average dose per day. In some health care data management systems, prescriptions written but never filled can also be monitored. Dispensing data also can be matched with medical record and health care utilization databases to provide integrated analyses of the antecedents and consequences of patient adherence behaviors.

Studies using this methodology have examined patient adherence across a wide range of regimens and diseases, including depression (Lin et al., 1995), glaucoma (Gurwitz et al., 1993), hypertension (Halpren, Irwin, Brown, Clouse, & Hatziandreu, 1993; Maronde et al., 1989; Steiner et al., 1991) hyperlipidemia (Schectman, Hiatt, & Hartz, 1994), and asthma (Kelloway, Wyatt, & Adlis, 1994). Review of automated pharmacy records also can allow large-scale population studies of patient adherence with medications. Spitzer and colleagues (1992) examined the potential relationship between beta-agonist use in pulmonary patients and the risk of death and near-death from asthma by examining computerized prescription-refill records of residents of Saskatchewan, Canada. Their study suggested that regular use or overuse of beta-agonist medications (based on refill patterns) was associated with an increased risk of death or near-death. Although this provocative study could not determine if this increased risk results directly from toxic properties of the pharmacological agent itself or indirectly from patient overreliance on the symptom-relieving properties of the drugs—resulting in delayed treatment—its publication sparked intense debate on the relationship between patient adherence patterns and asthma mortality.

Pharmacy data review can reveal refill-based adherence patterns for different classes of medication or dosing regimens. Kelloway and colleagues (1994) examined pharmacy claims data within a health maintenance organization and found that asthmatic patients were significantly more adherent to prescribed tablet medication (theophylline) than to two commonly prescribed inhaled anti-inflammatory medications (inhaled corticosteroid and inhaled cromolyn). Review of pharmacy and medical records can also determine the risks associated with nonadherence. Maronde and colleagues (1989) reviewed records of patients being treated for hypertension who had been admitted to an acute -care hospital in the previous 6 months with a diagnosis of hypertension, and found that poor compliance was associated with a higher risk of rehospitalization within a year. In contrast, Steiner and colleagues (1991) reviewed the automated pharmacy records of hypertensive patients enrolled in a medication step-down program in a VA hospital and found that patients with histories of partial compliance were more likely to be successful in reducing their anti-hypertensive medication regimens, suggesting that some patients may have been successfully self-regulating their medication dosages. They note that the review of centralized pharmacy records to identify partial compliers with normal blood pressure would allow reductions in unnecessarily high doses of medication.

Pharmacy database review to identify nonadherence has several limitations. First, adherence estimates can only be calculated for patients who exclusively rely on the target pharmacy system for all prescriptions and refills. Patients who use "out-of-network" pharmacies will have incomplete refill data. Second, pharmacy data can determine when a prescription was filled; however, it provides no confirmation of consumption or appropriate consumption patterns. Pharmacy database review cannot determine if medications sit unused, are hoarded for future use, are shared or given to family and friends, or are taken inappropriately. Nevertheless, as more pharmacy data go online, this adherence measuring strategy has great potential to "be applied comprehensively, inexpensively and unobtrusively to a large number of individuals" (Steiner et al., 1991).

Electronic Medication Monitors

In the past 10 years, the increased availability of computer-based technology has introduced a new strategy for adherence monitoring. Electronic monitoring devices record and store the date (and in the case of some devices, the time) of each medication use. Devices have been developed to monitor medication adherence behaviors including, but not restricted to, opening a pill bottle, releasing a blister-pak pill, discharging inhaled medications, and releasing eyedrops. Behaviors important to medical outcomes, such as home apnea monitoring for premature infants (Cordero, Morehead, & Miller, 1993), self-monitoring of blood glucose for patients with diabetes (Wysocki, Green, & Huxtable, 1989) and the use of removable appliance wear in orthodontic patients (Bartsch, Witt, Sahm, & Schneider, 1993), also have been targeted for electronic monitoring.

Two electronic devices that have been widely investigated are the Medication Event Monitoring System (MEMS—Aprex Corp., Fremont, CA) and the Nebulizer Chronolog (NC—Medtrac Technologies, Inc., Lakewood, CO). The MEMS can be used in conjunction with any regimen that includes the use of pills or tablets. A microprocessor in the MEMS cap electronically records each time the bottle is opened and stores the date, time, and duration of opening for subsequent downloading and retrieval via computer. The NC replaces the plastic mouthpiece on metered dose inhalers (MDIs) and records each depression of the MDIs as an actuation (or use). The NC unit stores the date and time for every actuation and can store up to 2000 events.

While neither the MEMS or the NC provides actual data on medication use, these devices do provide a unique opportunity to investigate long-term patterns of presumptive adherence which were heretofore unavailable in such detail. Waterhouse and colleagues (1993) used the MEMS to study the discrepancies between traditional measures of compliance and those of the MEMS. Participants in this study received oral tamoxifen and were masked to the monitoring ability of the MEMS. In the population studied, both self-report and pill counts suggested significantly higher adherence rates than the MEMS monitoring. Matsuyama, Mason, and Jue (1993) compared the MEMS data with pill counts to assisting pharmacists in making recommendations regarding diabetes therapy. The MEMS data resulted in different types of recommendations (pharmacological and/or educational) than did pill counts. This was significant because pharmacists could first make specific recommendations regarding patient education before resorting to pharmacologic manipulations. The MEMS also was also used by Brun (1994) to compare a once-daily and twice-daily dosing schedule of oral formulations of 5-isosorbide monitrate in patients with stable angina pectoris. Not surprisingly, adherence was better with the once-daily than with the twice-daily formulation.

Mason and colleagues (1995) used several measures of adherence in addition to the MEMS to determine which most closely assessed metabolic control in patients with non-insulin dependent diabetes mellitus. Assessment of medication adherence by provider, patient, and pill count did not explain metabolic control as closely or as accurately as assessment by the MEMS. Additionally, Cramer, Scheyer, and Mattson (1990) have used the MEMS to document that adherence to anti-epilepsy medications declines between follow-up visits.

Adherence studies conducted as a part of the Lung Health Study (Rand et al., 1992) using the Nebulizer Chronolog also have demonstrated the limitations of self-report and medication measurement seen with many of the studies using the MEMS. However, the NC was better able to capture a phenomenon called "dumping". In the Lung Health Study, participant self-report and canister weighing overestimated participant adherence by more than 30%. In addition, this study indicated that there were a subset of participants who appeared to discard medication deliberately before follow-up visits. The phenomenon of medication "dumping" is nearly impossible to detect by traditional methods of adherence assessment, and inclusion of dumping data into a dose-response analysis can yield counterintuitive results; highly adherent subjects show poorer response than moderately adherent subjects. This phenomenon is likely to be present in any situation in which medication use is being monitored, and should be taken into consideration when making medication recommendations.

In recent years the number of published studies using electronic adherence monitoring devices has increased dramatically. The primary benefit of this type of monitoring is clear: electronic monitoring methods can provide a continuous record of timing of presumptive doses over periods of months.

Assessments of adherence made by provider, self-report, pill counts, or canister weights can be inaccurate because of recall, demand characteristics, deception, and provider biases. These methods are also insensitive to daily patterns of use over time. Marker methods, usually the "gold standards" of adherence, reveal medication ingestion, but do not reveal the timing of doses.

While this trend towards high-tech computer-based monitoring devices continues, these systems are not without their limitations. The cost for wide-scale use can be prohibitive for a small practice and may only be feasible in a clinical trial setting. The up-front cost can be thousands of dollars for a MEMS or NC setup. Additionally, there is a failure rate associated with the use of any type of electronic device. The failure rate in electronic devices can be caused by patient misuse, device failure or computer hardware/software problems. In a study by Cramer, Vachon, Desforges, Sussman (1995), participants at eight out of ten sites did not use MEMS properly, thereby voiding their data for analyses. It also may be argued that the monitoring devices themselves, or the awareness that one is being monitored electronically, may alter adherence behavior.

Direct Measures

Biochemical Analysis

Clinical analysis of blood, urine, or other bodily excretions has frequently been used to objectively measure medication or byproduct levels (Berg et al., 1993; Gordis, 1976; Schaub et al., 1993). This is the only method of adherence measurement that confirms that medications have actually been taken by a patient, and for this reason biochemical analysis is one of the most valuable techniques available for assessing adherence. Unfortunately, this strategy is available for only a few drugs, and individual variations in absorption patterns may limit interpretation. Investigators can sometimes measure adherence with drugs that are not directly evaluable by biochemical assays by adding tracer substances that can be monitored. Riboflavin (Dubbert et al., 1985), digoxin (Maenpaa, Manninen, & Heinonen, 1992), phenobarbitone (Hatton et al., 1996), and deuterium oxide (Rodewald & Pichichero, 1993) have all been used as added biochemical adherence markers.

While biochemical analysis allows a very direct assessment of drug use, it also has some limitations. In order for the excretion pattern of the drug, tracer, or byproduct to be clearly understood, drug adherence is best assessed by repeated measures and analyses. This type of repeated assessment is probably clinically practical only when the monitoring is also necessary for determining appropriate therapeutic levels of medication (i.e. theophylline levels). Repeated measures solely for confirming adherence are usually impractical; particularly when biochemical analysis requires the use of an invasive procedure to collect a sample. Even when biochemical monitoring is feasible, not all medications can be easily detected or tagged with tracer substances. Biochemical analysis can provide a measure of adherence for a single test, or for multiple tests, but it cannot realistically be used to measure day-to-day adherence with long-term medication. And finally, even this technique can be compromised if a patient deliberately or inadvertently begins taking his or her medication just prior to the clinical analysis.

Directly Observed Therapy (DOT)

Other than biochemical analysis, observed therapy is the only other direct measure of patient adherence with therapy. Directly observed therapy (DOT) requires that patients be monitored for each dose or treatment to confirm adherence. DOT was pioneered in the treatment of tuberculosis because 1) poor patient adherence had been identified as the major barrier to effective treatment; 2) as a highly infectious disease, TB posed a major public health threat, and 3) those populations with the highest incidence of TB (I.V. drug abusers, recent immigrants, homeless people) were historically the most transient and difficult to retain in conventional therapy. DOT has been shown to be feasible and sustainable to significantly improve patient adherence with both treatment for active disease and prophylactic therapy. Schluger, Ciotoli, Cohen, Johnson, and Rom (1995) treated 113 patients in whom HIV infection, alcoholism, homelessness, and illicit drug use were common, using DOT, and achieved a 99% bacteriologic cure in the 102 patients retained in follow-up. Bayer and Dupuis (1995) have noted that DOT is a potentially coercive strategy, particularly when used for society's most indigent, disenfranchised members, and, as such, raises important issues of public health policy, medical ethics, and civil liberties.

ISSUES IN ADHERENCE MEASUREMENT

No one measure of adherence is appropriate for all settings. When considering the most appropriate strategy to apply the following issues should be considered:

Reactivity

When adherence behavior is monitored by methods that are known by both the clinician and the patient to be both accurate and revealing, there is a strong possibility that the patient's adherence behavior will meet the demand characteristics of the monitoring situation. In fact, studies suggest that there can be a direct relationship between the detail and precision of any measurement strategy and its impact on adherence (Nides et al., 1993). How troublesome this reactivity will be will depend upon the goals of the study or clinical interaction. When the focus of a study is on the ability to generalize the study's conclusions (i.e., will most patients use enough bronchodilator to achieve therapeutic goals?) then the use of a specialized, highly reactive measurement methodology would be inappropriate (Dunbar, 1980). If, however, the goal is improved adherence for either research purposes (i.e., is this bronchodilator efficacious?) or clinical purposes, then the use of reactive measurement techniques may be desirable. It is therefore important to clarify the goals of adherence assessment in each research or clinical application and then to select the most appropriate measurement strategies.

Measuring Children's Adherence

Assessing medication adherence in children presents unique challenges that require evaluating and considering both the family context in which medication use occurs and the level of communication between the healthcare provider and the family.

This communication starts with identifying the family member responsible for delivering medications to the child and who is the most reliable source of adherence information. Responsibility for medication administration generally shifts as a child grows, from total parent management for a young child, to shared medication management for the school-age child, to complete self-management for the adolescent. As parents transfer responsibility for medication management, they generally become less accurate reporters of the child's medication adherence. Studies which have examined the concordance between parent-child reports of other health variables, such as symptoms, have found relatively poor agreement (Britten, 1994; Spector et al., 1986).

There can be great diversity among families in how medication management is implemented. Daycare providers, grandparents, and siblings may assume responsibility for regular medication delivery in some households. Because of the highly variable and often shifting family responsibility for a child's medication use, it is necessary for the health care provider to review medication-use habits with the parent and the child in order to develop an adherence profile.

Multiple Measures

Because of the relative strengths and weaknesses of each of the adherence measures discussed, the optimal strategy for assessing adherence will usually involve the use of multiple measures. Patient contacts in both clinical and research settings should almost certainly include eliciting self-report information. Skillfully collected, these data not only will identify adherence difficulties and barriers, but also will provide the investigator with information about the circumstances of nonadherence. The correction of adherence difficulties may well depend upon the investigator understanding the "whys of nonadherence" and working with the patient toward a solution. The inclusion of one or more objective measures when assessing adherence will confirm patients' self-reports, but potential reactive effect of the measures should be weighed. Self-report and an unannounced biochemical analysis of a urine sample are unlikely to have any impact on patients' adherence behavior, while self-report and electronic medication monitoring and repeated drug-screening urinalysis probably will alter either the patient's adherence behavior, the self-report, or both.

The Use of Adherence Data

Clinicians interested in assessing patient adherence should clarify to themselves and then in turn, to their patients, why this information is being collected and how the information will be used. In a research context, where the value of a drug or therapeutic regimen is being evaluated, the purpose of adherence assessment may be well-defined for the investigator, but unclear to the participant. In clinical care, adherence assessment can easily be interpreted by patients as paternalistic intrusion; the doctor checking for who's been "naughty" or "nice". Unfortunately, for some clinicians, that is exactly the intent and tone of their adherence assessment, with patients categorized as "good" adherers or "bad" adherers. Such classifications fail to consider the barriers to patient adherence and the role of the provider in facilitating appropriate adherence (Dunbar-Jacob, 1993; Ross, 1991; Waitzkin, 1984). If the goal of adherence determination is to evaluate a treatment's efficacy, rather than to judge the patient's reliability or trustworthiness, then this goal should be both explicit and implicit in the patient-physician interaction.

FUTURE DIRECTIONS FOR ADHERENCE RESEARCH

The better a behavior can be observed, the more complete will be our understanding of that behavior. The recent explosion in microcomputer technology has opened up remarkable new opportunities to incorporate adherence monitoring technology into everyday patient care. Similar opportunities are possible with the increased access to sophisticated, integrated pharmacy and healthcare databases. The possibility now exists for both the clinicians and investigator to examine real-life adherence behavior and directly correlate this behavior with patient response to therapy. While automated healthcare databases and specialized electronic adherence monitors are hardly a panacea for patient adherence difficulties, incorporating their use in both clinical and research settings would not only improve measurement precision, but also would offer increased opportunities for adherence-promoting interventions.

Whether sophisticated new technology or a simple clinical interview is used to measure and promote adherence, the patient or subject should be recognized as an active partner in the patient-provider exchange. No technology, now or in the future, will replace the good listening and sincere concern of a first-rate therapeutic relationship.

REFERENCES

Bartsch, A., Witt, E., Sahm, G., & Schneider, S. (1993). Correlates of objective patient compliance with removable appliance wear. *American Journal of Orthodontics & Dentofacial Orthopedics, 104*, 378–386.

Bayer, R., & Dupuis, L. (1995). Tuberculosis, public health, and civil liberties. *Annual Review of Public Health, 16*, 307–326.

Berg, J. S., Dischler, J., Wagner, D. J., Raia, J. J., & Palmer-Shevlin, N. (1993). Medication compliance: a healthcare problem. *Annals of Pharmacotherapy, 27*, S1–S24.

Besch, C. L. (1995). Compliance in clinical trials. *AIDS 9*, 1–10.

Britten, N. (1994). Patients' ideas about medicines: A qualitative study in a general practice population. *British Journal of General Practice, 44*, 465–468.

Brownell, K. D., Marlatt, G. A., Lichtenstein, E., & Wilson, G. T. (1986). Understanding and preventing relapse. *American Psychologist, 41*, 765–782.

Brun, J. (1994). Patient compliance with once-daily and twice-daily oral formulations of 5-isosorbide mononitrate: A comparative study. *Journal of International Medical Research, 22*, 266–272.

Christensen, D. B. (1978). Drug-taking compliance: A review and synthesis. *Health Services Research,13*, 841–848.

Cordero, L., Morehead, S., & Miller, R. (1993). Parental compliance with home apnea monitoring. *Journal of Perinatology, 13*, 448–452.

Coutts, J. A. P., Gibson, N. A., & Paton, J. Y. (1992). Measuring compliance with inhaled medication in asthma. *Archives of Disease in Childhood, 67*, 332–333.

Cramer, J. A., Mattson, R. H., Prevey, M. L., Scheyer, R. D., & Oullette, V. L. (1989). How often is medication taken as prescribed? A novel assessment technique. *JAMA, 261*, 3273–3277.

Cramer, J., Scheyer, R. D., & Mattson, R. H. (1990). Compliance declines between clinic visits. *Archives of Internal Medicine, 150*, 1509–1510.

Cramer, J., Vachon, L., Desforges, C., & Sussman, N. M. (1995). Dose frequency and dose interval compliance with multiple antilepileptic medications during a controlled clinical trial. *Epilepsia, 36*, 1111–1117.

Cromer, B. A., Steinberg, K., Gardner, L., Thornton, D., & Shannon, B. (1989). Psychosocial determinants of compliance in adolescents with iron deficiency. *American Journal of Dis Child, 143*, 55–58.

Davis, M. S. (1966). Variations in patients' compliance with doctors' orders: Analysis of congruence between survey responses and results of empirical investigations. *Journal of Medical Education, 41*, 1037–1048.

De Geest, S., Borgermans, L., Gemoets, H., Abraham, I., Vlaminck, H., Evers, G., & Vanrenterghem, Y. (1995). Incidence, determinants, and consequences of subclinical noncompliance with immunosuppressive therapy in renal transplant recipients. *Transplantation, 59*, 340–347.

Dimatteo, M. R., Sherbourne, C. D., Hays, R. D., Ordway, L., Kravitz, R. L., McGlynn, E. A., Kaplan, S., & Rogers, W. H. (1993). Physicians' characteristics influence patients' adherence to medical treatment: Results from the medical outcomes study. *Health Psychology, 12*, 93–102.

Dolce, J., Crisp, C., Manzella, B., Richards, J. M., Hardin, M., & Bailey, W. C. (1991). Medication adherence patterns in chronic obstructive pulmonary disease. *Chest, 99*, 837–841.

Donovan, J. L., & Blake, D. R. (1992). Patient non-compliance: Deviance or reasoned decision-making? *Social Science and Medicine, 34*, 507–513.

DuBard, M. B., Goldenberg, R. L., Copper, R. L., & Hauth, J. C. (1993). Are pill counts valid measures of compliance in clinical obstetric trials? *American Journal of Obstetrics and Gynecology, 169*, 1181–1182.

Dubbert, P. M., King, A., Rapp, S. R., Brief, D., Martin, J. E., & Lake, M. (1985). Riboflavin as a tracer of medication compliance. *Journal of Behavioral Medicine, 8*, 287–299.

Dunbar, J. M. (1980). Assessment of medication compliance: A review. In R. B. Haynes, M. E. Mattson, & T. O. Engebretson, Jr. (Eds.), *Patient compliance to prescribed antihypertensive medication regimens: A report to the National Heart, Lung, and Blood Institute* NIH Publication No. 81-2102 (pps. 59–82). Washington, DC: U.S. Government Printing Office.

Dunbar-Jacob, J. (1993). Contributions to patient adherence: Is it time to share the blame? *Health Psychology, 12*, 91–92.

Gibson, N. A., Ferguson, A. E., Aitchison, T. C., & Paton, J. Y. (1995). Compliance with inhaled asthma medication in preschool children. *Thorax, 50*, 1274–1279.

Gonder-Frederick, L. A., Julian, D. M., Cox, D. J., Clarke, W. L., & Carter, W. R. (1988). Self-measurement of blood glucose: Accuracy of self-reported data and adherence to recommended regimen. *Diabetes Care, 11*, 579–585.

Gordis, L. (1976). Methodologic issues in the measurement of patient compliance. In D. L. Sackett & R. B. Haynes (Eds.), *Compliance with therapeutic regimens* (pp. 51–66). Baltimore, MD: Johns Hopkins University Press.

Gurwitz, J. H., Glynn, R. J., Monane, M., Everitt, D. E., Gilden, D., Smith, N., & Avorn, J. (1993). Treatment for glaucoma: Adherence by the elderly. *American Journal of Public Health, 83*, 711–716.

Halpren, M. T., Irwin, D. E., Brown, R. E., Clouse, J., & Hatziandreu, E. J. (1993). Patient adherence to prescribed potassium supplement therapy. *Clinical Therapy, 15*, 1133–1145.

Hatton, M. Q. F., Allen, M. B., Vathenen, S. V., Feely, M. P., & Cooke, N. J. (1996).

Compliance with oral corticosteroids during steroid trials in chronic airways obstruction. *Thorax, 51*, 323–324.

Heszen-Klemens, I., & Lapinska, E. (1984). Doctor-patient interaction, patients' health behavior and effects of treatment. *Social Science and Medicine, 19*, 9–18.

Hilbrands, L. B., Hoitsma, A., & Koene, R. A. P. (1995). Medication compliance after renal transplantation. *Transplantation, 60*, 914–920.

Holloway, R. L., Rogers, J. C., & Gershenhorn, S. L. (1992). Differences between patient and physician perceptions of predicted compliance. *Family Practice, 9*, 318–322.

Kasl, S. V. (1975). Issues in patient adherence to health care regimens. *Journal of Human Stress, 1*, 5–17.

Kelloway, J. S., Wyatt, R. A., & Adlis, S. A. (1994). Comparison of patients' compliance with prescribed oral and inhaled asthma medications. *Archives of Internal Medicine, 154*, 1349–1352.

Koch, D. A., Giardina, P. J., Ryan, M., MacQueen, M., & Hilgartner, M. W. (1993). Behavioral contracting to improve adherence in patients with thalassemia. *Journal of Pediatric Nursing, 8*, 106–111.

Kraag, G. R., Gordon, D. A., Menard, H-A., Russell, A. S., & Kalish, G. H. (1994). Patient compliance with tenoxicam in family practice. *Clinical Therapy, 16*, 581–593.

Lin, E. H. B., Von Korff, M., Katon, W., Bush, T., Simon, G. E., Walker, E., & Robinson, P. (1995). The role of the primary care physician in patients' adherence to antidepressant therapy. *Medical Care, 33*, 67–74.

Maenpaa, H., Manninen, V., & Heinonen, O. P. (1992). Compliance with medication in the Helsinki Heart Study. *European Journal of Clinical Pharmacology, 42*, 15–19.

Maronde, R. F., Chan, L. S., Larsen, F. J., Strandberg, L. R., Laventurier, M. F., & Sullivan, S. R. (1989). Underutilization of antihypertensive drugs and associated hospitalization. *Medical Care, 27*, 1159–1166.

Mason, B. J., Matsuyama, J. R., & Jue, S. G. (1995). Assessment of sulfonylurea adherence and metabolic control. *Diabetes Educator, 21*, 52–57.

Masur, F. T. (1981). Adherence to health care regimens. In C. K. Prolop & L. A. Bradley (Eds.), *Medical psychology* (pp. 441–470). New York: Academic Press.

Matsui, D., Hermann, C., Klein, J., Berkovitch, M., Olivieri, N., & Koren, G. (1994). Critical comparison of novel and existing methods of compliance assessment during a clinical trial of an oral iron chelator. *Journal of Clinical Pharmacology, 34*, 944–949.

Matsuyama, J. R., Mason, B. J., & Jue, S. G. (1993). Pharmacists' interventions using an electronic medication-event monitoring device's adherence data versus pill counts. *Annals of Pharmacotherapy, 27*, 851–855.

Mawhinney, H., Spector, S. L., Kinsman, R. A., Siegel, S. C., Rachelefsky, G. S., Katz, R. M., & Rohr, A. S. (1991). Compliance in clinical trials of two non-bronchodilator, antiasthma medications. *Annals of Allergy, 66*, 294–299.

Melnikow, J., & Kiefe, C. (1994). Patient compliance and medical research: Issues in methodology. *Journal of General Internal Medicine, 9*, 96–105.

Morgan, M. (1995). The significance of ethnicity for health promotion: Patients' use of anti-hypertensive drugs in inner London. *International Journal of Epidemiology, 24(Suppl.1)*, S79–S84.

Moriskey, D., Green, L., & Levine, D. (1986). Concurrent and predictive validity of a self reported measure of medication adherence. *Medical Care, 24*, 67–74.

Mushlin, A. I., & Appel, F. A. (1977). Diagnosing potential non-compliance: Physician's ability in a behavioral dimension of medical care. *Archives of Internal Medicine, 137*, 318–321.

Nides, M. A., Tashkin, D. P., Simmons, M. S., Wise, R. A., Li, V. C., & Rand, C. S. (1993). Improving inhaler adherence in a clinical trial through the use of the nebulizer chronolog. *Chest, 104*, 501–507.

Pachter, L. M., & Weller, S. C. (1993). Acculturation and compliance with medical therapy. *Journal of Developmental and Behavioral Pediatrics, 14*, 163–168.

Paulson, S. M., Krause, S., & Iber, R. (1977). Development and evaluation of a compliance test for patients taking disulfiram. *Johns Hopkins Medical Journal, 141*, 119–125.

Rand, C. S. (1990). Issues in the measurement of adherence. In S. Shumaker, E. Schron, & J. Ockene (Eds), *The Handbook of Health Behavior Change* (pp. 102–110). New York: Springer Publishing Co.

Rand, C. S., & Wise, R. A. (1994). Measuring adherence to asthma medication regimens. *American Journal of Respiratory Critical Care & Medicine, 149*, S69–S76.

Rand, C. S., Wise, R. A., Nides, M., Simmons, M. S., Bleecker, E. R., Kusek, J. W., Li, V. C., & Tashkin, D. P. (1992). MDI adherence in a clinical trial. *American Review of Respiratory Disorders, 146*, 1559–1564.

Renouf, A. G., & Kovacs, M. (1994). Concordance between mothers' reports and children's self-reports of depressive symptoms: A longitudinal study. *Journal of the American Academy of Child and Adolescent Psychiatry, 33*, 208–216.

Rodewald, L. E., & Pichichero, M. E. (1993). Compliance with antibiotic therapy: A comparison of deuterium oxide tracer, urine bioassay, bottle weights, and parental reports. *Journal of Pediatrics, 123*, 143–147.

Ross, F. M. (1991). Patient compliance: Whose responsibility? *Social Science and Medicine, 32*, 89–94.

Rudd, P., Byyny, R. L., Zachary, V., LoVerde, M. E., Titus, C., Mitchell, W. D., & Marshall, G. (1989). The natural history of medication compliance in a drug trial: Limitations of pill counts. *Clinical & Pharmacological Therapy, 46*, 169–176.

Sackett, D. L., & Haynes, R. B. (1976). *Compliance with therapeutic regimens.* Baltimore, MD: Johns Hopkins University Press.

Schaub, A. F., Steiner, A., & Vetter, W. (1993). Compliance to treatment. *Clinical and Experimental Hypertension, 15*, 1121–1130.

Schectman, G., Hiatt, J., & Hartz, A. (1994). Telephone contacts do not improve adherence to niacin or bile acid sequestrant therapy. *Annals of Pharmacotherapy, 28*, 29–35.

Schluger, N., Ciotoli, C., Cohen, D., Johnson, H., & Rom, W. N. (1995). Comprehensive tuberculosis control for patients at high risk for noncompliance. *American Journal of Respiratory and Critical Care Medicine, 151*, 1486–1490.

Sears, M. R., & Rea, H. H. (1987). Patients at risk for dying of asthma: New Zealand experience. *Journal of Allergy & Clinical Immunology, 80*, 477–481.

Sheiner, L. B., Rosenberg, B., Marathe, V. V., & Peck, C. (1974). Differences in serum digoxin concentrations between outpatients and inpatients: An effect of compliance? *Clinical & Pharmacological Therapy, 15*, 239–246.

Spector, S. L., Kinsman, R., Mawhinney, H., Siegel, S. C., Rachelefsky, G. S., Katz, R. M., & Rohr, A. S. (1986). Compliance of patients with asthma with an experimental aerosolized medication: Implications for controlled clinical trials. *Journal of Allergy & Clinical Immunology, 77*, 65–70.

Spitzer, W. O., Suissa, S., Ernst, P., Horwitz, R. I., Habbick, B., Cockcroft, D., Boivin, J., McNutt, M., Buist, A. S., & Rebuck, A. S. (1992). The use of B-agonists and the risk of death and near death from asthma. *New England Journal of Medicine, 326*, 501–506.

Steele, D. J., Jackson, T. C., & Gutmann, M. C. (1990). Have you been taking your pill? The adherence-monitoring sequence in the medical interview. *The Journal of Family Practice, 30*, 294–299.

Steiner, J. F., Fihn, S. D., Blair, B., & Inui, T. S. (1991). Appropriate reductions in compliance among well-controlled hypertensive patients. *Journal of Clinical Epidemiology, 44*, 1361–1371.

Urquhart, J. (1991). Patient compliance as an explanatory variable in four selected cardiovascular studies. In J. A. Cramer & B. Spilker (Eds.), *Patient compliance in medical practice and clinical trials*, (pp. 301–322). New York: Raven.

Waitzkin, H. (1984). Doctor-patient communication. Clinical implications of social scientific research. *JAMA, 252*, 2441–2446.

Waterhouse, D. M., Calzone, K. A., Mele, C., & Brenner, D. E. (1993). Adherence to oral tamoxifen: A comparison of patient self-report, pill counts, and microelectronic monitoring. *Journal of Clinical Oncology, 11*, 1189–1197.

Wysocki, T., Green, L., & Huxtable, K. (1989). Blood glucose monitoring by diabetic dolescents: Compliance and metabolic control. *Health Psychology, 8*, 267–284.

SECTION II
Lifestyle Interventions and Maintenance of Behaviors

Judith K. Ockene, Editor

There has been a growing recognition in medicine and public health that many acute and chronic diseases can be prevented, or at least have their impact lessened, by increased attention to the adoption and maintenance of behaviors for optimal health. This recognition grows out of the many epidemiologic investigations that demonstrate the existence of a strong relationship between the onset, progression, and exacerbation of disease and subsequent quality of life, and alterable lifestyles such as stopping smoking, changing eating behavior, taking medications, practicing safe sex, and using stress-reducing strategies. This section focuses on intervention strategies designed to facilitate health-promoting and disease-preventing behaviors and the maintenance of these behaviors. Many of the adherence-enhancing strategies discussed in the chapters in Section II have been developed and tested using the theories and models presented in Section I, as well as theories addressing factors at the organizational and community levels. The strategies presented demonstrate the important link between theory, research, and practice.

A chapter that does not appear in this section but which eventually needs to be written would address the integration of interventions for working with individuals who have multiple risk factors or comorbidities. There is a void in the application of theories to address this problem in research and practice. Providers in all disciplines are faced each day with patients who come to us with a clustering of disease-promoting or comorbid behaviors. Health practitioners need integrated approaches that can be applied to most patients, rather than a collection of disparate single-behavior interventions. There are several theories, models, and frameworks which can be applied to the patient with multiple risk factors or comorbidities. However, such as application remains to be designed, implemented, and evaluated.

The chapters in Section II demonstrate that while we have learned much in the last several decades about facilitating the maintenance of healthy behaviors, such endeavors are still a challenge to health practitioners and researchers. Individuals with relatively low levels of education or income continue to present a challenge to practitioners and researchers. This group of patients is addressed in each of the chapters in Section II. However, we have only begun to understand how to work with these individuals to help them enhance and, even more challenging, maintain health-promoting behaviors.

Researchers Abrams and colleagues, in discussing "Adherence to Treatment for Nicotine Dependence" (Chapter 6), and Marcus and colleagues, in discussing "Adherence to Physical Activity Recommendations and Interventions" (Chapter 8) ask us to give strong consideration to Patient-Treatment Matching models as a way of responding to the differences patients bring with them. Abrams and colleagues go further with a stepped-care approach plus patient-treatment matching. McCann and Bovbjerg, in Chapter 7, "Promoting Dietary Change," stress the importance of community and organizational change for facilitating nutritional and other health-related interventions, and the complimentarity of individual and organizational change. Naughton and Ellis, in Chapter 9, "Adoption and Maintenance of Safer Sexual Practices," emphasize that the diversity of the population groups affected by unsafe sexual practices makes developing effective strategies for this population extremely challenging, and that societal norms and interpersonal relationships play a strong role in this behavior. The state of the science in this area is younger (only the last 10 years) than most of the other health-promoting behaviors which have been addressed, and it has not progressed from predictors and effective strategies "to where factors connected with adherence to safer sexual practices are clearly understood and defined." Salmon, Santorelli, and Kabat-Zinn remind us in Chapter 10 that we must be ever mindful of the "point of view" of the patient when caring for him or her. To do this, we must be "intentionally mindful when listening to and speaking with the patient." The authors of each of the chapters agree that long-term change is yet another challenge and one that often feels elusive.

6

Adherence to Treatment for Nicotine Dependence

David B. Abrams, Belinda Borrelli, William G. Shadel, Teresa King, Beth Bock, and Raymond Niaura

INDIVIDUAL AND POPULATION PERSPECTIVES ON ADHERENCE

Cigarette smoking contributes to nearly half a million deaths annually and is the leading preventable cause of death, disability, and excess health care costs in the United States (United States Department of Health and Human Services [USDHHS], 1989). Despite the steady decrease in the overall percentage of smokers in the population from 1965 to 1990 (Center for Disease Control [CDC], 1994), and the variety of clinical and public health interventions presently available to help smokers quit, (Abrams, Emmons, Niaura, Goldstein, & Sherman, 1991; Law & Teng, 1995; Lichtenstein & Glasgow, 1992; Schwartz, 1987; Shiffman, 1993) during the 1990s, population cessation rates have leveled off.

Supported in part by National Institute of Health grants P01CA38309, National Cancer Institute; R01HL32318 National Heart, Lung, and Blood Institute. The authors thank Barbara Doll for exceptional skill in preparing this manuscript for publication.

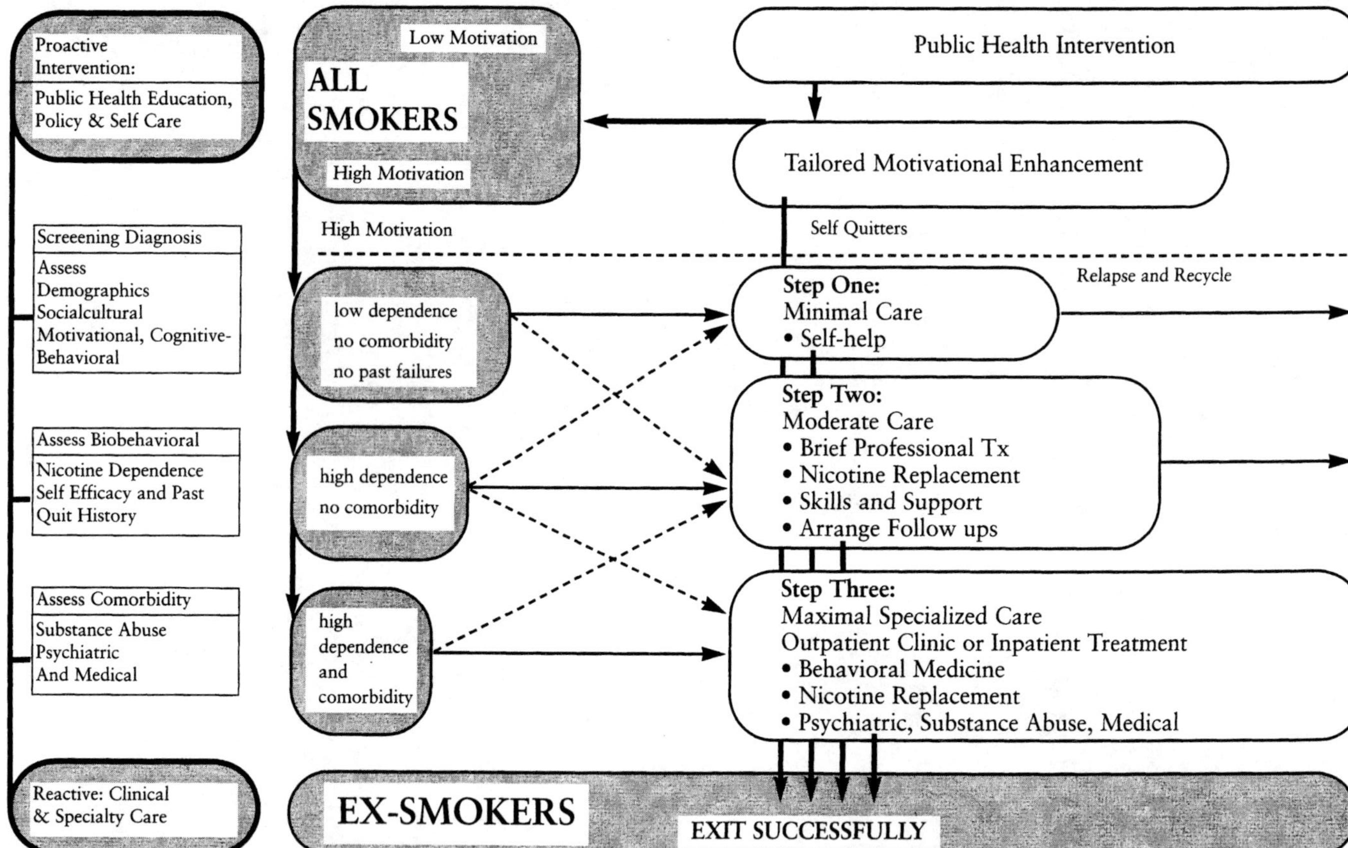

Reprinted with permission, Annals of Behavioral Medicine

Figure 6.1 Comprehensive stepped-care model.

Abrams, D. B., Orleans, C. T., Niaura, R. S., Goldstein, M. G., Prochaska, J. O., & Velicer, W. (1996). Integrating individual and public health perspective for treatment of tobacco dependence under managed health care: a combined stepped care and matching model. *Annals of Behavioral Medicine, 18*(4), 290–304. Reprinted with permission.

These static cessation rates are due to many factors that can broadly be construed as related to adherence issues, including:

1. Many smokers may not adhere adequately to the components of treatments which, in principle, are effective;
2. New "breakthrough" treatments that could be more effective at meeting certain smokers' needs are lacking;
3. Appropriate interventions are not proactively delivered to the majority of smokers who are not currently motivated to quit; and
4. Intervention delivery systems, economic, and other societal factors pose barriers to access to optimal treatment.

These factors, therefore, make it less likely that smokers will be adherent, that is, motivated to initiate cessation or achieve long-term maintenance of cessation. Thus, both individual and population or public health perspectives are relevant within this broader framework for conceptualizing adherence.

We have advanced a stepped-care plus patient-treatment matching model as one potential approach to bridge the individual and public health perspectives (Abrams et al., 1993, 1996). Neither stepped-care nor matching are new ideas (Hughes, 1994; Orleans, 1993), but these concepts rarely have been combined in a comprehensive approach. This model addresses adherence among smokers along a continuum from the individual level to group, organizational and population levels.

Stepped care involves the delivery of interventions in a graded fashion from least intensive and least costly to most intensive and most costly. Usually, the least costly interventions are also the least intensive, least effective, and most standardized, for example, self-help manuals or pamphlets. This improves adherence at the population level by optimizing the use of limited resources. Thus, the vast majority of people receive the least costly interventions, reserving the more costly interventions for those who are unsuccessful.

A treatment-matching model directly assigns smokers to a specific treatment. Such matching is presumed to improve adherence and outcomes (Agency for Health Care Policy and Research [AHCPR], 1996). For example, at the population level, groups of individuals may be matched to their population segment by gender, delivery channel (e.g., worksite, physician office), culture, ethnic group, age, or other sociodemographic variable. This strategy is sometimes referred to as "*targeted*" intervention (Rimer et al., 1994). Smokers could also be matched to qualitatively different treatments, such as a motivational intervention to prepare for cessation (Miller & Rollnick, 1991), or a pharmacological-plus-behavioral intervention for prevention of relapse (Marlatt & Gordon, 1985; Niaura, Goldstein & Abrams, 1994). Patient treatment-matching might also address individual differences (idiographic) within smokers over time, such as presence of comorbid depression or substance abuse (Abrams, 1995). Idiographic matching is referred to as "*tailored*" rather than targeted intervention (Strecher et al., 1994). Patient-treatment tailoring can, therefore, further improve adherence by "fine-tuning" population-level targeting.

A hybrid model that combines elements of stepped care and treatment matching may have advantages over either strategy alone. Based on past history of cessation attempts and other individual factors (e.g., comorbidity), some smokers may benefit from more intensive treatment without first having to cycle through the least intensive level of stepped care. A combined stepped-care plus treatment-matching model also permits an algorithm that views smoking cessation as a process in which, for example, recalcitrant smokers can be either recycled to different treatments with the same level of intensity, or "stepped up" to more intensive treatments. The combined stepped care-plus-matching model serves as the overarching conceptual approach to broadening our perspective on adherence (Abrams et al., 1993, 1996).

This chapter focuses on adult smokers and is based on cognitive social learning theory (Bandura, 1986). We begin by reviewing selected conceptual perspectives of most relevance to adherence. Next, we provide specific examples of the application of the stepped care-plus-treatment-matching model (Abrams et al., 1993, 1996). We segment stepped care into three broad divisions, ranging from the most intensive or maximal treatments (clinic-based), through moderate levels of intervention (brief treatments), to the most broad or minimal population-level interventions (self-change and community-based). Moreover, we discuss special issues which cut across the levels of stepped care, including ethnic/minority issues, comorbidity, and using computer-tailored interventions. The chapter concludes by exploring future directions.

BROADENING THE DEFINITION OF ADHERENCE

Based on the need to bridge individual and public health perspectives, "adherence" must be broadly defined to include not only the traditional viewpoint—the degree to which a smoker adheres to treatment and thereby maintains abstinence—but also the degree to which:

(a) an interventionist and/or
(b) the treatment "delivery system" adheres to a specific protocol (e.g., "best practice guidelines"), and/or

(c) the extent to which the treatment was proactively delivered to, and successfully reached, a specific population (e.g., an underserved population of smokers who were not motivated to consider cessation).

This broader definition of adherence includes contextual factors beyond traditional conceptualizations that assumes a motivated patient seeking clinical treatment from a trained specialist (for reviews, see Carmody, 1992; Lichtenstein & Glasgow, 1992). From this perspective, then, adherence may be defined more generally as the degree to which individuals and groups carry out strategies in the context of a range of interventions along the individual-population continuum, which facilitates the ultimate goal of individual smoking cessation and also has sufficient impact on the population. The criterion for adherence is to reduce the population prevalence of smoking over time. Thus, adherence addresses all the essential components that result in maximal impact on populations (reach or penetration χ efficacy or cost-effectiveness).

Adherence requires a solid match of multiple variables from three levels: *person variables* (i.e., individual differences in the biological, motivational and other cognitive-affective mediating mechanisms underlying the change process); *treatment (intervention) variables* (i.e., program content, provider training and skills); and *systems variables* (i.e., access to appropriate care, service delivery channels, reimbursement, policy, and other organizational or community factors). The interaction among the person, treatment, and systems variables produces a confluence of implicit and explicit factors that can increase or decrease the probability of producing optimal adherence.

We further expand the definition of adherence to include the concept of change as a process over time, comprising motivation, action coping skills, and maintenance or relapse prevention skills (Abrams et al., 1991). For those smokers who are low in motivational readiness to quit, adherence may be defined as the degree to which individual differences, intervention components, and systems level variables increase smokers' likelihood of considering quitting (i.e., changing motivation from low to high readiness is the outcome measure of successful adherence). Among smokers who are motivated and have begun to quit (e.g., cutting down, set a quit date), adherence may be defined as the degree to which the three levels of variables increase the likelihood that they will execute specific strategies to facilitate short-term cessation (24 hours to 7 days of continuous abstinence). Finally, for recently quit ex-smokers, adherence may be defined as the degree to which the above three levels of variables increase the likelihood that they will avoid lapses and will remain abstinent for the mid-term (8 days to 12 months) and longer term (12 months to lifetime) (Marlatt & Gordon, 1985).

TOWARD A STEPPED-CARE-MATCHING MODEL OF ADHERENCE

Population variables, motivation or readiness to quit, cognitive-behavioral mediators (e.g., self-efficacy), degree of nicotine dependence, past history of cessation attempts, and presence of comorbidity form the major cornerstones for optimal treatment of adult smokers (see Figure 6.1). While empirical evidence provides some support for the key stepped-care-matching parameters (AHCPR, 1996; Lichtenstein & Glasgow, 1992; Schwartz, 1987; Shiffman, 1993; USDHHS, 1989), few, if any, studies provide an empirical test of the value of a comprehensive stepped-care-matching hypothesis, tested on a defined population over a relatively long period of time. In any case, the model provides a necessary framework within which to discuss our broadened definition of adherence.

The essential elements in the stepped-care-matching model are briefly summarized below, with more details in Abrams et al. (1996). The model assumes an overall public health perspective where the goal is to accelerate the rate of reduction in smoking prevalence by targeting all smokers, including those who are hard to reach, or those who are low in motivation to quit. If the smoker is low in motivation, then an intervention tailored to increase motivation is delivered until high motivation to quit is achieved (Abrams & Biener, 1992; Velicer, Prochaska, Rossi, & Snow, 1992). This initial matching of the intervention to the smoker's motivation state assures that action-oriented treatments (focused on quitting and relapse prevention coping skills) are not used prematurely on those who are not ready to quit, which could result in nonadherence and a poor cessation outcome.

Once the smoker is ready to quit, the proposed stepped-care-matching model has three broad levels of care related to the intervention program type, intensity, and cost:

1. *minimal*: self-change/self-help;
2. *moderate*: brief (often tailored) counseling plus follow-up; and
3. *maximal*: specialized formal clinic treatment with both outpatient and inpatient options (Figure 6.1).

The stepped-care part of the model is designed so that the largest possible population impact is first achieved with the least costly, most easily disseminable interventions (steps 1 and 2), while the matching component ensures that a smaller number of smokers who need the more expensive, intensive clinical interventions (step 3) do indeed receive these interventions without the need to try the lower levels of care first. Generally, the first-time quitter, without clear signs of having any complications (e.g., comorbidity of depression, alcoholism) will first receive the minimal level of intervention intensity—Step 1 self-help materials. Smokers with a moderate level of dependence and a past history of failed cessation attempts, but no comorbidity, would receive a step 2 intervention of moderate intensity. Step 2 involves brief treatments and support group treatments provided by generalists such as non-doctoral level counselors, other health professionals, and physicians in general practice, such as in general internal medicine, pediatrics, and family medicine services. Step 3 includes highly specialized professionals in behavioral medicine or addiction and formal clinical treatment services, both inpatient and outpatient. Both Steps 2 and 3 can include nicotine replacement, but vary dramatically in intensity and expertise.

The stepped-care-matching approach can also help to address directly the challenge to adherence that comes from smokers who relapse following a serious quit attempt (Marlatt & Gordon, 1985). It is well known that relapse rates are high (40% within 30 days; over 65% within 3 months) among smokers who quit. Failure to quit at a lower level of stepped care ideally would be another variable that can be used in the decision algorithm to ensure that the smoker is "stepped up" to more intensive treatment, rather than "recycled" at the same level ad infinitum. Repeated failure damages self-efficacy, and the smoker can become demoralized. Research is needed to examine whether "stepping up" is more efficacious than recycling at the same level and what patient characteristics are most predictive of differential outcomes when patients are not matched to the appropriate level of stepped care for their individual profile. Such questions expand our view of treatment as a long-term process of persistent engagement with the smoker.

In this stepped-care matching model, nonadherence is seen as the problem of either the treatment approach or the system of delivery, rather than as something inherent within the smoker. At the population level, nonadherence could be viewed as a failure to (a) reach all the smokers; (b) motivate those reached to consider quitting; (c) address patient needs during treatment or relapse prevention; or (d) follow up with patients who relapse to encourage recycling. Smoking cessation should be approached within a stepped-care-matching model as an ongoing and potentially long-term process, much like the management of a chronic disease such as diabetes or hypertension. Encouragement and counseling to quit should be provided over the entire lifespan of the patient if necessary.

With continued failure at cessation, the treatment emphasis may eventually have to change from the goal of complete abstinence to a harm-reduction counseling approach (Marlatt & Tapert, 1993) that utilizes safer nicotine replacement therapies in place of tobacco product use. Since smoking at any level is harmful, it is hoped that continued engagement in treatment (and the message that there is always something else to offer the smoker) will lead to permanent abstinence and less harm over the long run. As the era of effective and safer nicotine replacement and alternative nicotine delivery systems approaches (e.g., transdermal nicotine patch, nicotine containing gum, and nicotine inhaler or nasal spray), harm reduction for recalcitrant smokers becomes an alternative option of last resort to improve adherence for some smokers. Thus, a stepped-care model is consistent with the harm-reduction perspective within public health.

THE ROLE OF COGNITIVE SOCIAL LEARNING THEORY IN PROMOTING ADHERENCE TO SMOKING CESSATION

Cognitive Social Learning Theory (CSLT; Bandura, 1986) forms the backbone of the stepped-care-plus-matching approach to improve adherence to smoking cessation. Reciprocal determinism, proximal goal-setting, self-efficacy, and outcome expectancies are crucial pathways leading to the initiation of, and adherence to, behavior change (Bandura, 1986, 1995). These self-regulatory mechanisms can serve to facilitate adherence at both individual and population levels of social structure (Abrams, Elder, Carleton, Lasater, & Artz, 1986; Abrams et al., 1991). In this section, we will discuss the role of several key components of CSLT—goal-setting, self-efficacy, and feedback—in promoting adherence.

Motivation, conceptualized as cognitions involved in proximal goal-setting (Bandura, 1995), is important for adherence to the initial decision to change the behavior, as well as for carrying out the tasks (i.e., the goals) required to complete the behavior change. For example, smokers not only need to make the decision about whether they are ready to quit, but also need to set goals consistent with this objective, such as gathering knowledge, changing attitudes, or setting a quit day (Borrelli & Mermelstein, 1994; Kamark & Lichtenstein, 1988). Motivation for smoking cessation also refers to both smokers' reasons for quitting and the strength of their desire to quit (Curry, Wagner, & Grothaus, 1990). Tailoring treatment to the smokers' cognitions that reflect their current motivational level can increase adherence to change (Miller & Rollnick, 1991). A number of options exist for increasing adherence to strategies that will increase motivation to quit. Miller and Rollnick (1991) have developed a method of client-centered techniques designed to increase motivation, primarily among substance abuse patients, who are often ambivalent about changing their addictive behavior(s) (Baer, 1995; Brown & Miller, 1993). The key intervention components involved in this approach are designed to decrease patient resistance to the idea of quitting smoking, thereby increasing their adherence to particular treatment strategies necessary for quitting (Emmons & Goldstein, 1992; Emmons, Abrams, & Linnan, 1995). For example, examining both the short- and long-term positive and negative outcome expectancies and guiding smokers through a decisional balance exercise (i.e., review the pros and cons of quitting versus continuing to smoke; Velicer, DiClemente, Prochaska, & Brandenburg, 1985; see also Janis & Mann, 1977) has the potential to affect adherence through changing smokers' attitudes about quitting. Smokers should approach the tasks inherent with quitting more readily if they perceive quitting as a valued outcome (see Cacioppo, Claiborn, Petty, & Heesacker, 1990; Marlatt & Gordon, 1985). These are many interventions directed at reaching and motivating the vast majority of smokers who are low in motivation to quit. These should call our attention to the need to focus on more sensitive measures of early movement towards change, in addition to cessation attempts and continuous abstinence. Prochaska and colleagues, using a stage-of-change model (Prochaska, DiClemente, Velicer, & Rossi, 1993), have shown that tailoring interventions to motivational level may increase smoking cessation among less motivated smokers.

There is some debate over the ultimate utility of a stage model of change (e.g., Sutton, 1996). Continuous measures to assess motivation, such as the Contemplation Ladder, have been developed and validated with respect to other mediators of adherence, such as intentions to quit, sociodemographics, and level of nicotine dependence (Biener & Abrams, 1991). Populations can be classified along a continuum of motivational readiness to change, with over 70% of current smokers being very low in readiness to change (Abrams & Biener, 1992; Velicer et al., 1995). Focusing on abstinence as the only goal could be overwhelming, and contradicts the principle of setting small proximal goals (Bandura & Schunk, 1981; Borrelli & Mermelstein, 1994). Also, when change is conceptualized as a dichotomous outcome (quit/not quit)—rather than as a continuous variable (degree of motivation) or as a series of states (Sutton, 1996; Weinstein, 1993)—one may erroneously label the smoker as nonadherent. In fact, a smoker who has moved from low to high motivation could be considered successful and adherent to the proximal goal.

Another CSLT construct that is important for promoting adherence is self-efficacy. Self-efficacy is the belief in one's capability to perform a particular behavior (Bandura, 1986). Self-efficacy judgments not only determine one's choice of activities (i.e., goals) but also how much effort is expended in these activities, and how long one will persist in the face of adversity. Self-efficacy appears to be inherently linked to proximal goal-setting and to motivation, and is central to adherence. Very high levels of self-efficacy coupled with low motivation may produce unrealistic optimism and an overconfidence that may inhibit adherence (e.g., Haaga & Stewart, 1992). In general, there is abundant support for the association between high levels of self-efficacy at the end of smoking treatment and abstinence at follow-up (Baer, Holt, & Lichtenstein, 1986; Borrelli & Mermelstein, 1994; Condiotte & Lichtenstein, 1981).

Self-efficacy, in combination with specific and challenging goals, can enhance motivation (Bandura & Cervone, 1986; Bandura & Schunk, 1981; Locke, Shaw, Saari, & Latham, 1981). When an individual perceives a discrepancy between where they are and where they would like to be (i.e., their goals), self-dissatisfaction is created, serving as a motivator to increase effort (Bandura & Cervone, 1986; Festinger, 1957; see also Higgins, 1987). However, whether or not this discrepancy is motivating or discouraging depends on the strength of one's perceived capability to attain the goal, or self-efficacy (Bandura, 1986; Bandura & Cervone, 1986). Self-efficacy affects goal choice, task performance, and goal commitment, even after controlling for performance and ability (Locke, Frederick, Lee, & Bobko, 1984). Self-efficacy, challenging goals, and feedback regarding progress towards goals have all been shown to enhance motivation, even if prior goals were not achieved (Bandura & Cervone, 1986; Locke et al., 1984). In fact, Borrelli and Mermelstein (1994) found that the achievement of specific subgoals in smoking cessation treatment (e.g., self-monitoring cigarette consumption, nicotine fading to a specific level) predicted abstinence through its effect on levels of self-efficacy. Taken together, these results suggest that self-efficacy, outcome expectations, goal-setting, and feedback are integral to the initiation and maintenance of behavior change and hence to adherence. Thus, CSLT constructs form the basis for bridging the gap between individual and public health perspectives within a stepped-care model. The following section is organized around the three levels of treatment intensity within the stepped-care framework, from the most complex, intensive, and costly (step 3—clinic) to the least intensive and costly (step 1—self-help).

SPECIFIC APPLICATIONS

Adherence and Intensive Clinic-Based Treatment (Step 3)

Clinic-based programs are among the most effective types of treatments available for smoking cessation, but typically do not have a broad public health impact, due to the expense and the limited population that seeks clinic treatment for nicotine dependence. Clinic-based interventions are directed at the smokers most difficult to treat or "hard-core" (e.g., due to comorbidity issues), and smokers who are referred by professionals, pressured by family, and/or have failed to quit with less intensive treatments.

Intensive clinic programs typically are composed of multiple sessions which include a psychoeducational component (e.g., reviewing the health risks of smoking); self-management training and instruction in stimulus control; coping skills training; social support; follow-up counseling (i.e., "booster") sessions; nicotine fading; nicotine replacement (gum or patch); and relapse-prevention training (Marlatt & Gordon, 1985; Schwartz, 1987; Shiffman, 1993). Such programs appear to have reached an asymptote in their ability to promote cessation among clinic participants (30% quit rates at one year; Law & Teng, 1995; Lichtenstein & Glasgow, 1992). Intensive clinic-based treatment may be the only viable option for the highly dependent smoker, for smokers for whom no other treatments have been effective in helping them to quit, or for smokers with psychiatric comorbidity (e.g., Major Depressive Disorder).

Adherence in the context of intensive clinic-based treatment generally involves two of the previously mentioned definitions of adherence: adhering to strategies which will promote and maintain quitting, and adherence to abstinence. Thus, adherence to treatment may be defined as task persistence, which is a function of two social learning constructs: goals and self-efficacy appraisals. Increasing adherence to treatment strategies among smokers in a clinic program may rely on the interventionist collaboratively constructing cessation plans and strategies with smokers, and increasing their perceptions of self-efficacy that they can execute those strategies.

One study of self-efficacy and goal-setting in a clinic-based sample of smokers found that completing a greater number of behavioral assignments predicted increases in self-efficacy, which, in turn, prospectively predicted an increased likelihood of abstinence at follow-up (Borrelli & Mermelstein, 1994; see also Kamark & Lichtenstein, 1988). Current self-efficacy appraisals of performance also can be increased through review of past personal successes with executing behavioral strategies (reminiscence challenge; see Rybarczyk & Auerbach, 1990). Thus, setting reachable and manageable treatment strategy goals during the initial phases of cessation treatment should lead to increases in adherence to those strategies.

Within the context of the clinic-based program, additional treatment matching can occur to further increase smokers' adherence (Abrams et al., 1993). For example, matching treatments to smokers' level of depressive symptoms or to a past history of affective disturbance (Hall, Munoz, Reus, & Sees, 1993), or to their level of nicotine dependence (Niaura et al., 1994) can improve adherence and cessation rates. Fear of weight gain following cessation, especially among women, also has been viewed as an important individual difference variable by which to match smoking cessation treatment (Hall, Ginsberg, & Jones, 1986). Use of physical activity, as part of a relapse prevention strategy to improve adherence to smoking cessation and prevent relapse, has been shown to have promise in promoting cessation among women in recent small-scale studies (Marcus et al., 1995).

Specialized treatment is also relevant for alcoholics and substance abusers, who have extremely high smoking rates and will likely require smoking cessation treatments adapted for use in alcohol and drug abuse treatment programs (Abrams, 1995; Monti, Rohsenow, & Abrams, 1995). However, aside from some select studies (e.g., Hall et al., 1993; Niaura et al., 1994), patient treatment matching is the exception, rather than the rule, in smoking treatment (Shadel & Mermelstein, 1996; Shiffman, 1993). Indeed, given its potential to improve adherence to treatment and thus increase long-term abstinence rates, future clinical research should adopt and test theoretically derived treatment-matching models.

Adherence and Nicotine Replacement Therapies (Steps 3 and 2)

The goal of using nicotine replacement therapies to aid in smoking cessation is to gradually wean the smoker from cigarettes by replacing blood levels of nicotine and decreasing the reinforcing value of smoking in response to particular internal and external stimuli. In this section, we will discuss the role of two replacement therapies, nicotine-containing gum (NCG), and the transdermal nicotine patch (TNP), in promoting adherence to smoking cessation, and in contributing to a stepped-care model. We also will discuss the facilitators and barriers to adherence to each form of therapy.

Nicotine-Containing Gum

Numerous studies have demonstrated the clinical efficacy of NCG in helping smokers quit. A meta-analysis of 14 randomized controlled studies of smokers in clinic-based programs showed that NCG produced a 27% quit rate at 6 months post-treatment, vs. an 18% quit rate for placebo subjects (Lam, Sze, Sacks, & Chalmers, 1987). However, NCG confers almost no benefit over placebo when utilized in medical practice settings without a behavioral program (e.g., 10% NCG, vs. 7% placebo at 11-month follow-up; Hughes, Gust, Keenan, Fenwick, & Healey, 1989).

There are several barriers to adhering to NCG use. First, smokers may use NCG improperly, either by chewing less than the 12–15 pieces per day recommended by the manufacturer (Fortmann, Killen, Telch, & Newman, 1988), or by chewing the gum too quickly, rather than use the correct "chew and park" technique. The latter may result in the swallowing of nicotine, which could lead to gastric upset and decreased absorption through the buccal mucosa (D. P. Sachs, 1989). Second, side effects are relatively common in NCG vs. placebo, and include the following: burning in the throat (76% vs. 53%), eructation (49% vs. 21%), hiccups (37% vs. 14%), dizziness (34% vs. 17%), nausea (33% vs. 17%), stomach ache (31% vs. 17%), and jaw ache (68% vs. 67%; Hughes et al., 1989). Finally, Fiore, Jorenby, Baker, and Kenford (1992) point out that while smokers can use NCG to cope with high-risk situations by chewing a piece of gum as a coping response, this may reinforce the use of gum and inhibit the development of alternative coping responses. Given this, it is not surprising that 8% to 25% of abstainers who use NCG continue their use beyond the recommended length of therapy (6 months; Hajek, Jackson, & Belcher, 1988).

There are several factors that may promote adherence to NCG. First, NCG decreases post-cessation weight gain in a dose-response manner, although this weight-suppression effect remains only during active NCG treatment (Gross, Johnson, Sigler, & Stitzer, 1995; Nides, et al., 1994). The delay in weight gain would allow the weight-concerned smoker to adjust to quitting and cope with withdrawal first, before undertaking weight-control strategies. Second, NCG has been shown to decrease the number and intensity of withdrawal symptoms (Hughes & Hatsukami, 1985; Hughes et al., 1984), and decreased withdrawal symptoms are related to better smoking cessation outcomes (Gross et al., 1995). Third, NCG is now available over the counter, which may translate to increased use among wider population segments who have little or no access to obtaining a physician prescription for NCG.

NCG can be an important component of a comprehensive stepped-care model. It appears that the use of NCG may be best suited for those who are in formal clinic-based treatment programs, where adherence and outcomes are more optimal. It also may be effective when properly integrated with briefer behavioral counseling in moderate-intensity treatments (e.g., primary care) (Ockene et al., 1991). However, it does not appear to be more effective than placebo when used in clinical practice without concomitant behavioral interventions (Cepeda-Benito, 1993). Group or clinic-based behavioral treatment, on the other hand, enables smokers to develop alternative coping responses to high-risk situations as they gradually wean from chewing gum. Furthermore, behavioral treatment allows for the enhancement of motivation and self-efficacy, and promotes internal, rather than external, attributions for success. Finally, highly dependent smokers appear to benefit the most from NCG in a dose-response fashion (Niaura, et al., 1994).

The Nicotine Patch

The transdermal nicotine patch (TNP) enhances both the initiation and maintenance of abstinence from cigarettes. A recent meta-analysis of 17 studies (N = 5,098) indicated that TNP produced quit rates of 27.1% at the end of treatment and 21.8% at 6-month follow-up compared to 13.1% and 8.4% for placebo (Fiore, Smith, Jorenby, & Baker, 1994). Unlike NCG, the patch demonstrates efficacy in both intensive and brief intervention formats. Studies examining the effect of physician advice to quit smoking with or without nurse follow-up have shown a doubling of quit rates for patch users vs. placebo at one-year follow-ups (Hurt et al., 1994; D. P.

Sachs, Sawe, & Leischow, 1993; Stapleton, et al., 1995). In addition, the meta-analysis by Fiore and colleagues (1994) found that those who received more intensive behavioral counseling were twice as likely to be abstinent at end of treatment and 6-month follow-up than those who received less intensive counseling.

The TNP has few barriers to adherence. Some of the most common side effects include erythema, pruritus, or burning (35–54%), edema (3–8%), mild to moderate insomnia (1–23%), diarrhea (1–9%), dyspepsia (1–9%), nervousness (3–9%), and abnormal dreams (1–9%). Although side effects concerning the skin are relatively common, one study found only a 1.3% drop-out rate due to skin irritation (Westman, Levin, & Rose, 1993). Like NCG, the TNP reduces withdrawal symptoms, such as craving (Tonnesen, Norregaard, Simonsen, & Sawe, 1991). However, unlike NCG, TNP does not appear to prevent post-cessation weight gain (Fiore et al., 1992; Tonnesen et al., 1991). This may be of some concern to those smokers who are concerned about post-cessation weight gain. Combination therapy may be indicated in such cases. For example, one study showed that the addition of NCG to TNP improved quit rates at 24 weeks (27.5% patch plus gum vs. 15.3% patch plus placebo gum; Kornitzer, Boutsen, Dramaix, Thijs, & Gustavsson, 1995). One final barrier to patch use is cost, which may be prohibitive for some smokers; insurance companies typically do not reimburse for TNP until the smoker has been abstinent for 1 year after treatment. TNP generally costs between $3–4 per day, resulting in $250–$300 to complete treatment. This may be especially daunting for the underserved smoker, who would probably benefit the most from TNP, given that the high rates of nicotine dependence and psychiatric comorbidity found in this population may make it especially difficult for them to quit.

TNP appears to be more flexible than NCG in that it appears to promote adherence at any level of the stepped-care model. The patch appears to be twice as cost-effective as the 2-mg gum in terms of quality-adjusted life years saved (QALYs), but equal to the 4-mg NCG (Fiscella & Franks, 1996). The fact that both TNP and NCG are now available over the counter may increase use among those who had previously not had access to physician prescription.

Enhancing Adherence Through Moderate/Brief Interventions (Step 2)

Moderate-level interventions, such as those conducted in medical office settings, have great potential to reach a wide range of smokers, since more than 70% of smokers see their physician each year (Prochaska & Goldstein, 1991). Indeed, from a stepped-care approach, these interventions have moderate efficacy in promoting cessation, and clearly can have moderate-to-high reach to the general population of smokers (Abrams et al., 1996). However, interventions conducted in medical settings pose special problems for patient adherence. In contrast to clinic-based settings, in which the clinician typically has an extended time frame of many weeks to implement intervention techniques, interventions delivered in the medical setting may be limited by their comparatively brief duration. In general, then, there may be less opportunity to conduct an adequate matching assessment, and to provide specific goal-setting and social support. Gilpin and colleagues (1992) reported that in population-based surveys, less than 50% of smokers said that they had ever been advised to quit by a physician.

Nonetheless, some of the same social learning principles reviewed above for clinic-based treatments may be applied to increasing adherence to cessation interventions in medical settings as well. The 4-A guidelines (Ask, Advise, Assist, Arrange), already effective in increasing abstinence rates at one year (about 4%; Kottke, Battista, Defriese, & Brekke, 1988; Manley, Epps, & Glynn, 1992; Ockene, 1987), allow physicians and other health professionals to set specific strategy and quit-day goals and to provide follow-up in a brief treatment context.

Given limitations on physician time, it may be most efficient and effective to employ the services of an allied health care provider (e.g., nurse practitioner, respiratory therapist, health educator), trained in brief cessation techniques, to deliver the bulk of the cessation intervention and follow-up. For example, brief motivational messages from the physician followed by interventions delivered by an allied health professional can increase significantly cessation rates compared with brief physician advice alone (about 7%; Hollis, Lichenstein, Vogt, Stevens, & Biglan, 1993). One mechanism which may mediate increases in cessation rates may be that motivational interventions increase a smoker's willingness to adhere to subsequent cessation strategy information provided by the allied health professional (e.g., read cessation information; see Orleans et al., 1991). In addition, the degree to which the physician can tailor the motivational messages to individual smokers may further enhance these smokers' adherence to subsequently assigned treatment strategies (Fiore et al., 1996). Even in relatively brief physician-delivered counseling interventions, physicians can be taught to help smokers to assess their own motivations to stop smoking (Ockene et al., 1988). Follow-up visits, which can increase the effectiveness of physician-delivered interventions (Kottke et al., 1988; Manley et al., 1992; Ockene, 1987; Ockene et al., 1991, 1994), also should increase adherence to cessation treatment protocols, through additional social support and opportunities to collaboratively set specific goals with the smoker.

However, if in the medical setting a pre-intervention matching assessment reveals that the smoker is in need of more intensive treatment for smoking (i.e., due to high levels of nicotine dependence or comorbidity) or if the smoker fails to quit with this moderate level of intervention, health care professionals should have at their disposal referral lists for more intensive programs with which to provide the smoker, if he or she appears ready to make a more formal attempt to quit. Furthermore, the degree to which the health care service provider can be specific about the goal of referring the smoker to an alternative and more intensive program (e.g., schedule a specific date and time for the patient to call about the visit) the greater the likelihood of a greater level of adherence with this next "step-up" for more intensive treatment. In any case, whether the smoker is ready to move to this next level of treatment, or is ambivalent about the decision to try to quit again (due to a recent failure to quit, for example), the provider would be advised to conduct a brief motivational intervention based on the smoker's readiness (Miller & Rollnick, 1991).

Adherence and Minimal Interventions in the Community (Step 1)

A central feature of community-based programs is that they provide self-change and self-help intervention for a large segment of the smoking population. An exemplar of such programs is the Community Intervention Trial for Smoking Cessation (COMMIT) (e.g., Glasgow, Sorensen, & Corbett, 1992). The COMMIT trial randomly assigned communities to the intervention or control groups. Quit rates among heavy smokers did not differ between targeted vs. control communities (Cohen, Lichtenstein, Prochaska, Rossi, & Gritz, 1995). However, smoking rates declined among light-to-moderate smokers in targeted communities, compared to control communities with most of the decline occurring in the less educated segment of the population (i.e., 12th grade or less education). Such programs have typically shown only modest efficacy, but are attractive in that they reach large proportions of the population (Fisher, 1995). The efficacy of community-based trials is often strongest within particular subgroups of smokers, such as light smokers (Cohen et al., 1989), and only minimally effective or ineffective with other groups such as highly dependent, heavy smokers, those with psychiatric comorbidity, and minority ethnic groups (Lando et al., 1995). The biggest challenge to increasing adherence in population-based interventions is that the typical self-help treatment is geared to quitting and relapse prevention skills, whereas the vast majority of the smokers in a population are low in motivation to quit, resulting in a mismatch between smoker readiness and treatment content.

Stepped-care methods are hypothesized to increase patient adherence and abstinence in community-based programs by proactively reaching and providing access to treatment and by directing individuals into the most appropriate treatment modality. Studies which provide a rigorous test of stepped-care versus less comprehensive community approaches are greatly needed.

In addition to triaging smokers to maximize patient-treatment matching, a cornerstone of the stepped-care approach is the recycling of unsuccessful smokers into increasingly intensive treatments. A community-wide intervention that employs patient recycling would assign smokers who were unsuccessful at achieving abstinence into progressively more intensive treatments until abstinence is achieved (Kviz, Crittenden, & Warnecke, 1992). Unfortunately, few if any studies have examined the efficacy of patient recycling in smoking cessation.

The degree of overall community awareness of smoking and health issues, or presence of other community-wide health initiatives, also could be used to assign communities to more or less intensive smoking cessation programs. More comprehensive stepped-care approaches could include several layers of intervention, from those targeted to raise public awareness (e.g., billboards, television advertising), to self-help programs, to maximally intensive clinic-based programs. Clearly, environmental, systems factors and legislative policies can directly and indirectly influence individual adherence (Abrams et al., 1991). A well-developed communication system linking the various layers of treatment for purposes of referral should be considered as an integral part of community-based stepped-care programs to improve overall population adherence to community-level interventions.

USING THE STEPPED-CARE MODEL TO PROMOTE ADHERENCE AMONG ETHNIC MINORITIES

Certain populations of smokers represent special challenges when attempting to design effective smoking cessation interventions. Ethnic minorities are one such population. The factors which are related to increased smoking prevalence in the general population, such as low education (Escobedo & Peddicord, 1996) and income (Shea et al., 1991) are especially prevalent among many ethnic populations. For example, only slightly more than one half (50.9%) of all Hispanics compared with 78.4% of Whites have completed high school (U.S. Bureau of the Census, 1991), and as many as 25% of Hispanics are below poverty level versus 10% of Whites (U.S. Bureau of the Census, 1984). In addition, participation rates for ethnic minorities in smoking cessation trials and clinic-based programs are low, especially among those of lower education (Marcus, King, Pinto, & Albrecht, 1994; Nevid & Javier, 1993). Thus, smoking cessation interventions which do not address economic barriers or low education levels, or which lack appreciation of the cultural beliefs and values of particular subgroups, may be contributing to these low participation rates. A stepped-care approach tailored to the treatment needs of the smoker and recognizant of the special needs of underserved groups may be more effective at increasing adherence.

A stepped-care approach asserts that the intensity of the treatment should depend on the degree of nicotine dependence and psychological factors. When assessing nicotine dependence in minority smokers, multiple measures of dependency may be needed, as patterns of cigarette use can vary dramatically from White Americans. For example, while African-Americans tend to smoke fewer cigarettes per day than White Americans, the cigarettes they smoke tend to be higher in tar and nicotine (Kabat, Morabia, & Wynder, 1991). In addition, certain ethnic groups have elevated rates of physical and psychiatric comorbidity, thus suggesting a need for a higher level of care.

Step one of the stepped-care approach consists of self-help with the possible addition of some motivational enhancements. Self-help methods may not be a particularly effective strategy with this population. For example, one study of methods of quitting for Native Americans found that the least popular method of quitting was following instructions in a book or pamphlet (Hodge et al., 1995). However, given that self-help materials are developed for the majority culture, specifically targeting for ethnicity in the material may increase acceptance. Self-help materials targeted to a specific population have been found to improve quit rates over generic materials (Rimer et al., 1986). Minorities with low educational attainment may not be able to benefit from self-help materials to quit smoking because of illiteracy or language barriers (Orleans et al., 1989).

Motivational enhancements typically focus on the smokers' personal health risks. Strategies to increase motivation should also be derived from information about each ethnic group's relevant motivations to quit. For example, Southeast Asian men have indicated saving money as a major motivation not to smoke, suggesting that a disease-focused anti-smoking message may not be sufficiently effective for this group (Chen et al., 1993). More exploration of the factors that different ethnicities find motivating is needed. Assessing knowledge of smoking risk factors may also be important when intervening with ethnic minorities.

Step 2 emphasizes more interaction by the interventionist with the smoker, treatment tailoring, and social support. For many underserved groups, this is likely to be the minimum level of care able to bring about effective results. Group-based treatments may be beneficial in that certain populations of ethnic minority smokers may lack support for quitting in their natural environments. For example, smoking tends to be more accepted in many Native American societies, this may be a function of both the ceremonial significance of tobacco and profit from the sale of tobacco on reservations. Studies of urban, low-income African-American women indicate that they also lack support for quitting (Lacey, 1993; Lacey et al., 1993; Manfredi, Lacey, Warnecke, & Buis, 1992). One potential problem with cognitive behavioral group-based treatments is their resemblance to school (e.g., homework assignments). Ethnic minorities with low educational attainment may reject this treatment format, as it may represent an area at which they feel ineffectual.

An important assessment for step 2 interventions with ethnic minorities is the presence of practical barriers. In a recent community-based, culturally specific smoking cessation program for Hispanic smokers, lower income was found to be predictive of attrition (Nevid, Javier, & Moulton, 1996). Attending to economic issues may be the only way to intervene effectively with individuals who are economically deprived. For example, preliminary research suggests that addressing practical and logistic barriers, such as child care and transportation, is beneficial in increasing participation rates of minority women (King, Marcus, & Borrelli, 1996).

Step 3 approaches are for those smokers who have repeatedly failed to quit smoking with steps 1 and 2 or who have psychiatric or medical comorbidity. Factors that may warrant a higher level of treatment intensity among ethnic minorities include psychiatric comorbidity, lower levels of education, and substance abuse. Minorities are at greater risk for the development of depression (Anda et al., 1990; Blazer, Kessler, McGonagle, & Swartz, 1994); therefore, depression may be a significant barrier to smoking cessation among these populations. Focus group data suggests that the content of programs may need to address a broad spectrum of issues in order to be of interest to African-American women who identify stress, not smoking, as their biggest health problem (Lacey, 1993; Lacey et al., 1993; Manfredi et al., 1992; Shervington, 1986). Thus, it appears that an appropriate level of care for many minority groups may be fairly intensive. However, cost represents a true barrier to the appropriate level of care which may include expensive, pharmacologic, and inpatient options.

In conclusion, adherence rates for ethnic minorities would likely improve if social marketing strategies were targeted to the population; if qualitative methodologies, such as focus groups, were used to ensure appropriate tailoring of the intervention; and social policies allowed access to the appropriate level of intervention by removing economic barriers. It is also important to determine what theoretical models for smoking cessation are effective for different minorities. Are theoretical frameworks such as Social-Cognitive Theory (Bandura, 1986) and the Stages of Change Model (Prochaska & DiClemente, 1983), which have been applied to smokers in general, applicable and effective among different minority groups? Answering this question is difficult, however, since procedures for determining whether theoretical concepts have cross-cultural consistency have not yet been developed (Johnson et al., 1995).

EXPERT SYSTEMS

Advances in computer technology, and the increasing complexity of both medical information and medical decision making, have combined with growing pressure under managed care for the development of low-cost, high-outreach interventions to create an increased interest in the utilization of computer expert systems in health care delivery. Expert systems have been designed to provide behavioral health interventions including assisting individuals to quit smoking and to adopt a more physically active lifestyle (Marcus et al., 1995). The foundation underlying expert systems interventions is the provision of personalized feedback to the individual patient/user. The type of feedback provided by these systems includes professionally developed intervention strategies which address problems detected from patient data.

Interactive expert systems are capable of tailoring assessment procedures based on information obtained during early parts of the assessment (Strecher et al., 1994). For example, a general health screening assessment which detects smoking may cue the system to request additional assessment from the user regarding prior quit attempts, motivation for making another quit attempt, depressive symptoms, or other pertinent information not required of nonsmoking users. This has the advantage of maximizing the thoroughness of the assessment while minimizing assessment length across all users. In addition, expert systems can alter the nature of the intervention based upon key characteristics of the individual user, such as psychological status (e.g., depressed, nondepressed, motivational level); behavioral status (e.g., nicotine dependence, smoking rate); or user-identified goals or problem areas (e.g., habit, emotional smoking). For example, items assessing participant self-efficacy can be compared to previously established norms (e.g. Bock, Marcus, Bock, & Abrams, 1996). Decision rules within the system can select the appropriate prewritten counseling message addressing the smoker's situation and incorporate this into a feedback report.

The utilization of computer expert systems has produced encouraging results in interventions for smoking cessation (e.g., Curry, Wagner, & Grothaus, 1991; Strecher et al., 1994), and exercise adoption (Bock et al., 1996).

The utilization of computer expert systems can enhance patient adherence by increasing the relevancy of treatment to match individual concerns and by reducing patient burden. Expert systems interventions can be delivered via remote systems (e.g., mail, phone) which remove transportation, time, and convenience as barriers to treatment adherence. Once development costs are covered, the cost per smoker is relatively inexpensive. Thus, expert systems can improve the reach and the efficacy of large-scale, population-focused interventions (step 1) by combining the advantages of mass dissemination to the community with the kind of individual tailoring that was previously limited to the more intensive face-to-face counseling interventions (Steps 2 and 3).

CONCLUSION

Research in the last decade has revealed promising new directions to improve adherence and outcomes at both individual and population levels. Bridging the gap between more traditional conceptualizations of adherence within the clinical context to the broader community and public health arena opens up new arenas for future research. Increasing adherence will have its greatest impact when intervention components and contextual systems variables are both incorporated into a more comprehensive approach to accelerating the annual reduction in population prevalence of adult smoking. Adherence improvement can be viewed as improved tailoring of intervention components to smoker characteristics along the continuum of care that includes proactive reaching out to the vast majority of smokers who are low in motivation to quit. Public health strategies to reach and provide access and choice of the whole range of smoking cessation tools to hard-to-reach and underserved populations is one of the central challenges to improving community-level adherence and, ultimately, improving treatment outcome, better relapse prevention, and overall prevalence reduction.

A broader definition of adherence was proposed to include microlevel individual matching components as well as macrolevel stepped-care and delivery system issues; and to proactively reach and motivate whole populations, as well as to improve outcomes for reactively recruited clinic volunteers who are already motivated to quit. New technologies in informatics and the electronic communications revolution provide unprecedented opportunities to optimize mass communication and public health models with fine-grained tailoring to unique individual needs and also with continuity of follow-up. Computer expert systems provide one example of how stepped-care plus matching, public health models, and algorithms derived from clinical models of best practices can begin to be combined to improve adherence to reach, motivate, improve cessation, and prevent relapse in whole populations of smokers.

REFERENCES

Abrams, D. B. (1995). Integrating basic, clinical, and public health research for alcohol-tobacco interactions. In J. Fertig (Ed.), *Alcohol and tobacco: From basic science to policy* (pp. 3–16). NIAAA Alcohol Research Monograph. Bethesda, MD: NIH, National Institute on Alcohol Abuse & Alcoholism.

Abrams, D. B., & Biener, L. (1992). Motivational characteristics of smokers at the worksite: A public health challenge. *Preventive Medicine, 21*, 679–687.

Abrams, D. B., Elder, J. P., Carleton, R. A., Lasater, T. M., & Artz, L. M. (1986). Social learning principles for organizational health promotion: An integrated approach. In M. F. Cataldo & T. J. Coates (Eds.), *Health and industry: A behavioral medicine perspective* (pp. 28–51). New York: John Wiley.

Abrams, D. B., Emmons, K. M., Niaura, R. S., Goldstein, M. G., & Sherman, C. E. (1991). Tobacco dependence: An integration of individual and public health perspectives. In P. E. Nathan, J. W. Langenbucher, B. S. McCrady, & W. Frankenstein (Eds.), *Annual review of addictions treatment and research (Vol. 1, pp. 391–436)*. New York: Pergamon.

Abrams, D. B., Orleans, C. T., Niaura, R., Goldstein, M., Prochaska, J., & Velicer, W. (1996). Integrating individual and public health perspectives for treatment of tobacco dependence under managed health care: A combined stepped-care and matching model. *Annals of Behavioral Medicine, 18*, 290–304.

Abrams, D. B., Orleans, C. T., Niaura, R. N., Goldstein, M., Velicer, W., & Prochaska, J. O. (1993). Treatment issues: Towards a stepped-care model. *Tobacco Control, 2*(Suppl), S17–S37.

Agency for Health Care Policy and Research. (1996). Smoking cessation clinical practice guidelines. *Journal of the American Medical Association, 275*, 1270–1280.

Anda, R. F., Williamson, D. F., Escobedo, L. G., Mast, E. E., Giovino, G. A., & Remington, P. L. (1990). Depression and the dynamics of smoking: A national perspective. *Journal of the American Medical Association, 264*, 1541–1545.

Baer, J. S. (1995). Secondary prevention of alcohol and tobacco use: Recommendations based on efforts with heavy drinking college students. In J. Fertig (Ed.), *Alcohol and tobacco: From basic science to policy*. (NIAAA Alcohol Research Monograph. pp. 265–280). Bethesda, MD: NIH, National Institute on Alcohol Abuse and Alcoholism.

Baer, J. S., Holt, C. S., & Lichtenstein, E. (1986). Self-efficacy and smoking re-examined: Construct validity and clinical utility. *Journal of Consulting and Clinical Psychology, 54*, 846–852.

Bandura, A. (1986). *Social foundations of thought and action: A social cognitive theory*. Englewood Cliffs, NJ: Prentice-Hall.

Bandura, A. (1995, March). *Moving in forward gear in health promotion and disease prevention.* Paper presented at the annual meeting of the Society of Behavioral Medicine, San Diego, CA.

Bandura, A., & Cervone, D. (1986). Differential engagement of self-reactive influences in cognitive motivation. *Organizational Behavior and Human Decision Processes, 38*, 92–113.

Bandura, A., & Schunk, D. H. (1981). Cultivating competence, self-efficacy, and intrinsic interest through proximal self-motivation. *Journal of Personal and Social Psychology, 41*, 586–598.

Biener, L., & Abrams, D. B. (1991). The contemplation ladder: Validation of a measure of readiness to consider smoking cessation. *Health Psychology, 10*, 360–365.

Blazer, D., Kessler, R., McGonagle, K., & Swartz, S. (1994). The prevalence and distribution of major depression in a national community sample: The National Comorbidity Survey. *American Journal of Psychiatry, 151*, 979–986.

Bock, B. C., Marcus, B. H., Bock, F. R., & Abrams, D. B. (1996). Designing expert system interventions: Lessons learned from a physical activity intervention. Submitted to International Journal of Behavioral Medicine.

Borrelli, B., & Mermelstein, R. (1994). Goal setting and behavior change in a smoking cessation program. *Cognitive Therapy and Research, 18*, 69–83.

Brown, J. M., & Miller, W. R. (1993). Impact of motivational interviewing on participation and outcome in residential alcoholism treatment. *Psychology of Addictive Behaviors, 7*, 211–218.

Cacioppo, J., Claiborn, C., Petty, R., & Heesacker, M. (1990). General framework for the study of attitude change in psychotherapy. In C. Snyder & D. Forsyth (Eds.), *Handbook of social and clinical psychology* (pp. 523–539). New York: Pergamon.

Carmody, T. (1992). Preventing relapse in the treatment of nicotine addiction: Current issues and future directions. *Journal of Psychoactive Drugs, 24*, 131–158.

Centers for Disease Control [CDC]. (1994). Cigarette smoking among adults: 1993. *Morbidity and Mortality Weekly Report, 43*, 925–930.

Cepeda-Benito, A. (1993). A meta-analytic review of the efficacy of nicotine chewing gum in smoking treatment programs. *Journal of Consulting and Clinical Psychology, 61*, 822–830.

Chen, M. S. (1993). Cardiovascular health among Asian Americans/Pacific Islanders: An examination of health status and intervention approaches. *American Journal of Health Promotion, 7*, 199–207.

Chen, M. S., Guthrie, R., Moeschberger, M., Wewers, M. E., Anderson, J., Kuun, P., & Nguyen, H. (1993). Lessons learned and baseline data from initiating smoking cessation research with Southeast Asian adults. *Asian American and Pacific Islander Journal of Health, 1*, 194–214.

Cohen, S., Lichtenstein, E., Prochaska, J. O., Rossi, J. S., Gritz, E. R., & The COMMIT Research Group. (1995). Community intervention trial for smoking cessation (COMMIT): I. Cohort results from a four-year community intervention. *American Journal of Public Health, 85*, 183–192.

Condiotte, M. M., & Lichtenstein, E. (1981). Self-efficacy and relapse in smoking cessation programs. *Journal of Consulting and Clinical Psychology, 49*, 648–658.

Curry, S., Wagner, E. H., & Grothaus, L. C. (1990). Intrinsic and extrinsic motivation for smoking cessation. *Journal of Consulting and Clinical Psychology, 58*, 310–316.

Curry, S. J., Wagner, E. H., & Grothaus, L. C. (1991). Evaluation of intrinsic and extrinsic motivation interventions with a self-help smoking cessation program. *Journal of Consulting and Clinical Psychology, 59*, 318–324.

Emmons, K., Abrams, D. B., & Linnan, L. (1995, March). *Motivation for smoking cessation: To quit or not to quit is not the question.* Paper presented at the meeting of the Society of Behavioral Medicine, San Diego, CA.

Emmons, K. M., & Goldstein, M. G. (1992). Smokers who are hospitalized: A window of opportunity for cessation interventions. *Preventive Medicine, 21*, 262–269.

Escobedo, L. G., & Peddicord, J. P. (1996). Smoking prevalence in US birth cohorts: The influence of gender and education. *American Journal of Public Health, 86*, 231–236.

Festinger, L. (1957). *A theory of cognitive dissonance*. Stanford, CA: Stanford University Press.

Fiore, M. C., Bailey, W. C., Cohen, S. J., et al. (1996). Smoking cessation Clinical Practice Guideline No. 18, AHCPR Publication No. 96–0692. Rockville, MD: AHCPR.

Fiore, M. C., Jorenby, D. E., Baker, T. B., & Kenford, S. L. (1992). Tobacco dependence and the nicotine patch: Clinical guidelines for effective use. *Journal of the American Medical Association, 268*, 2687–2694.

Fiore, M. C., Smith, S. S., Jorenby, D. E., & Baker, T. B. (1994). The effectiveness of the nicotine patch for smoking cessation. *Journal of the American Medical Association, 271*, 1940–1947.

Fiscella, K., & Franks, P. (1996). Cost-effectiveness of the transdermal nicotine patch as an adjunct to physicians' smoking cessation counseling. *Journal of the American Medical Association, 275*, 1247–1251.

Fisher, E. B. (1995). Editorial: The results of the COMMIT trial. *American Journal of Public Health, 85*, 159–160.

Fortmann, S. P., Killen, J. D., Telch, M. J., & Newman, B. (1988). Minimal contact treatment for smoking cessation: A placebo controlled trial of nicotine polacrilex and self-directed relapse prevention: Initial results of the Stanford Stop Smoking Project. *Journal of the American Medical Association, 260*, 1575–1580.

Gilpin, E., Pierce, J. Goodman, J., Giovino, G., Berry, C., & Burns, D. (1992). Trends in physicians' giving advice to stop smoking: United States, 1974–1987. *Tobacco Control, 1*, 31–36.

Glasgow, R. E., Sorensen, G., & Corbett, K. (1992). Worksite smoking control activities: Prevalence and related worksite characteristics from the COMMIT study, 1990. *Preventive Medicine, 21*, 688–700.

Gross, J., Johnson, J., Sigler, L., & Stitzer, M. L. (1995). Dose effects of nicotine gum. *Addictive Behaviors, 20*, 371–381.

Haaga, D. A. F., & Stewart, B. L. (1992). Self-efficacy for recovery from a lapse after smoking cessation. *Journal of Consulting & Clinical Psychology, 60*, 24–28.

Hajek, P., Jackson, P., & Belcher, M. (1988). Long-term use of nicotine chewing gum. *Journal of the American Medical Association, 260*, 1593–1596.

Hall, S. M., Ginsberg, D., & Jones, R. T. (1986). Smoking cessation and weight gain. *Journal of Consulting and Clinical Psychology, 54*, 342–346.

Hall, S. M., Munoz, R., Reus, V., & Sees, K. (1993). Nicotine, negative affect and depression. *Journal of Consulting and Clinical Psychology, 61*, 761–767.

Higgins, E. T. (1987). Self-discrepancy: A theory relating to self and affect. *Journal of Personality and Social Psychology, 94*, 319–340.

Hodge, F. S., Cummings, S., Fredericks, L., Kipnis, P., Williams, M., & Teehee, K. (1995). Prevalence of smoking among adult American Indian clinic users in Northern California. *Preventive Medicine, 24*, 441–446.

Hollis, J. F., Lichenstein, E., Vogt, T. M., Stevens, V. J., & Biglan, A. (1993). Nurse-assisted counseling for smokers in primary care. *Annals of Internal Medicine,*

118, 521–525.

Hughes, J. R. (1994). An algorithm for smoking cessation. *Archives of Family Medicine, 3*, 280–285.

Hughes, J. R., Gust, S. W., Keenan, R. M., Fenwick, J. W., & Healey, M. L. (1989). Nicotine vs. placebo gum in general medical practice. *Journal of the American Medical Association, 261*, 1300–1305.

Hughes, J. R., & Hatsukami, D. (1985). Short-term effects of nicotine gum. In J. Grabowski & S. M. Hall (Eds.), *Pharmacological adjuncts in smoking cessation* (NIDA Research Monograph No. 53), (pp. 68–82). Rockville, MD: National Institute on Drug Abuse.

Hughes, J. R., Hatsukami, D. K., Pickens, R. W., Krahn, D., Malin, S., & Lukmic, A. (1984). Effect of nicotine on the tobacco withdrawal syndrome. *Psychopharmacology, 83*, 82–87.

Hurt, R. D., Dale, L. C., Fredrickson, P. A., Caldwell, C. C., Lee, G. A., Offord, K. P., Lauger, G. G., Marusic, Z., Neese, L. W., & Lundberg, T. G. (1994). Nicotine patch therapy for smoking cessation combined with physician advice and nurse follow-up. *Journal of the American Medical Association, 271*, 595–600.

Janis, I. L., & Mann, L. (1977). *Decision making: A psychological analysis of conflict, choice and commitment*. New York: Collier Macmillan.

Johnson, K. W., Anderson, N. B., Bastida, E., Kramer, B. J., Williams, D., & Wong, M. (1995). Panel II: Macrosocial and environmental influences on minority health. *Health Psychology, 14*, 601–612.

Kabat, G. C., Morabia, A., & Wynder, E. L. (1991). Comparison of smoking habits of Blacks and Whites in a case-control study. *American Journal of Public Health, 81*, 1483–1486.

Kamark, T., & Lichtenstein, E. (1988). Program adherence and coping strategies as predictors of success in a smoking treatment program. *Health Psychology, 7*, 557–574.

King, T. K., Marcus, B. H., & Borrelli, B. (1996, March). *Evaluation of recruitment strategies to increase participation rates of underserved women in smoking cessation treatment*. Paper presented at the 17th annual meeting of the Society for Behavioral Medicine/Fourth International Congress of Behavioral Medicine, Washington, DC.

Kornitzer, M., Boutsen, M., Dramaix, M., Thijs, J., & Gustavsson, G. (1995). Combined use of nicotine patch and gum in smoking cessation: A placebo-controlled clinical trial. *Preventive Medicine, 24*, 41–47.

Kottke, T. E., Defriese, G. H., & Brekke, M. L. (1988). Attributes of successful smoking interventions in medical practice. A meta-analysis of 39 controlled trials. *Journal of the American Medical Association, 259*, 2883–2889.

Kviz, F. J., Crittenden, K. S., & Warnecke, R. B. (1992). Factors associated with nonparticipation among registrants for a self-help, community-based smoking cessation intervention. *Addictive Behaviors, 17*, 533–542.

Lacey, L. (1993). Cancer prevention and early detection strategies for reaching underserved urban, low-income Black women: Barriers and objectives. *Cancer, 72*, 1078–1083.

Lacey, L. P., Manfredi, C., Balch, G., Warnecke, R. B., Allen, K., & Edwards, C. (1993). Social support in smoking cessation among Black women in Chicago public housing. *Public Health Reports, 108*, 387–394.

Lam, W., Sze, P. C., Sacks, H. S., & Chalmers, T. C. (1987). Meta-analysis of randomized controlled trials of nicotine gum. *Lancet, 2*, 27–30.

Lando, H. A., Pechacek, T. F., Pirie, P. L., Murray, D. M., Mittelmark, M.B., Lichtenstein, E., Nothwehr, F., & Gray, C. (1995). Changes in adult cigarette smoking in the Minnesota Heart Health Program. *American Journal of Public Health, 85*, 201–208.

Law, M., & Teng, J. L. (1995). An analysis of the effectiveness of interventions intended to help people stop smoking. *Archives of Internal Medicine, 155*, 1933–1941.

Lichtenstein, E., & Glasgow, R. (1992). Smoking cessation: What have we learned over the past decade? *Journal of Consulting and Clinical Psychology, 60*, 518–527.

Locke, E. A., Frederick, E., Lee, C., & Bobko, P. (1984). Effect of self-efficacy, goals, and task strategies on task performance. *Journal of Applied Psychology, 69*, 241–251.

Locke, E. A., Shaw, K. N., Saari, L. M., & Latham, G. P. (1981). Goal setting and task performance: 1969–1980. *Psychological Bulletin, 90*, 125–152.

Manfredi, C., Lacey, L., Warnecke, R., & Buis, M. (1992). Smoking-related behavior, beliefs, and social environment of young Black women in subsidized public housing in Chicago. *American Journal of Public Health, 82*, 267–272.

Manley, M. W., Epps, R. P., & Glynn, T. J. (1992). The clinician's role in promoting smoking cessation among clinic patients. *Medical Clinics of North America, 76*, 477–494.

Marcus, B. H., Albrecht, A. E., Niaura, R. S., Taylor, E. R., Simkin, L. R., Feder, S. I., Abrams, D. B., & Thompson, P. D. (1995). Exercise enhances the maintenance of smoking cessation in women. *Addictive Behaviors, 20*, 87–92.

Marcus, B. H., King, T. K., Pinto, B. M., & Albrecht, A. E. (1994, March). Barriers to women's participation in smoking cessation treatment. Poster presented at the 16th annual meeting of the Society for Behavioral Medicine, San Diego, CA.

Marlatt, G. A., & Gordon, J. R. (1985). *Relapse prevention*. New York: Guilford.

Marlatt, G. A., & Tapert, S. F. (1993). Harm reduction: Reducing the risks of addictive behaviors. In J. S. Baer, G. A. Marlatt, & R. McMahon (Eds.), *Addictive behaviors across the lifespan*. Newbury Park, CA: Sage.

Miller, W. R., & Rollnick, S. (1991). *Motivational interviewing: preparing people to change addictive behavior*. New York, NY: Guilford.

Monti, P. M., Rohsenow, D. J., & Colby, S. M., Abrams, D. B. (1995). Smoking among alcoholics during and after treatment: Implications for models, treatment, strategies and policy. In J. B. Fertig (Ed.), *Alcohol and tobacco: From basic science to policy*. NIAAA Alcohol Research Monograph, pp. 187–206. Bethesda, MD: NIH, National Institute on Alcohol Abuse and Alcoholism.

Nevid, J. S., & Javier, R. A. (1993, August). Factors predicting participation in a minority-specific intervention program for Hispanic smokers. Paper presented at the 101st meeting of the American Psychological Association, Toronto, Canada.

Nevid, J. S., Javier, R. A., & Moulton, J. L. (1996). Factors predicting participation attrition in a community-based, culturally-specific smoking-cessation program for Hispanic smokers. *Health Psychology, 15*, 226–229.

Niaura, R. S., Goldstein, M. G., & Abrams, D. B. (1994). Matching high- and low-dependence smokers to self-help treatment with or without nicotine replacement. *International Journal of Preventive Medicine, 23*, 1–8.

Nides, M., Rand, C., Dolce, J., Murray, R., O'Hara, P., Voelker, H., & Connett, J. (1994). Weight gain as a function of smoking cessation and 2-mg nicotine gum use among middle-aged smokers with mild lung impairment in the first 2 years of the Lung Health Study. *Health Psychology, 13*, 354–361.

Ockene, J. K. (1987). Physician-delivered interventions for smoking cessation: Strategies for increasing effectiveness. *Preventive Medicine, 16*, 723–737.

Ockene, J. K., Kristeller, J., Goldberg, R., Amick, T. L., Penelope, P. S., Hermer, D., Quirk, M., & Kalan, K. (1991). Increasing the efficacy of physician-delivered smoking interventions: A randomized clinical trial. *Journal of General Internal Medicine, 6*, 1–8.

Ockene, J. K., Kristeller, J., Pbert, L., Hebert, J. R., Luippold, R., Goldberg, R. J., Landon, & Kalan, K. (1994). The physician-delivered smoking intervention projects: Can short-term interventions produce long-term effects for a general outpatient population? *Health Psychology, 13*, 278–281.

Ockene, J. K., Quirk, M., Goldberg, R. J., Kristeller, J., Donnelly, G., Kalan, K. L., Gould, B., Greene, H., Harrison-Atlas, R., Pease, J., Pickens, S., & Williams, J. (1988). A residents' training program for the development of smoking intervention skills. *Archives of Internal Medicine, 148*, 1039–1045.

Orleans, C. T. (1993). Treating nicotine dependence in medical settings: A stepped care model. In C. T. Orleans & J. Slade (Eds.), *Nicotine dependence: Principles and management*. New York: Oxford University Press.

Orleans, C. T., Schoenbach, V. J., Salmon, M. A., Strecher, V. J., Kalsbeek, W., Quade, D., Brooks, E. F., Konrad, T. R., Blackmon, C., & Watts, C. D. (1989). A survey of smoking and quitting patterns among black Americans. *American Journal of Public Health, 79*, 176–81.

Orleans, C. T., Schoenbach, V. J., Wagner, E., Quade, D., Salmon, M. A., Pearson, D. C., Fiedler, J., Porter, C. Q., & Kaplan, B. H. (1991). Self-help quit smoking interventions: Effects of self-help materials, social support instructions and telephone counseling. *Journal of Consulting and Clinical Psychology, 3*, 439–448.

Prochaska, J. O., & DiClemente, C. C. (1983). Stages and processes of self-change of smoking: Toward an integrative model of change. *Journal of Consulting and Clinical Psychology, 51*, 390–395.

Prochaska, J. O., DiClemente, C. C., Velicer, W. F., & Rossi, J. S. (1993). Standardized, individualized, interactive, and personalized self-help programs for smoking cessation. *Health Psychology, 12*, 399–405.

Prochaska, J. O., & Goldstein, M. G. (1991). Process of smoking cessation: Implications for clinicians. *Clinics in Chest Medicine, 12*, 727–735.

Rimer, B. K., Strecher, V. J., Keintz, M. K., & Engstrom, P. F. (1986). A survey of physicians' views and practices on patient education for smoking cessation. *Preventive Medicine, 15*, 92–98.

Rimer, B. K., Orleans, C. T., Fleisher, L., Cristinzio, S., Resch, N., Telepchak, J., & Keintz, M. K. (1994). Does tailoring matter? The impact of a tailored guide on ratings and short-term smoking-related outcomes for older smokers. *Health Education Research, 9*, 69–84.

Rybarczyk, B., & Auerbach, S. (1990). Reminiscence interviews as stress management interventions for older patients undergoing surgery. *The Gerontologist, 30*, 522–528.

Sachs, D. P. (1989). Nicotine polacrilex: Practical use requirements. *Current Pulmonology, 10*, 141–158.

Sachs, D. P., Sawe, U., & Leischow, S. J. (1993). Effectiveness of a 16-hour transdermal nicotine patch in a medical practice setting, without intensive group counseling. *Archives of Internal Medicine, 153*, 1881–1890.

Schwartz, J. L. (1987). *Review and dvaluation of smoking cessation methods: United States and Canada, 1978–1985*. (CDC Publication No. 79–8369). Bethesda, MD: Public Health Service.

Shadel, W. G., & Mermelstein, R. (1996). Individual differences in self-concept among smokers attempting to quit: Validation and predictive utility of measures of the Smoker Self-concept and Abstainer Self-concept. *Annals of Behavioral Medicine, 18*, 151–156.

Shea, S., Stein, A. D., Basch, C. E., Lantigua, R., Maylahn, C., Strogatz, D. S., & Novick, L. (1991). Independent associations of educational attainment and ethnicity with behavioral risk factors for cardiovascular disease. *American Journal of Epidemiology, 134*, 567–582.

Shervington, D. O. (1986). Attitudes and practices of African-American women regarding cigarette smoking: Implications for interventions. *Journal of the National Medical Association, 86*, 337–343.

Shiffman, S. (1993). Smoking cessation treatment: Any progress? *Journal of Consulting and Clinical Psychology, 61*, 718–722.

Stapleton, J. A., Russell, M. A., Feyerabend, C., Wiseman, S. M., Gustavsson, G., Sawe, U., & Wiseman, D. (1995). Dose effects and predictors of outcome in a randomized trial of transdermal nicotine patches in general practice. *Addiction, 90*, 31–42.

Strecher, V. J., Kreuter, M., Den Boer, D., Kobrin, S., Hospers, H. J., & Skinner, C. S. (1994). The effects of computer-tailored smoking cessation messages in family practice settings. *The Journal of Family Practice, 39*, 262–268.

Sutton, S. (1996). Can "stages of change" provide guidance in the treatment of addictions? A critical examination of Prochaska and DiClemente's model. In G. Edwards & C. Dare (Eds.), *Psychotherapy, psychological treatments and the addictions* (pp. 189–205). Cambridge: Cambridge University Press.

Tonnesen, P., Norregaard, J., Simonsen, K., & Sawe, U. (1991). A double-blind trial of a 16-hour transdermal nicotine patch. *New England Journal of Medicine, 325*, 311–315.

U.S. Bureau of the Census. *1984 U.S. Census*. Washington, DC: U.S. Government Printing Office.

U.S. Bureau of the Census. (1991). The Hispanic population in the U.S.: March 1991 (Current Population Reports, Series P-20, No. 455). Washington, DC: U.S. Government Printing Office.

U.S. Department of Health and Human Services. (1989). *Reducing the health consequences of smoking: A Report of the Surgeon General* (DHHS Publication No. CDC–89–8411). Washington, DC: U.S. Government Printing Office.

Velicer, W. F., DiClemente, C. C., Prochaska, J. O., & Brandenburg, N. (1985). A decisional balance measure of predicting smoking cessation. *Journal of Personality and Social Psychology, 48*, 1279–1289.

Velicer, W., Fava, J. L., Prochaska, J. O., Abrams, D. B., Emmons, K. M., & Pierce, J. P. (1995). Distribution of smokers by stage in three representative samples. *Preventive Medicine, 24*, 401–411.

Velicer, W. F., Prochaska, J. O., Rossi, J. S., & Snow, M. G. (1992). Assessing outcome in smoking cessation studies. *Psychological Bulletin, 111*, 23–41.

Weinstein, N. (1993). Testing four competing theories of health-protective behavior. *Health Psychology, 12*, 324–333.

Westman, E. C., Levin, E. D., & Rose, J. E. (1993). The nicotine patch in smoking cessation. A randomized trial with telephone counseling. *Archives of Internal Medicine, 153*, 1917–1923.

7

Promoting Dietary Change

Barbara S. McCann and Viktor E. Bovbjerg

Chronic diseases are the leading cause of death and disability in the United States, accounting for greater morbidity and mortality than acute infectious diseases and deaths from injury or other traumatic causes. Diet is assuming increasing importance in the prevention and management of a variety of diseases (Institute of Medicine Committee on Dietary Guidelines Implementation, 1991; National Research Council Committee on Diet and Health, 1989). The most prevalent conditions in which diet plays a prominent role include cardiovascular diseases, diabetes, and cancers. These conditions rank high among the 15 leading causes of death in the United States (National Center for Health Statistics (NCHS), 1994).

This chapter provides a brief overview of the chronic illnesses in which dietary change assumes a role in prevention or management. Interventions which promote dietary change have targeted patients seen in groups or individually (e.g., Bourn, Mann, McSkimming, Waldron, & Wishart, 1994), in worksites (e.g., Hebert et al., 1993), and entire communities (e.g. Carleton, Lasater, Assaf, Feldman, & McKinlay, 1995; Winkleby, Flora, & Kraemer,

Preparation of this chapter was supported in part by a grant from the National Institute of Diabetes, Digestive, and Kidney Diseases (DK-35816, Clinical Nutrition Research Unit).

1994). While a review of all of these intervention targets is beyond the scope of this chapter, we will examine illustrative examples of interventions which promote dietary change at the level of the individual and at the community level. The more promising approaches to promoting dietary change in individuals and communities will be identified.

THE ROLE OF DIET IN CHRONIC DISEASE

Much of the evidence for the role of diet in chronic diseases has received a comprehensive review by the Committee on Diet and Health of the National Research Council's Food and Nutrition Board. In the *Diet and Health* Report (National Research Council Committee on Diet and Health, 1989), this committee concluded there was strong evidence for a role of diet in atherosclerotic cardiovascular diseases and hypertension. Overwhelming evidence implicates excess caloric intake in obesity and non-insulin-dependent diabetes mellitus (NIDDM). The Committee noted modest evidence to support a role of diet in certain cancers (esophagus, stomach, large bowel, breast, lung, and prostate).

Atherosclerotic cardiovascular diseases include coronary heart disease (CHD), stroke, and peripheral arterial disease. In its efforts to promote the prevention of CHD, The National Cholesterol Education Program (NCEP) Expert Panel on Detection, Evaluation, and Treatment of High Blood Cholesterol in Adults (1993) has recommended that a dietary approach to cholesterol lowering be taken in individuals with low density lipoprotein (LDL) cholesterol levels exceeding 130 mg/dL and either CHD or two additional CHD risk factors (approximately corresponding total cholesterol above 200 mg/dL), and further, that otherwise healthy individuals with LDL cholesterol exceeding 160 mg/dL (total cholesterol of approximately 240 mg/dL) should modify their diet. The NCEP recommends a Step I diet initially, which includes intake of less than 30% of calories as total fat, 10% as saturated fat, and less than 300 mg/day of dietary cholesterol. If the response to diet is inadequate, the Step II diet is recommended: reduction of saturated fat intake to less than 7% of calories, and dietary cholesterol intake less than 200 mg/day. There is considerable evidence that these dietary changes can reduce blood cholesterol levels by as much as 10–20% (Grundy & Denke, 1990). The American Heart Association also advocates the Step II diet as a means of preventing myocardial infarction and death in individuals with coronary and other vascular diseases (S. C. Smith et al., 1995).

The National High Blood Pressure Education Program Working Group (1993) recommended that the public lose weight, reduce sodium intake, and reduce consumption of alcohol to prevent the development of hypertension. It is estimated that over half of hypertensive patients are salt-sensitive, particularly African Americans and the elderly and will respond to reductions in sodium intake with decreased blood pressure (Purdon et al., 1993). Recent clinical trials indicate that weight loss through caloric restriction, often in combination with sodium reductions and reductions in alcohol use, can produce beneficial changes in blood pressure among hypertensives (Elmer et al., 1995; Stamler et al., 1987), can decrease the need for antihypertensive medication (Davis et al., 1993), and can produce reductions in blood pressure among individuals with borderline elevated blood pressure levels (Hypertension Prevention Trial Research Group, 1990). It was recently reported that dietary changes among hypertensives were as effective in reducing left ventricular mass as dietary changes plus the addition of pharmacological approaches to blood pressure reduction (Liebson et al., 1995).

Over 4% of the U.S. population has diagnosed diabetes (Harris, 1995). The majority of these cases of diabetes are non-insulin dependent diabetes mellitus (NIDDM), or Type II diabetes. Obesity is a risk factor for the development of NIDDM, and dietary intervention figures prominently in its control. The American Diabetes Association recommends that individuals with NIDDM consume up to 55–60% of calories as carbohydrates, and limit fat intake to less than 30% of calories, with weight loss as the primary goal in obese patients (American Diabetes Association, 1992).

In addition to atherosclerotic disease, hypertension, and diabetes, diet plays a role in the prevention and management of a number of other diseases. Diet has been implicated in several forms of cancer (Garfinkel, 1985), although the supporting data are more equivocal (American Medical Association Council on Scientific Affairs, 1993; National Research Council Committee on Diet and Health, 1989). Nonetheless, a multicenter NIH study of fat reduction to decrease breast cancer risk in women is underway (Henderson, 1995). Osteoporosis is common among postmenopausal women and the elderly. Osteoporosis is characterized by decreased bone mass, which leaves afflicted individuals susceptible to fractures. There is some weak evidence that high calcium intake may help prevent osteoporosis (National Research Council Committee on Diet and Health, 1989). A recent report from the Framingham Study found that consumption of fruits and vegetables appears to lessen the likelihood of stroke in men (Gillman et al., 1995). Chronic renal disease requires lifelong changes in protein consumption and fluid intake (Caggiula & Milas, 1993), and there is some evidence that such changes delay decline in renal function in individuals with moderate renal insufficiency (Klahr et al., 1994). Phenylalanine hydroxylase deficiency phenylketonuria (PKU) occurs in only 1 of 10,000 births in the U.S., but widespread screening at birth is practiced because it is manageable through diet, and left untreated causes brain damage, motor deficits, and mental retardation. Excess phenylalaline in the diet is avoided through limiting protein intake. At one time, dietary restrictions were deemed necessary only until approximately 6–10 years of age. However, it has been shown that optimal management of PKU requires a lifetime of dietary management, and is particularly important during pregnancy (Potocnik & Widhalm, 1994).

Finally, obesity is associated with a number of diseases, including hypertension, hyperlipidemia, coronary heart disease, diabetes, gallbladder disease, respiratory disease, cancer, gout, and arthritis (Pi-Sunyer, 1993). Weight loss is a common goal in the management of many chronic diseases (D'Eramo-Melkus & Hagan, 1991). Data from the National Health and Nutrition Examination Surveys (NHANES) indicate that 24.2% of men and 27.1 % of women ages 20–74 years are overweight (Kuczmarski, 1992), defined as a body mass index exceeding the 85th percentile. The usual dietary approach to weight loss is caloric restriction, but most studies report significant regaining of weight among successful dieters (Wadden, 1993b).

RECOMMENDED DIETARY GUIDELINES

From the foregoing overview, it should be evident that many of the dietary changes recommended for preventing and managing illnesses are similar, emphasizing weight loss and the reduction of fat intake. The accumulated evidence regarding diet and chronic disease has led to the development of a number of recommendations and guidelines for the American public. Recommendations from *Diet and Health* (National Research Council Committee on Diet and Health, 1989) and the U.S. Departments of Agriculture and Health and Human Services (U.S. Department of Agriculture and U.S. Department of Health and Human Services, 1995) are presented in Table 7.1 and Table 7.2. These recommendations have a number of striking similarities, including emphasis on lowered fat and cholesterol intake; emphasis on fruits, vegetables, and complex carbohydrates; limited alcohol consumption for individuals who drink; limited salt intake; and maintenance of appropriate body weight.

ADHERENCE TO DIETARY RECOMMENDATIONS

It is difficult for people to make dietary changes and maintain them (Brownell & Cohen, 1995a). Recent reviews and studies confirm that initial adherence and subsequent maintenance are difficult to achieve in the dietary management of diabetes (Glasgow, McCaul, & Schafer, 1987), hyperlipidemia (McCann, Retzlaff, Dowdy, Walden, & Knopp, 1990), obesity (Wadden, 1993b), hypertension (Elmer, Grimm, Flack, & Laing, 1991; Stevens et al., 1993), renal disease (Kluge, Wildberger, & Wallmeier, 1989),

TABLE 7.1 Summary of Recent Dietary Guidelines for Americans

Recommendations from the Diet and Health Report

1. Reduce total fat intake to 30% or less of calories. Reduce saturated fatty acid intake to less than 10% of calories and the intake of cholesterol to less than 300 mg daily. The intake of fat and cholesterol can be reduced by substituting fish, poultry without skin, lean meats, and low- or nonfat dairy products for fatty meats and whole-milk dairy products; by choosing more vegetables, fruits, cereals, and legumes; and by limiting oils, fat, egg yolks, and fried or other fatty foods. (p. 13)
2. Every day eat five or more servings of a combination of vegetables and fruits, especially green and yellow vegetables and citrus fruits. Also, increase intake of starches and other complex carbohydrates by eating six or more daily servings of a combination of breads, cereals, and legumes. (p. 15)
3. Maintain protein intake at moderate levels. (p. 15)
4. Balance food intake and physical activity to maintain appropriate body weight. (p. 16)
5. The committee does not recommend alcohol consumption. For those who drink alcoholic beverages, the committee recommends limiting consumption to the equivalent of less than 1 ounce of pure alcohol in a single day. This is the equivalent of two cans of beer, two small glasses of wine, or two average cocktails. Pregnant women should avoid alcoholic beverages. (p. 16)
6. Limit total daily intake of salt (sodium chloride) to 6 g or less. Limit the use of salt in cooking and avoid adding it to food at the table. Salty, highly processed salty, salt-preserved, and salt-pickled foods should be consumed sparingly. (p. 16)
7. Maintain adequate calcium intake. (p. 17)
8. Avoid taking dietary supplements in excess of the RDA in any one day. (p. 17)
9. Maintain an optimal intake of fluoride, particularly during the years of primary and secondary tooth formation and growth. (p. 17)

Note. Adapted from *Diet and Health: Implications for Reducing Chronic Diease Risk* (pp. 13–17), by the Committee on Diet and Health, Food and Nutrition Board, Commission on Life Sciences, National Research Council, 1989, Washington, DC: National Academy Press.

TABLE 7.2 Dietary Guidelines for Americans

1. Eat a variety of foods.
2. Maintain healthy weight.
3. Choose a diet low in fat, saturated fat, and cholesterol.
4. Choose a diet with plenty of vegetables, fruits, and grain products.
5. Use sugars only in moderation.
6. Use salt and sodium only in moderation.
7. If you drink alcoholic beverages, do so only in moderation.

Note. Adapted from *Nutrition and Your Health-Dietary Guidelines for Americans* (4th ed.) (Home and Garden Bulletin No. 232) by U.S. Department of Agriculture and U.S. Department of Health and Human Services. Washington, DC: Authors.

and maternal PKU (Waisbren, Hamilton, St. James, Shiloh & Levy, 1995).

Precise estimates of the degree to which individuals are able to maintain long-term adherence to dietary changes are difficult to obtain (McCann, Retzlaff, Walden, & Knopp, 1990). Unreliability of self-reported food intake contributes to the lack of definitive data on the ability of people to adhere to dietary advice (Lowe, Kopyt, & Buchwald, 1996). Women appear to underreport dietary intake more than do men, and underreporting is also associated with greater adiposity (Johnson, Goran, & Poehlman, 1994). High levels of social desirability, or the tendency to present oneself favorably and as a follower of social norms, also has been linked to underreporting of food intake (Hebert, Clemow, Pbert, Ockene, & Ockene, 1995). Data on hypertensives comparing self-reported sodium intake with urinary excretion of sodium indicate that hypertensive patients frequently underreport salt intake (Forster, Jeffery, VanNatta, & Pirie, 1990; Wing, Caggiula, Nowalk, Koeske, Lee, & Langford, 1984).

PROMOTING DIETARY CHANGE IN INDIVIDUALS

A review of numerous research studies (Elmer et al., 1995; Hypertension Prevention Trial Research Group, 1990; McCann, Retzlaff, Dowdy et al., 1990; McNabb et al., 1993; Milas et al., 1995), overviews (Brownell & Cohen, 1995b; Foreyt & Goodrick, 1993; Wadden, 1993a), and treatment materials (Brownell, 1990; Dowdy et al., 1990; LeBow, 1989), reveals a number of common components designed to promote dietary change in individuals and maximize maintenance.

The cornerstone of all dietary interventions with individuals is nutrition education. This often consists of nutritionist-led individual or group sessions covering recipe modification, grocery shopping, and concrete recommendations regarding foods to eat and foods to avoid (e.g., Elmer et al., 1995; Walden, Retzlaff, Buck, McCann, & Knopp, 1996). Sometimes the health care provider, rather than the patient, is targeted for nutrition education. One such example is the training of primary care physicians in the Worcester Area Trial for Counseling in Hyperlipidemia (Ockene et al., 1995).

Identifying patient readiness to make dietary changes may be useful in planning interventions. The stage model of behavior change developed by Prochaska and DiClemente (Prochaska, DiClemente, & Norcross, 1992) proposes that behavior change occurs in stages: precontemplation (not considering behavior change); contemplation (thinking about behavior change); preparation (planning to change); action (initiating behavior change); and maintenance of behavior change. An individual may move from any stage along this process to an earlier or later stage. We have found that the stages-of-change model predicts whether men and women with elevated cholesterol levels will join a dietary intervention trial (McCann et al., 1996).

The initial assessment of dietary intake, before initiating a dietary intervention, enables the clinician to determine the individual participant's "starting point". As noted previously, though, underreporting of intake is the rule, rather than the exception (Schoeller, 1995). Traditional methods of dietary assessment include multiday food diaries, 24-hour recalls, and food frequency questionnaires. On the basis of this assessment, individually tailored goals can be established.

Goals may be based on current recommendations for specific conditions, such as the National Cholesterol Education Program guidelines, or general guidelines such as the *Dietary Guidelines for Americans*. When weight loss is a goal of the intervention, specific calorie and fat intakes may be recommended based on ideal body weight, desired percentage of weight loss, or the participant's desired target. Other goals may target maximum intakes of calories, fats, sodium, or protein. In the National Cancer Institute's "5 a Day" program, participants are simply encouraged to consume 5 (or more) servings of fruits and vegetables per day (Heimendinger & Van Duyn, 1995).

Self-monitoring of dietary intake is an essential component of programs promoting dietary change. Self-monitoring generally takes one of two forms: recording of certain macronutrients, such as grams of fat (e.g., White et al., 1992) calories (e.g., Smith & Wing, 1991), sodium (e.g., Elmer et al., 1995), or protein content (e.g., Milas et al., 1995); or an exchange system, in which participants are given a recommended daily number of servings of various food groups, along with examples of serving sizes (e.g., Knopp et al., 1996).

Stimulus control training refers to limiting exposure to settings or situations which are associated with eating inappropriate foods or inappropriate quantities. A number of studies have used stimulus control techniques as part of the overall treatment package (e.g., McNabb et al., 1993; Wing et al., 1988). Generally, stimulus control training is used early in treatment.

Many programs employ problem-solving training to facilitate long-term maintenance of dietary changes (e.g., McNabb et al., 1993; Stevens et al., 1993; Wing et al., 1988). Problem-solving training generally entails clinician- or patient-generated descriptions of scenarios in which adherence may be problematic, followed by discussion of ways in which adherence can be maintained in such situations. An important element of problem-solving training is to encourage participants to use these skills whenever they encounter situations which threaten adherence.

According to the Relapse Prevention Model (Marlatt & George, 1984), individuals maintain perceived control over behavior until they encounter a high-risk situation which threatens control and increases the risk of relapse. Inclusion of relapse prevention training has become increasingly common in dietary interventions (e.g., Elmer et al., 1995; McCann, Retzlaff, Dowdy et al., 1990; Stevens et al., 1993; Wing et al., 1988). Within interventions, relapse prevention training consists of assisting participants in identifying personally salient high-risk situations, and developing strategies for dealing with such situations. Encouraging participants to regard lapses in dietary adherence as opportunities to avoid future lapses is a key component of the training.

Social support, and support from spouses, is an important factor in dietary adherence. Active inclusion of the patient's spouse or the household cook in treatment programs has been a feature of dietary interventions for hyperlipidemia (Knopp et al., 1996; Walden et al., 1996) and obesity (Black, Gleser, & Kooyers, 1990). Individuals with high levels of support from their spouses are more likely to attain their dietary goals than those with weak levels of spouse support (Bovbjerg et al., 1995). Changing the diet of one family member may have beneficial effects on other family members as well (Shattuck, White, & Kristal, 1992).

Self-efficacy refers to the belief that one can execute a certain behavior required to produce particular outcomes (Bandura, 1991), and has been shown to predict the ability to initiate and maintain changes in a variety of health-related behaviors. Self-efficacy predicts extent of weight loss in overweight individuals (Bernier & Avard, 1986; Edell, Edington, Herd, O'Brien, & Witkin, 1987; Forster & Jeffery, 1986), extent of lipid lowering in hyperlipidemia (McCann et al., 1995), and dietary adherence in NIDDM (Skelly, Marshall, Haughey, Davis, & Dunford, 1995). The most critical components to enhance self-efficacy for long-term maintenance include relapse prevention and problem solving. During the active phases of the intervention, participants should be encouraged to test new skills (e.g., ordering low-fat food in a restaurant) to enhance their confidence in their ability to maintain dietary changes.

Finally, ongoing program contact is associated with better maintenance of dietary changes. Wing and colleagues have obtained good results by having Type II diabetic patients attend weekly meetings for 1 year to facilitate weight loss and maintenance (Smith & Wing, 1991; Wing, Blair, Marcus, Epstein, & Harvey, 1994). Perri's studies on weight loss maintenance in obese patients (generally, these patients are not diabetic) support the use of extended contact in maintaining weight loss (Perri, Sears, & Clark, 1993). A variety of approaches to achieving extended contact have been used: telephone contact, mail contact, contact in person, and even having patients form their own support networks for ongoing monitoring of weight loss (peer support). These studies generally make use of extensive periods of biweekly (e.g., every other week) therapist contact to achieve weight-loss maintenance (Perri et al., 1993).

RESULTS OF INDIVIDUAL-LEVEL INTERVENTIONS

A number of dietary intervention results for a variety of chronic conditions have appeared since the first edition of *The Handbook of Health Behavior Change* was published. Programs aimed at hypertension prevention and management through nonpharmacologic means have generally emphasized weight reduction, although reductions in sodium and alcohol intake are also encouraged. Initial weight reductions of approximately 5 kg are achieved, with gradual increases in weight during extended periods of follow-up (e.g., Davis et al., 1993; Elmer et al., 1995; Neaton et al., 1993). Decreases in blood pressure are on the order of 8-9 mmHg systolic and 7-8 mmHg diastolic (Applegate et al., 1992; Elmer et al., 1995; Neaton et al., 1993). Trials aimed at hypertension prevention (rather than management) have achieved modest but encouraging results in promoting weight loss and achieving blood pressure reductions (Hypertension Prevention Trial Research Group, 1990; Stevens et al., 1993).

Reductions in fat intake, generally expressed as percent of calories from fat, have resulted in modest improvements in lipids in a number of studies (Henkin, Garber, Osterlund, & Darnell, 1992; Knopp et al., 1996; Walden et al., 1996; Wood, Stefanick, Williams, & Haskell, 1991). Weight loss in recent studies of diabetics has ranged from 4–14 kg (Eriksson & Lindgärde, 1991; McNabb et al., 1993; Wing et al., 1994). Maintenance of initial weight loss has been difficult, however, in virtually all studies to date.

A 2-year randomized feasibility study provides an illustrative example of how well women can adhere to dietary recommendations to prevent breast cancer (Insull et al., 1990). Women randomized to a low-fat diet (20% of calories from fat) were able to reduce the percentage of calories from fat to 20.9% (from 39.1%) at 6 months, and sustain these reductions at 12 and 24 months. Their initial weight reduction averaged 3.1 kg; this remained stable through 12 months, but by 24 months, weight increased by 1.4 kg.

Individual-level dietary interventions, many of which are aimed at weight loss, produce initial decreases in body weight and improvements in other biological parameters of interest, such as lipids and glucose tolerance. However, these improvements are generally not sustained during long-term follow-up. Interestingly, where food records have provided more direct evidence of dietary adherence, initial reductions in fat and calorie intake appear to be sustained. This may reflect underreporting of food intake.

Individual-level interventions may be most suitable for well-educated individuals, and it has been argued that these interventions focus inappropriately on individual responsibility for acquiring and maintaining poor health practices (Green & Raeburn, 1990). Community interventions, which typically are developed in cooperation with communities and employ many channels of communication, may stand a better chance at reaching all segments of the community. Furthermore, institutional and environmental changes promoting healthful diets may be more likely to have equal effects across social strata.

Finally, individual-level dietary interventions seldom address dietary change issues in the population at large (Susser, 1995). Individual interventions typically recruit highly motivated and often high-risk individuals. Large reductions in individual risk factors can be brought about this way, but the extent to which these subjects' experience generalizes to the community as a whole is very limited.

Community interventions promote dietary changes among all residents of a given community. Traditional definitions of community have focused on geography and physical proximity, while taking for granted common social and cultural bonds among members of the community. A broader definition emphasizes social ties, defining community as " a group of people sharing values and institutions" (Thompson & Kinne, 1990). The term "community" can thus be applied to many different settings, including traditional geopolitically defined areas, worksites, churches, and even well-organized and purposeful Internet newsgroups. In this section, we will describe community interventions to reduce risk of cancer and cardiovascular disease through dietary change. We will also discuss the special issues involved in community-level interventions carried out at worksites and other organizations.

PROMOTING DIETARY CHANGE IN COMMUNITIES

The stimulation or activation of a community to make health-related change involves identification of an important health concern within the community, establishing the concern as an important target for action, instigating programs to modify the condition, and institutionalizing the mechanisms for maintaining the new status quo. At each step, the community should be intimately involved in the decision making and implementation, to build local commitment and "ownership" of the program.

It is useful to think of community organization as taking place in five sequential stages: 1) community analysis, 2) design-initiation, 3) implementation, 4) maintenance-consolidation, and 5) dissemination-reassessment (Bracht & Kingsbury, 1990). Community analysis identifies the needs, opportunities, and resources for community health programs, and has been referred to as needs assessment, needs mapping, and health education planning (Haglund, Weisbrod, & Bracht, 1990). Community analysis should focus on the assets communities have to initiate and maintain dietary programs, what social or physical barriers might hinder program development or implementation, the history of other health promotion efforts in the community, and setting priorities for intervention (Bracht & Kingsbury, 1990). While an idealized model of community analysis involves determining interventions based on community-identified needs, large-scale community projects are often initiated with the express purpose to intervene in a specific area (e.g., CHD prevention) by specific means (e.g., worksite intervention). The Minnesota Heart Health Program (MHHP) exemplifies the combination of community analysis with predetermined research goals. Despite being funded specifically for heart disease prevention, the MHHP allotted over 12 months for community analysis, laying the foundation for the education program that followed. The community analysis involved extensive assessment and involvement of community residents and organizations, and culminated in the initiation of community task forces and the organization of a community advisory board.

Unlike individual-level dietary interventions, community health promotion projects treat intact communities as the units of intervention. During design-initiation, one or more communities are designated as intervention (or education) communities, and one or more communities are designated as comparison communities. Investigators have attempted to circumvent the inability to randomly assign communities by matching similar communities or restricting the communities to assure similarity. Once selected, communities are assessed on disease states, biological and behavioral risk factors, and other important indices of health prior to the intervention. Following one or more baseline assessments, the intervention is initiated in the designated communities. Additional assessments take place during and after the intervention, and changes in the intervention communities are contrasted with changes in the comparison communities to determine whether the program has induced important levels of change above that expected due to chance or secular trends.

Implementation involves assuring that leaders, personnel, and programs are prepared, and carrying out the intervention as planned (Bracht & Kingsbury, 1990). Because resources are limited, even in well-funded community level projects, choices must be made among possible intervention strategies. Those selected must be relatively inexpensive per contact, be able to reach large segments of the community, and have the potential to change behavior (Finnegan, Murray, Kurth, & McCarthy, 1989). Programs emphasizing individual-level interventions may focus on the development and dissemination of class materials to individual community members through traditional health education methods. The Pawtucket Heart Health Program (PHHP) trained individual community members to modify their diets, relying on diffusion of behavior from trained individuals to others in their social networks (Elder et al., 1986).

The Coronary Risk Factor Study (CORIS) intervention included a high-intensity individual-level intervention for one of its communities, supplemented by a number of community-level activities (Rossouw et al., 1993). Programs emphasizing mass media and persuasion, such as the Stanford Five Cities Project (FCP) (Farquhar et al., 1990) and the MHHP (Luepker et al., 1994), may concentrate on the development of print and broadcast materials designed to reach many segments of the community and provide specific advice on dietary change.

Maintenance-consolidation reflects the degree to which communities maintain the programs, policies, and structures put in place during the intervention, and is one good measure of the effectiveness of the program implementation (Weisbrod et al., 1992). The maintenance of structures and organizations created during interventions is particularly important for community-level dietary change efforts. To have any meaningful impact on chronic diseases related to diet, community interventions must foster permanent changes in the communities in which they intervene.

In addition to assessing community-level mortality and morbidity and changes in biological and behavioral risk factors, community-level programs must assess the effectiveness of the implementation strategies used to encourage change (Weisbrod et al., 1992). Assessment must be made of both individual changes, using familiar tools such as food records and changes in blood pressure or cholesterol, and community changes, which demand tools developed specifically to measure changes at organizational or community levels. For example, in the MHHP, diet-related risk factors assessed included blood pressure and blood total and HDL cholesterol. Dietary habits were assessed, along with health behavior-specific behavioral intentions, knowledge, attitudes and beliefs. The FCP assessed dietary patterns using questionnaires which included items assessing perceived cardiovascular disease risk and self-efficacy for diet change (Winkleby et al., 1994). Dietary intake was also assessed in the FCP through 24-hour diet recalls. The Pawtucket HHP surveyed communities cross-sectionally, and collected information on CHD risk knowledge, health habits, blood pressure, and cholesterol (Carleton et al., 1995).

Because community interventions are generally conducted at the environmental as well as individual level, a number of community-level measures of program evaluation have been proposed, and termed environmental indicators (Cheadle, Wagner, Koepsell, Kristal, & Patrick, 1992). These tools are derived from observation of the physical, legal, social, and economic environments. Examples of potential community-level measures of dietary change include changes in food label regulations, changes in the percentage of grocery store shelves devoted to healthful foods, changes in prominence of healthful items in grocery store displays, or proportion of restaurants featuring and promoting healthful menu items (Cheadle et al., 1992).

The broad definition of community encompasses a wide variety of organizations, including worksites. Examples of worksite interventions include the Take Heart Project (Glasgow et al., 1994), a worksite-based clinical trial designed to reduce CHD risk, and the Wellworks prevention study, which promoted dietary changes and smoking cessation to improve CHD risk (Sorensen, Stoddard, Ockene, Hunt, & Youngstrom, 1996). Worksite interventions are often incorporated into larger community-level health promotion efforts. As part of larger efforts, worksites can assist with the sponsorship of community-wide events and reinforce dietary change messages conveyed in mass media (Sorensen, Glasgow, & Corbett, 1990). Representatives from worksites can participate in community needs assessments and implementation of programs. Many of the same considerations in conducting larger community-level interventions apply also to worksites. However, the social environment of worksites can vary considerably from that of larger communities. Often, employers and employees have different perspectives on worksite health policies, and the nature of the power relationship between employer and employee can influence the implementation and success of programs. For employers, health promotion efforts hold out the possibility of decreased health care costs, fewer sick days, improved morale and productivity, better retention of staff, and an enhanced corporate image. On the other hand, employers may be concerned about costs, liability, and diversion of employee attention from other pressing matters. Employees may perceive worksite programs as convenient and inexpensive compared to options in the larger community, and may enjoy programs more when friends and co-workers are involved as well. Employees may also view the program as interference in personal behavior, a diversion of attention from more important worksite health issues, potentially violating confidentiality, and difficult to schedule around work (Sorensen et al., 1990).

RESULTS OF COMMUNITY INTERVENTIONS

Changes in both behavioral and physiological measures of disease risk have been disappointing when intervention communities are placed alongside comparison communities. The North American trials described in this review have reported either few or no lasting clinically significant reductions in risk factors and disease endpoints. All of the interventions were able to influence CHD risk factor knowledge to some degree, but outcomes related to dietary changes, notably cholesterol levels, did not differ between intervention and control communities (Carleton et al., 1995; Farquhar et al., 1990; Luepker et al., 1994). Only the North Karelia project observed substantial reductions in CHD risk factors which were consistently greater in the intervention community than in the comparison community (Puska et al., 1979), but no significant differences in CHD morbidity and mortality were obtained. Given the short follow-up period and the relatively moderate changes in CHD risk observed in North Karelia as a result of the project, the initially null results may not be surprising.

In contrast to risk factor changes, indicators of program implementation suggest successful implementation of programs in general. For example, over 60% of residents in the intervention communities in the MHHP received risk factor assessments, education, or counseling. Virtually all primary care physicians took part in MHHP training programs, along with many other health professionals (Luepker et al., 1994).

CONCLUDING COMMENTS

Many of the interventions designed to promote dietary change in individuals contain similar components: nutrition education, assessing readiness, initial assessment of diet, establishing dietary goals, self-monitoring, stimulus control training, training in problem solving, relapse prevention training, enlisting social support (particularly from family members), enhancing self-efficacy, and ongoing contact with program staff. Several recent clinical trials on a variety of conditions report reasonably good initial changes in diet and physiologic outcomes using these strategies. However, long-term changes remain elusive, even though participants in clinical trials generally report maintaining their changes in diet.

Despite the initial success of many individual-level interventions, they are limited, first, by their inability to reach all individuals at risk, and, second, by the tendency for gains in risk factor reduction to be lost after exposure to social and environmental pressures away from healthful diets. Individual skills and behavior change can be accomplished through intense education strategies such as classes, but seldom reach large segments of the population, and do not address the social and physical environment which plays a large role in shaping dietary behavior (Finnegan et al., 1989). Because of this, their ability to change the risk profile of large groups is limited.

The growing use of community-level interventions recognizes the intimate relationship between the social and physical environments and individual behavior. By changing both individual behavior and the environment in which behavior occurs, it is hoped that individual-level dietary changes can be promoted and sustained in a supportive social and physical setting. Community involvement in the design and implementation of the intervention makes it more likely that the programs initiated will continue after the departure of the research team and that organizational changes promoting health will become a permanent part of the community.

Despite considerable resources expended, effective community- and individual-level intervention techniques, and enormous efforts on the part of researchers and community organizations, results from community trials to date have been disappointing. These modest outcomes could be due to a number of factors, including poor design, inappropriate interventions, exposures that are too weak or brief, deferred intervention effects, and contamination of comparison communities (Susser, 1995). The failure of state-of-the-art community intervention programs to achieve substantial and lasting changes in diet and other risk should not deter further development of community-level interventions. Compared to the wealth of knowledge about individual-level interventions, knowledge about the conditions under which community change can be expected to influence health and the means by which to induce community change is scarce (Bruce, 1995).

Although we have presented individual-level and community-level interventions separately, and weighed the merits of each, these approaches to promoting dietary change are complementary. The extent to which individuals make successful changes in their diet will be due to attributes of the individual, interactions between individuals and their social network (including family and community), influence of health care professionals and resources, and the compatibility between the behaviors the individual must adopt in order to make changes and the environment in which the behaviors must take place (McCann, Retzlaff, Walden et al., 1990). While we have focused our comments on only two approaches to promoting dietary change, we recognize that dietary changes are easiest to make and maintain when all of these factors work together in a coordinated effort.

REFERENCES

American Diabetes Association. (1992). Nutritional recommendations and principles for individuals with diabetes mellitus. *Diabetes Care, 15 (Suppl. 2)*, 21–28.

American Medical Association, Council on Scientific Affairs. (1993). Report of the Council on Scientific Affairs: Diet and cancer: Where do matters stand? *Archives of Internal Medicine, 153*, 50–56.

Applegate, W. B., Miller, S. T., Elam, J. T., Cushman, W. C., El Derwi, D., Brewer, A., & Graney, M. J. (1992). Nonpharmacologic intervention to reduce blood pressure in older patients with mild hypertension. *Archives of Internal Medicine, 152*, 1162–1166.

Bandura, A. (1991). Self-efficacy mechanisms in physiological activation and health-promoting behavior. In J. Madden, (Ed.), *Neurobiology of Learning, Emotion, and Affect* (pp. 229–270). New York: Raven Press.

Bernier, M., & Avard, J. (1986). Self-efficacy, outcome, and attrition in a weight-reduction program. *Cognitive Therapy and Research, 10*, 319–338.

Black, D. R., Gleser, L. J., & Kooyers, K. J. (1990). A meta-analytic evaluation of couples weight-loss programs. *Health Psychology, 9*, 330–347.

Bourn, D. M., Mann, J. I., McSkimming, B. J., Waldron, M. A., & Wishart, J. D. (1994). Impaired glucose tolerance and NIDDM: Does a lifestyle intervention program have an effect? *Diabetes Care, 17*, 1311–1319.

Bovbjerg, V. E., McCann, B. S., Brief, D. J., Follette, W. C., Retzlaff, B. M., Dowdy, A. A., Walden, C. E., & Knopp, R. H. (1995). Spouse support and long-term adherence to lipid-lowering diets. *American Journal of Epidemiology, 141*, 451–460.

Bracht, N., & Kingsbury, L. (1990). Community organization principles in health promotion: A five-stage model. In N. Bracht (Ed.), *Health promotion at the community level* (pp. 66–88). Newbury Park, CA: Sage.

Brownell, K. D. (1990). *The LEARN Program for weight control.* Dallas: American Health.

Brownell, K. D., & Cohen, L. R. (1995a). Adherence to dietary regimens: 1. An overview of research. *Behavioral Medicine, 20*, 149–154.

Brownell, K. D., & Cohen, L. R. (1995b). Adherence to dietary regimens: 2. Components of effective interventions. *Behavioral Medicine, 20*, 155–164.

Bruce, T. A. (1995). Community health science: A discipline whose time has already come. *American Journal of Preventive Medicine, 11 (Suppl. 3)*, 7.

Caggiula, A. W., & Milas, N. C. (1993). Approaches to successful nutrition intervention in renal disease. In W. Mitch and S. Klahr (Eds.), *Nutrition and the kidney* (pp. 365–387). Boston: Little, Brown.

Carleton, R. A., Lasater, T. M., Assaf, A. R., Feldman, H. A., & McKinlay, S. (1995). The Pawtucket Heart Health Program: Community changes in cardiovascular risk factors and projected disease risk. *American Journal of Public Health, 85*, 777–785.

Centers for Disease Control. (1994). Mortality patterns: United States, 1992. *Morbidity and Mortality Weekly Report, 43*, 916–920.

Cheadle, A., Wagner, E., Koepsell, T., Kristal, A., & Patrick, D. (1992). Environmental indicators: A tool for evaluating community-based health-promotion

programs. *American Journal of Preventive Medicine, 8*, 345–350.
Curry, S. J., Kristal, A. R., & Bowen, D. J. (1992). An application of the stage model of behavior change to dietary fat reduction. *Health Education Research, 7*, 97–105.
Davis, B. R., Blaufox, M. D., Oberman, A., Wassertheil-Smoller, S., Zimbaldi, N., Cutler, J. A., Kirchner, K., & Langford, H. G. (1993). Reduction in long-term antihypertensive medication requirements: Effects of weight reduction by dietary intervention in overweight persons with mild hypertension. *Archives of Internal Medicine, 153*, 1773–1782.
D'Eramo-Melkus, G., & Hagan, J. A. (1991). Weight reduction interventions for persons with a chronic illness: Findings and factors for consideration. *Journal of the American Dietetic Association, 91*, 1093–96, 1099.
Dowdy, A., Retzlaff, B., McCann, B., O'Leary, M., Kaplan, C., Burgher, B., Buck, B., Wilson, C., & Knopp, R. (1990). *Cholesterol Counts: A course to promote good health with good food: Instructor's and student's manuals*. Seattle, WA: Health Sciences Center for Educational Resources Distribution Services, University of Washington.
Drapkin, R. G., Wing, R. R., & Shiffman, S. (1995). Responses to hypothetical high risk situations: Do they predict weight loss in a behavioral treatment program or the context of dietary lapses? *Health Psychology, 14*, 427–434.
Edell, B. H., Edington, S., Herd, B., O'Brien, R. M., & Witkin, G. (1987). Self-efficacy and self-motivation as predictors of weight loss. *Addictive Behaviors, 12*, 63–66.
Elder, J. P., McGraw, S. A., Abrams, D. B., Ferreira, A., Lasater, T. M., Longpre, H., Peterson, G. S., Schwertfeger, R., & Carleton, R. A. (1986). Organizational and community approaches to community-wide prevention of heart disease: The first two years of the Pawtucket Heart Health Program. *Preventive Medicine, 15*, 107–117.
Elmer, P. J., Grimm, R. H. J., Flack, J., & Laing, B. (1991). Dietary sodium reduction for hypertension prevention and treatment. *Hypertension, 17*, I182–I189.
Elmer, P.J., Grimm, R., Laing, B., Grandits, G., Svendsen, K., Van Heel, N., Betz, E., Raines, J., Link, M., Stamler, J., & Neaton, J. (1995). Lifestyle intervention: Results of the Treatment of Mild Hypertension Study (TOMHS). *Preventive Medicine, 24*, 378–88.
Eriksson, K.-F., & Lindgärde, F. (1991). Prevention of Type 2 (non-insulin-dependent) diabetes mellitus by diet and physical exercise: The 6-year Malmö feasibility study. *Diabetologia, 34*, 891–898.
Farquhar, J. W., Fortmann, S.P., Flora, J. A., Taylor, C. B., Haskell, W. L., Williams, P. T., MacCoby, N., & Wood, P. D. (1990). Effects of communitywide education on cardiovascular disease risk factors: The Stanford Five-City Project. *Journal of the American Medical Association, 264*, 359–365.
Farquhar, J. W., Fortmann, S. P., MacCoby, N., Haskell, W. L., Williams, P. T., Flora, J. A., Taylor, C. B., Brown, B. W., Soloman, D. S., & Hulley, S. B. (1985). The Stanford Five-City Project: Design and methods. *American Journal of Epidemiology, 122*, 323–334.
Finnegan, J. R., Murray, D. M., Kurth, C., & McCarthy, P. (1989). Measuring and tracking education program implementation: The Minnesota Heart Health

Program experience. *Health Education Quarterly, 16*, 77–90.
Foreyt, J. P., & Goodrick, G. K. (1993). Evidence for success of behavior modification in weight loss and control. *Annals of Internal Medicine, 119*, 698–701.
Forster, J. L., & Jeffery, R. W. (1986). Gender differences related to weight history, eating patterns, efficacy expectations, self-esteem, and weight loss among participants in a weight reduction program. *Addictive Behaviors, 11*, 141–147.
Forster, J. L., Jeffery, R. W., VanNatta, M., & Pirie, P. (1990). Hypertension prevention trial: Do 24-h food records capture usual eating behavior in a dietary change study? *American Journal of Clinical Nutrition, 51*, 253–257.
Garfinkel, L. (1985). Overweight and cancer. *Annals of Internal Medicine, 103*, 1034–1036.
Gillman, M. W., Cupples, L. A., Gagnon, D., Posner, B. M., Ellison, R. C., Castelli, W. P., & Wolf, P. A. (1995). Protective effects of fruits and vegetables on development of stroke in men. *Journal of the American Medical Association, 273*, 1113–1117.
Glanz, K., Patterson, R. E., Kristal, A. R., DiClemente, C. C., Heimendinger, J., Linnan, L., & McLerran, D. F. (1994). Stages of change in adopting healthy diets: Fat, fiber, and correlates of nutrient intake. *Health Education Quarterly, 21*, 499–519.
Glasgow, R. E., McCaul, K. D., & Schafer, L. C. (1987). Self-care behaviors and glycemic control in type I diabetes. *Journal of Chronic Diseases, 40*, 399–412.
Glasgow, R. E., Terborg, J. R., Hollis, J. F., Severson, H. H., Fischer, K. J., Boles, S. M., Pettigrew, E. L., Foster, L. S., Strycker, L. A., & Bischoff, S. (1994). Modifying dietary and tobacco use patterns in the worksite: The Take Heart Project. *Health Education Quarterly, 21*, 69–82.
Green, L. W., & Raeburn, J. (1990). Contemporary developments in health promotion: Definitions and challenges. In N. Bracht (Ed.), *Health promotion at the community level* (pp. 29–44). Newbury Park, CA: Sage.
Grilo, C. M., Shiffman, S., & Wing, R. R. (1989). Relapse crises and coping among dieters. *Journal of Consulting & Clinical Psychology, 57*, 488–495.
Grundy, S. M., & Denke, M. A. (1990). Dietary influences on serum lipids and lipoproteins. *Journal of Lipid Research, 31*, 1149–1172.
Haglund, B., Weisbrod, R. R., & Bracht, N. (1990). Assessing the community: Its services, needs, leadership, and readiness. In N. Bracht (Ed.), *Health promotion at the community level*. Newbury Park, CA: Sage.
Harris, M. I. (1995). Epidemiologic studies on the pathogenesis of non-insulin-dependent diabetes mellitus (NIDDM). *Clinical and Investigative Medicine, 18*, 231–239.
Hebert, J. R., Clemow, L., Pbert, L., Ockene, I. S., & Ockene, J. K. (1995). Social desirability bias in dietary self-report may compromise the validity of dietary intake measures. *International Journal of Epidemiology, 24*, 389–398.
Hebert, J. R., Harris, D. R., Sorensen, G., Stoddard, A. M., Hunt, M. K., & Morris, D. H. (1993). A work-site nutrition intervention: Its effects on the consumption of cancer-related nutrients. *American Journal of Public Health, 83*, 391–394.
Heimendinger, J., & Van Duyn, M. A. (1995). Dietary behavior change: The challenge of recasting the role of fruit and vegetables in the American diet. *American Journal of Clinical Nutrition, 61 (Suppl)*, 1397S–1401S.

Henderson, M. M. (1995). Nutritional aspects of breast cancer. *Cancer, 76 (Suppl 10)*, 2053–2058.

Henkin, Y., Garber, D. W., Osterlund, L. C., & Darnell, B. E. (1992). Saturated fats, cholesterol, and dietary compliance. *Archives of Internal Medicine, 152*, 1167–1174.

Hypertension Prevention Trial Research Group. (1990). The Hypertension Prevention Trial: three-year effects of dietary changes on blood pressure. *Archives of Internal Medicine, 150*, 153–162.

Institute of Medicine Committee on Dietary Guidelines Implementation. (1991). *Improving America's diet and health: From recommendations to action.* Washington, DC: National Academy Press.

Jackson, C., Winkleby, M. A., Flora, J. A., & Fortmann, S. P. (1991). Use of educational resources for cardiovascular risk reduction in the Stanford Five-City Project. *American Journal of Preventive Medicine, 7*, 82–88.

Johnson, R. K., Goran, M. I., & Poehlman, E. T. (1994). Correlates of over- and under reporting of energy intake in healthy older men and women. *American Journal of Clinical Nutrition, 59*, 1286–1290.

Klahr, S., Levey, A. S., Beck, G. J., Caggiula, A. W., Hunsicker, L., Kusek, J. W., & Striker, G. (1994). The effects of dietary protein restriction and blood-pressure control on the progression of chronic renal disease: Modification of Diet in Renal Disease Study Group. *New England Journal of Medicine, 330*, 877–884.

Kluge, R., Wildberger, D., & Wallmeier, K. (1989). Dietary protein restriction in renal insufficiency in private practice. *Blood Purification, 7*, 43–45.

Knopp, R. H., Walden, C. E., Retzlaff, B. M., McCann, B. S., Dowdy, A. A., Albers, J. J., Gey, G. O., & Cooper, M. N. (1996). *Long-term cholesterol lowering effects of four different fat restricted diets in hypercholesterolemic and combined hyperlipidemic men: The Dietary Alternatives Study*. Manuscript submitted for publication.

Kravitz, R. L., Hays, R. D., Sherbourne, C. D., DiMatteo, M. R., Rogers, W. H., Ordway, L., & Greenfield, S. (1993). Recall of recommendations and adherence to advice among patients with chronic medical conditions. *Archives of Internal Medicine, 153*, 1869–1878.

Kuczmarski, R. J. (1992). Prevalence of overweight and weight gain in the United States. *American Journal of Clinical Nutrition, 55 (Suppl. 2)*, 495S–502S.

LeBow, M. D. (1989). *Adult obesity therapy*. New York: Pergamon.

Liebson, P. R., Grandits, G. A., Dianzumba, S., Prineas, R. J., Grimm, R. H., Neaton, J. D., & Stamler, J. (1995). Comparison of five antihypertensive monotherapies and placebo for change in left ventricular mass in patients receiving nutritional-hygienic therapy in the Treatment of Mild Hypertension Study (TOMHS). *Circulation, 91*, 698–706.

Life Sciences Research Office, Federation of American Societies for Experimental Biology. (1995). *Third Report on Nutrition Monitoring in the United States: Executive Summary* Washington, DC: U.S. Government Printing Office.

Lowe, M. R., Kopyt, D., & Buchwald, J. (1996). Food intake underestimation: Its nature and impact on obesity treatment. *The Behavior Therapist, 19*, 17–20.

Luepker, R. V., Murray, D. M., Jacobs, D. R., Mittelmark, M. B., Bracht, N., Carlaw, R., Crow, R., Elmer, P., Finnegan, J., Folsom, A. R., Grimm, R., Hannan, P. J.,

Jeffrey, R., Lando, H., McGovern, P., Mullis, R., Perry, C. L., Pechacek, T., Pirie, P., Sprafka, J. M., Weisbrod, R., & Blackburn, H. (1994). Community education for cardiovascular disease prevention: Risk factor changes in the Minnesota Heart Health Program. *American Journal of Public Health, 84*, 1383–1393.

Marlatt, G. A., & George, W. H. (1984). Relapse prevention: Introduction and overview of the model. *British Journal of Addictions, 79*, 261–273.

McCann, B. S., Bovbjerg, V. E., Brief, D. J., Turner, C., Follette, W. C., Fitzpatrick, V., Dowdy, A., Retzlaff, B., Walden, C. E., & Knopp, R. H. (1995). Relationship of self-efficacy to cholesterol lowering and dietary change in hyperlipidemia. *Annals of Behavioral Medicine, 17*, 221–226.

McCann, B. S., Bovbjerg, V. E., Curry, S. J., Retzlaff, B. M., Walden, C. E., & Knopp, R. H. (1996). Predicting participation in a dietary intervention to lower cholesterol among individuals with hyperlipidemia. *Health Psychology, 15*, 61–64.

McCann, B. S., Retzlaff, B. M., Dowdy, A. A., Walden, C. E., & Knopp, R. H. (1990). Promoting adherence to low-fat, low-cholesterol diets: review and recommendations. *Journal of the American Dietetic Association, 90*, 1408–1415,1417.

McCann, B. S., Retzlaff, B. M., Walden, C. E., & Knopp, R. H. (1990). Dietary intervention for coronary heart disease prevention. In S. A. Shumaker, E. B. Schron, & J. K. Ockene (Eds.), *The Handbook of Health Behavior Change*. (pp. 191–215). New York: Springer Publishing Co.

McNabb, W. L., Quinn, M. T. & Rosing, L. (1993). Weight loss program for inner-city black women with non-insulin-dependent diabetes mellitus: PATHWAYS. *Journal of the American Dietetic Association, 93*, 75–77.

Milas, N. C., Nowalk, M.P., Akpele, L., Castaldo, L., Coyne, T., Doroshenko, L., Kigawa, L., Korzec-Ramirez, D., Scherch, L. K., & Snetselaar, L. (1995). Factors associated with adherence to the dietary protein intervention in the Modification of Diet in Renal Disease Study. *Journal of the American Dietetic Association, 95*, 1295–1230.

Modification of Diet in Renal Disease Study Group. (1994). Reduction of dietary protein and phosphorus in the Modification of Diet in Renal Disease Feasibility Study: The MDRD Study Group. *Journal of the American Dietetic Association, 94*, 986–990.

National Cholesterol Education Program Expert Panel on Detection, Evaluation, and Treatment of High Blood Cholesterol in Adults. (1993). Summary of the second report of the National Cholesterol Education Program (NCEP) Expert Panel on Detection, Evaluation, and Treatment of High Blood Cholesterol in Adults (Adult Treatment Panel II). *Journal of the American Medical Association, 269*, 3015–3023.

National High Blood Pressure Education Program Working Group. (1993). *Working group report on primary prevention of hypertension*. Bethesda, MD: National Institutes of Health.

National Research Council Committee on Diet and Health. (1989). *Diet and health: Implications for reducing chronic disease risk*. Washington, DC: National Academy Press.

Neaton, J. D., Grimm, R. H., Prineas, R. J., Stamler, J., Grandits, G. A., Elmer, P. J., Cutler, J. A., Flack, J. M., Schoenberger, J. A., McDonald, R., Lewis, C. E., &

Liebson, P. R. (1993). Treatment of Mild Hypertension Study: Final results. *Journal of the American Medical Association, 270*, 713–724.

Ockene, J. K., Ockene, I. S., Quirk, M. E., Hebert, J. R., Saperia, G. M., Luippold, R. S., Merriam, P. A., & Ellis, S. (1995). Physician training for patient-centered nutrition counseling in a lipid intervention trial. *Preventive Medicine, 24*, 563–570.

Perri, M. G., Sears, S. F., & Clark, J. E. (1993). Strategies for improving maintenance of weight loss: Toward a continuous care model of obesity management. *Diabetes Care, 16*, 200–209.

Pi-Sunyer, F. X. (1993). Medical hazards of obesity. *Annals of Internal Medicine, 119*, 655–660.

Potocnik, U., & Widhalm, K. (1994). Long-term follow-up of children with classical phenylketonuria after diet discontinuation: A review. *Journal of the American College of Nutrition, 13*, 232–236.

Prochaska, J. O., DiClemente, C. C., & Norcross, J. C. (1992). In search of how people change: Applications to addictive behaviors. *American Psychologist, 47*, 1102–1114.

Prochaska, J. O., Norcross, J. C., Fowler, J. L., Follick, M. J., & Abrams, D. B. (1992). Attendance and outcome in a work site weight control program: Processes and stages of change as process and predictor variables. *Addictive Behaviors, 17*, 35–45.

Purdon, C., Brousson, M., Nyveen, S. L., Miles, P. D. G., Halter, J. B., Vranic, M., & Marliss, E. B. (1993). The roles of insulin and catecholamines in the glucoregulatory response during intense exercise and early recovery in insulin-dependent diabetic and control subjects. *Journal of Clinical Endocrinology and Metabolism, 76*, 566–573.

Puska, P., Tuomilehto, J., Salonen, J., Neittaanmaki, L., Maki, J., Virtamo, J., Nissinen, A., Koskela, K., & Takalo, T. (1979). Changes in coronary risk factors during comprehensive five-year community programme to control cardiovascular diseases (North Karelia project). *British Medical Journal, 2*, 1173–1178.

Rossouw, J. E., Jooste, P. L., Chalton, D. O., Jordaan, E. R., Langenhoven, M. L., Jordaan, P. C. J., Steyn, M., Swanepoel, A. S. P., & Rossouw, L. J. (1993). Community-based intervention: The Coronary Risk Factor Study (CORIS). *International Journal of Epidemiology, 22*, 428–438.

Schoeller, D. A. (1995). Limitations in the assessment of dietary energy intake by self-report. *Metabolism, 44 Suppl. 2*, 18–22.

Shattuck, A. L., White, E., & Kristal, A. R. (1992). How women's adopted low-fat diets affect their husbands. *American Journal of Public Health, 82*, 1244–1250.

Skelly, A. H., Marshall, J. R., Haughey, B. P., Davis, P. J., & Dunford, R. G. (1995). Self-efficacy and confidence in outcomes as determinants of self-care practices in inner-city, African-American women with non-insulin-dependent diabetes. *Diabetes Educator, 21*, 38–46.

Smith, D. E., & Wing, R. R. (1991). Diminished weight loss and behavioral compliance during repeated diets in obese patients with type II diabetes. *Health Psychology, 10*, 378–383.

Smith, S. C., Blair, S. N., Criqui, M. H., Fletcher, G. F., Fuster, V., Gersh, B. J., Gotto, A. M., Gould, K. L., Greenland, P., Grundy, S. M., Hill, M. N., Hlatky, M. A.,

Houston-Miller, N., Krauss, R. M., LaRosa, J., Ockene, I. S., Oparil, S., Pearson, T. A., Rapaport, E., & Starke, R. D. (1995). Preventing heart attack and death in patients with coronary disease. *Circulation, 92*, 2–4.

Sorensen, G., Glasgow, R. E., & Corbett, K. (1990). Involving worksites and other organizations. In N. Bracht (Ed.), *Health promotion at the community level* (pp. 158–184). Newbury Park, CA: Sage.

Sorensen, G., Morris, D. M., Hunt, M. K., Hebert, J. R., Harris, D. R., Stoddard, A., & Ockene, J. K. (1992). Work-site nutrition intervention and employees' dietary habits: The Treatwell Program. *American Journal of Public Health, 82*, 877–880.

Sorensen, G., Stoddard, A., Ockene, J.A., Hunt, M.K., & Youngstrom, R. (1996). Worker participation in an integrated health promotion/health protection program: Results from the WellWorks Project. *Health Education Quarterly, 23*, 191–203.

Stamler, R., Stamler, J., Grimm, R., Gosch, F. C., Elmer, P., Dyer, A., Berman, R., Fishman, J., Van Heel, N., Civinelli, J., & McDonald, A. (1987). Nutritional therapy for high blood pressure. Final report of a four-year randomized controlled trial: the Hypertension Control Program. *Journal of the American Medical Association, 257*, 1484–91.

Stevens, V. J., Corrigan, S. A., Obarzanek, E., Bernauer, E., Cook, N. R., Hebert, P., Mattfeldt-Beman, M., Oberman, A., Sugars, C., Dalcin, A. T., & Whelton, P. K. (1993). Weight loss intervention in phase 1 of the trials of hypertension prevention. *Archives of Internal Medicine, 153*, 849–858.

Susser, M. (1995). Editorial: The tribulations of trials: interventions in communities. *American Journal of Public Health, 85*, 156–158.

Thompson, B., & Kinne, S. (1990). Social change theory: Applications to community health. In N. Bracht (Ed.), *Health promotion at the community level* (pp. 45–65). Newbury Park, CA: Sage.

U.S. Department of Agriculture and U.S. Department of Health and Human Services, 1995. *Nutrition and your health: Dietary guidelines for Americans*, (4th ed.). (Home & Garden Bulletin No. 232). Washington, DC: Author.

Wadden, T. A. (1993a). The treatment of obesity: An overview. In A. J. Stunkard & T. A. Wadden (Eds.), *Obesity: Theory and therapy* (pp. 197–217). New York: Raven.

Wadden, T. A. (1993b). Treatment of obesity by moderate and severe caloric restriction. Results of clinical research trials. *Annals of Internal Medicine, 119*, 688–693.

Waisbren, S. E., Hamilton, B. D., St. James, P. J., Shiloh, S., & Levy, H. L. (1995). Psychosocial factors in maternal phenylketonuria: Women's adherence to medical recommendations. *American Journal of Public Health, 85*, 1636–1641.

Walden, C. E., Retzlaff, B. M., Buck, B. L., McCann, B. S., & Knopp, R. H. (1996). *Lipoprotein lipid response to the National Cholesterol Education Program Step II diet by hypercholesterolemic and combined hyperlipidemic women and men.* Manuscript submitted for publication.

Weisbrod, R. R., Pirie, P. L., & Bracht, N. F. (1992). Impact of a community health promotion program on existing organizations: The Minnesota Heart Health Program. *Social Science and Medicine, 34*, 639–648.

White, E., Shattuck, A. L., Kristal, A. R., Urban, N., Prentice, R. L., Henderson, M.

M., Insull, W., Moskowitz, M., Goldman, S. & Woods, M. N. (1992). Maintenance of a low-fat diet: Follow-up of the Women's Health Trial. *Cancer Epidemiology, Biomarkers and Prevention, 1*, 315–323.

Wing, R. R., Blair, E., Marcus, M., Epstein, L. H., & Harvey, J. (1994). Year-long weight loss treatment for obese patients with type II diabetes: Does including an intermittent very-low-calorie diet improve outcome? *American Journal of Medicine, 97*, 354–362.

Wing, R. R., Caggiula, A. W., Nowalk, M. P., Koeske, R., Lee, S., & Langford, H. (1984). Dietary approaches to the reduction of blood pressure: the independence of weight and sodium/potassium interventions. *Preventive Medicine, 13*, 233–244.

Wing, R. R., Epstein, L. H., Paternostro-Bayles, M., Kriska, A., Nowalk, M. P., & Gooding, W. (1988). Exercise in a behavioural weight control programme for obese patients with Type 2 (non-insulin-dependent) diabetes. *Diabetologia, 31*, 902–909.

Winkleby, M. A., Flora, J. A., & Kraemer, H. C. (1994). A community-based heart disease intervention: Predictors of change. *American Journal of Public Health, 84*, 767–772.

Wood, P. D., Stefanick, M. L., Williams, P. T., & Haskell, W. L. (1991). The effects on plasma lipoproteins of a prudent weight-reducing diet, with or without exercise, in overweight men and women. *New England Journal of Medicine, 325*, 461–466.

8

Adherence to Physical Activity Recommendations and Interventions

Bess H. Marcus, Teresa K. King, Beth C. Bock, Belinda Borrelli, and Matthew M. Clark

INTRODUCTION

Understanding how to facilitate the maintenance of healthy behaviors represents a major challenge for health practitioners and researchers. Physical activity is particularly challenging as it takes more time and effort than most other preventive health behaviors (Dishman, 1996). The difficulty of adhering to regular physical activity is reflected in the high proportion of individuals who are sedentary or irregularly active and thus not physically active at the level needed to achieve health benefits. Difficulty adhering to physical activity also is reflected by the high relapse rates from physical activity programs, which have been estimated at approximately 50% (Dishman, 1990). Regular physical activity yields tremendous benefits, and

This work was partially supported by Grants KO7CA01757 and R29CA59660 from the National Cancer Institute, a supplement to R29CA59660 from the Office of Research on Women's Health, and Grant 9407826S from the American Heart Association, Rhode Island Affiliate, to Dr. Marcus. The authors wish to express their appreciation to Barbara Doll and Regina Traficante for technical assistance. The authors thank Leigh Ann Forsyth for her comments on an earlier draft of this chapter.

additional benefits continue to be discovered. Therefore, adherence to physical activity is a critical issue.

Adherence is difficult to define, as it can be discussed in very specific or very general terms and can apply to all phases of physical activity : initiating, maintaining, relapsing from, and resuming physical activity. Thus, there is much inconsistency in the literature as to how physical activity adherence is defined. Some authors choose to define adherence as fulfillment of predetermined goals (Dubbert, Rappaport, & Martin, 1987; Robison & Rogers, 1994). This definition is acceptable, as it can be adapted to include goals set by public health initiatives such as Healthy People 2000 (United States Department of Health and Human Services [USDHHS], 1991). In this chapter, adherence is considered more broadly to include physical activity behaviors as they relate to both physical activity programs and national objectives. *Exercise* is typically used to refer to programmed activity, and *physical activity* usually refers more broadly to bodily movement. Therefore, we will generally refer to physical activity throughout this text, but we will refer to exercise when it is more descriptive of the research being presented.

This chapter focuses on recent studies examining the impact of various interventions on the exercise patterns of healthy adults. Several of these studies were theoretically conceptualized, therefore, theories which have been used in the exercise literature are presented. Next, specific intervention studies organized by the channel utilized (i.e., provider-delivered, worksites, communities) are discussed. It should be noted that the discussion of interventions is not an exhaustive review, which would go beyond the scope of this chapter (see Dishman, 1991; Dubbert, 1992).

PHYSICAL ACTIVITY RECOMMENDATIONS

Despite the mounting evidence regarding the benefits of physical activity (Blair et al., 1995), data from the Behavioral Risk Factor Surveillance System show that 58% of the U.S. population are sedentary (Center for Disease Control (CDC), 1993). Sedentary individuals are those who do not meet the minimum physical activity recommendations for vigorous or moderate activity. For vigorous physical activity, the minimum physical activity recommendation is exercise performed at 60 to 80% of maximum heart rate for 20 minutes or more 3 or more days per week (American College of Sports Medicine [ACSM], 1990). The Centers for Disease Control (CDC) and American College of Sports Medicine (ACSM)'s new joint recommendation for physical activity (1993) is an accumulation of 30 minutes or more of moderate-intensity physical activity on most (preferably all) days of the week (Pate et al., 1995). One brisk, 2-mile walk daily is a specific way to meet the new standard. The new standard has important implications for adherence, as research has demonstrated that individuals are more likely to adopt and maintain moderate, as opposed to vigorous, physical activity (Sallis et al., 1986).

USEFUL PSYCHOLOGICAL FRAMEWORKS

Understanding complex behavior, such as physical activity behavior, is facilitated through theories and models identifying important constructs (see Marcus, King, Clark, Pinto, & Bock, 1996 for a review). Theories such as learning theory (Skinner, 1953), social-cognitive theory (Bandura, 1977, 1986), the stages-of-change model (Prochaska & DiClemente, 1983) and the relapse prevention model (Marlatt & Gordon, 1985) are especially useful because of their inclusion of both personal and environmental factors and their explicit implications for interventions (Marcus & Sallis, 1997; USDHHS, 1996).

Learning Theory

Applications of operant learning have been widely used in physical activity interventions. Physical activity is conceived as a response that can be acquired and maintained by controlling or modifying the antecedents and consequences associated with physical activity participation. Behavior modification strategies such as stimulus control and contingency management have been found to increase physical activity adherence 10–75% above no-treatment control groups (see reviews by King et al., 1992; Leith & Taylor, 1992). Stimulus control involves increasing the cues for physical activity and/or decreasing the cues prompting sedentary behavior. Contingency management utilizes reinforcements to increase physical activity adherence, and may include strategies such as contracts, incentives, lotteries, and competitions. A recent review of behavior modification strategies reported that most of the various behavior modification strategies were effective at improving adherence; however, which particular strategy was utilized did not appear important (Leith & Taylor, 1995).

Social-Cognitive Theory

Social-cognitive theory (Bandura, 1977, 1986) focuses on the importance of the interaction between the person and their environment and stresses an individual's ability to control his or her behavior. Self-efficacy is a central concept within social-cognitive theory (Bandura, 1977, 1986) and involves individuals' degree of confidence that they can perform a particular behavior. Self-efficacy is one of the most frequently identified psychosocial determinants of adherence to physical activity among adults, and numerous studies demonstrate that high levels of self-efficacy prospectively predict physical activity behavior (e.g., McAuley, Courneya, Rudolph & Lox, 1994; Reynolds et al., 1990; Rodgers & Brawley, 1993; Sallis et al., 1990; Sallis, Hovell, & Hofstetter, 1992). Other components of social-cognitive theory applied to physical activity behavior include goal setting, feedback, problem solving, self-monitoring, and self-reinforcement (e.g., Dishman, 1991; King, Haskell, Taylor, Kraemer, & DeBusk, 1991; Knapp, 1988; Martin et al., 1984).

Stages-of-Change Model

The stages-of-change or transtheoretical model integrates a person's current behavior with their intention to maintain or change this pattern of behavior (DiClemente et al., 1991; Prochaska & DiClemente, 1983). According to the model, individuals progress through a series of stages of readiness for change. As applied to physical activity, precontemplation includes individuals who do not participate in physical activity and do not intend to start. People in the contemplation stage do not participate in physical activity, but intend to start. Those in preparation participate in some physical activity, but not regularly. Regular activity is defined as vigorous activity at least three times per week for at least 20 minutes each time (ACSM, 1990) or accumulating at least 30 minutes of moderate physical activity on most, preferably all, days of the week (Pate et al., 1995). The action stage includes individuals who currently participate in regular activity, but have done so for less than 6 months, whereas maintenance entails participation in regular physical activity for 6 months or longer (Marcus, Rossi, Selby, Niaura, & Abrams, 1992). The concepts of self-efficacy (Bandura, 1977) and decisional balance (e.g., pros and cons of initiating exercise) (Janis & Mann, 1977) are often used in conjunction with the stages of change in terms of both intervention content and outcomes. Interventions based on the transtheoretical model utilize the concept of tailoring treatment to the individual's stage of readiness for change (e.g., Marcus et al., 1992; Marcus, Bock, et al., in press; Marcus, Emmons, et al., in press; Marcus, Goldstein, et al., 1997). A stage-matched physical activity promotion intervention for individuals in the early stages of change (precontemplation and contemplation) would focus on increasing awareness of the benefits of physical activity and would encourage thinking about becoming active. Materials designed for individuals in the later stages would focus more on encouraging the individual to begin physical activity and on strategies for maintaining an active lifestyle.

Relapse Prevention

The relapse-prevention model posits that maintenance of a new behavior is influenced by an individual's ability to cognitively and behaviorally cope with relapses back to the undesirable behavior (Marlatt & Gordon, 1980) (see also Chapter 2). One concept from the relapse-prevention model, the abstinence violation effect (AVE), applies to a broad range of behaviors, and is a maladaptive belief that once the abstinence rule has been broken, total relapse is inevitable. One goal of the model is to teach individuals to distinguish a lapse from a relapse in order to prevent a lapse from physical activity (e.g., missing a physical activity session) from escalating into a complete relapse (e.g., return to a sedentary lifestyle). The individual is encouraged to identify situations that are likely to lead to a lapse, and then receives training in appropriate cognitive and behavioral skills to cope with the lapse. Interventions utilizing the relapse prevention model may also include a "planned" relapse (e.g., not being physically active for a specified period) to give the individual an opportunity to experience the AVE and apply the learned cognitive and behavioral skills. Data suggest that physical activity relapsers have fewer strategies for coping with high-risk situations than do physical activity maintainers (Simkin & Gross, 1994) and that relapse-prevention strategies are effective for increasing adherence to a physical activity program (Belisle, Roskies, & Levesque, 1987; King & Frederiksen, 1984). However, studies incorporating a planned relapse as part of the intervention have been less effective (Marcus & Stanton, 1993; Martin et al., 1984).

GROUP-BASED INTERVENTIONS

The majority of physical activity adherence research has focused on the identification of individual factors that are predictive of activity level (King, 1994). However, in light of the prevalence of a sedentary lifestyle and the costs associated with delivering individualized treatments, effective strategies need to be identified which can be applied at a group level. Some group interventions merely try to apply techniques obtained from research examining individual behavior to a group setting. However, group interventions can differ from individual treatment on a number of dimensions. Group interventions can focus on social support, peer groups, and observational learning. This section will review recent research which has examined predictors of adherence in group settings, and then discuss strategies which enhance physical activity adoption and maintenance.

Most of the research on group-based interventions has utilized on-site facilities. For example, Klonoff, Annechild, and Landrine (1994) examined predictors of adherence to a 10-week aerobic class program. Three classes were scheduled daily over the 10 weeks to maximize convenience. The study found that overweight, physically uncomfortable, and mildly anxious (not extremely stressed) subjects attended more sessions. The researchers speculated that focus on the immediate weight-reduction, symptom-relief, and anxiety-reduction benefits of physical activity may enhance its initiation and adoption. This is an interesting finding, given that many studies suggest that the overweight are less likely to participate in physical activity.

Other researchers (Morey et al., 1989) have examined the role of health problems (arthritis, hypertension, heart disease, chronic lung disease, and diabetes) on physical-activity adherence. A 4-month outpatient exercise program was established at a VA medical center, this consisted of a 3-day-per-week supervised exercise program. Subjects demonstrated improvements in MET (metabolic equivalent) level, weight, treadmill time, and resting heart rate. Eighteen (26%) of the 69 subjects dropped out of treatment. Patients who dropped out of treatment had an average of 2.3 chronic diseases, compared to an average of 1.6 for the completers. Thus, complex health problems may be a barrier to exercise adoption and maintenance in a group setting. Support and guidance from a primary care physician may be beneficial in problem-solving solutions to these barriers.

As reviewed earlier in this chapter, self-efficacy is predictive of behavior, and exercise self-efficacy is related to activity level. Researchers (McAuley et al., 1994) recently investigated the effectiveness of a self-efficacy intervention on participation in a walking program. One hundred and fourteen healthy middle-aged men and women participated in a 20 week on-site 3-times-per-week walking program. In addition to the physical activity intervention, subjects were assigned randomly to a self-efficacy intervention or an attention control group. The self-efficacy intervention consisted of (1) mastery accomplishments: focusing on improvements in duration and intensity of exercise; (2) social modeling: watching videotapes of others succeeding at adopting a walking program; (3) social persuasion: forming "buddy groups" of two to three individuals; and (4) the physiological system: learning how the body adapts to exercise. Subjects in the intervention group exercised more frequently and walked more miles per week than the control group. Additionally, subjects assigned to the self-efficacy intervention attended 67% of the sessions, compared to 55% for the control group. Thus, a group intervention designed to enhance self-efficacy improved attendance and adherence to a supervised walking program.

Researchers also have examined the efficacy of group-based versus home-based interventions. In a year-long community-based trial (King, Haskell, Taylor, Kraemer, & DeBusk, 1991), healthy sedentary men and women were randomly assigned to one of four experimental conditions: (1) high intensity group-based physical activity training at a community center consisting of 3 days per week of on-site physical activity; (2) high-intensity home-based physical activity with weekly phone contact, written information, and activity logs; (3) low-intensity home-based physical activity; or (4) a control group. Subjects in all three physical activity conditions showed significant improvements in fitness (VO2 max). Subjects who adhered to physical activity also demonstrated reductions in anxiety and symptoms of depression (King, Taylor, & Haskell, 1993). However, physical-activity adherence was about 75% in the home-based conditions, but only about 50% in the community-based condition. Thus, home-based physical activity programs, which are more convenient, may enhance maintenance of physical-activity behavior.

Researchers have also examined the effectiveness of adding low-cost strategies to enhance adherence to group interventions. In particular, mailings and phone contact have been examined as strategies to increase physical-activity adherence. Researchers (Lombard, Lombard, & Winett, 1995) examined the effects of telephone contact on the initiation and maintenance of a walking program. Subjects attended a 15-minute group session at which they received American College of Sports Medicine (ACSM) guidelines to walk at least 3 times per week for at least 20 minutes each time. Subjects also received walking maps, handouts on how to enlist walking partners, and instructions on how to slowly start a walking program. Subjects were encouraged to organize walking groups or to find walking partners. Subjects were then randomly assigned to receive, over the next 12 weeks, phone calls once each week or once every three weeks, or to a control group receiving no phone calls. At week 24, 46% of those receiving once-per-week phone contacts, 13% of those receiving phone contact once every three weeks, and 4% in the control condition were walking at a level to meet the ACSM goal. Given that the phone contacts took a mean of 1–5 minutes at a staff cost of $1.00, the researchers concluded that frequent prompting appears to be an effective behavioral strategy that could be used to enhance adherence to group exercise interventions and could be easily applied in health maintenance organizations or other primary care settings.

Another study examined the impact of receiving monthly mailings and brief phone contact on exercise adherence following participation in a 1-year exercise program for weight loss (King, Frey-Hewitt, Dreon, & Wood, 1989). Following participation in a supervised 3-times-per-week aerobic exercise program, subjects were assigned to either a maintenance condition with contact, or an assessment-only condition. Subjects who received the intervention reported a greater amount of time spent in vigorous activity and maintained a greater weight loss compared to subjects in the control condition.

In summary, investigators have learned that home-based interventions appear to achieve higher adherence rates, and that strategies to enhance self-efficacy are efficacious for increasing physical-activity adoption and adherence. Many of these interventions are costly, and in light of high relapse rates, researchers have begun to re-examine lower-cost maintenance strategies such as prompts and cues. Brief telephone contacts have proven effective in prompting physical-activity maintenance. Healthy individuals may be appropriately treated with lower-cost interventions such as educational materials, phone calls, and computerized prompts. However, it may be that individuals with complex health problems will need professionally delivered multidisciplinary home visits to foster physical-activity adoption, suggesting that treatment may need to be matched to the individual's motivational and physiological readiness to maximally increase physical activity adherence.

PUBLIC HEALTH APPROACHES TO PHYSICAL ACTIVITY PROMOTION

Individual and small-group approaches to enhancing adherence to physical activity have met with some success. However, these approaches, while important, are unlikely to make a significant impact in the achievement of the national physical activity goals outlined in Healthy People 2000 (USDHHS, 1991). A primary goal of these objectives is to increase the proportion of adults who engage in regular moderate or vigorous physical activity. Individual and small-group approaches only reach a small segment of the population, who may be self-selected and somewhat motivated to change their behavior. Thus, higher-level and more macro-level approaches may be needed to achieve these goals. Public health interventions extend their reach to the 20–30% of the population who are most sedentary and are at greatest risk for diseases preventable by increases in physical activity. These more macro approaches utilize worksites, primary care settings, and communities as both the target of intervention and the unit of analysis, and aim for environmental, organizational, and policy changes. Thus, public health approaches widen the scope of intervention delivery by proactively targeting at-risk groups, often through pre-existing channels. In the following section, we will discuss the role of public health interventions in enhancing adherence to physical activity in whole communities and in special subgroups within communities, such as worksites and physician's offices. We will also discuss the policy and environmental changes that can facilitate the adoption and maintenance of the behavior change.

Worksite Interventions

One approach to increasing participation in physical activity has been to provide programs at the worksite (Blair, Piserchia, Wilbur, & Crowder,

1986; Fielding, 1984; Godin & Shephard, 1990). Worksites offer an accessible and often diverse population base, convenience, potential avenues for group support, and existing communication and health care delivery channels (Winette, King, & Altman, 1989). Recent years have witnessed increasing interest in providing health-promotion programs at the worksite. Employers cite a number of reasons for offering worksite physical activity programs, including improvement of employee health, reduced health care costs, improvements in productivity and absenteeism, and strengthening the company's ability to recruit and retain employees (Fielding & Knight, 1994). Companies sponsoring these programs often hope to reduce costs to their business, such as costs associated with health insurance and absenteeism (Shephard, 1988, 1992).

The presence of worksite-based physical activity programs, together with flexible work schedules which permit physical activity participation, have resulted in increased rates of physical-activity participation among employees (King et al., 1992; Shephard, 1992). However, overall dropout rates and differential rates of usage among employee groups (male/female, blue-collar, middle and upper white-collar, healthy/at risk) remain a significant concern.

Overall, men tend to utilize worksite programs more frequently than do women (Lynch & Main, 1993). For example, one prospective study of 949 employees showed that women were 50% more likely to drop out of worksite physical-activity programs than men (Lynch & Main, 1993). Women who do utilize worksite physical-activity programs tend to be those who are already physically active, suggesting that current workplace physical activity programs do not serve the needs of the women who may need such programs the most (Verhoef, Hamm, & Love, 1993).

Across a number of studies, higher socioeconomic status, including education and income level and type of job (white-collar), is positively associated with participation in leisure-time physical activity (Dishman & Sallis, 1994). For example, a recent study demonstrated that white-collar employees tend to utilize worksite physical-activity programs more frequently than do blue-collar employees (Lynch & Main, 1993). However, worksite physical-activity programs which have specifically targeted traditionally hard-to-reach blue-collar workers also have shown significant improvements in physical-activity participation (King, 1994). In addition, worksite programs utilizing videotaped messages regarding barriers to physical activity followed by structured assignments addressing barrier reduction have resulted in physical-activity frequency and intensity rates at twice that of controls (Huddy, Hebert, Hyner, & Johnson, 1995).

Worksite interventions should be behaviorally focused. Educational interventions work well to increase an individual's knowledge base regarding physical activity. However, if the goal is to increase actual physical activity participation, behaviorally tailored interventions are more effective (Gomel, Oldenburg, Simpson, & Owen, 1993). Some successful programs including the Team Health Program (Knadler & Rogers, 1987), and the Stanford Coming Alive Program (Altman et al., 1986) have utilized contests which incorporate behavior change techniques such as goal-setting, regular tracking of physical activity, feedback, and incentives. The Team Health project was able to maintain good participation after initial recruitment by using a very accessible form of physical activity (stair-climbing), forming stair-climbing clubs, and continued utilization of low-cost incentives. Efforts targeted at recruiting a typically hard-to-reach segment (blue-collar workers) produced a 25% increase in physical activity participation among that group (King, Taylor, Haskell, & DeBusk, 1988).

One successful method of tailoring worksite interventions to meet the needs of employees is to tailor program content to match the individual's motivational readiness for physical-activity adoption. Worksite surveys indicate that only 10% of workers are ready to take action to change their activity patterns (Marcus, Rossi, Selby, Niaura, & Abrams, 1992). Further, data from a worksite sample of women indicate that approximately 40% of respondents had no plans to begin being physically active in the near future, and another 34% were not regularly active (Marcus, Pinto, Simkin, Audrain, & Taylor, 1994). Designing separate interventions specifically to meet the needs of individuals at each stage has demonstrated superior efficacy in helping people to change sedentary lifestyles (Marcus, Banspach, et al., 1992; Marcus, Emmons, et al., in press).

For example, in one such study (Marcus, Emmons et al., in press), employees were randomized to a self-help intervention tailored to their motivational readiness for physical-activity adoption or a standard non-tailored self-help intervention. Printed self-help materials were delivered at baseline and again 1 month later. Results showed significantly greater gains in readiness for physical-activity participation among subjects given the tailored intervention compared to those given the standard intervention.

In conclusion, worksite health promotion and physical activity campaigns have been used successfully to increase physical activity adoption among employees (Blair et al., 1986; Brill et al., 1991; King et al., 1988). Employee participation can be maximized through offering a variety of physical activities, tailoring the intervention to employee's level of motivation for change, maximizing convenience, permitting employees to be physically active on company time, and/or allowing flexible time schedules to use facilities (e.g., Brill et al., 1991). While educational campaigns can aid recruitment, employee involvement in program setup and administration also may be important to program success (King, 1994). Incentives and awards for regular participation also have been used to enhance continued participation (e.g., Stoffelmayr et al., 1992).

Additional work is needed to determine the most effective methods for increasing physical activity among employees. Thus far, the majority of studies in these settings have enrolled self-selected samples of people who volunteer to participate in a physical-activity program. This does not reach the majority of individuals who are most sedentary and would stand to benefit most from these interventions.

Provider-Delivered Interventions

Physicians play an important role in the promotion of healthy lifestyle behaviors such as physical activity. The U.S. Preventive Services Task Force has recommended that physicians counsel all patients to engage in a program of regular physical activity, tailored to their health status and personal lifestyle (U.S. Preventive Services Task Force, 1989). The National Health Promotion and Disease Prevention Objectives for the year 2000 (USDHHS, 1991) include the objective: increase to at least 50% the proportion of primary care providers who routinely assess and counsel their patients regarding their physical activity practices.

Physicians are a potentially influential group for effecting change in the activity habits of individuals, since a majority of people visit physicians frequently and patients look to physicians for advice regarding preventive behavior (Wallace, Brennan, & Haines, 1987; Godin & Shephard, 1990). Although physicians are likely to have a positive effect on patients' level of activity, the rate of physical-activity counseling by physicians is generally low (Gemson & Elinson, 1986; Lewis, C. E., Wells, & Ware, 1986; Wechsler, Levine, Idelson, Rohman, & Taylor, 1983). For example, in one study, only 29% of physicians surveyed reported that they usually counsel on physical activity during a preventive checkup (Rosen, Logson, & Demak, 1984). Studies that have surveyed patients report even lower rates of physical activity counseling by physicians than those utilizing data from physician self-report (C. E. Lewis, 1988; Russell & Roter, 1993).

There is some evidence to suggest that physician-delivered counseling can change patient activity levels. In a multi-site, multi-behavior intervention by primary care physicians, Logsdon and colleagues (Logsdon, Lazaro, & Meier, 1989) found that 33.8% of the intervention vs. 24.1% of the control patients ($p < .05$) reported starting to exercise (comparisons adjusted for age, gender, and location by group status interaction). Positive results have also been obtained in other studies (e.g., B. S. Lewis & Lynch, 1993; Washburn, Janney, & Caswell, 1990).

Project PACE (Provider-Based Assessment and Counseling for Exercise), a multi-site field trial of a medical office-based exercise counseling intervention, was based on the transtheoretical model of behavior change and social cognitive theory (Long et al., 1996). Twenty-seven primary care physicians in four locations throughout the United States were trained in physical-activity counseling tailored to patient's stage of readiness for physical-activity adoption. Physicians were provided with an assessment form to identify a patient's level of activity and to determine the appropriate counseling protocol. In addition, they were trained to provide specific suggestions for changing factors that influence physical-activity adoption, such as social support, perceived barriers, and self-efficacy, and to use goal setting, contracting, problem solving, and self-reward to help their patients. Results revealed that 75% of physicians reported they would recommend PACE to other physicians, and that over 80% of their patients were receptive to the intervention. Assessment of physical activity in patients revealed that 50% of precontemplators considered beginning an activity program. Sixty-six percent of contemplators reported making recommended changes in activity, and 89% of patients in action continued their current level of activity. In a randomized trial evaluating the efficacy of Project PACE, experimental patients significantly increased their duration of walking and demonstrated a greater increase in readiness to become physically active than did control patients (Calfas et al., 1996).

The transtheoretical model and social-cognitive theory also were used in a pilot study on the feasibility of training physicians in activity-counseling techniques for middle-aged and older adults (Marcus et al., 1997). Four physicians in one community-based primary care office practice participated. Physicians were instructed to counsel their patients according to stage of activity adoption, provide their patients with a written activity prescription and a stage-matched self-help manual supplied by the research team, and schedule a follow-up visit to discuss physical activity. Experimental patients significantly increased their scores on the Physical Activity Scale for the Elderly (PASE). Physicians were enthusiastic about the counseling approach and delivered it to their designated patients. The effect was strongest for those patients who reported receiving more specific counseling from their physician. A randomized clinical trial to more clearly evaluate this research question is now in the field and entitled Project PAL (Physically Active for Life).

A 5-year (1994–1999) multicenter trial funded by the National Heart, Lung, and Blood Institute entitled ACT (Activity Counseling Trial) is also in the field. This trial utilizes health educators in addition to physicians to deliver the counseling message. This is a hierarchical design with patients receiving physician advice or advice plus a media-based intervention or physician advice, media-based intervention, and health-educator counseling and classes. This trial is also based on social cognitive theory and the transtheoretical model. Change in physical activity, physical fitness, and various psychological and quality-of-life parameters will be evaluated.

In summary, the efficacy of physician-delivered interventions in physical activity needs further study. From a public-health perspective, however, the impact of physician counseling on inactivity could be significant. Trials examining minimal and optimal doses of physician and other allied health professionals' time to produce the desired behavior change in patients are extremely important at this time.

Randomized Community Trials

Few large-scale national trials have focused exclusively on the promotion of physical activity. Rather, enhancement of physical activity has been embedded within larger multiple risk-factor interventions. The Stanford Five-City Multiple Risk Reduction Project (Farquhar et al., 1990), for example, was a 5-year randomized community trial to reduce cardiovascular disease risk factors through community organization and education to reduce cholesterol, blood pressure, cigarette use, obesity, and sedentary behavior. With regard to the latter, residents in the treatment cities were encouraged to build physical activity into their daily routines (e.g., walk to the store, take stairs), to increase participation in recreational activities, and to enroll in exercise classes (Young, Haskell, Taylor, & Fortmann, 1996). Furthermore, educational messages promoting the benefits of exercise were given through multiple channels and settings, and community walking events were established. While overall mortality and CHD risk were significantly reduced in intervention communities (Farquhar et al., 1990), changes in knowledge, attitudes, and behavior regarding physical activity were modest. Although numerous analyses were conducted, the only significant findings were from cross-sectional analyses, which indicated that men in the treatment cities increased daily energy expenditure and percent participation in vigorous activities; women in the treatment cities who were prospectively followed demonstrated an increase in the number of moderate activities (Young et al., 1996). The authors posit that the lack of strong results may have been a function of a weak physical-activity intervention effort relative to the delivery of other health promotion messages. However, in a representative community sample of the Stanford project, increases in physical activity (both moderate and vigorous) over a 5-year period were associated with an increase in HDL cholesterol in both men and women, and decreases in BMI and CHD risk in men (Young, Haskell, Taylor, & Fortmann, 1993). Taken together, these results suggest that 1) public health messages that convey the benefits of increasing moderate activities can propel sedentary people to increase their levels of physical activity, since messages that promote moderate activity may provide the additional flexibility that is needed when targeting large groups of people; and 2) widespread efforts to increase physical activity can reduce cardiovascular risk. Whether or not increases in physical activity can be maintained over the long term is unclear.

The Minnesota Heart Health Program (MHHP; Crow et al., 1986) involved the delivery of a multicomponent health education campaign to reduce risk factors for cardiovascular disease in three matched pairs of communities over 5 years. The three intervention communities received multiple strategies, including physical activity campaigns, environmental changes (e.g., provision of bike racks), media education, physical-activity screening, adult education, and education for physicians and other health professionals with the goal of increasing motivation and reducing barriers to physical activity. The emphasis of the program was to increase levels of low-to-moderate-physical activity. Cross-sectional analyses of the data over time indicated a positive effect of the intervention on leisure time activity (representing moderate activity, in this study), and exposure to the intervention increased knowledge about physical activity and health (Blake et al., 1987). However, there were no differences between intervention and control communities in levels of general physical activity (Nothwehr, Elmer, & Hannan, 1994). A process evaluation of the facilitators of increased physical activity indicated that programs in schools and worksites were more effective than community events in increasing levels of physical activity (Blake et al., 1987).

Both the Stanford and MHHP results suggest that recommendations for low-to-moderate activity may increase adherence to physical activity. While these results are encouraging, they continue to fall short of national activity goals. One possible explanation may be that these studies utilize broad-based approaches with little accounting for differences between individual segments of the population. Although both studies penetrated the population at a variety of different levels vertically (from the microlevel face-to-face intervention to the macrolevel of mass media interventions), there was little attempt to account for differences between individuals within these different levels, horizontally (sociodemographic, psychosocial, and biobehavioral parameters).

A substudy within The Pawtucket Heart Health Program (Elder et al., 1986) was one of the first attempts to integrate an individual-level behavior-change model (the stages-of-change model; Prochaska & DiClemente, 1983) with a public-health approach (Marcus, Banspach et al., 1992). The stage of change of 610 sedentary individuals was assessed at baseline, followed by a 6-week stage-matched self-help manual and community-based intervention. Although this was not a controlled trial, the results were encouraging: 30% of those who were thinking about changing their behavior (contemplation stage) at baseline, and 60% of those who were occasional exercisers (preparation stage), had initiated regular physical-activity participation post-intervention. Computerized expert systems may facilitate population-wide approaches to patient-treatment matching (Marcus, Bock et al., in press). Future randomized trials of the use of the stages-of-change model to facilitate physical activity behavior change and adherence at the population level are needed. Therefore, population approaches and patient-treatment matching may not be mutually exclusive, and a hybrid of both approaches may increase physical-activity adherence. Effective community-level health promotion campaigns may need to, first, account for individual differences in sociodemographic and psychosocial variables; second, segment populations according to these differences; and third, develop interventions that would target these specific subgroups and accelerate the acceptance of behavior change (King, 1994).

Targeting At-Risk Populations Within the Community

One characteristic of public-health approaches is that they adopt a "seeking," rather than a "waiting," stance (King, 1994). The seeking stance is especially important for high-risk groups who are unlikely to respond proactively to interventions or traditional recruitment strategies. The Bootheel Heart Health Project was a 3-year, multicomponent cardiovascular risk reduction project targeting the rural population of southeastern Missouri, an area with high rates of poverty, low educational levels, and the highest population of African-Americans in the state (Brownson et al., 1996). Intervention activities included walking clubs, health promotion during church sermons, and environmental changes (e.g., fitness paths). Although the study lacked a true experimental design and comparison groups (data from the Behavioral Risk Factor Surveillance System were used for comparison), communities which actively promoted intervention activities through coalitions demonstrated significant improvements in the levels of physical activity. Since community coalitions can form a stable structure in the community, they may facilitate physical-activity adherence as well.

While the previous study focused on promoting a variety of health behaviors, there are at least two trials that focus exclusively on the promotion of physical activity among low-SES African-Americans: The Community Health Assessment and Promotion Project (CHAPP; Lasco et al., 1989) and the Physical Activity Risk Reduction Project (PARR; B. S. Lewis et al., 1993). The goal of CHAPP was to promote nutrition and moderate physical activity among African-American females in Atlanta using culturally sensitive intervention methods at several levels (individual, environmental, and policy) while addressing practical needs of this group (e.g., security escorts for walkers in high-crime neighborhoods, free transportation and child care). Adherence to physical-activity recommendations were measured by client participation, which at the end of 4 months was over 60%.

The PARR project was a randomized community trial to increase physical activity in public-housing communities in Alabama. Intervention communities received pamphlets written at a 6th-grade reading level. The PARR project tested two interventions: 1) a basic intervention, which involved a community-based physical activity program and pamphlets on a home-based physical activity program; and 2) an enhanced intervention, which involved the basic program plus behavioral interventions to increase participation and adherence (competitions, support of community church leaders, training leaders in behavioral concepts to motivate individuals, and overcoming barriers such as child care). There were no significant differences in change in physical activity from pre- to post- intervention between the intervention groups, or between the control and intervention groups.

Although the PARR intervention was not successful despite its tailoring to a particular high-risk population, other studies have shown a diffusion effect for physical activity messages. For example, the Zuni Indians Diabetes Project sought to increase physical-activity participation as a means of controlling diabetes using culturally similar physical-activity instructors. Diabetic participants significantly reduced their weight relative to diabetic nonparticipants, and importantly, 18% of inactive diabetic individuals who did not participate in the program initiated a home-based physical activity program (Heath, Wilson, Smith, & Leonard, 1991). Thus, changes in community norms and the creation of stable structures in the community may be important for the initiation of behavior change and adherence to that change.

In conclusion, public-health approaches to increasing physical activity have produced modest results. This may be due to the fact that few interventions have focused exclusively on the promotion of physical activity. Instead, physical activity interventions have been embedded within multiple risk-factor interventions, some of which contain stronger messages to change other health-risk behaviors that may overshadow the importance of initiating and adhering to physical activity.

DISCUSSION

While physical activity is positively associated with numerous physiological and psychological benefits, the majority of the population continues to be sedentary and therefore at increased risk for morbidity and mortality. While past research on the health benefits of physical activity has been concerned with vigorous exercise, there is accumulating evidence that moderate activity is also associated positively with improvements in health. The new CDC/ACSM physical activity guidelines recommending moderate and/or vigorous activity are more flexible, and given that research suggests improved adherence to moderate activity, these guidelines could result in a higher proportion of individuals who are regularly active.

It is clear that sedentary behavior is more characteristic of minorities, the elderly, and individuals with lower education and income levels (CDC, 1993). Physical activity interventions need to accommodate the current needs of these individuals and address potential barriers to physical-activity participation, recognizing that different individuals may have different needs and face different barriers to becoming physically active. For example, while certain barriers such as time, money, and access to child care are frequently cited by both genders (Sallis, Hovell, & Hofstetter, 1992), these barriers tend to have a greater impact among women and low-income individuals (Etkin, 1994; Verhoef et al., 1993; Zakarian, Hovell, Hofstetter, Sallis, & Keating, 1994). Programs should be designed with these potential barriers in mind.

Worksite-based physical-activity programs can reduce several common barriers to physical-activity participation, such as the convenience of facilities, financial considerations, and both work and child-care schedules. In addition, two frequently cited barriers to participation, time and accessibility (Dishman & Sallis, 1994), may be most readily addressed by providing interventions in the workplace.

The issue of physical-activity adherence, independent of initiation, has been neglected in large-scale community and public-health level studies. This may be due to the fact that it is difficult to promote the initiation even of physical activity, let alone adherence. Public-health interventions need to deliver interventions at all levels of analysis (from micro-individual to macro policy changes) while accounting for psychosocial and demographic factors within each level of analysis. In this way, patient-treatment matching does not have to lie exclusively within the realm of clinic-based programs.

Recent advances in computer technology have enabled health-care delivery services to provide low-cost, yet highly individualized interventions. Computer "expert systems" have been developed to deliver professional-level counseling and interventions for smoking cessation (e.g., Strecher et al., 1994) and physical-activity adoption (Marcus, Bock, et al., in press). An expert system is a computer program which mimics the reasoning or advice-giving capabilities of a human expert (Negotia, 1985). These systems can be used to supplement behavioral treatments and can enhance interventions provided by health-care workers. Expert systems also may differ in their acceptability and accessibility among different socioeconomic and ethnic groups. Expert systems can provide inexpensive, tailored interventions, and are capable of modifying the intervention to match the needs and interests of the user (Slack, Safran, Kowaloff, Pearce, & Delbanco, 1995). Computers cannot and should not be used in contexts where "high-touch" is a distinct advantage, to create redundancy with the existing functions of human interviewers, or in situations where computers are not acceptable to patients. However, with the increase in the number of home computers in this country, the possibility for computerized prompts and interactions appears to be an important area for investigation.

In conclusion, research on physical-activity interventions highlights the importance of increasing our understanding of the factors related to physical-activity adherence so that more effective interventions can be developed. Most investigators in behavior change have identified the importance of individual factors and thus support patient-treatment matching models; this appears to hold in the physical activity realm as well. Theories such as the stages-of-change model are particularly useful in treatment-matching, as they provide a framework for tailoring the intervention to the motivation level of the individual.

REFERENCES

American College of Sports Medicine. (1990). Position statement on the recommended quantity and quality of exercise for developing and maintaining cardiorespiratory and muscular fitness in healthy adults. *Medicine and Science in Sports and Exercise, 22*, 265–74.

Altman, D. G., Evans, A. J., Flora, J. A., Benjamin, L., Albright, C. L., King, A. C., Blaskovich, L. G., Schneider, M., & Fortmann, S .P. (1986). A worksite exercise contest. In *Proceedings of the Society of Behavioral Medicine's Seventh Annual Scientific Sessions* (p. 38). Washington, DC: Society of Behavioral Medicine.

Bandura, A. (1977). Self-efficacy. Toward a unifying theory of behavioral change. *Psychological Review, 84*, 191–215.

Bandura, A. (1986). *Social foundations of thought and action. A social cognitive theory*. Englewood Cliffs, NJ: Prentice-Hall.

Belisle, M., Roskies, E., & Levesque, J. (1987). Improving adherence to physical activity. *Health Psychology, 2*, 159–172.

Blair, S. N., Piserchia, P. V., Wilbur, C. S., & Crowder, J. H. (1986). A public health intervention model for work-site health promotion: Impact on exercise and physical fitness in a health promotion plan after 24 months. *Journal of the American Medical Association, 255*, 921–926.

Blake, S. M., Jeffery, R. W., Finnegan, J. R., Crow, R. S., Pirie, P. L., Ringhofer, K. R., Fruetel, J. R., Caspersen, C. J., & Mittelmark, M. B. (1987). Process evaluation of a community-based physical activity campaign: The Minnesota Heart Health Program experience. *Health Education Research, 2*, 115–121.

Brill, P. A., Kohl, W. H., Rogers, T., Collingwood, T. R., Sterling, C. L., & Blair, S. N. (1991). Recruitment, retention and success in worksite health promotion: Association with demographic characteristics. *American Journal of Health Promotion, 5*, 215–221.

Brownson, R. C., Smith, C. A., Pratt, M., Mack, N. E., Jackson-Thompson, J., Dean, C. G., Dabney, S., & Wilkerson, J. C. (1996). Preventing cardiovascular disease through community-based risk reduction: The Bootheel Heart Health Project. *American Journal of Public Health, 86*, 206–213.

Calfas, K. J., Long, B. J., Sallis, J. F., Wooten, W. J., Pratt, M., & Patrick, K. (1996). A controlled trial of physician counseling to promote the adoption of physical activity. *Preventive Medicine, 25*, 225–233.

Centers for Disease Control. (1993). Prevalence of sedentary lifestyle-behavioral risk factor surveillance system, United States, 1991. *Morbidity and Mortality Weekly Report, 42*, 576–579.

Centers for Disease Control and American College of Sports Medicine. (1993). Summary statement: Workshop on physical activity and public health. *Sports Medicine Bulletin, 28*, 7.

Crow, R., Blackburn, H., Jacobs, D., Hannan, P., Pirie, P., Mittelmark, M., Murray, D., & Luepker, R. (1986). Population strategies to enhance physical activity: The Minnesota Heart Health Program. *Acta Medica Scandinavica*, Suppl 711, 93–112.

DiClemente, C. C., Prochaska, J. O., Fairhurst, S. K., Velicer, W. F., Velasquez, M. M., & Rossi, J. S. (1991). The process of smoking cessation: An analysis of precontemplation, contemplation, and preparation stages of change. *Journal of Consulting and Clinical Psychology, 59*, 295–304.

Dirkin, G. (1994). Technological supports for sustaining exercise. In R. K. Dishman (Ed.), *Advances in exercise adherence* (pp. 237–247). Champaign, IL: Human Kinetics.

Dishman, R. K. (1990). Determinants of participation in physical activity. In C. Bouchard, R. J. Shephard, T. Stephens, J. R. Sutton, & B. D. McPherson (Eds.), *Exercise, fitness and health* (pp. 75–102). Champaign, IL: Human Kinetics.

Dishman, R. K. (1991). Increasing and maintaining physical activity and exercise. *Behavior Therapy, 41*, 3–15.

Dishman, R. K. (1996 March). *Helping people succeed when exercise programs fail.* Paper presented at the New England Chapter of the American College of Sports Medicine, Amherst, MA.

Dishman, R. K., & Sallis, J. F. (1994). Determinants and interventions for physical activity and exercise. In B. Bouchard, R. J Shephard, & T. Stephens (Eds.), *Physical activity, fitness, and health: International proceedings and consensus statement* (pp. 214–238). Champaign, IL: Human Kinetics.

Dubbert, P. M. (1992). Exercise in behavioral medicine. *Journal of Consulting and Clinical Psychology, 60*, 613–618.

Dubbert, P. M., Rappaport, N. B., & Martin, J. E. (1987). Exercise in cardiovascular disease. *Behavior Modification, 11*, 329–347.

Elder, J. P., McGraw, S. A., Abrams, D. B., Ferreira, A., Lasater, T.M., Longpre, H., Peterson, G.S., Schwertfeger, R., & Carleton, R.A. (1986). Organizational and community approaches to community-wide prevention of heart disease: The first two years of the Pawtucket Heart Health Program. *Preventive Medicine, 15*, 107–117.

Etkin, S. E. (1994). Reaching the hard to reach: Active living programs for low socioeconomic individuals. In H. A. Quinney, L. Gauvin, & A. E. T. Wall (Eds.), *Toward active living* (pp. 263–268). Champaign, IL: Human Kinetics.

Farquhar, J. W., Fortmann, S. P., Flora, J. A., Taylor, C. B., Haskell, W. L., Williams, P. T., Maccoby, N., & Wood, P. D. (1990). The Stanford Five-City Project: Effects of community-wide education on cardiovascular disease risk factors. *Journal of the American Medical Association, 264*, 359–365.

Fielding, J. E. (1984). Health promotion and disease prevention at the worksite. *Annual Review of Public Health, 5*, 237–265.

Fielding, J. E., & Knight, K. K. (1994). Cost-benefit analysis of workplace active living programs: The employer perspective. In H. A. Quinney, L. Gauvin, & A. E. T. Wall (Eds.), *Toward active living* (pp. 187–192). Champaign, IL: Human Kinetics.

Gemson, D. H., & Elinson, J. (1986). Prevention in primary care: Variability in physician practice patterns in New York City. *American Journal of Preventive Medicine, 2*, 226–234.

Godin, G., & Shephard, R. J. (1990). An evaluation of the potential role of the physician in influencing community exercise behavior. *American Journal of Health Promotion, 4*, 255–259.

Gomel, M., Oldenburg, B., Simpson, J., & Owen, N. (1993). Work-site cardiovascular risk reduction: A randomized trial of health risk assessment, education, counseling, and incentives. *American Journal of Public Health, 83*, 1231–1238.

Heath, G. W., Wilson, R. H., Smith, J., & Leonard, B. E. (1991). Community-based exercise and weight control: Diabetes risk reduction and glycemic control in Zuni Indians. *American Journal of Clinical Nutrition, 53*, 1642S–1646S.

Huddy, D. C., Hebert, J. L., Hyner, G. C., & Johnson, R. L. (1995). Facilitating changes in exercise behavior: Effect of structured statements of intention on perceived barriers to action. *Psychological Reports, 76*, 867–875.

Janis, I. L., & Mann, L. (1977). *Decision making: A psychological analysis of conflict, choice and commitment.* New York: Free Press.

King, A. C. (1994). Clinical and community interventions to promote and support physical activity participation. In R. Dishman (Ed), *Advances in exercise adherence* (pp.183–212). Champaign, IL: Human Kinetics.

King, A. C., Blair, S. N., Bild, D., Dubbert, P. M., Marcus, B. H., Oldridge, N. B., Paffenbarger, R. S., Powell, K. E., & Yeager, K. (1992). Determinants of physical activity and interventions in adults. *Medicine and Science in Sports and Exercise, 24*(suppl), S221–S236.

King, A. C., & Frederiksen, L. W. (1984). Low-cost strategies for increasing exercise behavior. *Behavior Modification, 8*, 3–21.

King, A. C., Frey-Hewitt, B., Dreon, D. M., & Wood, P. D. (1989). Diet exercise in weight maintenance: The effects of minimal intervention strategies of long-term outcomes in men. *Archives of Internal Medicine, 149*, 2741–2746.

King, A. C., Haskell, W. L., Taylor, C. B., Kraemer, H. C., & Debusk, R. F. (1991). Group vs. home-based exercise training in healthy older men and women. *Journal of the American Medical Association, 266*, 1535–1542.

King, A. C., Taylor, C. B., & Haskell, W. L. (1993). Effects of differing intensities and formats of 12 months of exercise training on psychological outcomes in older adults. *Health Psychology, 12*, 292–300.

King, A. C., Taylor, C. B., Haskell, W. L., & DeBusk, R. F. (1988). Strategies for increasing early adherence to and long-term maintenance of home-based exercise training in healthy middle-aged men and women. *American Journal of Cardiology, 61*, 628–632.

Klonoff, E. A., Annechild, A., & Landrine, H. (1994). Predicting exercise adherence in women: The role of psychological and physiological factors. *Preventive Medicine, 23*, 257–262.

Knadler, G. F., & Rogers, T. (1987). Mountain climb month program: A low-cost exercise intervention program a high-rise worksite. *Fitness in Business*, October, 64–67.

Knapp, D. N. (1988). Behavioral management techniques and exercise promotion. In R. K. Dishman (Ed.), *Exercise adherence: Its impact on public health* (pp. 203–236). Champaign, IL: Human Kinetics.

Lasco, R. A., Curry, R. H., Dickson, V. J., Powers, J., Menes, S., & Merritt, R. K. (1989). Participation rates, weight loss, and blood pressure changes among obese women in a nutrition-exercise program. *Public Health Reports, 101*, 125–131.

Leith, L. M., & Taylor, A. H. (1992). Behavior modification and exercise adherence: A literature review. *Journal of Sport Behavior, 15*, 60–74.

Lewis, B. S., & Lynch, W. D. (1993). The effect of physician advice on exercise behavior. *Preventive Medicine, 22*, 110–121.

Lewis, C. E. (1988). Disease prevention and health promotion practices of primary care physicians in the United States. *American Journal of Preventive Medicine, 4*(suppl.), 9–16.

Lewis, C. E., Raczynski, J. M., Heath, G. W., Levinson, R., Hilyer, J. C., & Cutter, G. R. (1993). Promoting physical activity in low-income African-American communities: The PARR project. *Ethnicity & Disease, 3*, 106–118.

Lewis, C. E., Wells, K. B., & Ware, J. (1986). A model for predicting the counseling practices of physicians. *Journal of General Internal Medicine, 1*, 14–19.

Logsdon, D. N., Lazaro, C. M., & Meier, R. V. (1989). The feasibility of behavioral risk reduction in primary medical care. *American Journal of Preventive Medicine, 5*, 249–256.

Lombard, D. N., Lombard, T. N., & Winett, R. A. (1995). Walking to meet health guidelines: The effect of prompting frequency and prompt structure. *Health Psychology, 14*, 164–170.

Long, B. J., Calfas, K. J., Patrick, K., Sallis, J. F., Wooten, W. J., Goldstein, M., Marcus, B., Schwenk, T., Carter, R., Torez, T., Polinkas, L., & Heath, G. (1996). Acceptability, usability and practicality of physician counseling for physical activity promotion: Project PACE. *American Journal of Preventive Medicine, 12*, 73–81.

Luepker, R. (1994). Community trials. *Preventive Medicine, 23*, 602–605.

Lynch, W. D., & Main, D. S. (1993). Frequency of exercise and dropouts in a worksite program. Correlates of 6-month activity patterns. *Journal of Occupational Medicine, 35*, 1147–1151.

Marcus, B. H., Banspach, S. W., Lefebvre, R. C., Rossi, J. S., Carleton, R. C., & Abrams, D. B. (1992). Using the stages of change model to increase the adoption of physical activity among community participants. *American Journal of Health Promotion, 6*, 424–429.

Marcus, B. H., Bock, B. C., Pinto, B. M., Forsyth, L. H., Roberts, M. B., & Troficoate, R. (in press). Efficacy of an individualized motivationally tailored physical activity intervention. *Annals of Behavioral Medicine.*

Marcus, B. H., Eaton, C. A., Rossi, J. S., & Harlow, L. L. (1994). Self-efficacy, decision making and stages of change: An integrative model of physical exercise. *Journal of Applied Social Psychology, 24*, 489–508.

Marcus, B. H., Emmons, K. M., Simkin-Silverman, L. R., Linnan, L., Taylor, E. R.,

Bock, B. C., Roberts, M. B., Rossi, J. S., & Abrams, D. B. (in press). Evaluation of motivationally tailored versus standard self-help physical activity interventions at the workplace. *American Journal of Health Promotion.*

Marcus, B. H., Goldstein, M. G., Jeffe, A., Simkin-Silverman, L., Pinto, B. M., Milan, F., Washburn, R., Smith, K., Rakowski, W. & Dube, C. (1997). Training physicians to conduct physical activity counselling. *Preventive Medicine, 26,* 382–388.

Marcus, B. H., King, T. K., Clark, M. M., Pinto, B. M., & Bock, B. C. (1996). Theories and techniques for promoting physical activity behaviors. *Sports Medicine, 22,* 321–331.

Marcus, B. H., Pinto, B. M., Simkin, L. R., Audrain, J. E., & Taylor, E. R. (1994). Application of theoretical models to exercise behavior among employed women. *American Journal of Health Promotion, 9,* 49–55.

Marcus, B. H., Rossi, J. S., Selby, V. C., Niaura, R. S., & Abrams, D. B. (1992). The stages of processes of exercise adoption and maintenance in a worksite sample. *Health Psychology, 11,* 386–395.

Marcus, B. H., & Sallis, J. F. (1997). Determinants of physical activity behavior and implication for intervention. In A. S. Lean (Ed.) *Physical Activity and Cardiovascular Health* (pp. 192–201). Champaign, IL: Human Kinetics.

Marcus, B. H., & Stanton, A. L. (1993). Evaluation of relapse prevention and reinforcement interventions to promote exercise adherence in sedentary females. *Research Quarterly for Exercise and Sport, 64,* 447–452.

Marlatt, G. A., & Gordon, J. R. (1980). Determinants of relapse: Implications for the maintenance of behavior change. In P. O. Davidson (Eds.), *Behavioral medicine: Changing health lifestyles* (pp. 410–452). Elmsford, NY: Pergamon.

Marlatt, G. A., & Gordon, J. R. (1985). *Relapse prevention: Maintenance strategies in addictive behavior change.* New York: Guilford.

Martin, J. E., Dubbert, P. M., Katell, A. D., Thompson, J. K., Raczynski, J. R., Lake, M., Smith, P. O., Webster, J. S., Sikora, T., & Cohen, R. E. (1984). Behavioral control of exercise in sedentary adults: Studies 1 through 6. *Journal of Consulting and Clinical Psychology, 52,* 795–811.

McAuley, E., Courneya, K. S., Rudolph, D. L., & Lox, C. L. (1994). Enhancing exercise adherence in middle-aged males and females. *Preventive Medicine, 23,* 498–506.

Morey, M. C., Cowper, P. A., Feussner, J. R., DiPasquale, R. C., Crowley, G. M., Kitzman, D. W., & Sullivan, R. J., Jr. (1989). Evaluation of a supervised exercise program in a geriatric population. *Journal of the American Geriatric Society, 37,* 348–354.

Negotia, U. N. (1985). *Expert systems and fuzzy systems.* Menlo Park, CA: Benjamin/Cummings.

Nothwehr, M. A., Elmer, P., & Hannan, P. (1994). Prevalence of health behaviors related to hypertension in three blood pressure treatment groups: The Minnesota Heart Health Program. *Preventive Medicine, 23,* 362–368.

Ossip-Klein, D. J., Doyne, E. J., Bowman, E. D., Osborn, K. M., McDougall-Wilson, J. B., & Neimeyer, R. A. (1989). Effects of running or weight lifting on self- concept in clinically depressed women. *Journal of Consulting and Clinical Psychology, 57,* 158–161.

Pappas, G. P., Golin, S., & Meyer, D. L. (1990). Reducing symptoms of depression with exercise. *Psychosomatics, 31*, 112–113.

Pate, R. R., Pratt, M., Blair, S. N., Haskell, W. L., Macera, C. A., Bouchard, C., Buchner, D., Ettinger, W., Heath, G. W., King, A. C., Kriska, A., Leon, A. S., Marcus, B. H., Morris, J., Paffenbarger, R. S., Patrick, K., Pollock, M. L., Rippe, J. M., Sallis, J., & Wilmore, J. H. (1995). Physical activity and public health: A recommendation from the Centers for Disease Control and the American College of Sports Medicine. *Journal of the American Medical Association, 273*, 402–407.

Prochaska, J. O., & DiClemente, C. C. (1983). Stages and processes of self-change of smoking: Toward an integrative model of change. *Journal of Consulting and Clinical Psychology, 51*, 390–395.

Reynolds, K. D., Killen, J. D., Bryson, S. W., Maron, D.J., Taylor, C.B., Maccoby, N., & Farquhar, J.W. (1990). Psychosocial predictors of physical activity in adolescents. *Preventive Medicine, 19*, 541–551.

Robison, J. I., & Rogers, M. A. (1994). Adherence to exercise programmes. *Sports Medicine, 17*, 39–52.

Rodgers, W. M., & Brawley, L. R. (1993). Using both self-efficacy theory and the theory of planned behavior to discriminate adherers and dropouts from structured programs. *Journal of Applied Sports Psychology, 5*, 195–206.

Rosen, M. A., Logson, D. N., & Demak, M. M. (1984). Prevention and health promotion in primary care: Baseline results on physicians from the INSURE project on lifecycle preventive health services. *Preventive Medicine, 13*, 535–548.

Russell, N. K., & Roter, D. L. (1993). Health promotion counseling of chronic-disease patients during primary care visits. *American Journal of Public Health, 83*, 979–982.

Sallis, J. F., Haskell, W. L., Fortmann, S. P., Vranizan, K. M., Taylor, C. B., & Solomon, D. S. (1986). Predictors of adoption and maintenance of physical activity in a community sample. *Preventive Medicine, 15*, 331–341.

Sallis, J. F., Hovell, M. F., & Hofstetter, C. R. (1992). Predictors of adoption and maintenance of vigorous physical activity in men and women. *Preventive Medicine, 21*, 237–251.

Sallis, J. F., Hovell, M. F., Hofstetter, C. R., Elder, J. P., Hackley, M., Caspersen, C. J., & Powell, K. E. (1990). Distance between homes and exercise facilities related to frequency of exercise among San Diego residents. *Public Health Reports, 105*, 179–185.

Sallis, J. F., Hovell, M. F., Hofstetter, C. R., & Faucher, P. (1989). A multivariate study of determinants of vigorous exercise in a community sample. *Preventive Medicine, 18*, 20–34.

Shephard, R. J. (1988). Exercise adherence in corporate settings: Personal traits and program barriers. In R. K. Dishman (Ed.), *Exercise adherence: Its impact on public health* (pp. 305–320). Champaign, IL: Human Kinetics.

Shephard, R. J. (1992). A critical analysis of work-site fitness programs and their postulated economic benefits. *Medicine and Science in Sports and Exercise, 24*, 354–370.

Simkin, L. R., & Gross, A. M. (1994). Assessment of coping with high-risk situations for exercise relapse among healthy women. *Health Psychology, 13*, 274–277.

Skinner, B. F. (1953). *Science and human behavior*. New York: Macmillan.

Slack, W. V., Safran, C., Kowaloff, H. B., Pearce, J., & Delbanco, T. L. (1995). A computer administered health screening interview for hospital personnel. *MD Computer, 12*, 25–30.

Stoffelmayr, B. E., Mavis, B. E., Stachnik, T., Robison, J., Rogers, M., VanHuss, W., & Carlson, J. (1992). A program model to enhance adherence in worksite based fitness programs. *Journal of Occupational Medicine, 34*, 157–161.

Strecher V. J., Kreuter, M., Den Boer D., Kobrin, S., Hospers, H. J., & Skinner, C. S. (1994). The effects of computer-tailored smoking cessation messages in family practice settings. *Journal of Family Practice, 39*, 262–268.

United States Department of Health and Human Services (1991). *Healthy people 2000: National health promotion and disease prevention objectives* (DHHS Publication No. [PHS] 91–50212). Washington, DC: U.S. Government Printing Office.

United States Department of Health and Human Services. (1996). *Physical activity and health*. A report of the Surgeon General. Centers for Disease Control and Prevention. National Center for Chronic Disease Prevention and Health Promotion.

United States Preventive Services Task Force. (1989). *Guide to clinical preventive services: An assessment of the effectiveness of 169 interventions* (pp. 297–304). Baltimore, MD: Williams & Wilkins.

Verhoef, M. J., Hamm, R. D., & Love, E. J. (1993). Exercising at work: Barriers to women's participation. *American Association of Occupational Health Nurses, 41*, 275–281.

Wallace, P. G., Brennan, P. J., & Haines, A. P. (1987). Are general practitioners doing enough to promote healthy lifestyle? Findings of the Medical Research Council's General Practice Research Framework study on lifestyle and health. *British Medical Journal, 294*, 940–942.

Washburn, R. A., Janney, C. A., & Caswell, C. (1990). Physicians recommendation influences walking for exercise in older people. *Medicine and Science in Sports and Exercise, 22*, 546.

Wechsler, H., Levine, S., Idelson, R. K., Rohman, M., & Taylor, J. O. (1983). The physician's role in health promotion—A survey of primary-care practitioners. *New England Journal of Medicine, 308*, 97–100.

Winette, R. A., King, A. C., & Altman, D. G. (1989). *Health psychology and public health: An integrative approach*. Elmsford, NY: Pergamon.

Young, D. R., Haskell, W. L., Taylor, C. B., & Fortmann, S. P. (1993). Effect of community health education on physical activity knowledge, attitudes, and behavior: The Stanford Five-City Project. *American Journal of Epidemiology, 144*, 264–274.

Zakarian, J. M., Hovell, M. F., Hofstetter, C. R., Sallis, J. F., & Keating, K. J. (1994). Correlates of vigorous exercise in a predominantly low SES and minority school population. *Preventive Medicine, 23*, 314–321.

9

Adoption and Maintenance of Safer Sexual Practices

Michelle J. Naughton and Shellie D. Ellis

INTRODUCTION

Unsafe sexual practices are a leading cause of morbidity in the U.S. and the world. Consequences of such behaviors include the contraction of sexually transmitted diseases, including HIV infection, and unintended pregnancies. Sexual behavior is directly intertwined in the contraction of these conditions, and there is a burgeoning need for the development and evaluation of strategies to reduce unsafe sexual practices that may lead to undesirable health consequences. Barrier methods of contraception, particularly latex condoms, have been shown to be effective in reducing the spread of sexually transmitted diseases and in preventing unplanned pregnancies (Carey et al., 1992; Centers for Disease Control [CDC], 1988). Therefore, the majority of safer sex prevention programs have been aimed at increasing condom use and in eliminating or decreasing risky sexual behaviors. In this chapter, we present an overview of safer sexual intervention strategies that have been used with men who have sex with men, injecting drug users, and adolescents and young adults. Recommendations for further research are provided.

MEN WHO HAVE SEX WITH MEN

The sexual practices and relative risks of sexual consequences are different for men who have sex with men than for heterosexuals and adolescents. Estimates of the prevalence of homosexuality in the United States have ranged from 2% to 20% (R. C. Friedman & Downey, 1994). A recent review of homosexual behaviors throughout the world, however, concluded that approximately 6% of men and 3% of women have engaged in same-sex behaviors since adolescence (Diamond, 1993). Gay males are more likely than heterosexual males to initiate sexual activities at a younger age (12.7 versus 15.7 years, respectively), and to have multiple sexual partners (R. C. Friedman & Downey, 1994). In contrast, lesbians and heterosexual females report similar ages at the time of their first sexual experiences (Rotheram-Borus & Gwadz, 1993). The majority of homosexual men have had 20 or fewer sexual partners in their lifetime, which is similar to the numbers of partners of heterosexual males (Fay, Turner, Klassen, Gagnon 1989; R. C. Friedman & Downey, 1994). A small subgroup of homosexual males, however, may engage in sexual behaviors with a high number of sexual partners, placing them at increased risk for negative health consequences (R. C. Friedman & Downey, 1994).

In male-male sex there is no risk of pregnancy, which is a primary motivation for condom use among heterosexuals (Tanfer, Grady, Klepinger, & Billy, 1993). Condom use was initially low among gay men, and thus, HIV infection became prevalent in industrialized countries before condom use was established as an efficient means of prevention. Consequently, the risk of having sex with an infected person has been greater for these individuals, and men who have sex with men continue to account for the major mode of transmission in the United States (CDC, 1995). Cases of AIDS are increasing more rapidly, however, among injecting drug-users, and through heterosexual contact (CDC, 1994).

The stigma of homosexuality has engendered a different context for behavioral interventions and adherence. Once effective HIV prevention methods were determined, many intervention programs were developed to change sexual behavior among gay men. While public health programs were slow to address prevention in this population (R. L. Miller, 1995), significant resources in the gay community made grassroots organization and intervention possible. Public health campaigns focused on HIV testing, providing information, and modeling safer sexual behaviors (Robert & Rosser, 1990). Gay community-based interventions concentrated on risk counseling with HIV testing, eroticizing safer sex, modeling social and behavior change through community organization, and condom skills training (R. L. Miller, 1995; Robert & Rosser, 1990). Because of the urgency of the impending epidemic, little time was available for determining efficacy of methods prior to the interventions (Valdiserri, Lyter, Leviton, Stoner, & Silvestre, 1987), and little evaluation of such programs has been completed. Since the majority of programs are provided by community-based organizations, they are rarely documented. Program effectiveness and the processes by which these programs work are unknown (R. L. Miller, 1995). The effects of widespread media campaigns conducted by public health professionals are difficult to measure. However, despite the limited understanding of intervention efficacy (Robert & Rosser, 1990), and methodological problems of measurement such as the use of serial cross-sectional studies instead of longitudinal studies (R. L. Miller, 1995), much research on men who have sex with men focuses on behavior maintenance and relapse prevention.

Although bisexual or homosexual men are more likely than heterosexual men to report condom use (Tanfer et al., 1993), the frequency of consistent condom use is low among men who have sex with men. Estimates of consistent condom use range from less than 20% in Scotland (Gruer & Ssembatya-Lule, 1993) to 39 and 43% in England and Wales for insertive and receptive anal intercourse, respectively (Weatherburn, Hunt, Davies, Coxon, & Manus, 1991). Condom use varies by sexual activity, too; it is much higher for anal sex than for oral sex (Hunt et al., 1993). Attempts to identify predictors of condom use lack consensus and often provide contradictory results. Catania et al. (1991) found consistent condom use to be associated with higher levels of social support from informal sources of help, more positive expectations that condoms will have positive interpersonal and personal consequences, and HIV-positive serostatus. Cultural and social circumstances may also affect correlates of condom use. For example, African-American gay men may have less social support, and therefore lower condom use, because of the strong stigma associated with homosexuality in the African American community. In another study of gay and bisexual African American men, unprotected anal intercourse was associated with low income, sex for payment, and drug injection (Peterson et al., 1992).

Relationship type also seems to bear on safer sexual practices. Anal intercourse is more common in coupled relationships (Meyer & Dean, 1995), and condom use is more prevalent with casual rather than regular partners (Hunt et al., 1993). Although some studies indicate that alcohol and other drug use are associated with unsafe sex (Meyer & Dean, 1995), other research indicates that gay men are no more likely to engage in risky behaviors after consuming alcohol (Weatherburn et al., 1993). Gay and bisexual men who do consistently have unprotected anal intercourse while under the influence of alcohol or other drugs are more likely to have less than a college education, to have an income of less than $20,000, to use amyl nitrite and cocaine, and to report a higher frequency of anal sex. Interestingly enough, these men are also less likely to approve of sex without love, less likely to perceive that safe sex is the community norm, and to have little encouragement from friends to practice safer sex (Crosby, Stall, Paul, Barrett, & Midanik, 1996). Research based on the theory of reasoned action provides contradictory findings as well. Attitudes and norms were the most significant correlates of intentions to use condoms and actual condom use behaviors among both heterosexual and homosexual men (Fisher, Fisher, & Rye, 1995; Treffke, Tiggemann, & Ross, 1992). However, in another study of homosexual men in Australia, attitudes were poor predictors of intentions, whereas subjective norms were good predictors of intentions to use condoms (Ross & McLaws, 1992).

Both intervention-specific and population-based evaluations of interventions demonstrate initial success. Condom use among gay men in Denver increased from 63% to 71% following a CDC Demonstration Project for HIV prevention (Cohn et al., 1992) Other population-based studies suggest that gay men have dramatically changed their sexual behavior in the face of the AIDS crisis. Condom use has increased (Catania et al., 1991; Hunt et al., 1993; Kelly, St. Lawrence, & Brasfield, 1991), as has abstinence of both receptive and insertive anal sex (Adib, Joseph, Ostrow, Tal, Schwartz, 1991; Kelly et al., 1991). Sex with one-time or occasional partners was discontinued at higher rates than relapse (Cohn et al., 1992), and the number of sexual partners also has decreased (Kelly et al., 1991). Even though these changes have been remarkable, epidemiological studies have indicated other disturbing trends (Miller, 1995). Rates of HIV infection have leveled off among gay men, but rates of infection with other STDs have begun to rise. Gonorrhea diagnoses increased among STD clients in Amsterdam and among American homosexual men (CDC, 1989; de Wit, vanden Hack, Sandfort, & van Griensven, 1993).

Few intervention programs have been evaluated long-term. Of the evaluations which have been done, one study in New Zealand demonstrated little difference in global safer sexual practices across four different intervention strategies, although targeted strategies influenced specific safer sexual behaviors in different ways (Robert & Rosser, 1990). Another program effectively reduced participants' frequency of risky sexual practices and increased knowledge, behavioral skills, and safer sex practices by providing a combination of an AIDS risk educational program, cognitive-behavioral self-management training, sexual assertion training, and assistance in developing social support (Kelly, St. Lawrence, Hood, & Brasfield, 1989).

Based on assumptions of intervention effectiveness, recent research has focused on the "relapse" of risky sexual behavior among gay men (Adib, Joseph, Ostrow et al., 1991; Adib, Joseph, Ostrow, Tal et al., 1991; Kelly et al., 1991; McCusker, Stoddard, McDonald, & Zapka, Mayer, 1992). Rates of unsafe sex dubbed "relapse" are estimated to be 31% for receptive anal sex and 35% for insertive anal sex in one evaluation of a coping and change study (Adib, Joseph, Ostrow, Tal et al., 1991). Exceptions to safe sex, or relapse, are associated with younger age, earlier history of frequent unprotected receptive anal intercourse with multiple partners, greater number of past sex partners, reinforcement value levels of high-risk practices and condom use, intoxication preceding sex, lower scores on a depression measure, greater belief that HIV infection is largely determined by external factors such as chance or luck, and homosexuality "outness" (Kelly et al., 1991). Monogamous relationships, less peer support, and less assertiveness in negotiating safer sex were noted as predictors of relapse in another study (Adib, Joseph, Ostrow et al., 1991). Among gay and bisexual men in Sweden, exceptions to safe sex were linked with particular circumstances such as holidays, poor emotional state, and situations in which proposing condom use might jeopardize the relationship (Dubois-Arber, Masur, Hausser, Zimmerman, & Paccaud, 1993).

Although much attention is ultimately focused on relapse, little research looks at the barriers to maintenance of safe behaviors among men who have sex with men. The studies which have examined maintenance have identified uncertainty about the actual risks of particular behaviors, such as oral sex, rimming, and some sado-masochistic practices, as well as the anxiety which the uncertainty of risk provokes, as barriers to condom use. Such research has also addressed men's fear of being assumed to be seropositive because of proposing to use a condom and subsequent rejection by a partner (Dubois-Arber et al., 1993). One community-based program, "Keep it Up!" was effective in positively affecting men's condom attitudes, safer sex beliefs, and self-efficacy expectations, but did not result in behavior change after 4 months (R. L. Miller, 1995). Evaluation of the program was problematic, since participants in the program were not necessarily consistent condom users at baseline. Dubois-Arber et al. (1993), found that for the Swedish cohort, proximity to AIDS and being reminded of the need for protection by a close friend or someone with whom it is possible to identify, engenders the commitment to change and maintain preventive behavior.

More recent research in relapse examines the context of risky behavior (Donovan, Mearns, McEwan, & Sugden, 1994; Dubois-Arber et al., 1993) the relationship type (McLean et al., 1994; Meyer & Dean, 1995), relationship characteristics (Julien, Chartrand, & Begin, 1996), and sexual networks (Morris, Zavisca, & Dean, 1995) for clues to effective and long-lasting behavior change. The effects of some of these strategies look promising, but are only now beginning to be evaluated.

INJECTING-DRUG AND OTHER SUBSTANCE USE

The second leading cause of HIV infection is injecting-drug use (Center for Disease Control and Prevention [CDCP], 1996). This includes not only those individuals who are injecting-drug users (IDUs), but their sexual partners, and children whose mothers are drug users or sex partners of IDUs. In 1995, two-thirds of AIDS cases among women and 85% of cases among heterosexual men with an identified exposure were associated with injecting-drug use (CDCP, 1996). Only 10% of gay men with AIDS had a history of IDU. Persons of color are disproportionately represented among IDU-associated HIV/AIDS cases, with 50% occurring in African Americans, and 25% in Hispanics (CDCP, 1996). Ethnic differences in these rates most likely reflect socioeconomic characteristics and behavioral and other risk factors related to the use of such substances.

There appears to be a strong link between IDU and risky behaviors. Injecting drug users may be at higher risk for STDs and HIV/AIDS due to the sharing of unsterilized needles, increased numbers of sexual partners, the exchange of sex for drugs, engaging in sexual activities with an injecting-drug user, and through unprotected sexual activities (Bowen & Trotter, 1995). Similar patterns of behavior have been associated with addictions to noninjecting drugs, such as crack cocaine. Compounding the situation is the fact that multiple behavioral risks are associated with acquiring HIV among IDUs, such as unsterilized needles, unprotected intercourse, and multiple partners (CDCP, 1996).

Several types of interventions have been tried with injecting-drug users. These have included drug prevention programs to stop the initial and/or regular use of such substances, the promotion of safer injection practices, increasing opportunities for drug treatment, and promoting safer sexual practices (CDCP 1996; Des Jarlais et al., 1994). These programs have varied in their levels of sophistication and degree of evaluation.

Many cities/states throughout the world have instituted policies to provide needle exchange programs and/or clean syringes to injecting-drug users (CDC, 1995b; Coates et al., 1996; Groseclose et al., 1995). The focus of these programs is on reducing the spread of the disease and medicalizing the problem, rather than on criminalization, among persons who are likely to continue using injecting drugs (Coates et al., 1996). The most effective efforts have been shown in those programs that were implemented early on in the epidemic (Des Jarlais et al., 1994); cities which delayed in implementing preventive strategies have reported prevalence rates of 20% or more among their IDU population (Coates et al., 1996).

Intervention efforts using education materials and information dissemination also have been used with some moderate degree of success. In a study reported by Neaigus et al. (1990), IDUs were provided with information about the risk of AIDS, safer sexual practices, condoms, and referrals to drug treatment and testing sites. Follow-up conducted 4 to 5 months after the intervention indicated a decline in injecting drug use and unsafe sexual behaviors, such as sexual contact without a condom, less prostitution, and more abstinence. A program by Ginzburg and colleagues (1986) utilized a "peer counseling" approach to disseminate AIDS prevention information to IDUs. Former IDUs were trained to provide prevention information to current IDUs at actual drug use sites. However, only approximately 17% of 577 IDUs questioned postintervention reported receiving information from an IDU educator, although informal observations suggested an increase in the street demand and cost of new needles and syringes. Other programs combining information about AIDS risk reduction, needle exchange, and referrals for testing and counseling have resulted in higher rates of needle exchange, single use of needles, and a reduction in needle borrowing (Newcombe & Parry, 1989; van den Hoek, van Haastrecht, & Coutinho, 1989). Informational programs, however, have not always been found to provide significant effects in terms of changing either drug use or sexual behaviors (Fisher & Fisher, 1992).

Programs which have focused primarily on modifying sexual practices have centered around the promotion of condom use and reducing the number of sexual partners. Estimates of the use of condoms by IDUs have been hard to measure accurately. Investigations by Chitwood, McCoy, & Cornerfield (1990) indicated that 91% of IDU cocaine and opiate users were sexually active, although 70% never used condoms, and only 10% used condoms at least half of the time. Furthermore, in a study of male IDUs in stable relationships, 83% reported two or more partners in the previous 5 years (Lewis, Watters, & Case, 1990). S. R. Friedman and colleagues (1994) examined how condom use differed according to the HIV status of the IDUs, and as to whether their sex partner was also an IDU. Overall, they found that 33% of the IDUs always used condoms during sex. The use of condoms, however, was less common with IDU sex partners than non-IDU sex partners (26 and 51%, respectively). IDUs who were seropositive reported always using condoms 46% of the time, in contrast to seronegative IDUs who used condoms in 27% of their sexual encounters. When the IDU was seropositive, but the partner did not inject drugs, condom use was 68%. The reasons for increased condom use in the relationships between seropositive IDU and noninjecting sex partners were not explored in the study, but it was speculated that the increase may be due to two primary factors: altruism on the part of the IDU in wanting to protect the partner from being infected with HIV, and the actions of the sex partner. Sex partners who are not IDUs may be more proactive in the use of condoms if they know or suspect that they are having sex with an individual who is an IDU or who is HIV-seropositive.

Partner factors also have been identified as crucial elements in other studies of HIV risk reduction among IDUs. Bowen and Trotter (1995) used the Transtheoretical Model of Change and the AIDS Risk Reduction Model for predicting condom use among crack cocaine smokers and IDUs who were not currently in treatment. Participants were grouped as to whether they had casual partners or main sexual partners, and into one of three stages of change: precontemplation, contemplation, and action. The results indicated that condom use behaviors differed between main partners and casual partners. The barriers to using condoms were not found to be significant in predicting use with casual partners; the positive aspects may be all that is necessary for condom use. Persons in more permanent relationships, however, required an increase in the positive aspects of condom use, and a decrease in the perceived disadvantages of using condoms. Persons aged 18–24, however, reported more condom use in both casual and main partner relationships. Risks for relapse were perceived to be greater with casual partners, however, where over time, responsibility and safety may become less of an issue as the relationship becomes more stable and exclusive. Assertiveness was found to be an important component of the progression from precontemplation to action, and in condom use with both casual and main partners. Consistent condom use with main partners may depend on the ability to discuss the issue, and to develop methods to reduce negative perceptions of condom use.

Similar results were found in a study of condom use in high-risk heterosexual adults. Morrison, Gillmore, and Baker (1995) extended the Theory of Reasoned Action to include measures of self-efficacy. The results indicated that self-efficacy was significantly related to intentions to use condoms with steady partners, but was not as strong for casual partners. The factors influencing condom use were also not the same for men and women. Women's intentions to use condoms were strongly shaped by societal norms, whereas attitudes towards condom use were a stronger determinant for men. Persons holding less power in the relationship were more likely to acquiesce to the partner's wishes, regardless of whether the person was male or female. These results suggest that interventions aimed at women with steady partners should focus more on changing social norms about condom use, whereas interventions aimed at men should focus on changing negative attitudes about the use of condoms.

For all these intervention efforts, the incidence of HIV related to IDU continues to rise in regions of the United States and Europe, particularly among persons aged 30–49 (WHO Regional Office for Europe, 1995). This suggests that the most effective strategies have not been implemented and that there is an important residual of risk behaviors engaged in among IDUs (Coates et al., 1996). More sophisticated research designs that would enable the measurement of multiple risk behaviors, as well as the factors that may mediate risk reduction, are needed (Fisher & Fisher, 1992). Interventions are also needed to decrease relapse and increase the maintenance of safer drug and sexual practices among IDUs. Few studies have addressed these issues comprehensively, and from a longitudinal perspective.

ADOLESCENTS AND YOUNG ADULTS

In the past few decades there has been an increase in the initiation of sexual behaviors among teenagers and young adults. Trends in the age at first premarital, vaginal intercourse have increased from 28.6% of young women aged 15–19 to 51.5% in 1988 (CDC, 1991). African-American females are more likely to have their initial sexual encounter at younger ages than White females, although by age 19, there are no significant differences between White and African-American females in rates of ever having vaginal intercourse, (72.6% versus 75.6%, respectively) (CDC, 1991b). Among adolescent males, 79% have had vaginal intercourse at least once by age 19. African-American males are more likely to initiate intercourse earlier than White or Hispanic males, with approximately 48% of African-American males indicating they have had intercourse by age 15 in contrast to 16% of White and 19% of Hispanic males (Sonenstein, Pleck, & Ku, 1991). Persons who initiate sexual intercourse at younger ages report a higher number of sexual partners in their lifetime, and are at greater risk for an unintended pregnancy and/or contracting a sexually transmitted disease, largely due to higher rates of unprotected intercourse. Approximately 13 million persons in the United States are newly infected with at least one STD each year (Althaus, 1991; Healy, 1995). Eighty-six percent of these cases occur in persons between the ages of 15 and 29 years of age (CDC, 1991a). The majority of persons with HIV/AIDS are also between 20 and 45 years of age, suggesting that these individuals were infected as adolescents or young adults. African Americans and Hispanics are overrepresented in the proportion of persons with HIV/AIDS (CDC, 1995a), and infection through heterosexual contact is rising (CDC, 1994).

Safer-sex interventions in adolescents and young adults are aimed primarily at reducing the incidence of STDs, including AIDS, and/or unplanned pregnancies. Although the behaviors to be initiated or sustained are basically the same for the prevention of STDs and for pregnancy (e.g., condom use; reduction in the number of sexual partners; discontinuing risky sexual behaviors), the focus of the interventions and the information provided vary.

Among adolescents and college students, the consistent use of condoms is low. Several studies have shown that one-third or less of young adults college students use condoms consistently (Ford, Rubinstein, & Norris, 1994; Hinkle, Johnson, Gilbert, Jackson, & Lollis, 1992; Johnson et al., 1992; Marin, Tschaum, Gomez, & Kegeles, 1993). Condom use also appears to be higher in casual relationships or those of shorter duration than in long-term and/or exclusive sexual relationships (Carroll, 1991; Doval, Duran, O'Donnell, & O'Donnell, 1995; Ku, Sonenstein, & Pleck, 1994; Plichta, Weisman, Nahanson, Ensminger, & Robinson, 1992; Reisen & Poppen, 1995). The movement away from consistent use of condoms in long-term relationships may reflect the progression to a more stable, exclusive status, where there is perceived trust in the partner, as well as a decision to use an unobtrusive or more effective method of contraception, such as oral contraceptives. The higher use of nonbarrier methods of contraception, however, has increased the risk of acquiring a STD among young adults who are not in exclusive sexual relationships and do not also use condoms for the prevention of disease. Several studies have indicated that both men and women who use oral contraceptives are less likely to perceive a need to use condoms (Catania et al., 1989; MacDonald et al., 1990; Wendt & Solomon, 1995), suggesting that condoms are viewed primarily as a means of contraception, not as protection against STDs.

Similar results have been found in surveys of young and middle-aged adults. The national AIDS Behavioral Survey examined changes in risk factors for HIV and other STDs, as well as prevention practices among heterosexual adults, aged 18 to 49, from 1990 to 1992 (Catania, Stone, Binson, & Dolcini, 1995). In general, little reduction was observed in the overall prevalence of HIV risk factors nationally or in high-risk cities. There also was no significant change in HIV test-seeking for any at-risk group. There was a significant increase in consistent condom use with secondary sexual partners, although there was little change in consistent condom use with primary partners, suggesting that some individuals may be placing their primary sexual partners at risk for STDs. Black heterosexual adults with multiple sexual partners reported the largest increase in condom use from 1990 to 1992. Additional data from two independent, representative samples of the U.S. population indicated that consistent condom use was significantly increased from 11% in 1990/1991 to 20% in 1992 (Choi & Catania, 1996). This increase, however, did not occur in all groups. Women, Whites, persons in their 20s and 40s, the college-educated, and those who had ever married made little change in their use of condoms. People with less than a high-school education modified their sexual behavior by increasing the use of condoms rather than by reducing the number of sexual partners.

Despite increasing knowledge of the transmission of STDs and HIV, many persons underestimate their vulnerability to contracting a STD. Younger people who are just becoming sexually active are particularly apt to believe they are invincible to these risks (Baldwin & Baldwin, 1988; DiClemente, Zorn, & Temoshok, 1986; Strunin & Hingson, 1987). Several factors may contribute to this misperception, including that few people see themselves as the "type" of person who gets an STD or AIDS (Pinkerton & Abramson, 1992). Furthermore, this philosophy may extend to partners, in that appropriate precautions may not be taken during sexual activity because the partner does not "seem" like the type of person who could be infected. Another factor that may lower the sense of personal vulnerability is that people tend to view themselves as luckier than the norm (Pinkerton & Abramson, 1992). A result of this belief is that with each sexual encounter that does not result in an unwanted health consequence, an individual's sense of security might be reinforced, despite the fact that the consequences of a particular sexual encounter are completely uncorrelated with those of subsequent acts. This effect also operates at the cohort level: the risky experiences of friends who do not encounter negative consequences are sometimes taken as additional evidence that unsafe sexual behavior is not really as risky as it is purported to be. This is particularly unfortunate given the long latency of HIV infection and the prevalence of asymptomatic HIV and other STDs, as well as the long-term life consequences of an unplanned pregnancy (Pinkerton & Abramson, 1992). The lack of perceived vulnerability to an undesirable health consequence as a result of sexual behavior is further complicated by the fact that adolescents and young adults may engage in relatively short-term sexual relationships with different partners (B. C. Miller, Christopherson, & King, 1993). A higher number of sexual partners increases the vulnerability to infection with an STD, particularly if sexual activity is begun at a young age. The need for education and intervention with adolescents and young adults is particularly crucial, as it is in this period of life that patterns of sexual behavior are tried and adopted, and may frame subsequent behavior and practices during adulthood (Krahe & Reiss, 1995).

Many studies have investigated barriers to condom use among adolescents and young adults. Some of the most frequently mentioned barriers are the cost of condoms (Stiffman, Dore, & Cunningham, 1994); their interference with pleasure and spontaneity (Kline & VanLandingham, 1994; Libbus, 1995); embarrassment about purchasing condoms (Libbus, 1995; MacDonald et al., 1990); difficulty negotiating condom use with partners (De Bro, Campbell, & Peplau, 1994; Helweg-Larsen & Collins, 1994; MacDonald et al., 1990); alcohol and other substance use (Fortenberry, 1995; Kline & Van Landingham, 1994; Mahoney, Thombs, & Ford, 1995; Millstein & Moscicki, 1995); lack of partner support (Cohen, Dent, MacKinnin, & Hahn, 1992; Eldridge, St. Lawrence, Little, Shelby, & Brasfeild, 1995; Kline & VanLandingham, 1994); involvement with only one partner believed not to be infected with a STD (Hobfall, Jackson, Lavin, Britton, & Shephard, 1993; Sacco, Rickman, Thompson, Levine, & Reed, 1993); and low perceived need (Detzer et al., 1995; Wendt & Solomon, 1995). Other factors that have not been predictive of condom use are fears of contracting AIDS, and knowledge about STDs (Krahe & Reiss, 1995; Wulfert & Wan, 1993). Prior investigations also show that increased numbers of sexual partners and the use of oral contraceptives are associated with decreased condom use among women (MacDonald et al., 1990; Upchurch et al., 1992; Wendt & Solomon, 1995). Interestingly, a history of STDs is not related to the consistent use of condoms (Catania et al., 1994; MacDonald et al., 1990; Stiffman et al., 1994).

Factors related to the partner relationship and the ability to communicate with one another have been identified as crucial factors in consistent condom use. Differences with respect to gender and socialization play a critical role in the negotiation of the use of condoms, as well as the types of sexual behaviors in which a couple engages. Women's choices with regard to safer sexual practices are often constrained by the context of differential power relations between men and women. Minority women's choices may be further constrained by broader social forces (Catania et al, 1992; Marin et al., 1993). In casual or short-term sexual relationships, the balance of power is generally more equal between partners. The power differential may become greater in long-term relationships, however, as financial, emotional, or social dependence on the male increases (Maxwell & Boyle, 1995). Studies of African American women, in particular, have reported that the higher ratio of females to males has resulted in a greater power imbalance in interpersonal relationships and a greater tolerance of nonmonogamous behaviors (Fullilove, Fullilove, Haynes, & Gross, 1990). Economic shifts in African American communities further aggravate communication, and thus, safe sexual practices.

An additional concern is that the condom is a male-dependent method of contraception and STD prevention, and the female does not have ultimate control over its use. Studies have indicated that women may feel uncomfortable in broaching the subject of condom use due to embarrassment or beliefs that their partner will perceive that they do not trust them, or alternatively, may think that they have a STD (MacDonald et al., 1990). Trust and social acceptability are barriers related to condom use in primary relationships among Hispanics (Doval et al., 1995; Moore, Kay, Deren, & Doll, 1995). Males also report more negative beliefs regarding the use of condoms than do females (Campbell, Peplau, & De Bro, 1992; Sacco et al., 1993), and may show more reluctance to wear a condom. Women who are in the subordinate power position within a sexual relationship are less likely to be able to negotiate the use of condoms effectively (Kline & VanLandingham, 1994), and are more prone to acquiesce to the desires of their partners. Sexual coercion may also play a more significant role in younger women's sexual behavior than has been thought previously (Biglan, Noell, Ochs, Smolkowski, & Metzler, 1995). Incidents of rape, sexual assault, and emotional coercion place women at increased risk for negative health outcomes.

A variety of different interventions has been used with adolescents and young adults to encourage condom use, safer sexual practices, and effective methods of contraception for those persons who are sexually active. Strategies that have been developed include peer education programs, didactic lectures, patient education in student health or community health centers, school-based clinics, brochures, increasing condom availability, skills training, and presentations by print and broadcast media (Turner, Korpita,

Mohn, & Hill, 1993). Providing safer-sex interventions to adolescents has been a very socially sensitive issue (St. Lawrence et al., 1995). Concerns have been expressed that providing explicit information or skills training may serve to condone or promote sexual activity. Others, however, have advocated a more explicit and interactive approach due to the high rates of sexual activity among adolescents, and the fact that sexual activity is rarely followed by a return to abstinence once it has been initiated (DiClemente, 1993). This dichotomy in beliefs about appropriate sexual behavior for adolescents and young adults has hindered the development of effective prevention strategies, and as a result, both infection with STDs and unplanned pregnancies continue to rise.

Informational programs are the most widely used interventions with adolescents and young adults (St. Lawrence et al., 1995). These approaches alone, however, have not been successful in motivating behavior change (Bellingham & Gillies, 1993; Geringer, Marks, Allen, & Armstrong, 1993; Hinkle et al., 1992; Jemmott & Jemmott, 1992; Johnson et al., 1992; Kirby, Barth, Leland, & Fetro, 1991), although increases in knowledge about STDs have been observed (Ruder, Flam, Flatto, & Curran, 1990). Education alone appears to be unrelated to behavior change without skills training or modification in attitudes, beliefs, and situational determinants of risky behavior (Ross & Rosser, 1989). Skills training aimed at addressing social interactions provides young adults with methods to increase interpersonal competencies to resist coercion and peer pressure, and increase skills to manage and negotiate their preferences successfully (St. Lawrence et al., 1995).

A number of studies with minority women have provided guidance on structuring intervention strategies to specific portions of the population. Focus group research with mainly Latina and Black women from high HIV-prevalence neighborhoods indicate that HIV interventions should consist of sex education, including anatomy and physiology, instruction of sex negotiation skills, and should consider many women's desire for pregnancy (Ehrhardt, Yingling, Zawadzi, & Martinez-Ramirez, 1992). Results of another focus group of low-income African American women suggest an emphasis on training in sexual negotiation, conflict resolution, and refusal skills in HIV-prevention programs for African-American women is needed (Wingood, Hunter-Gamble, & DiClemente, 1993). Qualitative research with inner-city Black women suggests that group discussion of HIV, a reduction of women's dependence on men, and adjustment of HIV-education curricula to better meet the needs of urban minority women are good ways to promote safer sex among these women (Sobo, 1993). Because recent economic shifts in the Black community have affected communication between men and women, Fullilove et al. (1990) recommend that AIDS prevention programs for African Americans try to improve communication between men and women, and work within the context of rebuilding the community.

Several factors characterize or predict condom use among Hispanics and should be considered in planning interventions. Highly acculturated Hispanics tend to have a more positive view of condoms (Norris & Ford, 1994). In a study of Hispanics aged 17–56, condom use was associated with men and with machismo practices, such as protecting the woman by using condoms (Mikawa et al., 1992). Among Hispanic adolescents, AIDS communication had a positive effect on condom predisposition (Norris & Ford, 1995). To capitalize on cultural beliefs, Mikawa and colleagues (1992) have suggested directing AIDS prevention messages to males and emphasizing the protection of women through their use.

There are several examples of comprehensive safer-sex interventions in the published literature. Risk behaviors of first-year college students were examined before and 3 months after a health education intervention that included information about STDs, safer sex, values, decision-making, and assertiveness skills (Turner et al., 1993). Compared with students who had not received the intervention, men reported increased sexual abstinence, but no change in consistent condom use. Women in the intervention, however, reported no change in sexual abstinence, but an increase in consistent condom use at 3 months. Fewer women who had participated in the program reported never using a condom, as compared to women who had not received the intervention. McLean (1994) reported on the effects of the Ujima Project at Syracuse University. This program used peer educators/mentors to provide first-year African-American students with accurate information about HIV, and how to build life skills for STD prevention that enhance self-esteem and provide ongoing social support. Short-term evaluation of the program indicated significant increases in the students' knowledge about STDs, a decrease in risky behaviors, and increases in students' self-esteem and talking with a partner about their past sexual history.

In another investigation, St. Lawrence and colleagues (1995) examined the use of combined education and behavior skills training to reduce the risk of STD infection among low-income, African American adolescents. Participants were recruited from a community health clinic and were randomly assigned to an educational program or an 8-week intervention combining both educational materials and skills training. Skill-trained individuals reduced unprotected intercourse, increased the use of condoms during sexual activities, and displayed increased behavioral skills when compared to those in the education alone condition. These effects were maintained one year later. Thirty-one percent of adolescents in the education program who were abstinent at baseline had initiated sexual activity at the 1 year follow-up, in contrast to 11.5% of the skill-trained individuals. This suggests that adolescents who possess knowledge and skills regarding safer sexual practices can reduce their STD risks and can defer the onset of sexual activity. Other moderately successful intervention programs have focused on increasing knowledge of AIDS/STD transmission, fostering less favorable attitudes towards risky sexual behaviors and positive attitudes towards condom use, and increasing self-efficacy and interpersonal communication (DiClemente & Wingood, 1995; Jemmott & Jemmott, 1992; Jemmott, Jemmott, & Fong, 1992).

School-based contraceptive and STD clinics have become more common in the United States since the early 1990s. Comprehensive evaluations of these programs, however, have yet to be completed. Some school-based programs have been able to delay the onset of sexual activity, and to decrease the time from onset of sexual activity to initiating family planning services (Kirby, Waszak, & Ziegler, 1991; Zabin, 1986; 1988). Their effects on pregnancy rates, however, have been inconsistent (Bearss, Santelli, Papa, 1995; Kirby, Waszak, et al., 1991; Zabin, 1986).

In general, effective strategies to prevent risky sexual behaviors and undesirable health consequences in adolescents and young adults are at a premium. Long-term evaluations of successful interventions are needed in order to identify factors related to the adoption and maintenance of effective behavior changes, and to reduce the rising incidences of STDs and unplanned pregnancies in this age group.

ETHNIC CONSIDERATIONS

Just as the influence of gender differences influences the adoption of safer sex practices, ethnic differences in sexual behavior should also be considered. The disproportionate prevalence and incidence of STDS, including HIV, among African Americans and Hispanics also makes ethnic consideration imperative. Ethnicity, however, is a category which glosses a complex set of political, economic, and social interactions. To protect members of various ethnic groups effectively, these complex processes must be understood.

First, because of current and historical discriminatory practices, minority groups are at a disadvantage in the U.S. Reporting disease and behavior by ethnic categories obscures other correlates of risk, such as low socioeconomic status. Poverty is highly correlated with ethnicity and increased risk of disease (Wyatt, 1994), but cultural or ethnic differences should not be confused with differences engendered by political and economic forces. Second, the heterogeneity within ethnic groups, as well as gender differences among members of the same ethnic group, must be understood. There is likely more diversity within ethnic groups than across (Wyatt, 1994). Third, high-risk individuals may have characteristics and may act in ways unlike the rest of their ethnic group (Johnson et al., 1994). It is possible that "differences observed between whites and African Americans may not be the same as those that distinguish high-risk African Americans from African-Americans at low risk" (Johnson et al., 1994, p. 746). Finally, different research foci have been placed on different ethnic groups. Weeks, Singer, Grier, and Schensul (1996) point out that research on African American sexual behavior has been conducted from a strictly political and economic perspective, while research on Latino sexual behavior has been conducted with a limited understanding of the full range of cultural determinants. Both political-economic and community-influenced behaviors work to shape behavior among members of ethnic groups. Each factor, as well as the interaction of these forces, must be considered in measuring sexual behaviors and designing appropriate interventions for behavior change.

CONCEPTUAL CONSIDERATIONS

The adoption of safer sexual practices and STD prevention strategies is of critical importance. That this is a complex problem is unquestioned. Intervention strategies must largely focus on the modification of very intimate behaviors between individuals, which, in themselves, are shaped by the larger social environment. Societal norms and expectations for behavior, as well as attitudes, strongly influence sexual behaviors and the adoption and maintenance of preventive strategies. In addition, the diverse population groups affected by unsafe sexual practices make devising effective strategies extremely challenging.

The majority of research with regard to safer sexual practices has been completed in the past 10 years. Research across many subgroups is still focused on delineating predictors of safer sexual practices, and developing effective strategies to modify behavior. The state of the science has not progressed to the point that factors associated with adherence to safer sexual practices are clearly understood and defined.

During the course of reviewing research in this area, several cross-cutting themes emerged:

1. Sexual activities are often viewed as an individual act, rather than as a social act engaged in by two or more individuals. Interventions which have focused on changing the behavior of individuals without regard to the social relation of sexual behavior have been less effective. Condom use should be viewed as an attribute of a relationship rather than as an individual attribute, because condom use varies between relationships.

2. Sexual behavior is often viewed as monosemic. Sexual behavior has different meanings in different contexts, and consequently, different codes of behavior apply in different situations. Attention should be focused on the type of relationship in which sex is shared (e.g., casual or primary partner; the exchange of sex for drugs), and the factors that promote or reduce condom use and safer sexual practices in each of these contexts.

3. Power imbalances in relationships are often ignored in intervention strategies. Across all categories, the less powerful, whether they be the young, women, economically disadvantaged, or uneducated, seem to be the least successful in changing their behavior. Research has indicated that women, in particular, are often at a disadvantage in negotiating safer sexual practices, due to having less power and control in their sexual relationships. Strategies which attempt to modify sexual practices without examining the social and economic context in which such behavior occur are short-sighted. These observations also suggest the need for intervention efforts which target the empowered partner separately from, and in equal proportion to, the disempowered partner in the relationship.

4. Gender differences are also intricately entwined in sexual activities. Social norms and gender roles strongly influence the ability to implement and maintain safer sexual practices. Beliefs about appropriate behavior for males and females are strongly ingrained across subgroups of the population, and need to be considered in intervention efforts. Gender-specific interventions may be required in some instances.

5. Ethnic and cultural differences will influence the adoption of safer sexual practices. It is essential to understand ethnicity as a social category and to fully understand the diversity within ethnic groups. For interventions to be effective, it is essential to incorporate ethnic values and priorities into program efforts, as well as specific attitudes and behaviors toward condom use and safer sexual practices. Issues of ethnic-specific gender differences also need to be addressed and targeted in order to enact positive changes in behavior.

6. Results from many of the studies suggested that greater success in adopting and maintaining safer sexual behaviors was obtained when action was taken early. Research has also indicated that it is much easier and efficient to prevent the adoption of unsafe sexual practices than it is to attempt to modify existing patterns of behavior. For instance, middle-aged women who initiated sexual activity when the primary focus was on pregnancy prevention, primarily with the use of oral contraceptives, have had to reorient their view of "protected" intercourse to include not only contraception, but the prevention of STDs as well. Thus, adolescents and young adults should be targeted with efforts to establish safer sexual practices from the onset.

RESEARCH NEEDS

Several research needs, and unanswered questions posed by investigators in this area, were identified from this review:

1. There is an overreliance on cross-sectional data to infer trends in sexual behaviors, and success in modifying and maintaining safer sexual prac-

tices. More research is needed to follow cohorts of individuals in order to evaluate program effectiveness over time.

2. Limiting analyses of the predictors of sexual behavior to intrapersonal characteristics is missing the social nature of interpersonal interactions and the larger social context in which such interactions occur. Research could be improved by the inclusion of variables, such as the duration and nature of the relationship (e.g., casual, exclusive, sex, work), characteristics of the setting or social context in which the behavior occurs, or societal norms and expectations for appropriate behaviors regarding safer sexual practices.

3. More emphasis needs to be given to the partner aspects of the sexual relationship and how negotiations about safer sexual practices occur. For example, research across all subgroups has indicated that condom use is higher with casual partners than in long-term relationships. Studies are needed to address the decision to stop using condoms consistently with main partners, particularly if one or both partners is engaging in sexual activity or high-risk behaviors with another partner(s).

4. The power differential in sexual relationships needs further exploration in order to devise effective strategies to empower the low-power person in negotiating condom use and other behaviors. Examining past research and theoretical frameworks from the social sciences, which have investigated status, power and gender, would be particularly useful in this area.

5. Studies focused on identifying effective strategies to change the negative attitudes towards condoms, particularly among males, may prove to increase condom use.

6. Gender and ethnic differences in adopting and adhering to safer sexual practices need to be incorporated and evaluated in intervention programs. Both of these variables are critical factors in modifying behavior effectively.

7. More research regarding how social norms may vary in different social situations or contexts is needed. For instance, the leveling off of rates of HIV among men who have sex with men suggests that risk behaviors can be changed. However, the recent increases in other STDs suggests that behavior change is not total. Either a reservoir of risky actors still exists, or new members of the population are not yet practicing safe behaviors. More in line with recent conceptual innovations, it is likely that situations or contexts persist in which risky behavior is dictated. Studies to explore this hypothesis could be helpful in targeting interventions for men who have sex with men.

CONCLUSION

Research in the area of effecting and maintaining safer sexual practices is of the utmost importance, but is extremely challenging to complete. Research efforts in the past decade, however, have provided much needed information which can be used to guide and modify intervention efforts. Targeted, future research will only serve to enhance public health efforts to reduce the spread of undesirable health consequences associated with unsafe sexual practices and injecting drug use.

REFERENCES

Adib, S. M., Joseph, J. G., Ostrow, D. G., & James, S. (1991). Predictors of relapse in sexual practices among homosexual men. *AIDS Education and Prevention, 3*, 293–304.

Adib, S. M., Joseph, J. G., Ostrow, D. G., Tal, M., & Schwartz, S. A. (1991). Relapse in sexual behavior among homosexual men: A 2-year follow-up from the Chicago MACS/CCS. *AIDS, 5*, 757–760.

Althaus, F. A. (1991). An ounce of prevention...STDs and women's health. *Family Planning Perspectives, 23*, 173–177.

Baldwin, J. D., & Baldwin, J. I. (1988). Factors affecting AIDS-related sexual risk-taking behavior among college students. *Journal of Sex Research, 25*, 181–196.

Bearss, N., Santelli, J. S., & Papa, P. (1995). A pilot program of contraceptive continuation in six school-based clinics. *Journal of Adolescent Health, 17*, 178–183.

Bellingham, K., & Gillies, P. (1993). Evaluation of an AIDS education program for young adults. *Journal of Epidemiology and Community Health, 24*, 134–138.

Biglan, A., Noell, J., Ochs, L., Smolkowski, D., & Metzler, C. (1995). Does sexual coercion play a role in the high-risk behavior of adolescent and young adult women? *Journal of Behavioral Medicine, 18*, 549–568.

Bowen, A.M., & Trotter, R. (1995). HIV risk in intravenous drug users and crack cocaine smokers: Predicting stage of change for condom use. *Journal of Consulting and Clinical Psychology, 63*, 238–248.

Campbell, C. A., Peplau, I. A.,& DeBro, S. C. (1992). Women, men, and condoms: Attitudes and experiences of heterosexual college students. *Psychology of Women Quarterly, 16*, 273–288.

Carey, R. F., Herman, W. A., Retta, S. M., Rinaldi, J. E., Herman, B. A., & Athey, T. W. (1992). Effectiveness of latex condoms as a barrier to human immunodeficiency virus-sized particles under conditions of simulated use. *Sexually Transmitted Disease, 19*, 230– 234.

Carroll, L. (1991). Gender, knowledge about AIDS, reported behavioral change, and sexual behavior of college students. *Journal of American College Health, 40*, 5–12.

Catania, J. A., Coates. T. J., Golden, E. G., Dolcini, M. M., Peterson, J., Kegeles, S., Siegel, D., & Fullilove, M. T. (1994). Correlates of condom use among black, Hispanic and white heterosexuals in San Francisco: The AMEN longitudinal survey. *AIDS Education and Prevention, 26*, 12–26.

Catania, J. A., Coates, T. J., Kegeles, S., Fullilove, M. T., Peterson, J., Marin, B., Siegel, D., & Hulley, S. (1992). Condom use in multi-ethnic neighborhoods of San Francisco: The population-based AMEN (AIDS in multi-ethnic neighborhoods) study. *American Journal of Public Health, 82*, 284–287.

Catania, J. A., Coates, T. J., Stall, R., Bye, L., Kegeles, S. M., Capell, F., Henne, J., McKusick, L., Morin, S., Turner, H., & Pollack, L. (1991). Changes in condom use among homosexual men in San Francisco. *Health Psychology, 10*, 190–199.

Catania, J. A., Dolcini, M., Coates, T. J., Kegeles, S. M., Greenblatt, R., Puckett, S., Corman, M., & Miller, J. (1989). Predictors of condom use and multiple partner sex among sexually active adolescent women. Implications for AIDs-related health interventions. *Journal of Sex Research, 26*, 514–524.

Catania, J. A., Stone, V., Binson, D., & Dolcini, M. M. (1995). Changes in condom use among heterosexuals in Wave 3 of the AMEN survey. *Journal of Sex Research, 32*, 193–200.

Centers for Disease Control. (1988). Condoms for the prevention of sexually transmitted diseases. *Morbidity and Mortality Weekly Report, 37*, 133–137.

Centers for Disease Control. (1989). Trends in gonorrhea in homosexually active men: King County, Washington, 1989. *Morbidity & Mortality Weekly Report, 38*, 762–764.

Centers for Disease Control. (1991). *Division of STD/HIV Prevention Annual Report, 1990*. Atlanta: Author.

Centers for Disease Control. (1991b). Premarital sexual experience among adolescent women: United States, 1970–1988. *Morbidity and Mortality Weekly Report, 39*, 929–932.

Centers for Disease Control. (1994). Update: Trends in AIDS diagnosis and reporting under the expanded surveillance definition for adolescents and adults: United States, 1993. *Morbidity and Mortality Weekly Report, 43*, 826–831.

Centers for Disease Control. (1995a). First 500,000 AIDS cases: United States, 1995. *Morbidity and Mortality Weekly Report, 44*, 849–853.

Centers for Disease Control. (1995b). Syringe-exchange programs: United States, 1994–1995. *Morbidity and Mortality Weekly Report, 44*, 684–691.

Centers for Disease Control. (1995c). Update: Trends in AIDS among men who have sex with men: United States, 1989–1994. *Morbidity and Mortality Weekly Report, 44*, 401–404.

Centers for Disease Control and Prevention. (1996). AIDS associated with injecting-drug use: United States, 1995. *Morbidity and Mortality Weekly Report, 45*, 392–398.

Chitwood, D., McCoy, C., & Comerfield, M. (1990). Risk behavior of intravenous cocaine users: Implication for intervention. In C. G. Leukefeld, R. J. Battjes, & X. Amsel (Eds.), *AIDS and Intravenous Drug Use* (pp. 43–61). New York: Guilford.

Choi, K-H., & Catania, J. A. (1996). Changes in multiple sexual partnerships, HIV testing, and condom use among US heterosexuals 18 to 49 years of age, 1990 and 1992. *American Journal of Pubic Health, 86*, 554–556.

Coates, T. J., Aggleton, P., Gutzwiller, F., Des Jarlais, D, Kihara, M., Kippax, S., Schechter, M., & van den Hoek, J. A. R. (1996). HIV prevention in developed countries. *The Lancet, 348*, 1143–1148.

Cohen, D. A., Dent, C., MacKinnin, D., & Hahn, G. (1992). Condoms for men, not women. *Sexually Transmitted Diseases, 19*, 245–251.

Cohn, D. L., Rietmeijer, C. A. M., Kane, M. S., Cooper, S. G., Martindale, C. J., & Judson, F. N. (1992). Changes in sexual behavior and condom use associated with a risk-reduction program: Denver. *Journal of the American Medical Association, 268*, 184.

Crosby, G. M., Stall, R. D., Paul, J. P., Barrett, D. C., & Midanik, L. T. (1996). Condom use among gay/bisexual male substance abusers using the timeline follow-back method. *Addictive Behaviors, 21*, 249–257.

De Bro, S. C., Campbell, S. M., & Peplau, L. A. (1994). Influencing a partner to use a condom: A college student perspective. *Psychology of Women Quarterly, 18*, 165–182.

de Wit, J. B. F., van den Hoek, J. A. R., Sandfort, T. G. M., & van Griensven, G. J. P. (1993). Increase in unprotected anogenital intercourse among homosexual men. *American Journal of Public Health, 83*, 1451–1453.

Des Jarlais, D. C., Friedman, S. R., Sotheran, J. L., Wenston, J., Marmor, M., Yancovitz, S. R., Frank, B., Beatrice, S., & Mildvan, D. (1994). Continuity and change within an HIV epidemic: Injecting drug users in New York City, 1984 through 1992. *Journal of the American Medical Association, 271*, 121–127.

Detzer, M. J., Wendt, S. J., Solomon, L. J., Dorsch, E., Geller, B. M., Friedman, J, Hauser, H, Flynn, B. S., & Dorwaldt, A. L. (1995). Barriers to condom use among women attending planned parenthood clinics. *Women and Health, 23*(1), 91–102.

Diamond, M. (1993). Homosexuality and bisexuality in different populations. *Archives of Sexual Behavior, 22*, 291–310.

DiClemente, R. J. (1993). Preventing HIV/AIDS among adolescents: Schools as agents of behavior change. *Journal of the American Medical Association, 270*, 760–762.

DiClemente, R. J., & Wingood, G. M. (1995). A randomized controlled trial of an HIV sexual risk-reduction intervention for young African-American women. *JAMA, 274*, 1271–1276.

DiClemente, R. J., Zorn, J., & Temoshok, L. (1986). Adolescents and AIDS: A survey of knowledge, attitudes, and beliefs about AIDS in San Francisco. *American Journal of Public Health, 76*, 1443–1445.

Donovan, C., Mearns, C., McEwan, R., & Sugden, N. (1994). A review of the HIV-related sexual behavior of gay men and men who have sex with men. *AIDS Care, 6*, 605–617.

Doval, A. S., Duran, R., O'Donnell, L., & O'Donnell, C. R. (1995). Barriers to condom use in primary and nonprimary relationships among Hispanic STD clinic patients. *Hispanic Journal of Behavioral Sciences, 17*, 385–397.

Dubois-Arber, F., Masur, J. B., Hausser, D., Zimmerman, E., & Paccaud, F. (1993). Evaluation of AIDS prevention among homosexual and bisexual men in Switzerland. *Social Science and Medicine, 37*, 1539-1544.

Ehrhardt, A. A., Yingling, S., Zawadzi, R., & Martinez-Ramirez, M. (1992). Prevention of heterosexual transmission of HIV: Barriers for women. *Journal of Psychology and Human Sexuality, 5*, 37–67.

Eldridge, G. D., St. Lawrence, J. S., Little, C. E., Shelby, M. C., & Brasfield, T. L. (1995). Barriers to condom use and barrier method preferences among low-income African- American women. *Women and Health, 23*, 73–89.

Fay, R. E., Turner, C. F., Klassen, A. D., & Gagnon, J. H. (1989). Prevalence and patterns of same-gender sexual contact among men. *Science, 243*, 338–48.

Fisher, J. D., & Fisher, W. A. (1992). Changing AIDS-risk behavior. *Psychological Bulletin, 111*, 455–474.

Fisher, W. A., Fisher, J. D., & Rye, B. J. (1995). Understanding and promoting AIDS-preventive behavior: Insights from the theory of reasoned action. *Health Psychology, 14*, 255–264.

Ford, K., Rubinstein, S., & Norris, A. (1994). Sexual behavior and condom use among urban, low-income, African-American and Hispanic youth. *AIDS Education and Prevention, 6*, 219–229.

Fortenberry, J. D. (1995). Adolescent substance use and sexually transmitted diseases risk: A review. *Journal of Adolescent Health, 16*, 304–308.

Friedman, R. C., & Downey, J. I. (1994a). Homosexuality. *New England Journal of Medicine, 33*, 923–930.

Friedman, S. R., Jose, B., Neaigus, A., Goldstein, M., Curtis, R., Ildefonso, G., Mota, P., & Des Jarlais, D. C. (1994). Consistent condom use in relationships between seropositive injecting drug users and sex partners who do not inject drugs. *AIDS, 8*, 357–361.

Fullilove, M. T., Fullilove, R. E., Haynes, K., & Gross, S. (1990). Black women and AIDS prevention: A view towards understanding the gender rules. *The Journal of Sex Research, 27*, 47–64.

Geringer, W. M., Marks, S., Allen, W. J., & Armstrong, K. A. (1993). Knowledge, attitudes, and behavior related to condom use in a high risk population. *Journal of Sex Research, 30*, 75–83.

Ginzburg, H. M., French, J., Jackson, J., Hartsock, P. I., MacDonald, M. G., & Weiss, S. H. (1986). Health education and knowledge assessment of HTLV-III diseases among intravenous drug users. *Health Education Quarterly, 13*, 373–382.

Groseclose, S. L., Weinstein, B., Jones, T. S., Valleroy, L. A., Fehrs, L. J., & Kassler, W. J. (1995). Impact of increased legal access to needles and syringes on practices of injecting- drug users and police officers—Connecticut, 1992–1992. *Journal of Acquired Immune Deficiency Syndromes and Human Retrovirology, 10*, 82–89.

Gruer, L. D., & Ssembatya-Lule, G. (1993). Sexual behavior and use of the condom by men attending gay bars and clubs in Glasgow and Edinburgh. *International Journal of STD and AIDS, 4*, 95–98.

Healy, B. (1995). *A new prescription for women's health*. New York: Penguin.

Helweg-Larsen, M., & Collins, B. E. (1994). The UCLA multidimensional condom attitudes scale: Documenting the complex determinants of condom use in college students. *Health Psychology, 13*, 224–237.

Hinkle, Y. A., Johnson, E. H., Gilbert, D., Jackson, L., & Lollis, C. M. (1992). African- American women who always use condoms: Attitudes, knowledge about AIDS and sexual behavior. *Journal of the American Medical Women's Association, 47*, 230–237.

Hobfall, S. E., Jackson, A. P., Lavin, J., Britton, P. J., & Shephard, J. B. (1993). Safer sex knowledge, behavior, and attitudes of inner-city women. *Health Psychology, 69*, 481– 488.

Hunt, A. J., Weatherburn, P., Hickson, F. C., Davies, P. M., McManus, T. J., & Coxon, A. P. M. (1993). Changes in condom use by gay men. *AIDS Care, 5*, 439–448.

Jemmott, J. B., Jemmott, L. S., & Fong, G. T. (1992). Reductions in HIV risk-associated sexual behaviors among Black male adolescents: Effects of an AIDS prevention intervention. *American Journal of Public Health, 82*, 372–377.

Jemmott, L. S. & Jemmott, J. B. (1992). Increasing condom-use intentions among sexually active Black adolescent women. *Nursing Research, 41*, 273–279.

Johnson, E. H., Gant, L., Hinkle, Y. A., Gilbert, D., Willis, C., & Hoopwood, T. (1992). Do African-American men and women differ in their knowledge about AIDS, attitudes about condoms, and sexual behaviors? *Journal of the National Medical Association, 84*, 49–64.

Johnson, E. H., Jackson, L. A., Hinkle, Y., Gilbert, D., Hoopwood, T., Lollis, C. M., Willis, C., & Gant, L. (1994). What is the significance of black-white differences in risky sexual behavior? *Journal of the National Medical Association, 86*, 745–759.

Julien, D., Chartrand, E., & Begin, J. (1996). Male couples' dyadic adjustment and the use of safer sex within and outside of primary relationships. *Journal of Family Psychology, 10*, 89–96.

Kelly, J. A., St. Lawrence, J. S., & Brasfield, T. L. (1991). Predictors of vulnerability to AIDS risk behavior relapse. *Journal of Consulting and Clinical Psychology, 59*, 163–166.

Kelly, J. A., St. Lawrence, J. S., Hood, H. V., & Brasfield, T. L. (1989). Behavioral intervention to reduce AIDS risk activities. *Journal of Consulting and Clinical Psychology, 57*, 60– 67.

Kirby, D., Barth, R. P., Leland, N., & Fetro, J. V. (1991). Reducing the risk: Impact of a new curriculum on sexual risk-taking. *Family Planning Perspectives, 23*, 253–62.

Kirby, D., Waszak, C., & Ziegler, J. (1991). Six school-based clinics: Their reproductive health services and impact on sexual behavior. *Family Planning Perspectives, 23*, 6–16.

Kline, A., & Van Landingham, M. (1994). HIV-infected women and sexual risk reduction: The relevance of existing models of behavior change. *AIDS Education and Prevention, 6*, 390–402.

Krahe, B., & Reiss, C. (1995). Predicting intentions of AIDS-prevention behavior among adolescents. *Journal of Applied Social Psychology, 25*, 2118–2140.

Ku, L., Sonenstein, F. L., & Pleck, J. H. (1994). The dynamics of young men's condom use during and across relationships. *Family Planning Perspectives, 26*, 246–251.

Lewis, D., Watters, J., & Case, P. (1990). The prevalence of high-risk sexual behavior in male intravenous drug users with steady female partners. *American Journal of Public Health, 80*, 465–466.

Libbus, K. (1995). Women's beliefs concerning condom acquisition and use. *Public Health Nursing, 12*, 341–347.

MacDonald, N. E., Wells, G. A., Fisher, W. A., Warren, W. K., King, M. A., Doherty, J. A., & Bowie, W. R. (1990). High-risk STD/HIV behavior among college students. *Journal of the American Association, 263*, 3155–3159.

Mahoney, C. A., Thombs, D. L., & Ford, O. J. (1995). Health belief and self-efficacy models: Their utility in explaining college student condom use. *AIDS Education and Prevention, 7*, 32–49.

Marin, B., Tschann, J. M., Gomez, C. A., & Kegeles, S. M. (1993). Acculturation and gender differences in sexual attitudes and behaviors: Hispanic vs non-Hispanic White unmarried adults. *American Journal of Public Health, 83*, 1759–1761.

Maxwell, C., & Boyle, M. (1995). Risky heterosexual practices amongst women over 30: gender, power and long term relationships. *AIDS Care, 7*, 277–293.

McCusker, J., Stoddard, A. M., McDonald, M. Zapka, J. G., & Mayer, K. H. (1992). Maintenance of behavioral change in a cohort of homosexually active men. *AIDS, 6*, 861– 868.

McLean, J. (1994). A model for HIV risk reduction and prevention among African college students. *Journal of American College Health, 42*, 220–223.

McLean, J., Boulton, M., Brookes, M., Lakhani, D., Fitzpatrick, R., & Dawson, J. (1994). Regular partners and risky behaviour: Why do gay men have unprotected intercourse? *AIDS Care, 6*, 331–41.

Meyer, I. H., & Dean, L. (1995). Patterns of sexual behavior and risk taking among young New York City gay men. *AIDS Education and Prevention, 7* (Supplement), 13–23.

Mikawa, J. K., Morones, P. A., Gomez, A., Case, H. L., Olsen, D., & Gonzales-Huss, M. J. (1992). Cultural practices of Hispanics: implications for the prevention of AIDS. *Hispanic Journal of Behavioral Sciences, 14*, 421–433.

Miller, B. C., Christopherson, C. R., & King, P. K. (1993). Sexual behavior in adolescence. In T. P. Gullotta, G. R. Adams, & R. Montemayor (Eds.), *Adolescent sexuality* (pp. 57– 76). Newbury Park, CA: Sage.

Miller, R. L. (1995). Assisting gay men to maintain safer sex: An evaluation of an AIDS service organization's safer sex maintenance program. *AIDS Education and Prevention,* 7(5 Suppl), 48–63.

Millstein, S. G., & Moscicki, A. (1995). Sexually-transmitted disease in female adolescents: Effects of psychosocial factors and high risk behaviors. *Journal of Adolescent Health, 17*, 83–90.

Moore, J., Harrison, J. S., Kay, K. L., Deren, S., & Doll, L.S. (1995). Factors associated with Hispanic women's HIV-related communication and condom use with male partners. *AIDS Care, 7*, 415–427.

Morris, M. Zavisca, J., & Dean, L. (1995). Social and sexual networks: Their role in the spread of HIV/AIDS among young gay men. *AIDS Education and Prevention,* 7(Supplement), 24–35.

Morrison, D. M., Gillmore, M. R., & Baker, S. A. (1995). Determinants of condom use among high-risk heterosexual adults: A test of the Theory of Reasoned Action. *Journal of Applied Social Psychology, 25*, 651–676.

Neaigus, A., Sufian, M., Friedman, S. R., Goldsmith, D. S., Stepherson, B., Mota, P., Pascal, J., & Des Jarlais, D. C. (1990). Effects of outreach intervention on risk reduction among intravenous drug users. *AIDS Education and Prevention, 2*, 253–271.

Newcombe, R., & Parry, A. (1989). *Preventing the spread of HIV infection among and from injecting drug users in the UK: An overview with specific reference to the Mersey regional strategy*. Liverpool, England: The Maryland Centre.

Norris, A. E., & Ford, K. (1995). Condom use by low-income African American and Hispanic youth with a well-known partner: Integrating the health belief model, theory of reasoned action, and the construct accessibility model. *Journal of Applied Social Psychology, 25*, 1801–1830.

Norris, A. E., & Ford, K. (1994). Condom beliefs in urban, low income, African American and Hispanic youth. *Health Education Quarterly, 21*, 39–53.

Peterson, J. L., Coates, T. J. Catania, J. A., Middleton, L., Hilliard, B., & Hearst, N. (1992). High-risk sexual behavior and condom use among gay and bisexual African-American men. *American Journal of Public Health, 82*, 1490–1494.

Pinkerton, S. D., & Abramson, P. R. (1992). Is risky sex rational? *The Journal of Sex Research, 29*, 561–568.

Plichta, S. B., Weisman, C. S., Nahanson, C. A., Ensminger, M. E., & Robinson, J. C. (1992). Partner-specific condom use among adolescent women clients of a family planning clinic. *Journal of Adolescent Health, 13*, 506–513.

Reisen, C. A., & Poppen, P. J. (1995). College women and condom use: Importance of partner relationship. *Journal of Applied Social Psychology, 25*, 1485–1498.

Robert, B., & Rosser, S. (1990). Evaluation of the efficacy of AIDS education interventions for homosexually active men. *Health Education Research, 5*, 299–308.

Ross, M. W., & McLaws, M. L. (1992). Subjective norms about condoms are better predictors of use and intention to use than attitudes. *Health Education Research, 7*, 335–339.

Ross, M. W., & Rosser, B. R. S. (1989). Education and AIDS risks: A review. *Health Education Research, 4*, 273–284.

Rotheram-Borus, M. J., & Gwadz, M. (1993). Sexuality among youths at high risk. *Adolescent Psychiatric Clinics of North America, 2*, 215–431.

Ruder, A. M., Flam, R., Flatto, D., & Curran, A. S. (1990). AIDS education: Evaluation of school and worksite based presentations. *New York State Journal of Medicine, 90*, 129– 133.

Sacco, W. P., Rickman, R. L., Thompson, K., Levine, B., & Reed, D. L. (1993). Gender differences in AIDS-relevant condom attitudes and condom use. *AIDS Education and Prevention, 5*, 311–326.

Sobo, E. J. (1993). Inner-city women and AIDS: The psycho-social benefits of unsafe sex. *Culture, Medicine and Psychiatry, 17*, 455–485.

Sonenstein, F. L., Pleck, J. H., & Ku, L.C. (1991). Levels of sexual activity among adolescent males in the United States. *Family Planning Perspectives, 23*, 162–167.

St. Lawrence, J. S., Brasfield, T. L., Jefferson, K. W., Alleyne, E., O'Bannon, R. E., & Shirley, A. (1995). Cognitive-behavioral intervention to reduce African-American adolescents' risk for HIV infection. *Journal of Consulting and Clinical Psychology, 62*, 221–237.

Stiffman, A. R., Dore, P., & Cunningham, R. M. (1994). Inner-city youths and condom use: Health beliefs, clinic care, welfare, and the HIV epidemic. *Adolescence, 29*, 805–820.

Strunin, L., & Hingson, R. (1987). Acquired Immunodeficiency Syndrome and adolescents: Knowledge, beliefs, attitudes, and behaviors. *Pediatrics, 79*, 825–828.

Tanfer, K., Grady, W. R., Klepinger, D. H., & Billy, J. O. G. (1993). Condom use among U.S. Men, 1991. *Family Planning Perspectives, 25*, 61–66.

Treffke, H., Tiggemann, M., & Ross, M.W. (1992). The relationship between attitude, assertiveness and condom use. *Psychology and Health, 6*, 45–52.

Turner, J. C., Korpita, E., Mohn, L. A., & Hill, W. B. (1993). Reduction in sexual risk behaviors among college students following a comprehensive health education intervention. *Journal of American College Health, 42*, 187–193.

Upchurch, D. M., Ray, P., Reichart, C., Celentano, D. D., Quinn, T., & Hook, E. W. (1992). Prevalence and patterns of condom use among patients attending a sexually transmitted disease clinic. *Sexually Transmitted Diseases, 19*, 175–180.

van den Hoek, J. A. R., van Haastrecht, H. J. A., & Coutinho, R. A. (1989). Risk reduction among intravenous drug users in Amsterdam under the influence of AIDS. *American Journal of Public Health, 79*, 1355–1357.

Valdiserri, R. O., Lyter, D. W., Leviton, L. C., Stoner, K., & Silvestre, A. (1987). Applying the criteria for the development of health promotion and education programs to AIDS risk reduction programs for gay men. *Journal of Community Health, 12*, 199–212.

Weatherburn, P., Davies, P. M., Hicks on, F. C. I., Hunt, A. J., McManus, T. J., & Coxon, A. P. M. (1993). No connection between alcohol use and unsafe sex among gay and bisexual men. *AIDS, 7*, 115–119.

Weatherburn, P., Hunt, A. J., Davies, P. M., Coxon, A. P. M., & McManus, T. J. (1991). Condom use in a large cohort of homosexually active men in England and Wales. *AIDS Care, 3*, 31–41.

Weeks, M. R., Singer, M., Grier, M., & Schensul, J. J. (1996). Gender relations, sexuality, and AIDS risk among African American and Latina women. In C.F. Sargent & C.B. Brettell, (Eds.). *Gender and health: An international perspective* (pp. 338–370). Upper Saddle River, NJ: Prentice Hall.

Wendt, S. J., & Solomon, L. J. (1995). Barriers to condom use among heterosexual male and female college students. *Journal of American College Health, 44*, 105–110.

WHO Regional Office for Europe. (1995). The Global Programme on AIDS in the European Region, 1994 and 1995. Geneva: World Health Organization.

Wingood, G. M., Hunter-Gamble, D., & DiClemente, R. J. (1993). A pilot study of sexual communication and negotiation among young African American women. *Journal of Black Psychology, 19*, 190–203.

Wulfert, E., & Wan, C. K. (1993). Condom use: A self-efficacy model. *Health Psychology, 12*, 346–353.

Wyatt, G. E. (1994). The sociocultural relevance of sex research: Challenges for the 1990s and beyond. *American Psychologist, 49*, 748–754.

Zabin, L. S. (1986). Evaluation of a pregnancy prevention program for urban teenagers. *Family Planning Perspectives, 18*, 119–126.

Zabin, L. S. (1988). The Baltimore pregnancy prevention program for urban teenagers. I. How did it work? *Family Planning Perspectives, 20*, 182–190.

10

Intervention Elements Promoting Adherence to Mindfulness-Based Stress Reduction Programs in the Clinical Behavioral Medicine Setting

Paul G. Salmon, Saki F. Santorelli, and Jon Kabat-Zinn

INTRODUCTION

The medicine of the 21st century will be far more overtly participatory than its late 20th-century counterpart. While medicine has always been participatory to one degree or another in that its practice takes place at the intersection of two interacting worlds, that of the physician and that of the patient, the point of view of the patient in modern scientific medicine has frequently been considered less relevant to treatment than that of the physician or of the dictates of medicine itself. Sometimes the patient's point of view or feelings can be ignored completely and remain unknown (Toombs, 1993).

The process of caring for people in times of both health and illness increasingly involves active collaboration, problem solving, and decision-making between caregivers and the recipients of such care, most usually termed "patients" in the medical context. This greater level of participation by patients in managing their health and treatment during illness requires recognition and respect for the patient as a person, rather than merely as an interesting problem or case. This in turn requires some degree of sensitivity to the actual lived experience (Toombs, 1993) of the patient and an appreciation of its nature and embodiment in the context of the life of the patient, its relevance to treatment and outcome, and its value in mobilizing the inner resources of the patient for healing and coping with life-altering chronic medical conditions.

One manifestation of this more participatory trend in medicine is the rapid rise and proliferation of hospital and clinic-based Mindfulness-Based Stress Reduction (MBSR) programs. These are outpatient referral services based on a patient education rather than on a clinical treatment model, and structured to engage patients to learn how to take better care of themselves as a complement to whatever medical treatments they may be receiving (Kabat-Zinn, 1990, 1993a). There are presently over 240 hospitals and clinics nationwide and abroad that offer MBSR programs (Kabat-Zinn, 1997).

MBSR originated with the Stress Reduction Clinic at the University of Massachusetts Medical Center in 1979. Since its inception, more than 10,000 medical patients have been through its basic program, which takes the form of an 8-week-long course, based on intensive training in mindfulness meditation and its applications to daily living and to coping with stress, pain, and illness. Over 90% of all referrals are from physicians, with the rest deriving from other health professionals. Of particular note is the comparatively high rate of program completion and of other forms of adherence associated with the clinic, as documented in a series of outcome studies (Kabat-Zinn, 1982; Kabat-Zinn & Chapman-Waldrop, 1988; Kabat-Zinn, Lipworth, & Burney, 1985; Kabat-Zinn, Lipworth, Burney, & Sellers, 1986; Kabat-Zinn et al., 1992; Miller, Fletcher, & Kabat-Zinn, 1995). It is the purpose of this chapter to briefly describe the MBSR intervention and highlight some of its characteristic features which may positively influence patient participation and adherence. We devote special attention to those elements that appear particularly potent in both engaging and sustaining active participant involvement.

MINDFULNESS-BASED STRESS REDUCTION

MBSR is based on intensive training of medical patients in mindfulness meditation: the systematic cultivation of nonjudgmental, nonreactive, moment-to-moment attention. Following evaluation and enrollment, patients participate in 8 weekly 2.5 hour-long, instructor-taught classes, attended by approximately thirty individuals with a wide range of chronic conditions and levels of disability, including cancer, cardiac disease, hypertension, gastrointestinal problems, and chronic pain. The mix of patients with different diagnoses allows for a generic approach, focusing on several things: commonalities across diagnoses (stress, anxiety, suffering); what is "right" with a person rather than exclusively on what is "wrong"; shared experiences, such as breathing, proprioception, thoughts and emotions, work and family life, health and illness; and on seeing oneself as a whole person, rather than solely as a patient with a particular disease. There is a day-long silent meditation retreat during the sixth week attended by patients from the different classes, as well as by graduates of the program. This retreat is typically attended by approximately 150 participants on each of the two weekend days it is offered.

Prior to enrolling, each patient referred to the program has an hour-long individual meeting with a clinic staff member (the preintervention interview) in which the patient's story is heard, and the relevant medical history, reasons for the referral, and motivation for taking the program are explored by the patient and interviewer together. The patient is given a brief description of the course format and its requirements for class attendance and for "homework", which takes the form of various meditative practices and attentional exercises. Prior to the interview, data are obtained from patients using a battery of measures to assess individual and group clinical outcomes. Following completion of the program, all participants meet individually with their class instructor in hour-long interviews to review and discuss their experiences. Together, they develop strategies for maintaining continuity in the meditation practice and for ongoing support, if appropriate.

Both interviews are conducted with a high degree of intentional mindfulness on the part of the interviewer, both in listening and in speaking with the patient (Kabat-Zinn, 1993b). Participants can request additional individual time with instructors during the course as well so that private matters can be discussed outside of the class environment.

During the program itself, participants are exposed to three formal meditation techniques:

1. a body scan meditation, practiced lying down (supine if possible);
2. sitting meditation, practiced on straight-backed chairs or on the floor; and
3. mindful hatha yoga, which involves positioning the body in a range of postures that involve the development of full-body musculoskeletal strength, balance, and flexibility.

These techniques and the rationale for their use are described in detail elsewhere (Kabat-Zinn, 1990, 1994b). We believe that inclusion of a range of meditation practices with varying degrees of movement and stillness and different primary foci for attention is instrumental in connecting in personally meaningful ways with a broad range of individuals who have different dispositions and degrees of mobility and receptivity, and thus for achieving high levels of participant interest, engagement, satisfaction, and adherence.

As "homework", patients are required to practice a mix of these methods a minimum of six days per week for 45 minutes at a time, using audiotapes for guidance. In addition, "informal" mindfulness practices are assigned each week, and participants are encouraged to create their own ways to sustain mindfulness throughout the day. Informal practices include moment-to-moment, intentionally nonjudgmental awareness of different aspects of daily life experience such as breathing, walking, driving, cooking, eating, cleaning, ironing, showering, talking, listening, working, parenting, and playing. Informal mindfulness practices also include awareness of emotional states, thoughts, and perceptions during daily activities, as well as awareness of particularly stressful situations, options for responding to them mindfully, and the tendency to react automatically and unconsciously, especially when under stress. Because informal practice is intended to be woven into the fabric of a person's daily life, these intentional shifts in attention require little in the way of time and are rated as useful or highly useful by a majority of responders in long-term (3- and 4-year) follow-up studies, suggesting adherence to acquired skills well beyond the completion of the intervention (Kabat-Zinn et al., 1986; Miller et al., 1995).

In addition to practicing formal meditation together in the classes, participants and instructors spend considerable class time discussing various aspects of the participants' experiences with the meditation practice during the preceding week, and its potential relevance to what is happening in their lives. The instructor spends a great deal of time down on the floor with and among the participants, and conducts the classes in such a way that the energy, expertise, and creativity is identified as residing in all individuals, and is not the exclusive domain of the instructor.

ADHERENCE VERSUS COMPLIANCE

The establishment of a collaborative working relationship between healthcare providers and the people they serve is now widely acknowledged as a critical aspect of healthcare delivery (Tresolini et al., 1994). Greater personal engagement by those we sometimes call healthcare "recipients" can go far beyond simply complying with treatment regimens. As commonly used, the term "compliance" connotes a relatively passive relationship of obedience and acquiescence to a higher authority. "Adherence," by contrast, connotes sustained engagement in a mutually agreed-upon plan. In this chapter, we define adherence as an ongoing, dynamic process in which the patient's self-monitoring, self-exploration, and deepening self-knowledge interact with treatment directives, structure, and methods to facilitate potential positive changes in health and in overall adaptation (Santorelli, 1992).

Working within the framework of both Social Learning Theory and the Health Belief Model, Meichenbaum and Turk (1987) identified four broad factors that appear to reduce adherence in any intervention program:

1. Participants either do not know what to do, or else lack the skills and/or the resources to carry out the prescribed treatment program.
2. Participants either do not believe themselves capable of carrying out the program, or else are not convinced that doing so will make a difference (low "self-efficacy"; see Chapter 1, this volume).
3. Adherence is associated with aversive or nonreinforcing events, or else is seen as so demanding that participants do not believe that the benefits of adherence outweigh the costs ("Health Belief Model"; see Chapter 1, this volume; also Strecher and Rosenstock, 1997).
4. Enabling strategies are poor: The quality of the relationship between participants and the healthcare provider is poor, continuity of care is lacking, and/or the program itself is not oriented toward facilitating adherence.

The identification of potential impediments to adherence may shed light on the more difficult question of identifying and optimizing factors that might promote high levels of patient adherence with medical and lifestyle interventions. At minimum, an enumeration of some basic "red flags" related to adherence provides a context for analyzing high adherence-related elements of MBSR interventions. To this end, we will examine how both the structure and process of MBSR address the potential obstacles to treatment adherence articulated by Meichenbaum and Turk (1987).

We begin with an overview of a series of outcome studies of patients participating in the MBSR program of the Stress Reduction Clinic, and follow this with an analysis of factors integral to the structure of the program which we think contribute to the relatively high rates of adherence reported.

OUTCOME AND PROGRAM ADHERENCE IN MBSR

A series of outcome studies documenting the clinical effectiveness of MBSR and its high adherence rates have been reported. An initial study (Kabat-Zinn, 1982) evaluated the effects of the MBSR on 51 patients referred with chronic pain conditions and for whom traditional medical care had ceased to provide additional relief. The most common pain diagnoses in this population were low-back, shoulder, and neck pain, and tension and migraine headaches. Postintervention, nearly two thirds of the subjects (65%) reported reductions in pain ratings of 33% or greater, and for over half of the subjects, the reduction was greater than 50%. Similar reductions in general medical and psychiatric symptomatology also were noted. These effects were generally maintained at follow-up intervals of 2.5, 4, and 7 months. In terms of program adherence, over 90% of the patients screened for admission into the program in a 1-hour interview started the program, and more than 85% of those starting the program completed it. The pain reductions observed appeared to represent a generalized reduction in pain, not restricted to periods of formal meditation practice.

In a subsequent study (Kabat-Zinn et al., 1985) ninety patients with chronic pain undergoing MBSR, including the subset of 51 from the previous study, were compared to a diagnostically similar group of 21 chronic pain patients concurrently receiving traditional care (nerve blocks, TENS units, physical therapy, analgesics, and antidepressants) in a pain clinic. A definitive interpretation of the results was not possible because patient assignment to the two treatments was not random and the groups were not comparable in all respects demographically. However, the patients participating in MBSR exhibited significantly higher mean reductions in present-moment pain, pain-related activity inhibition, psychological and medical symptoms, and negative body image than the comparison group.

Fifty-six out of 72 patients contacted who underwent MBSR (78%) responded to a follow-up questionnaire. For all measures save "present moment pain", improvements noted immediately postprogram were maintained up to 15 months later. More than 70% of the 78% who responded to the follow-up study reported continued practicing some form of meditation after the program ended. This group included some individuals whose outcome data suggested only minimal symptom reduction or none at all. For chronic pain patients to maintain adherence to a treatment program in the absence of significant pain relief is notable, and suggests that program effects other than symptom reduction may be of value to at least some patients.

A subsequent study of 225 patients with chronic pain, including the 90 subjects cited above (Kabat-Zinn et al., 1986), provided additional evidence of the stability of the observed treatment effects as well as of substantial adherence rates. In this study, significant reductions in pain ratings as well as medical and psychiatric symptoms were found. Except for present-moment pain ratings (which could not be effectively measured without face-to-face interviewer administration), symptom reductions were sustained for up to 48 months post-treatment. At each follow-up time from 6 to 48 months, at least 93% of subjects reported that they were still practicing one of the three major MBSR techniques at some level.

A subsequent study (Kabat-Zinn & Chapman-Waldrop, 1988) measured program completion and compliance in a MBSR program over a 2-year period and explored factors influencing adherence. This study illustrates how each step in the referral, encounter, enrollment, attendance, and program completion process represents a phase during which adherence-related motivational factors come into play. Of 1,155 patients referred to the Stress Reduction Clinic for MBSR, 869 (75%) were interviewed. Of these, 784 (90%) enrolled; 716 (91% of those enrolled) began the program, and 598 (85% of those who started; 76% of those who enrolled) completed it, which constituted 52% of the original referral cohort (see Figure 10.1). The greatest loss (25% of subjects) occurred between the time patients were referred and the initial interview. These results have remained basically the same over the past 10 years in spite of periodic changes in teaching personnel. The relatively high levels of program completion and adherence to the meditation practices reported in the above studies probably stem, at least in part, from a level of motivational selectivity operative during the referral and initial interview phases.

Recently, program completion was studied in an inner-city, multiethnic and cross-cultural MBSR program (Kabat-Zinn et al., 1993c, Kabat-Zinn et al., 1994, 1997). This program is offered free of charge, with free on-site day care and free door-to-door taxi transportation when required, to reduce common barriers to participation in such interventions. In addition, the program is offered entirely in Spanish, as well as in English. Results from a 2-year study showed that of 745 people referred to the program, 492 (66%) attended a focus-group meeting to describe the program. (Focus groups were held in lieu of individual interviews because extremely low attendance rates at those interviews had persisted until after people had attended a focus group meeting). Of those attending the focus groups, 485 (99%) enrolled and filled out data forms. Of these, 333 (68%) attended the first class, and 200 (60% of those who started, and 27% of those who were referred) completed the program. The quantitative differences between these results and those for the more middle-class population seen at the main clinic suggest cultural differences which are important to consider when attempting to deliver interventions in a low-income, low-education, and high social and economic stress environment. These adherence factors are the subject of ongoing investigation. Outcomes for those individuals completing the inner city MBSR were qualitatively similar to those obtained in the main clinic (Kabat-Zinn et al., 1994, 1997).

Short and long-term measures of program adherence for patients with medical conditions who also have a diagnosed anxiety disorder have also been reported for the MBSR intervention (Kabat-Zinn et al., 1992; Miller et al., 1995). In an initial study of 24 subjects meeting DSM-III(R) criteria for Generalized Anxiety Disorder or Panic Disorder (with or without agoraphobia), in addition to their medical diagnoses, pre-, post-, and follow-up assessments using a range of standardized measures indicated a high completion rate (22 of the 24 subjects, 92%). There was also substantial reduction of symptoms on the Beck Anxiety and Beck Depression Scales following program completion and at a 3-month follow-up in 20 of the 22 subjects completing the program. At 3-month follow-up, 91% of those who completed the program (20 of 22) reported that they had been keeping up the practice of the stress reduction techniques, using either one specific formal technique or a combination of techniques. Moreover, 84% (N = 16) reported practicing three or more times per week. Almost all (21 of 22) indicated ongoing use of mindfulness of breathing in their daily lives (Kabat-Zinn et al., 1992).

The results of this study are consistent with previous research based on patients with chronic pain diagnoses in suggesting that MBSR tends to promote both high rates of program completion and continued meditative practice. A 3-year follow-up study of this cohort of patients (Miller et al., 1995) found that 18 of the original 22 program completers, plus a larger cohort of 99 program participants who also met study admission criteria, maintained significant reductions in anxiety, depression, and panic symptoms. Moreover, ongoing adherence with formal meditation practices was reported by a majority of responders (10 of 18). Sixteen of the eighteen responders reported continued use of the informal practice of mindfulness of breathing in daily life.

MBSR AND ADHERENCE: DESCRIPTIVE FACTORS

Results of these studies of MBSR show high rates of program completion and substantial ongoing adherence to formal and informal mediation practices (maintenance). The following characteristics of MBSR may contribute to these levels of adherence and ongoing compliance:

1. The approach employs a time-limited, group-based format in which the duration of treatment, as well as the length of the treatment sessions, are clearly specified;
2. The educational orientation, the courselike format, its overall structure and curriculum, and the interactive nature of the instruction are designed to evoke a sense of active participation and to ignite a passion for self-observation, inner exploration, and self-inquiry among the patients enrolled in the program;
3. A range of different methods and exercises are offered to cultivate mindfulness, so that people with different dispositions may find at least some aspects of the course compatible with their personal orientation and learning style;

4. High levels of competency, clarity, commitment, compassion, and effective communication are required of instructors;

5. The lived experience of each patient is accorded a profound importance and every attempt is made to honor it explicitly and implicitly in all aspects of the program;

6. The nature of the meditation practices themselves promote increasing sensitivity and appreciation for the many ways mind and body interact; increased experiences of self-efficacy regarding observing and coping more effectively with physical and emotional discomfort; and increased feelings of interconnectedness and the possibilities for personal transformation through sustained awareness in daily life;

7. Participation in the social setting of a course, in which people sit in a circle around a spacious room rather than "theater-style" and share their adventures in being mindful of the events unfolding in their lives from week to week, builds a strong sense of community, feelings of belonging, and of being listened to and respected;

8. The all-day silent retreat, in the 6th week of the course, provides a unique motivational element as patients engage in a range of meditation practices and mindfulness exercises over the course of an entire day with over 150 other patients and former patients; and finally

9. When one person experiences growth and learning, either in the form of pain reduction or symptom improvement, or from having encountered and coped effectively with an untoward and stressful situation, or from simply being able to stay awake during a body scan meditation, or from self-insight at a particular moment, that experience may positively influence the person's motivation to keep up attendance and to practice regularly the various forms of meditation assigned for homework each week. Reporting this experience in class can have a similar motivating influence on other members of the class who may be struggling, or who have not yet had such experiences themselves.

An analysis of the major factors influencing adherence in MBSR programs must consider the following aspects of the structure of the program: (1) the referral process and the preprogram interview; (2) the initial stage of the program, i.e. the first two classes and the intervening week; (3) an intermediate stage, i.e. the central core of the program and the all-day session; (4) the end-stage characteristics in weeks 7 and 8; and (5) the post-program interview and subsequent follow-up. These aspects are examined below, followed by a consideration of relapse.

Referral Procedures, Preprogram Interview, and Adherence

The preprogram interview serves two purposes. First, it provides an opportunity to screen referred patients for potential contraindications for participation. There are very few exclusionary criteria in MBSR; the principal one is active suicidality. Indications of severe psychopathology in which either reality-testing or ego boundaries appear to be substantially impaired would also warrant exclusion.

A network of referral sources developed during the years of the Stress Reduction Clinic's operation tends to limit inappropriate referrals. Some referring physicians have taken the course themselves or have attended programs designed to familiarize them with its characteristics. Most get a feeling for whom to refer based on the experiences of patients they have referred in the past, and from periodic updates sent to them from the clinic which characterize appropriate and inappropriate referrals (see discussion below). Moreover, since the focus of the program is primarily on patients with medical problems, the number of individuals with severe psychiatric symptomatology is low. There is, however, substantial psychiatric comorbidity, in that conditions such as anxiety and depression are common accompaniments of many of the medical conditions seen in the clinic.

Referral procedures can exert a strong influence on future adherence because they select and prepare appropriate candidates, who are then more likely to subscribe to the overall goals and requirements of the treatment program. The clinic communicates with its large pool of referring physicians, both within the hospital and in the greater community, through periodic announcements describing the program. Descriptions of appropriate categories of referral emphasize the participatory nature of the intervention and the need for self-motivation and discipline. Referring physicians are also sent periodic calendars showing the best times for referral. These links to the community of referring physicians increases the likelihood that the individuals referred will be appropriate candidates for the intervention.

In addition to providing an opportunity to screen prospective participants, the preprogram interview also serves important educational and motivational functions including, frequently, a patient's first exposure to the concept and practice of mindfulness meditation. All interviewers are long-term meditators who practice mindfulness meditation themselves on a daily basis. They are trained to listen mindfully and to bring a full range of mindfulness-based communications skills to the encounter. Included in the process is the interviewer's conscious intention to conduct the interview with an abiding, moment-to-moment awareness of the sacred quality—in the Hippocratic sense—of the encounter between patient and provider. The performance of the interviewers is periodically assessed through supervision and formal evaluation procedures to ensure high standards for this critical exchange.

The interview is long enough (typically lasting 1 hour) for the patient to be able to tell his or her story, experience an empathic and interested listener, speak about areas of particular concern that may underlie the referral itself, the diagnosis, or his or her life circumstances, and to be informed about the structure of the program and the requirements for acceptance. As part of the interview, each prospective participant is told about the program in detail. They are informed about the meditation and the yoga practices they will encounter; the need to attend class once a week with 25 to 35 other participants with a wide range of medical problems who are all referred by their physicians; and the requirement to attend an all-day silent "retreat" on the weekend in the 6th week of the program. The interview characterizes the program as a challenge to the patients to do something for themselves as a complement to what the health care system might be doing for them. Thus, patients who have completed the preprogram evaluation go into the 8-week program "with their eyes open"—informed not just about the program's structure and orientation, but also about the degree of participation expected of them and the forms that participation might take.

MBSR is, in fact, a highly demanding program, requiring considerable time and effort: 2.5 hours per week in class at the hospital; 8 weeks of classes; the all-day weekend session; and between 45 and 60 minutes of daily homework and practice 6 days per week. No attempt is made to "sell" the program or to convince prospective patients that it would be useful for them. In fact, prospective candidates are usually told that it is "stressful to take the stress reduction program," in part because of the immediate lifestyle change that it requires just to make the time to practice at home according to the required schedule. It is left to the patient to make the decision to enroll or not, and in which class (typically from a choice of 4 mornings and 4 evenings each week). Thus the entire interview acts as a potential turning point for the patient. It includes a frank and empathic look at the forces and circumstances that brought the individual to the clinic in the first place, and also an opportunity to take some level of responsibility for their own health and choose to do something that may have important and long-lasting beneficial consequences. It is emphasized, however, that there are no guaranteed outcomes, not even that people will feel better or be more relaxed or less stressed.

The detailed explanation of the program to prospective participants at its very outset is likely to have at least two screening effects that might influence subsequent adherence. First, it is likely to discourage enrollment on the part of individuals who are not up to the challenges posed by the program. For example, some patients believe strongly in the standard "medical model" treatment paradigm, which accords them a relatively passive role in the process of healing. Others may decline to participate because they are not able or willing to make the necessary commitment of time and energy.

Motivation and adherence related to attendance, program completion, and daily homework are also influenced by the way in which the program is presented to the patient and its highly participatory nature emphasized.

The program is framed as an opportunity to see if there might not be things one might do for oneself that no one else could do for you, and that would possibly contribute to a movement toward greater health and well-being.

In addition to the emphasis on time and energy demands, patients are exposed to an approach that explicitly emphasizes non-doing and non-striving, in accordance with the meditative approach itself (Kabat-Zinn, 1994b). In the interview, patients are cautioned against becoming overly invested in obtaining "results" such as an end to their pain, or relief from anxiety. Each patient is asked to state three goals that they would like to work towards after electing to enroll in the program at the close of the interview. These goals are recorded so they can be revisited at the completion of the program. However, the patients are also advised not to strive toward achieving these goals or persist in measuring their "progress" toward them each day while they are in the program, but instead to concentrate on simply doing what is being asked of them from day to day and from week to week. It is suggested that they suspend judgment as much as possible about the program and about whether or not they are making progress, and that, at the end, they can assess whether it was of any value or not.

In characterizing the commitment to keep up the regular daily practice of the meditation and yoga, prospective patients are typically informed, with a combination of humor and seriousness, that "You don't have to like it; you just have to do it". Thus, a strong suggestion is made "preemptively" that the meditation practice does not necessarily require or evoke pleasant feelings or immediately positive outcomes, and that one needs to suspend judgment and just do the work, remaining aware of all tendencies to judge and evaluate, but without either rejecting or pursuing these tendencies. This orientation is a reflection of the way in which all thought and emotion, regardless of content, is held in awareness during formal and informal mindfulness practice. The power of reducing mental distress through facing difficult experiences with openness, rather than with avoidance or suppression, is a well-established therapeutic effect, recently documented in a series of studies by Wegner and colleagues (Wegner, 1994).

The emphasis on just doing the work and not worrying about the results is thus explicitly established as part of the "contract" for enrollment in the very first encounter. Importantly, the statement "You don't have to like it; you just have to do it" is not used as an externally oriented directive, but as quite the opposite: a method for engaging each potential participant in an act of self-directed choice. This approach conveys to potential participants a clear understanding of what it will actually take to engage in the program. The choice to participate expresses a willingness to fulfill a mutually agreed upon "learning contract". More importantly, choosing to participate initiates the development of an "internal" contract leading to the formation of personal intention—a deliberate, self-motivating decision to "work" on one's own behalf during the program. It is our view that such intentionality, actively cultivated and reinforced through the ongoing practice of the various meditative methods during the program, and through the social support to which the emerging community of the class gives rise, can ignite a self-generating learning cycle in the patient, leading to increased adherence to the program.

Thus, the emphasis on changing behavior and working toward specific goals characteristic of cognitive/behavioral interventions is replaced in MBSR by an initial emphasis on careful self-observation and on learning . . . learning, for instance, what is actually involved in experiencing one's life from moment to moment, including times of discomfort, stress, pain, and anxiety. There is no emphasis in MBSR on trying to "fix" anything. The emphasis is rather to "work" consciously with one's situation as one finds it. Somewhat paradoxically, such an acceptance itself constitutes a profoundly positive change—an attitudinal shift for those who struggle constantly with the desire for things to be somehow different than they are. While not precluding behavioral change, the MBSR approach provides patients with an opportunity for active participation in a program that does not make overt change and goal achievement the litmus test for success, not unlike 'acceptance'-based psychotherapy models (Hayes, 1994).

In summary, the physician referral to the program, coupled with the initial interview as described above, serve as a multidimensional introduction to the intervention for the prospective patient, and provides clinic staff with an opportunity to carry out pretreatment screening and patient education. The physician referral (whether the original impulse to take the program comes from the physician or from the patient) and an educational orientation that ultimately rests on the inner resources of the patient for observation, concentration, relaxation, insight, acceptance, learning, growing, healing, and taking action are both critical factors influencing adherence to the program both while people are in it, and when participants are well beyond completion of the 8-week intervention.

Initial Stage of the Program and Adherence

As noted above, upon completion of the initial interview, 90% of patients enroll. Of these, 92% actually begin the program, and of those who start, 85% complete it (Kabat-Zinn & Chapman-Waldrop, 1988) see Figure 10.1). Thus, there is an overall completion rate of 76%, with a 9% no-show rate and a 15% drop-out rate.

Patients who drop out once the program has started tend to do so within the first 3 weeks. A number of factors are involved. Some patients encounter problems allotting the necessary time to attend class and practice daily. Some find that they are so uncomfortable with the relatively large classes that they choose to leave. A few simply find the methods either unsatisfying or too demanding.

During the program, patients are expected to call in if they have to miss a class, and to make it up if possible. If they do not call, the instructor calls the patient within a day of missing the class to see how he or she is doing, to give the homework assignment, and to suggest attendance at another class. Such immediate expressions of interest and concern can contribute to the development of a more personal connection between an instructor and a class member who may be feeling overwhelmed or unmotivated, or who may be experiencing a crisis. Such personal follow-up generally enhances a sense that the patient is valued and respected, and conveys as well the sense that the work the patient is doing is important. According this kind of attention to individuals when they do miss a class probably contributes in many cases to a resolve on the part of the patient to remain in the program in spite of difficulties.

The first class frequently progresses spontaneously to a substantial level of self-disclosure, as participants are invited to share their reasons for enter-

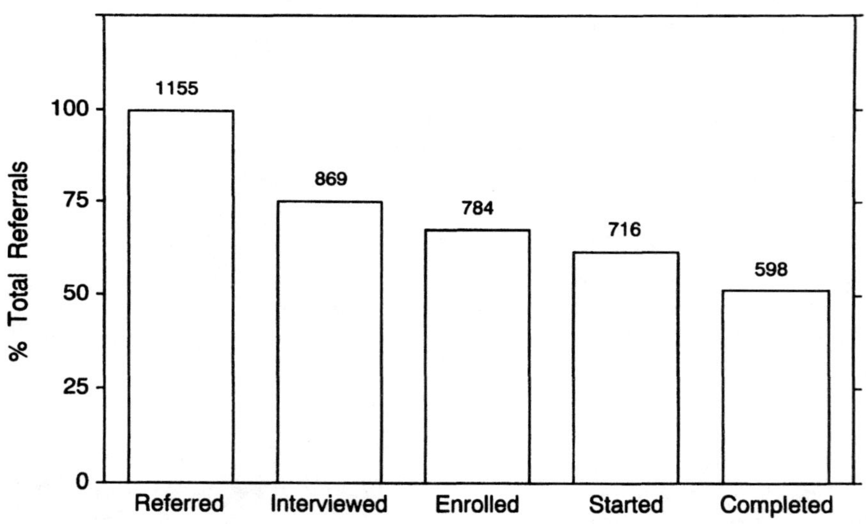

Figure 10.1 Population adherence to the stages of follow-through with a physician referral for MBSR training.

From "Compliance with an outpatient stress reduction program: Rates and predictors of completion," by J. Kabat-Zinn and A. Chapman-Waldrop, 1988, *Journal of Behavioral Medicine, 11,* p. 341. Copyright Plenum Press. Reprinted with permission.

ing the program. The willingness of at least some participants to spontaneously and openly express grief, fear, and pain has several effects. First, it makes apparent to the entire class that a broad range of human suffering is represented within the room. This, in turn, tends to place any one person's story or problems in a larger context. Some people, no matter how severe their own problems, respond to the first class by thinking that they do not belong there because they feel other people's problems are more serious. Second, powerful emotional forces are often generated as people begin to share with each other—many for the first time ever—burdens which have typically been accumulating for years, and which have now been compounded by some more recent stress event which may have catalyzed referral to the program. As some individuals spontaneously express such feelings, others may come to feel permission to express similar levels of emotion about their own circumstances, or perhaps to silently acknowledge similar emotions within themselves. One participant characterized the program as "the community of the afflicted" and found he could speak about things in the class and feel accepted in ways that he found unique and supportive (Kabat-Zinn, 1994a).

In the first class, participants are provided with a more detailed context and framework for participation in the program, which builds on the foundation established in the initial interview. The cultivation of a non-goal orientation and of a nonjudgmental, moment-to-moment attending to one's experience is emphasized, coupled with the explicit suggestion that "As long as you are breathing, there is more 'right' with you than 'wrong' with you", no matter what is "wrong," and no matter what the reasons for referral into the program.

Common misconceptions about meditation are that it is as a weird or mystical inner manoeuver that requires sitting in the full lotus posture and/or making one's mind a blank. To disabuse participants of such notions, the first meditation conducted in class is typically an "eating meditation". The exercise involves eating one raisin mindfully. With concurrent instructions, it can take from 5 or 10 minutes to eat one raisin. The sheer novelty and intensity of this experience, with a highly focused attention directed at the ordinary act of eating, including seeing the raisin, holding it in the hand, awareness of the arm and hand moving to place the raisin at the lips and of salivation in response to the anticipation of eating, the action of the tongue, the tasting, the chewing, and the swallowing, are sufficient to effectively illustrate that meditation involves a refined, open, and systematic attending that may be more relevant to the lives of program participants, and a lot more accessible and down-to-earth, than they might have previously thought. The experiential and highly participatory aspects of the program and the commonsensical orientation taken toward meditation characterize MBSR from the very first class.

The first class also stresses the disciplined, consistent, day-to-day, moment-to-moment nature of mindfulness meditation practice. Instructors portray their role as that of guide or coach, and do not assume an authoritarian stance or tone. One apt metaphor likens the program to a river rafting trip, which the guide has made many times, but still experiences uniquely on each occasion. Described in this manner, the program conveys an element of the unknown, like an adventure, perhaps even with some risk, as it is made clear that one cannot rely on the security of a completely predictable programmatic or manualized experience. It is also made clear that the teachers are not requiring anything of the participants that they do not also practice themselves to at least the same degree, and usually more, on a daily basis. The commitment on the part of the instructors to use the practice in their own lives can entrain a similar commitment on the part of the participants, and thus positively influence adherence.

ONGOING PARTICIPATION AND ADHERENCE

Perhaps the most powerful element leading to ongoing attendance in the MBSR classes and to strong engagement in the meditation practices assigned for homework, in spite of the time commitment and lifestyle changes required to follow through on the original commitment, is the deep feeling of well-being that can arise out of the practice of the body scan, sitting meditation, and the mindful hatha yoga. These feelings are related to an intentional willingness to reside in stillness and silence, observing the unfolding of one's experience from moment to moment, and intentionally, as best one can, assuming a nonreactive and nonjudgmental stance toward every experience during this time. While high degrees of discomfort, boredom, frustration, anxiety, irritability, and other mind states are a natural part of the interior landscape during periods of formal practice, the frame of intentional nonjudgmental awareness allows them to be seen merely as "events" in the field of awareness and to be attended to in such a way that feelings of relaxation, calmness, self-confidence, commitment, and self-efficacy can arise within the very process of observing. Such experiences are potentially available in each moment, without having to have anything change in the inner landscape itself, only in the way it is seen and held.

MBSR participants soon discover this potential within the practice, either from their own direct experience of it or from hearing others speak of it in class. The different formal techniques can be seen as different "doors" into the same room, from the point of view of experiencing feelings of stillness and well-being and their accessibility in any moment. Once a person has tasted the relaxation and calmness associated with inner stillness and wakefulness, these experiences themselves become powerful motivators for continued practice, since they act as a form of immediate "nourishment", whether relaxation, calmness, or any other particular potential feature of the practice is strong or not during any particular practice session. Typically, within a 45-minute period of time, the practitioner will experience at least some fleeting moments of relative peace; this experience can reinforce the motivation to continue the practice.

As the program continues from week to week, new factors potentially related to adherence come into play as well. The required daily practice for "homework" translates for many participants into behavior patterns that become embedded in daily life, reinforced by experiences similar to those described above. In contrast to some homework-oriented programs, where both content and structure may vary from week to week, MBSR emphasizes continuity in the cultivation of mindfulness throughout the course, both though specific homework assignments and by incorporating the ongoing changing life circumstances of a particular day or week into one's practice. Nevertheless, there is a very strong element of repetition, in that the same tapes are used over and over, and the meditation practice is always fundamentally the same: cultivating and sustaining mindfulness. This overriding factor of continuity in the practice itself lends coherence to the course as a whole and unifies the thrust of the homework assignments.

Elements of Western psychotherapeutic techniques such as "self-monitoring" and "nonreinforced exposure" used in cognitive and related therapies (Linehan, 1994), can be discerned within the orientation and practice of mindfulness meditation. Mindfulness provides participants with a unique means of responding effectively to doubt, fatigue, and other forces which can negatively affect adherence motivation. The intentional suspending of judging that is encouraged by the basic meditation instructions makes it less likely that any feelings of inadequacy or failure on the part of participants about how they are doing will have an adverse impact on adherence, since such perceptions are identified as merely more thinking, as events arising in the field of awareness, rather than as a true description of the practitioner's situation. Mindfulness thus makes it more likely that thoughts and feelings that may adversely affect practice motivation will be detected. It provides a conceptual framework and practical strategy for limiting the direct impact of such thoughts and feelings on behavior when they occur. It establishes an inner attitude of openness and curiosity, sometimes referred to as "putting out a welcome mat" for whatever arises in the field of awareness, thereby potentially reducing aversive reactions in the face of challenging intrapsychic material. And it encourages bringing nonjudgmental awareness to whatever one may be doing, which may minimize the degree to which troublesome thoughts and emotions occur.

A range of informal mindfulness practices is assigned and encouraged during the program. These provide an effective vehicle for generalizing treatment effects in a manner reminiscent of psychotherapeutic "exposure" or "inoculation" (see, for example, Meichenbaum, 1993). The characteristics of informal practice, as ascertained through text analysis of in-depth participant interviews conducted periodically through the 8-week program and at 2-month follow-up (Santorelli, 1992) suggests a progression of stages. These include: deliberate or planned strategies utilized when preparing for a usually stressful situation, e.g., "I decided to take three breaths before walking into the meeting with my boss"; spontaneous moments of mindfulness, e.g., reports of being aware of the rhythm of the breath "without thinking about it" or responding in a proactive, uncharacteristic manner in the midst of typically stressful situations; and trends of mindfulness in daily life, whereby participants reported their capacity to make deliberate, intentional shifts throughout the day as becoming more generalized and therefore less differentiated from formal practice periods.

The MBSR curriculum emphasizes both formal and informal mindfulness practices. Formal practice is typically conducted in a quiet place in the home during a period when one will not be disturbed or interrupted. Over time, through the type of attention characteristic of mindfulness and emphasized in the guided meditation instructions in class and on the audiotapes used to practice at home, formal practice cultivates and develops increased concentration, a refined sensitivity and greater equanimity regarding body sensations, perceptions, impulses, thoughts and feelings, and nonattachment, self-acceptance, feelings of compassion for others and for oneself, and deepening insight into what we think of as "self" and of self-in-relationship (Gunaratana, 1991; Kabat-Zinn, 1990; Kabat-Zinn, Skillings, & Salmon, 1996; Thera, 1962).

Informal mindfulness practice, which like formal practice, can take many forms, can be thought of as extensions of the practice into in vivo situations—analogous to behavioral exposure techniques—whereby mindfulness is brought to whatever arises in the course of one's life unfolding. This can include experiences that may be far more challenging than those encountered in the classroom or during periods of quiet practice at home. By teaching basic skills in the context of formal meditation practices and encouraging their development through daily practice, and by then expanding the field of objects of meditative awareness to include everyday activities, the program helps bridge the gap between in-class and in-vivo experience (Kabat-Zinn & Chapman-Waldrop, 1988; Santorelli, 1992). This, we contend, comprises a powerful mechanism for the optimizing of program adherence. It is one of the virtues and benefits of a once-a-week course format. The time between classes serves as an in-vivo laboratory for practice. In this way, practice becomes understood as a way of being, rather than a technique that one uses to "reduce one's stress", and living itself becomes seen as practice.

Preliminary research (Santorelli, 1992) suggests that a generative learning cycle develops from the reciprocal relationship between formal and informal meditation practices. For example, highly stressed participants initially reported periods of "being more relaxed" or "calm" during formal practice as a new or novel experiences for them. As the program progressed, they reported similar experience of well-being arising during informal meditation practice in everyday situations. Over time, both forms of meditation mutually reinforced each other, and led to reported increases in self-confidence in stressful situations (Santorelli, 1992).

To maximize adherence, it is essential for such a group-based intervention to have effective ways to accommodate individual differences and technique preferences. One study found a broad range of preferences among program participants for the three different formal practices, even though practice of all three was required, with the exception of yoga in the case of people who could not do it fully because of chronic pain (Kabat-Zinn et al., 1997). The degree to which those participants who had high levels of anxiety, as measured by the SCL-90-R (Derogatis, 1983) liked the individual techniques of the body scan, the sitting meditation, and the mindful hatha yoga was found to be dramatically related to the pattern that characterized their experience of anxiety. The cohort of individuals whose anxiety was experienced in a predominantly cognitive mode preferred the most physical (somatic) technique (yoga) and liked the sitting meditation least, while those who experienced anxiety in a predominantly somatic mode preferred the least physical and most "cognitive" technique (sitting meditation), and liked the yoga least. This study suggests that a range of methods can serve a heterogeneous population in providing at least one approach that resonates with the disposition of individual participants, and thus afford a sense of meaningful connection that may allow a patient to explore other practices that may not have held an initial attraction.

The high levels of adherence achieved in the program may also be due in part to a progressive shift in emphasis from careful adherence to the curriculum during the initial (learning) sessions, regardless of individual likes and dislikes, to an emphasis on "finding your own way" and "making the practice your own" by the time it is over. Self-exploration and self-responsibility are continually encouraged as a means of translating the suggestions of the instructor into personal terms for each participant, and for developing sensitivity to one's own body and its internal messages. As noted above, the emphasis throughout the program is not on achieving a particular result or outcome, but rather on engaging in an ongoing process of exploration. This orientation may be critical to achieving a high degree of adherence in programs aimed at mobilizing the inner resources of the patient to move towards greater levels of health, well-being, and effective living.

The MBSR approach to patient education, growth, and change represents an important contrast to many other treatment approaches, in relation to program adherence where the purpose of adhering to a specific regimen is commonly aimed at achieving a specific desirable goal or result. In MBSR, adherence simply asks that participants try to cultivate an awareness of what they are already doing, thinking, or experiencing in any particular moment, whatever it may be. Provided that one is willing to attempt to bring an attitude of nonjudgmental awareness to any moment, there is, paradoxically, little else that one might do or say or think that would somehow not reflect inherent adherence. The injunction to simply "pay attention" creates a broad and relatively permissive context within which change can occur. This approach is similar to that used in acceptance-based psychotherapy (Hayes, 1987, 1994; Linehan, 1994). Perhaps one of the strengths of MBSR is that mindfulness itself reduces potential resistance, because it can always focus on the resistance as an object of attention, thereby maintaining adherence to the practice and narrowing the range of what would otherwise be considered "nonadherent" behaviors.

Participation in the all-day session in week 6 can serve as a turning point for many program participants. The demands of an entire day of practice, in silence, and with large numbers of other people, helps build on everything that has been done in the preceding weeks in the program, and often results in a far deeper understanding of practice and its value. Small- and large-group dialogue at the end of the day often leads to an abiding sense of mindfulness practice as a lifetime's work, rather than something one does for 8 weeks to pick up some techniques and change one's lifestyle or habits. This can come in part from hearing former patients, who come to these sessions in large numbers and tend to share their experiences during the discussion period, and describe their learning trajectories with MBSR and the effects it has had on their lives and their health.

Concluding Program Phase and Adherence

In week 7, participants are encouraged to devise their own home schedule of meditation practice. Having now received training in all three formal methods, they are invited to work out their own combination of formal practices for the week (still adhering to the 45-minutes-per-day standard) and integrate this combination into their daily schedule. This may positively affect end-stage adherence in several ways. First, the element of choice reinforces the importance of personal responsibility emphasized throughout the course. Second, it takes advantage of the fact that, as noted above, many participants have strong preferences for specific techniques.

Thus, the last 2 weeks of the program provide opportunities for participants to explore and reinforce individual inclinations and initiatives, and to tailor the program to their own particular needs. This latitude may contribute to the high levels of commitment to maintain the practice commonly reported by program participants.

Post-Program Interview and Adherence

After a battery of postintervention assessment measures has been completed by the patient, a personal interview with the course instructor concludes the intervention. This interview serves two purposes. First, it provides each participant with an opportunity to review the program in its entirety, and to reflect upon his or her experience during the preceding 8 weeks. Goals that were articulated at the beginning and then set aside are now explicitly re-examined with the patient with an emphasis, not on "success" or "failure" in terms of attaining a goal, but to discern whether any degree of movement towards the self-set goals has been detected, and to explore the evidence for one's assessment of "progress". Second, and perhaps more importantly, this session is used to plan ways to integrate mindfulness into the individual's day-to-day life beyond the end of the program. In addressing this issue explicitly, the instructor sets the stage for longer-term adherence to the formal and informal practices and their applications in dealing with stress, pain, and illness. To this end, participants are asked for homework toward the end of the last class to identify three short-term (3-months) and three long-term (6-months) goals related to their own experiences and aspirations developed while in the program, and to elaborate explicit strategies for achieving them. They are asked to bring these new goals and strategies for achieving them to the post-program interview. The most common short- and long-term goal is to keep up the practice and deepen it.

Once the program is completed, graduates are eligible to attend free weekly "drop-in" meditation sessions that bring them into contact with other MBSR instructors and other graduates of the program on a regular basis. They are also eligible to attend any or all of the 6 day-long weekend sessions offered during the course of each year as an integral part of the regular MBSR program. These opportunities provide a significant way for graduates to maintain contact with both the philosophical and structural elements of the program, and may be seen as akin to "booster sessions" that have proven effective in other contexts at reducing drop-out and nonadherence rates (Meichenbaum, 1993).

The clinic also offers "advanced" or "graduate" classes on a regular basis. Program graduates receive notices three times per year announcing these offerings. Graduate classes typically meet one time per month for 5 months. They include extended periods of meditation practice using all the methods taught in the "basic" course, with an overarching focus on the application of mindfulness to stress, pain, illness, disability, health, and well-being. Homework includes both formal practice assignments and a focus on a specific theme. Additional materials and assignments are mailed out frequently to participants at the midway point between hospital sessions. These communications serve to build on the themes of previous classes and to generate a degree of anticipation and curiosity regarding the upcoming class. This approach encourages ongoing engagement of the participants over an extended period (5 weeks) between classes, and helps to keep the focus on continuously bringing mindfulness to the unfolding of daily life experience. It may thus offer participants who may have relapsed in a particular week something of an incentive to re-engage in the practice, or simply to encourage and further the systematic deepening of mindfulness for those who have continued to practice regularly.

Relapse

Relapse to one's original condition, mind-state, or behavior patterns always constitutes a significant impediment to long-term adherence, even following "successful" interventions for behavior change (see Chapter 2, this volume; Marlatt & Gordon, 1985). Teasdale, Segal, and Williams (1995) have recently suggested that mindfulness practice may help mitigate relapse tendencies in patients with chronic depression by enhancing sensitivity to initial, and often subtle, affective deterioration in time to activate previously learned cognitive coping strategies.

Since MBSR is offered to medical patients with a wide range of physical and psychological problems, relapse in MBSR may take a number of different forms. The most common is discontinuing the formal and informal practices adopted during the program. For some, the consequences of abandoning the behavioral framework of daily practice may entail an increased frequency of anxious feelings, panic, or depression; others may return to using high doses of medication in response to pain. Others may have a sort of "cognitive" relapse. Perhaps uncomfortable with the prospect of making the active, long-term commitment to their own health characteristic of MBSR, they may revert to the more passive "patient" role, seeking primarily to be cared for and helped through the efforts of others. In the process, they may cease formal practice entirely or practice at a very low level. They may abandon informal practice as well.

Relapse is a troublesome problem in many healthcare contexts. A single incident can trigger a cognitive and behavioral "chain reaction" leading to complete disengagement from program adherence, along with accompanying feelings of failure, unworthiness, or hopelessness. MBSR addresses relapse in a number of unique ways.

First, the nonjudgmental, nonstriving orientation of the practice itself tends to reframe ideas of "relapse" (and other comparably judgmental terms) in a more benign and accepting manner. Relapse in the form of ceasing to practice is seen as a natural and inevitable part of the learning process, and a phenomenon worthy of attention and interest in its own right. It is also remediable in the next moment simply by re-establishing mindfulness. Thus, one is always only one breath, one moment, one thought away from being back in the practice, especially if this shift in attention can be sustained over several moments and minutes.

Other implications of the MBSR conceptual framework also impinge on and influence the risk of relapse. In meditation, one readily experiences that things are changing from moment to moment, and that the present moment is constantly and continuously unfolding, presenting itself in new and unique configurations. One comes to experience directly that no two moments are the same, and that, while patterns of behavior do have, by definition, enduring and persistent qualities, they also contain the potential in any moment to chart a new way to being, to see a new opening, to ally oneself to the possibility of letting a new choice emerge, and to allow change to occur by itself out of one's tenaciously cultivated awareness. A common self-statement describing relapse, such as "I've fallen back into my old patterns again", has embedded in it the thought that one is at the mercy of old behaviors, simply repeated without variation. This is not only improbable, but as noted, it is virtually impossible, owing to the dynamic and fluid nature of experience itself. The components of the statement: "I", "have fallen back" "into my old patterns"; "again" contain a number of imprecise linguistic characterizations (i.e., thoughts) of a specific current experience that, in reality, has a unique potential and character and, therefore, cannot be identical with past experiences. Attending systematically to present-moment experience via the practice of mindfulness, rather than merely thinking about an experience or a moment, loosens "the dominance of evaluative languaging" (Hayes, 1994, p. 16).

Furthermore, within the mindfulness framework, a relapse incident can be viewed with generosity and self-compassion; more as an opportunity for refocusing one's attention, than as a setback. Experiences which might otherwise be interpreted in negative terms, or in ways that imply that progress toward treatment goals has been impeded, are framed and reframed in more benign terms. A period of relapse, as in having stopped meditating, or in the form of recurrence of a panic attack, or of strong feelings of anxiety or depression, can all be seen as opportunities to practice mindfulness. By framing events in this manner, mindfulness emphasizes, as do contemporary contextualist (Hayes, 1994), cognitive, and constructivist psychotherapies (Meichenbaum, 1993), and relapse prevention theory itself (Marlatt, 1985), the importance of taking a "fresh look" at commonly ignored, linguistically driven, interpretive biases. MBSR patients or former patients who report relapses in their practice are encouraged to "go into" the experience of "relapse" and see what might be learned from it. They might inquire whether it does actually entail a simple repetition of a previous behavior pattern. What are its unique qualities, its antecedents, its ensuing consequences? Casting problems as further "grist for the mill", seeing them as potential resources and opportunities, however unwanted, to practice being present and wakeful in the face of the actuality of one's life experience, helps restore balance in the face of the reflexive negative self-assessments that so typically accompany distressful experiences and emotions. If the overarching goal is to be more mindful in one's life, rather than confining the goal to a limited and highly specific objective, such as getting off addictive pain medications or stopping drinking, a relapse can be seen as one significant and potentially interesting event, embedded within the larger fabric of all events comprising moment-to-moment experience. Thus, the systematic, dispassionate observing of one's own episodes of relapse is a way to further learning, growth (i.e., adult development), and the process of change. By worrying less about what a relapse may signify, for example, and investing more time in simply observing the nature of the experience, one is in a better position to notice subtle elements that may signify that change is in fact occurring—as when, for example, one becomes aware that one is observing a particular behavior that previously was perhaps carried out unconsciously, such as reflexively reaching for medication in response to the first onset of pain.

The practice of mindfulness encourages getting behind, or beyond, static linguistic concepts ordinarily used unconsciously to describe experience (Hayes, 1994). The unconscious, habitual, reflexive use of verbal descriptors of illness tends to foreclose the seeing of new possibilities for adaptation and accommodation, for growth and change. We speak, for example, of "having" a disease or a "disability", of "getting" treatment, of "suffering" pain, and "worrying" about a relapse or recurrence. Such expressions encompass a vast array of unexamined beliefs that tend to escape systematic observation, owing to our reliance on conceptual labels to talk about and explain our experiences to ourselves and to others. By inviting participants in the program to become more observant of the ebb and flow of their own beliefs and experiences, and to question the accuracy of their thoughts and self-statements about their conditions, both voiced and silent, they are encouraged to find ways to move beyond what are often emotionally laden concepts capable of triggering a range of distressing emotional or physical reactions commonly associated with spirals of relapse.

In summary, the phenomenon of "relapse" is addressed within the MBSR intervention in the following ways:

1. By emphasizing the novelty and freshness of each moment, including behavior patterns that may seem old and habitual (e.g., breathing, health attitudes and behaviors, self-statements, impulses to revert to old habits).
2. By going beyond labels commonly associated with relapse events, such

as "habit", "backsliding", "reversal", even the term "relapse" itself, and simply treating the experience as an opportunity for the application of focused attention.

3. By emphasizing the phasic, changing nature of phenomena and experience in such a way that a "relapse" is construed as an event occurring in a flow of many other events, and not as a repetition of anything. "Relapses" can be seen as events with novel and unique qualities which are themselves potent opportunities for growth and change.

Of crucial importance here is the "phasic", nonlinear model of the cyclic nature of human development and learning. Relapse is commonly viewed as a discontinuity in a linear process of change. However, growth and change are dynamic, nonlinear processes. Psychological and behavioral change always involves cycles of regression, restructuring, and reintegration. This cyclic progression, documented by Kornfield (1979) in a study of mindfulness meditation practitioners, suggests that periods of what from one vantage point might be termed "relapse" or "regression" actually are experienced by participants as personal growth when they use "not practicing" as an object of attention and nondiscursive inquiry. This takes place within the larger developmental cycle comprised of alternating periods of regression, restructuring, and reintegration.

In one intensive case-analysis study, eight participants in the stress reduction clinic were selected randomly from a group of 15 people who had enrolled in a particular class and who had agreed to be studied if selected, and whose identity as study participants was not known to their MBSR instructor. All had experienced relapse within the first month of program completion. One participant described the experience as follows: "I think I resorted back, I think I was afraid of this new person emerging. I think I wanted to slip back, you feel surer of yourself the way you were. It's more familiar." He reinitiated regular practice after a few weeks because, "I don't want to go back to that old place . . . it's scary . . . to have the realization that I can be in control of myself, that I can be responsible for myself." In this study, all eight participants reported reengagement in formal practice following the reemergence of the medical and psychological symptoms for which they were initially referred. While this is not the pattern for all participants who stop practicing for a time, as we have seen, the phenomenon of "relapse" may be one critical, even essential, phase in a far more complex learning process within MBSR furthering ongoing human development in (Santorelli, 1992).

SUMMARY AND CONCLUSIONS

The mindfulness-based stress reduction intervention implicitly and explicitly promotes adherence at multiple levels, through its structure, through its theoretical base, and above all, through the character and affect of the MBSR instructors and through the qualities and requirements of the meditation practice itself. In this chapter, we have addressed adherence to the MBSR program primarily in a middle-class population. Studies conducted in an inner-city MBSR clinic with a diverse, multicultural clientele characterized by pervasive high levels of economic poverty and social stress have shown that both outcomes and adherence to the MBSR program elements in this population are qualitatively similar to adherence in the middle-class population seen in the main clinic. However, there are strong and important quantitative differences in adherence which may be related to cultural and social factors.

In general, MBSR appears to be highly effective in minimizing, from the outset, those factors—enumerated at the opening of this chapter—that are most commonly related to nonadherence in behavioral interventions (i.e., insufficient knowledge; lack of conviction; aversive or excessive demand qualities; poor working relationship). More positively, the overall simplicity of the message, in essence, to practice paying attention and to be present with whatever arises in the field of experience, is easily remembered and explored in a variety of contexts, through both formal and informal mindfulness practices. The behavioral changes associated with MBSR are generally simple and direct. Emphasis is placed on becoming more reflective and less reactive, focusing more on "being" and less on "doing." This orientation is attractive in its simplicity, although the practice that it requires is both rigorous and arduous. MBSR skills can be practiced at many levels of comprehension and awareness, but all have in common the commitment to cultivate nonattachment regarding notions of "success" or "failure" or "goal attainment."

Breathing and just sitting quietly are within the capabilities of virtually all persons, despite the fact that internal associative mind states vary widely from one individual to the next. Such meditative practices can lead to experiences of well-being and self-efficacy well beyond those that most program participants have previously experienced. They represent the discovery of a new form of nourishment and growth that is accessible through a commitment to living life with intentional awareness and through a kind of "rotation in consciousness" that can accompany the ongoing discipline of mindfulness practice.

REFERENCES

Derogatis, L. R. SCL-90-R Manual II. Towsend, MD: *Clinical Psychiatric Research*, 1983.

Gunaratana, H. (1991). *Mindfulness in plain English*. Boston: Wisdom.

Hayes, S. C. (1987). A contextual approach to therapeutic change. In N. Jacobson

(Ed.), *Psychotherapists in clinical practice: Cognitive and behavioral perspectives* (pp. 327–387). New York: Guilford.

Hayes, S. C. (1994). Content, context, and the types of psychological acceptance. In S. C. Hayes, N. S. Jacobson, V. M. Follette, & M. J. Dougher (Eds.), *Acceptance and change: Content and context in psychotherapy* (pp. 13–32). Reno, NV: Context.

Kabat-Zinn, J. (1982). An out-patient program in Behavioral Medicine for chronic pain patients based on the practice of mindfulness meditation: Theoretical considerations and preliminary results. *General Hospital Psychiatry, 4*, 33–47.

Kabat-Zinn, J. (1990). *Full catastrophe living: Using the wisdom of your body and mind to face stress, pain, and illness*. New York: Delacorte.

Kabat-Zinn, J. (1993a). Mindfulness meditation: Health benefits of an ancient Buddhist practice. In D. Goleman, & J. Gurin (Eds)., *Mind/body medicine* (pp. 259–275). Yonkers, NY: Consumer Reports.

Kabat-Zinn, J. (1993b). Psychosocial factors in coronary heart disease: Their importance and management. In I. S. Ockene & J. Ockene (Eds.), *Prevention of coronary heart disease* (pp. 299–333). Boston: Little, Brown.

Kabat-Zinn, J. (1994a). Forword. In M. Lerner, *Choices in healing* (p. xvi). Cambridge, MA:MIT Press.

Kabat-Zinn, J. (1994b). *Wherever you go, There you are: Mindfulness meditation in everyday life*. New York: Hyperion.

Kabat-Zinn, J. (1997). *Indra's net: The Bulletin of the Mindfulness-Based Stress Reduction Network* Volume 2, Number 2. Worcester, MA: U Mass Medical Center, Center for Mindfulness in Medicine, Health Care and Society.

Kabat-Zinn, J., & Chapman-Waldrop, A. (1988) Compliance with an outpatient stress reduction program: Rates and predictors of completion. *Journal of Behavioral Medicine*, 11, *333–352.*

Kabat-Zinn, J., Chapman, A., & Salmon, P. (1997). *Relationship of cognitive and somatic components of anxiety to patient preference for alternative meditation techniques.*

Kabat-Zinn, J., Lipworth, L., & Burney, R. (1985). The clinical use of mindfulness meditation for the self-regulation of chronic pain. *Journal of Behavioral Medicine, 8*, 63–190.

Kabat-Zinn, J., Lipworth, L., Burney, R., & Sellers, W. (1986). Four-year follow-up of a meditation-based program for the self-regulation of chronic pain: Treatment outcomes and compliance. *Clinical Journal of Pain, 2*, 159–173.

Kabat-Zinn, J., Massion, A. O., Kristeller, J., Peterson, L. G., Fletcher, K., Pbert, L., Linderking, W., & Santorelli, S. F. (1992). Effectiveness of a meditation-based stress reduction program in the treatment of anxiety disorders. *American Journal of Psychiatry, 149, 936–943.*

Kabat-Zinn, J., Mumford, G., Levi-Alvares, D., Santorelli, S., & Skillings, A. (1993, March). *A mindfulness-meditation based stress reduction clinic for low-income inner city residents: outcomes and receptivity*. Poster presented at the 14th Annual Meeting of the Society of Behavioral Medicine, San Francisco.

Kabat-Zinn, J., Skillings, A., & Salmon, P. (1996). *The effect of Mindfulness-Based Stress Reduction training on personality measures in medical patients: Short and long-term observations*. Unpublished study.

Kornfield, J. (1979) Intensive insight meditation: A phenomenological study. *Journal of Transpersonal Psychology, 11*, 41–58.

Linehan, M. (1994). Acceptance and change: The central dialectic in psychotherapy. In S. C. Hayes, N. S. Jacobson, V. M. Follette, & M. J. Dougher (Eds.) *Acceptance and change: Content and context in psychotherapy* (pp. 73–86). Reno, NV: Context.

Marlatt, A. (1985). Cognitive assessment and intervention procedures for relapse prevention. In A. Marlatt & J. R. Gordon (Eds.), *Relapse prevention: Maintenance strategies in the treatment of addictive behaviors* (pp. 201–279). New York: Guilford.

Marlatt, A., & Gordon, J. R. (1985). (Eds.) *Relapse prevention: Maintenance strategies in the treatment of addictive behaviors*. New York: Guilford.

Meichenbaum, D. (1993). Changing conceptions of cognitive behavior modification: Retrospect and prospect. *Journal of Consulting and Clinical Psychology, 61*, 202–204.

Meichenbaum, D., & Turk, D. C. (1987). *Facilitating treatment adherence: A practitioner's guidebook*. New York: Plenum.

Miller, J., Fletcher, K., & Kabat-Zinn, J. (1995). Three-year follow-up and clinical implications of a mindfulness-based stress reduction intervention in the treatment of anxiety disorders. *General Hospital Psychiatry, 17*, 192–200.

Santorelli, S. F. (1992). A qualitative case analysis of mindfulness meditation training in an outpatient stress reduction clinic and its implications for self-knowledge. Kalamazoo, MI: University Microfilms International. Doctoral Dissertation.

Strecher, V. J., & Rosenstock, I. M. (1997). In K. Glanz, F. M. Lewis, & B. K. Rimer (Eds.) *Health behavior and health education: Theory, research, and practice* (2nd ed.) (pp. 41–@59). San Francisco: Jossey-Bass.

Teasdale, J. D., Segal, Z., & Williams, J. M. (1995). How does cognitive therapy prevent depressive relapse and how should attentional control (mindfulness) training help? *Behavior Research and Therapy, 1*, 25–39.

Thera, N. (1962). *The heart of Buddhist meditation*. New York: Weiser.

Toombs, S. K. (1993). *The meaning of illness: A phenomenological account of the different perspectives of physician and patient* (pp. 1–29). Dordrecht (Netherlands): Kluwer.

Tresolini, C. P. (Ed) (1994). *Health professions education and relationship-centered care*. San Francisco: Fetzer/Pew Health Professions Commission.

Wegner, D. M. (1994). *White bears and other unwanted thoughts: Suppression, obsession, and the psychology of mental control*. New York: Guilford.

SECTION III
Obstacles to Lifestyle Change and Adherence

Eleanor B. Schron, Editor

Many factors can inhibit people's ability to change behaviors and to maintain healthier behavior patterns. In this section of the book, the authors address potential biological, health provider, and contextual obstacles to successful health behavior change.

In Chapter 11, "Biological Obstacles to Adoption and Maintenance of Health-Promoting Behaviors," Grunberg and Klein describe a framework for the categorization of biological obstacles that affect adoption and maintenance of health-promoting behaviors: (1) unpleasant biological side effects; (2) physical or cognitive problems; (3) interference of healthful behaviors with enjoyable behaviors; (4) absence or misinterpretation of biological cues; (5) substance abuse; and (6) contribution of behavioral genetics as a biological obstacle. In describing each of these categories, formerly considered biological "barriers", the authors establish that biological obstacles exist and are important to compliance with and adherence to health-promoting and illness-preventing behavior. The authors use the term "obstacles" to signal their belief that the biological variables that dissuade individuals from complying with medical and health-promoting behaviors are surmountable.

In Chapter 12, "Improving Physicians' Implementation of Clinical Practice Guidelines," Dugan and Cohen address critically important issues regarding the role of practice guidelines in clinical care. Clinical practice guidelines synthesize research findings and opinions of experts to assist practitioners in the prevention, diagnosis, treatment, and management of clinical conditions. However, factors relating to physicians, clinical practice settings, and the clinical guidelines present challenges to the implementation of guidelines. These factors are explored within the context of the expanding number of guidelines in a changing healthcare system.

Altman and Jackson's focus in Chapter 13, "Adolescent Tobacco Use and the Social Context," is on how environment, policy, and interpersonal factors influence tobacco use; the authors offer suggestions for preventing adolescent tobacco use. They review topics in the regulatory and policy domains that have been or might be targets of public policy and legislation at local, state, or federal levels. The influence of family socialization on adolescent tobacco use is examined. Altman and Jackson maintain that nicotine addiction is an important factor in the development and maintenance of tobacco use. The authors present a convincing picture of how tobacco-related behavior and the setting in which such behavior occurs are interdependent factors. While much has been accomplished to slow the epidemic of tobacco-related disease, Altman and Jackson detail future research issues worthy of consideration.

11

Biological Obstacles to Adoption and Maintenance of Health-Promoting Behaviors

Neil E. Grunberg and Laura Cousino Klein

INTRODUCTION

Hippocrates wrote, "keep aware of the fact that patients often lie when they state that they have taken certain medicines" (Haynes, Taylor, & Sackett, 1979). Despite remarkable advances in modern medicine, Hippocrates' words still hold true. Today, only 33% of patients correctly follow their physicians' advice, 50% of appointments with physicians are canceled, 20–60% of patients stop taking their medicine too early, but 75% of patient-initiated appointments are kept. It is valuable to understand why patients fail to comply and how to overcome obstacles to compliance (Eraker, Kirscht, & Becker, 1984; Gerber & Nehemkis, 1986; Haynes, Taylor, & Sackett, 1979).

Biological obstacles to patient compliance received little attention before the 1990s. Grunberg and Lord (1990) first highlighted this category of variables and offered a framework for categorization of so-called biological

The opinions or assertions contained herein are the private ones of the authors and are not to be construed as official or reflecting the views of the Department of Defense or the Uniformed Services University of the Health Sciences. We thank Virginia Minich for her help with this chapter.

barriers. Since then, the topic of compliance has received increased attention and has become a part of some medical and healthcare curricula. With regard to biological variables, they continue to be important on their face and they are beginning to receive increased attention. A computer literature search of MEDLINE and *Psychological Abstracts* on "compliance" or "adherence" currently will list almost 2,000 reports in the last 5 years. Of these many reports, dozens now consider biologically relevant aspects of compliance. It is beyond the scope and not the purpose of this chapter to review all of the available studies that investigate variables that are biological or that include variables that affect biological processes. Instead, this chapter reexamines the topic first presented by Grunberg and Lord (1990) in light of these and related developments.

Much of the information discussed in 1990 regarding biological variables and compliance still holds true today and is reiterated in this chapter. There also has been some expansion of examples within the categories of biological factors and some addition of new categories. One of the marked and purposeful changes that we have made in this chapter is to rename biological "barriers" as biological "obstacles." We have made this change to signal our opinion that the biological variables that dissuade individuals from complying with medical and health-promoting behaviors are surmountable. Whereas barriers block or prevent access, obstacles are deterrents that can be negotiated or navigated, as in an obstacle course. We offer this new nomenclature for several reasons. First, the mere identification of these variables allows a delineation of courses of behavior to get by these deterrents. Second, compliance, in general, has received increased attention in medical curricula, continued medical education, and general publications (such as this volume and its first edition) that help focus attention on variables that can deter compliance and potential ways to surmount these deterrents. Third, we believe that marked technological advances in biological sciences, substantial expansion of interdisciplinary and multidisciplinary consideration of health issues, and incorporation of multilevel analyses in behavior and health have worked together to result in a renewed monism. Cartesian monism seems to have become a truism in the 1990s, and developments in biobehavioral measurements, brain imaging, neurosciences, and molecular biology all seem to work in concert to emphasize that this approach that considers psychological and biological information is now truly possible. In the context of the present chapter and present volume, biological variables are part of the psychobiological and environmental milieu that affects compliance, but we emphasize biological factors in order that they continue to be included in studies of compliance and how best to enhance compliance.

A FRAMEWORK FOR CATEGORIZATION OF BIOLOGICAL OBSTACLES

The biological obstacles that affect adoption and maintenance of health-promoting behaviors can be categorized into six major groups:

1. unpleasant biological side effects of healthful behaviors or therapeutic regimens;
2. physical or cognitive problems;
3. interference of healthful behaviors with enjoyable behaviors;
4. absence or misinterpretation of biological cues;
5. substance abuse; and
6. contribution of behavioral genetics as a biological obstacle.

Each major category is addressed in order.

Unpleasant Biological Side Effects of Healthful Behaviors or Therapeutic Regimens

When a healthful behavior is physically unpleasant, painful, or causes discomfort, people are less likely to adhere to the healthful behavior. This category includes unpleasant biological side effects of nonmedicinal treatments; prescription medications; nonprescription medications; drug interactions with alcohol; and drug-drug interactions.

Non-Medicinal Treatments

Rehabilitation medicine has expanded dramatically in the United States over the past 10 years, and the role of physical therapy in medical treatment has earned respect. Unfortunately, physical therapy has a variety of effects that can be considered to be unpleasant biological effects (or psychobiological actions) that deter compliance.

For example, consider an individual who was rear-ended in rush-hour traffic and suffered whiplash but minor apparent bruises. The patient now receives muscle relaxants, analgesics, and several months to several years of physical therapy. This therapy includes traction, muscular and neural electrical stimulation; heat and cold packs; specific exercise routines; deep muscle manipulation (euphemistically called "massage"); muscular ultrasound; stretching exercises; and spinal disc manipulation. Although this therapeutic adjunct to pharmacotherapy is valuable and effective, it hurts, and has effects that can be characterized as biological obstacles that may deter patients from compliance. Specifically, physical therapy can result in headaches, numbness, nausea, muscle aches, muscle fatigue, pain, sleep disturbances, and a cascade of other physical discomforts as physical therapy and manipulation has a domino effect on other, presumably uninjured, parts of the body. As with other aspects of compliance, predictability, identification of the cause of problems, understanding of the time course of duration of discomfort, and communication among the healthcare team of physician, other healthcare specialists, and patient, all are likely to encourage compliance.

In addition to physical therapy, there are other nonmedical treatments that result in discomfort and may act as biological obstacles to compliance with a particular treatment or lifestyle change. For example, surgeries that are not required for survival are, indeed, unpleasant and frightening episodes that we all would prefer to avoid. Even when we become convinced that the benefits of surgery outweigh the risks, we also become aware of the impact of surgery on our comfort and regular routines. When we know someone who has gone through a similar experience and who reports being bedridden for weeks or who reports the resultant pain and discomfort, we often can come up with lots of "good" reasons to put that procedure off just a bit longer. Communication from healthcare providers that is credible in reporting the unpleasant side effects, yet which presents a convincing rationale for the benefits of the procedure, can go a long way to surmount the biological obstacles. Perhaps healthcare providers who are faced with such obstacles that obstruct the best procedures should consider the value of adopting a convincing and concerned advocacy position, rather than an authoritarian posture or a seemingly disinterested presentation. Moreover, the involvement of supportive significant others may help negotiate the real biological obstacles that exist.

Even rather innocuous changes, such as exercise and healthful dietary changes, may result in discomfort for individuals and, thereby, act as biological obstacles. In these cases, anything that can be done to make the healthful behaviors accessible, positive, and rewarding would help. Enhancement of motivation is likely to help with compliance, particularly when the consequences may be uncomfortable.

Prescription Medications

Pharmaceutical houses certainly aim to develop and market drugs with the widest possible therapeutic range and the fewest and weakest unpleasant side effects. Unfortunately, many therapeutically effective and lifesaving drugs have unpleasant biological effects that deter people from taking their medicine. These side effects range from the mildly irritating to the almost debilitating.

Unpleasant biological effects of drugs that could interfere with adherence to drug-taking therapies become clear when one consults the *Physicians' Desk Reference* (1994) or reference books about pharmacotherapeutics (e.g.,

Hardman, Limbird, Molinoff, Ruddon, & Gilman, 1996; Melmon, Morrelli, Hoffman, & Nierenberg, 1992; Silverman & Simon, 1982). There are many unpleasant side effects associated with a variety of drugs. For example, tricyclic antidepressants can cause hallucinations, disorientation, delusions, anxiety, restlessness, excitement, numbness and tingling in the extremities, lack of coordination, muscle spasms or tremors, seizures, confusion, convulsions, dry mouth, blurred vision, constipation, inability to urinate, rash, itching, sensitivity to bright light or sunlight, retention of fluids, fever, allergy, nausea, vomiting, loss of appetite, stomach upset, diarrhea, agitation, sleep disturbances, nightmares, panic, peculiar taste in the mouth, stomach cramps, black coloration of the tongue, yellowing of the eyes or skin, perspiration, flushing, frequent urination, drowsiness, dizziness, weakness, headache, and loss of hair. A brief examination of this list reveals why a patient might not comply with this medication regimen.

Lifesaving antineoplastic drugs also can cause many unpleasant side effects that can interfere with a patient's willingness to undergo cancer chemotherapy. These effects include nausea and vomiting, peripheral neuropathies, cerebral blindness, loss of taste and hearing, and seizures (e.g., cisplatin or Platinol®); leukopenia, thrombocytopenia, anemia, anorexia, nausea, vomiting, and diarrhea (e.g., cyclophosphamide or Cytoxan®); pain, scarring, suppuration, alopecia, diarrhea, anorexia, nausea, vomiting, toxic granulation, eosinophilia, thrombocytopenia, and contact dermatitis (e.g., fluorouracil or Efudex®); hepatotoxicity, fibrosis, cirrhosis, fetal death and/or congenital anomalies, methotrexate-induced lung disease, anemia, leukopenia, thrombocytopenia, diarrhea, ulcerative stomatitis, nausea, vomiting and anorexia (e.g., Methotrexate®, formerly Amethopterin®). Consequently, there are obvious reasons why a patient might fail to completely follow a regimen of even a lifesaving drug.

Drugs taken to improve cardiovascular function can manifest a variety of unpleasant effects that may deter patients from adhering to their medication schedules. For example, digitalis administration may cause abdominal discomfort, pain, and headaches; hydralazine administration may cause headaches, angina, myalgia, arthralgia, or chest pain; methyldopa administration can cause diarrhea, blurred vision, dizziness, mental lassitude, impaired concentration, and nightmares; propranolol can cause insomnia or sexual impairment; and metoprolol administration can cause fatigue and dizziness. These biological side effects can become obstacles to adherence to and compliance with prescribed pharmaceutical regimens, especially in those individuals whose condition is asymptomatic (i.e., hypertension).

Anti-HIV medications, such as the synthetic nucleoside analogues AZT (azidothymidine, Retrovir®), ddC (zalcitabine, Hivid®), ddI (didanosine, Videx®), d4T (stavudine, Zerit®), and 3TC (lamivudine, Epivir®), slow the progression of HIV disease, but do not cure AIDS. Long-term use of several of these drugs (ddC, ddI, and d4T in particular) may result in debilitating peripheral neuropathies, severe pain, and general toxicity (Berger et al., 1993; Border & Arcane, 1990; Dubinsky, Arcane, Dalakas, & Border, 1989; Merigan, Skowron, & ddC Study Group, 1990). All of these effects can seriously interfere with patient compliance.

Non-Prescription Medications

The over-the-counter (OTC) pharmacopeia is becoming more and more impressive every day. This development helps keep prices down and helps to make medications more available, but often makes the medicines seem like nonmedicines and the condition seem like a nonmedical condition. These medications, including bronchodilators, cough suppressants, antihistamines, painkillers, mild sympathomimetics, and treatments for yeast and fungal infections, can act to mask biological symptoms that otherwise would motivate individuals to seek medical attention. This desirable effect of treatment, therefore, can have the paradoxical effect to deter the seeking of and adoption of health-promoting actions. Conversely, these medications, in some cases, can have side effects (e.g., gastrointestinal irritation, dermatologic irritation, sleep disturbances, tachycardia) that can be categorized as biological obstacles to compliance.

Drug Interactions With Alcohol

In addition to these nonprescription medications, alcohol must be considered as a nonprescription drug that can interact with other drugs and medications to cause untoward side effects. It is noteworthy that negative interactions can occur with the use, and not necessarily the abuse, of alcohol. For example, many drugs which otherwise have a wide therapeutic range with few side effects can cause serious problems when taken along with alcohol. Alcohol with antianginal drugs (e.g., nitroglycerin) results in hypertension, dizziness, and syncope; alcohol with anticoagulants (e.g., Coumadin®, dicumarol, Panwarfin®) alters the anticoagulant action depending on acute or chronic alcohol ingestion. Also, alcohol with antidiabetic drugs (e.g., Diabinese®, Dymelor®, Orinase®) results in unpredictable blood sugar, disulfiram-like reactions, and angina pectoris; alcohol with antihypertensives has an additive hypotensive effect; alcohol with antitubercular drugs (e.g., isoniazid, rifampin) decreases the therapeutic response and increases the likelihood of hepatotoxicity; alcohol with salicylates (e.g., aspirin) leads to gastrointestinal bleeding. Alcohol plus some antibiotics (e.g., cephalosporins, furazolidone) produces disulfiram-like reactions. Alcohol self-administration with benzodiazepines also can contribute to adverse side effects such as vomiting and nausea.

Drug-Drug Interactions

Drug-drug interactions (besides alcohol) also may be dangerous or unpleasant. Administration of OTC nonsteroidal anti-inflammatory drugs (NSAIDs) like ibuprofen (Advil®) with concomitant administration of certain antineoplastics (e.g., methotrexate) can cause unexpected, sometimes fatal, bone marrow suppression and gastrointestinal toxicity. Even simple antacids can potentiate the effects of anticholinergics, inhibit the actions of anticoagulants, and potentiate the effects of antihistamines, antimalarials, and bronchodialators (e.g., albuterol or Proventil®, beclomethasone dipropionate or Vanceril®). Nicotine (other than that derived from tobacco products) now is a prescription and OTC medication that can interact with other drugs. Nicotine is the active pharmacological agent in several smoking cessation aids (e.g., nicotine polacrilex gum, nicotine patch, nicotine nasal spray) and is being tested as a medical agent for the treatment of several disorders (e.g., Parkinson's Disease, Tourette's Syndrome, and Attention Deficit Disorder with and without Hyperactivity). Nicotine is a powerful sympathomimetic that affects catecholamines, indoleamines (including serotonin), sex hormones, pro-opiomelanocorticotrophin hormones (including the endogenous opioid peptides), insulin, and other neurochemicals and hormones. There can be drug-drug interactions between nicotine and other medications that can result in uncomfortable effects and affect compliance.

There are many other undesirable side effects of drugs. This list is meant to provide an illustrative, rather than a comprehensive, review of biological effects that are unpleasant enough to become obstacles to compliance and adherence, particularly when weighed against the salience to the individual of the benefits of the given drugs.

Physical or Cognitive Problems

Another category of biological obstacles to adherence and compliance involves problems or deficiencies in physical or biologically based cognitive abilities of patients. For example, deafness interferes with ability to hear and, therefore, understand oral instructions about prescribed health behaviors. It also may make a patient more reticent to ask questions of the healthcare provider. Impaired vision interferes with the processing of written instructions about prescribed health behaviors. Difficulties in visual acuity, myopia, and hyperopia all can act to make objectively clear written instructions inaccessible to a given patient. Color deficiencies in an individual patient also can interfere with the patient's ability to adhere to medication regimens that require taking different colored pills, on different days, or at different times of the day. These types of problems occur in the elderly and also in the general population.

Physical barriers to adherence and compliance also include a variety of allergies. For example, food allergies may interfere with nutrition; drug allergies may prevent the administration of effective pharmacologic agents; and contact dermatologic reactions may interfere with the use of some medications and some soaps, and may prevent safe sex practices. Respiratory allergic responses, such as extrinsic asthma or allergic rhinitis, can inhibit an individual from exercise activities, eating certain foods, and compliance with immunotherapy (e.g., allergy shots).

There also are biologically based cognitive impairments that interfere with adoption and maintenance of healthy behaviors. These impairments include mental retardation, senile dementias, Alzheimer's Disease, injury-induced cognitive impairments, HIV-induced cognitive impairments, AIDS dementia, drug-induced dementias, and attentional disorders.

Interference of Healthful Behaviors With Enjoyable Behaviors

Restrictive diets designed to improve cardiovascular function (e.g., low-cholesterol diet), to decrease the likelihood of cancer (e.g., high-fiber diet), or to help lose weight (e.g., avoidance of sweet, high-caloric foods) promote health (Grunberg, 1987) but are generally unenjoyable. Daily rituals (e.g., morning coffee, a high-fat or high-cholesterol breakfast) may have biological actions to which we adapt, come to need, and enjoy. Undoubtedly, we miss such daily pleasures when they become unavailable. Perhaps the enjoyment associated with specific foods, such as salty or sweet foods, involves a biologically driven hedonic preference to consume foodstuffs needed by the body (Cabanac, 1971; Richter, 1943; Young, 1936, 1955). In this context, it is interesting to note that cigarette smokers prefer and consume more sweets after cessation of smoking (Grunberg, 1985, 1986a). Anecdotal reports indicate that similar phenomena accompany abstinence from habitual use of alcohol or narcotics. It has been hypothesized that the enjoyment derived from eating specific foods taps similar biological processes involved in self-administration of some drugs of dependence (Grunberg & Klein, in press; Grunberg & Baum, 1985). Specifically, the unpleasantness associated with withdrawal from habitual drug use can be attenuated by the consumption of sweets and carbohydrates (Grunberg, 1986b; Grunberg & Baum, 1985). Whether or not this hypothesis linking drugs of dependence to food preferences is correct, it is clear that consumption of specific foods is enjoyable, that restricted diets are not, and that people often cheat on their diets.

In addition to eating, people enjoy drinking, smoking, and using "recreational" drugs. Consumption of alcohol, nicotine, marijuana, cocaine, ecstasy, herbal extracts, and psychotropic drugs is reportedly enjoyable. These drugs have various effects and become desired by the users. Even when the health messages for these substances are well-known (e.g., smoking is responsible for 400,000 deaths annually in the United States [Lynch & Bonnie, 1994]; drinking while driving can be lethal), individuals are motivated by the pleasurable effects of psychotropic drugs or by the discomfort of abstinence or withdrawal and, therefore, continue to self-administer rather than to adopt more healthful behaviors.

Safe-sex practices are another example of healthy behaviors that interfere with biologically based enjoyment. Sexual intercourse with condoms and abstinence from sexual intercourse are recommended to decrease the likelihood of transmission of HIV and sexually transmitted diseases (STDs). Safe-sex practices, however, decrease or prevent sensuality and pleasures of sexual intimacy. They also take time and planning which can interfere with intimate, arousing moments.

Medication schedules also can interfere with biologically based enjoyable behaviors. Some medications require administration during the night or during a sleep period. Other medications require administration either an hour before or 2 hours after a meal. These modifications or inconveniences place the health-promoting behavior against a biologically necessary state. In addition to medication-dosing schedules, some drugs are associated with behavioral restrictions that many people find annoying or inconvenient. For example, medications that are accompanied by the instruction "Do not operate a motor vehicle or other large equipment" can be a nuisance that interferes with pleasures and conveniences, or this instruction can interfere with one's livelihood. Instructions to avoid strenuous activities (e.g., physical activity, exercise, lifting, sexual activity) can interfere with jobs, hobbies, and general enjoyment.

In all of these cases, the interference of healthful behaviors with enjoyable behaviors is surmountable. However, the incompatible relationship of these behaviors and the intensity of the pleasures that are lost must be addressed by the healthcare provider and cannot be ignored. For example, most people agree that safe-sex practices are important. However, the decreased pleasure and inconveniences associated with abstinence or condom use may offset concerns about STDs or AIDS, especially when the likelihood of contracting these infections is viewed as minimal. In order to optimize adherence to healthful behaviors, the balance between biological and psychological aspects of the healthful behaviors with their impact on quality of life needs to be addressed.

Absence or Misinterpretation of Biological Cues

Another factor that may affect compliance and adherence, but that does not receive appropriate attention in the research literature, is patients' failure to experience or correctly interpret symptoms of underlying disorders. Basically, the patients feel fine and conclude that they are fine. As a result, they believe that they do not need bed rest, medications, restricted activities, or dietary changes. Premature discontinuation of therapy can be dangerous, however. For example, a patient typically feels better (e.g., no fever, weakness, pain, cough) before a course of antibiotic treatment is finished. Symptomless diseases, such as hypertension or organ rejection (e.g., heart transplant recipients), require treatments (e.g., medication, regular medical tests and check-ups, dietary changes, exercise) with effects that will not be felt by the patient. Preventive treatment for asthma with daily inhalation of nonsteroidal medications (e.g., cromolyn sodium or Intal®) and peak flow meter evaluation is not directly or immediately felt by the patient, and prevention efficacy is measured by decreased number of asthma attacks weeks later. In addition, misinterpretation of symptoms (e.g., "I get headaches whenever my blood pressure is high" or "I feel anxious right before I have an asthma attack") may lead to inappropriate self-dosing or inappropriate abstinence (e.g.," I don't have a headache, so I don't need to take my pills" or "My chest doesn't feel tight, so I don't need to take my inhaler").

A variant of this misinterpretation obstacle to healthy behavior compliance is when a person feels fine and, therefore, does not feel the need to do anything special to promote or improve health. For example, because the person feels fine he or she assumes that it is unnecessary to exercise, be careful about cholesterol intake, quit smoking, or avoid excess sun exposure.

Adherence and compliance also are reduced when a given healthful behavior has no noticeable positive effects that are obvious to the individual. For example: "I've been exercising for weeks, but I don't feel any better (in fact, I feel worse);" "I've given up smoking for 3 months now, but I don't feel better (in fact, I've gained weight);" "I've quit eating eggs and putting mayonnaise on my sandwiches, but I feel the same as I did before;" "I take my pills regularly, but I don't feel any different—I bet the doctor gave me sugar pills because he thinks I'm not sick or to stop me from bugging him;" "I've been getting allergy shots twice a week for over a year and I still sneeze around cats." These experiences and lack of awareness of bodily states, therapeutic effects, or preventive effects should be addressed and explained to patients.

Patient expectations about treatments and illnesses can be wrong. It is this expectation, however, that affects the confidence in a given healthful behavior, the credibility of a healthcare provider, and the likelihood of adhering to and complying with healthy behaviors.

Substance Abuse

Cigarette smoking is the single most preventable cause of premature death and illness (United States Department of Health and Human Services [USD-

HHS], 1988). The health message is clear: Do not smoke. Quitting smoking, however, is far more difficult than this simple health message leads us to believe. Use of tobacco products is an addictive behavior that involves powerful psychological and biological reinforcers. Consequently, asking habitual smokers to abstain from smoking requires the cessation of self-administration of an addictive pharmacological agent, namely nicotine. Smoking cessation results in irritability, irascibility, anxiety, sleep disturbances, inability to concentrate, and body weight gains (Grunberg & Bowen, 1985; Shiffman, 1979). These biologically based abstinence effects are powerful obstacles to adopting and maintaining a healthy lifestyle. In addition, abstinence means that the smoker no longer will receive effects of nicotine that are considered positive, such as decreased body weight, focused attention, and stress modulation.

Other abused substances, including alcohol, opiates, and sympathomimetics, similarly have biological effects that are reinforcing and abstinence effects that are unpleasant. Therefore, abstinence from use and abuse of these substances is hindered by biological obstacles, and it is important that healthcare providers and patients' significant others become aware of the consequences of abstinence.

Moreover, some substances (e.g., alcohol, some tranquilizers), when used in excess, reduce motivation or competence to comply with instructions involving other healthful behaviors. Prodding, coercion, scare tactics, and hinting are minimally effective in changing a dazed, addicted individual into someone who exercises, eats right, and takes medications on schedule.

Contribution of Behavioral Genetics as a Biological Obstacle

Since 1990, there has been a remarkable explosion in knowledge about genetics and an increased emphasis on the importance of genetic contributions to health conditions. This development is relevant to the present topic in several ways.

1. There are likely to be biologically-based individual differences in susceptibility to each of the effects that we have delineated throughout this chapter. For example, certain individuals are more likely to experience a given side effect of particular medications or in response to a behavioral treatment.
2. There are likely to be marked biologically based differences in the likelihood of developing pathophysiologic conditions, psychopathologic conditions, and biobehavioral conditions that can become obstacles to compliance. For example, certain individuals are more likely to develop obesity, senile dementias, mood disorders, or substance abuse. These biologically

based differences in the likelihood of developing a particular condition can differentially contribute to the role of the condition as a biological obstacle to compliance.

3. There are likely to be genetically based differences in the moderation or mediation of a given set of variables (e.g., a given medication, dietary regimen, or physical activity) on the development of an adverse side effect, not simply because of individual differences in effect, but because of individual differences in interaction.

4. There are ethical dilemmas that emerge as genetic mapping may allow prediction of probabilistic development of particular pathophysiologic conditions (e.g., cardiovascular disease, stroke, lung cancer, breast cancer, chronic obstructive lung disease, diabetes); biobehavioral conditions (e.g., obesity, anorexia nervosa, substance abuse, sleep disorders, AIDS); and psychopathologic conditions (e.g., depression, anxiety, obsessive-compulsive disorder, schizophrenia). For example, should we know what we are prone to get, as a way to help prevent the unwanted condition and to enhance compliance with preventive measures and treatments? Or does such knowledge give us excuses for developing these conditions and, thereby, act to deter compliance?

At this point, this information may sound like science fiction, but the rate of information acquisition makes it all worthy of serious consideration. We suspect that the next time we revise this chapter, this section will merit substantial space.

CONCLUSIONS AND RECOMMENDATIONS

Biological obstacles are important and must be considered to make headway to increase compliance with and adherence to healthful behaviors. Psychological and behavioral factors certainly are important in compliance, but they do not consider the entire spectrum of relevant variables. This chapter categorizes biological variables that can alter likelihood of compliance. We consider these variables as obstacles because they are identifiable and are potentially surmountable.

Many of the biological obstacles that we have discussed merit attention from the health care team, including the patient. The discomfort and pain cannot be erased, but their negative impact on compliance is likely to be decreased by identifying the effects; alerting patients; alerting significant others; offering choices to patients; providing predictability; and increasing control. In addition, it is possible that increased understanding by patients and healthcare providers of the role of biological obstacles to compliance can assist in the development of optimal strategies that minimize the deterrent effects of particular variables. At this point, we remain speculative, but optimistic, because little work has directly evaluated how best to minimize the effects of biological obstacles to compliance. Perhaps, the next version of this chapter will be able to report on the successes of strategies and interventions that address biological obstacles to compliance.

REFERENCES

Berger, A. R., Arezzo, J. C., Schaumberg, H. H., Skowron, G., Merigan, T., Bozette, S., Richman, D., & Soo, W. (1993). 2',3'-dideoxycytidine (ddC) toxic neuropathy: A study of 52 patients. *Neurology, 43*, 358–362.

Border, S., & Arcane, R. (1990). Dideoxycytidine: Current clinical experience and future prospects. *The American Journal of Medicine, 88*(5B), 31S–33S.

Cabanac, M. (1971). Physiological role of pleasure. *Science, 173*, 1103–1107.

Dubinsky, R. M., Arcane, R., Dalakas, M., & Border, S. (1989). Reversible axonal neuropathy from the treatment of AIDS and related disorders with 2',3'-dideoxycytidine (ddC). *Muscle & Nerve, 12*, 856–860.

Eraker, S. A., Kirscht, J. P., & Becker, M. H. (1984). Understanding and improving patient compliance. *Annals of Internal Medicine, 100*, 258–268.

Gerber, K. E., & Nehemkis, A. M. (1986). (Eds.). *Compliance: The dilemma of the chronically ill.* New York: Springer Publishing Company, Inc.

Grunberg, N. E. (1985). Nicotine, cigarette smoking, and body weight. *British Journal of Addiction, 80*, 369–377.

Grunberg, N. E. (1986a). Behavioral and biological factors in the relationship between tobacco use and body weight. In E. S. Katkin & S. B. Manuck (Eds.), *Advances in behavioral medicine* (volume 2, pp. 97–129). Greenwich, CT: JAI.

Grunberg, N. E. (1986b). Nicotine as a psychoactive drug: Appetite regulation. *Psychopharmacology Bulletin, 22*, 875–881.

Grunberg, N. E. (1987). Behavioral factors in preventive medicine and health promotion. In W. Gordon, A. Herd, & A. Baum (Eds.), *Perspectives on behavioral medicine* (Vol. 3, pp. 1–41). New York: Academic.

Grunberg, N. E., & Baum, A. (1985). Biological commonalities of stress and substance abuse. In S. Shiffman & T.A. Wills (Eds.), *Coping and substance abuse* (pp. 25–62). New York: Academic.

Grunberg, N. E., & Bowen, D. J. (1985). Coping with the sequelae of smoking cessation. *Journal of Cardiopulmonary Rehabilitation, 5*, 285–289.

Grunberg, N. E., & Klein, L. C. (1998). The relevance of stress and eating to the study of gender and drugs. *NIDA Research Monograph Series.*

Grunberg, N. E., & Lord, D. (1990). Biological barriers to adoption and maintenance of health-promoting behaviors. In S. A. Shumaker, E. B. Schron, & J. K. Ockene (Eds.), *The handbook of health behavior change* (pp. 221–230). New York: Springer Publishing Company.

Hardman, J. G., Limbird, L. E., Molinoff, P. B., Ruddon, R. W., & Gilman, A. G. (1996). (Eds.). *Goodman and Gilman's pharmacological basics of therapeutics* (9th ed.). New York: McGraw-Hill.

Haynes, R. B., Taylor, D. W., & Sackett, D. L. (1979). (Eds.). *Compliance in health care*. Baltimore, MD: Johns Hopkins University Press.

Lynch, B. S., & Bonnie, R. J. (1994). (Eds.). Growing up tabacco free: Preventing nicotine addiction in children and youths. Washington, DC: National Academy Press.

Melmon, K. L., Morrelli, H. F., Hoffman, B. B., & Nierenberg, D. W. (1992). (Eds.). *Melmon and Morrelli's clinical pharmacology: Basic principles in therapeutics* (3rd ed.). New York: McGraw-Hill.

Merigan, T. C., Skowron, G., & ddC Study Group of the AIDS Clinical Trials Group of the National Institute of Allergy and Infectious Diseases. (1990). Safety and tolerance of dideoxycytosine as a single agent. *The American Journal of Medicine, 88*(5B), 11S–15S.

Physicians' desk reference (48th ed.). (1994). Montvale, NJ: Medical Economics.

Richter, C. P. (1943). Total self regulatory functions in animals and human beings. *Harvey Lecture Series, 38*, 63–103.

Shiffman, S. M. (1979). The tobacco withdrawal syndrome. In N. A. Krasnegor (Ed.), *Cigarette smoking as a dependence process* (NIDA Research Monograph 23) (pp. 158–184). Rockville, MD: Department of Health, Education, & Welfare: Alcohol, Drug Abuse, & Mental Health Administration.

Silverman, H. M., & Simon, G. I. (1982). *The pill book* (2nd ed.). New York: Bantam.

U.S. Department of Health and Human Services. (1988). *The health consequences of smoking: Nicotine addiction. A report of the Surgeon General.* (DHHS Pub. No. (CDC)88-8406). Washington, DC: U.S. Government Printing Office.

Young, P. T. (1936). *Motivation of behavior*. New York: Wiley.

Young, P. T. (1955). The role of hedonic processes in motivation. In M. R. Jones (Ed.), *Nebraska symposium on motivation* (pp. 193–238). Lincoln: University of Nebraska Press.

12

Improving Physicians' Implementation of Clinical Practice Guidelines: Enhancing Primary Care Practice

Elizabeth Dugan and Stuart J. Cohen

The title of this chapter reflects two assumptions: first, that human behavior *can* change; second, that clinical practice guidelines may be used to enhance the quality of care provided to patients. Guidelines are systematically developed documents to facilitate practitioner and patient decisions about appropriate health-care for specific clinical conditions. Clinical guidelines attempt to synthesize the latest research findings and opinions of experts to assist practitioners in the prevention, diagnosis, treatment, and management of clinical conditions (Fantl et al., 1996). We believe that evidence-based guidelines can promote good medical practice and thus focus on methods of enhancing guideline implementation. Nevertheless, there is often a gap between recommended levels of care as specified in clinical practice guidelines and the actual delivery of care. This chapter addresses some of the reasons for these gaps and potential ways to reduce them. While practice guidelines exist for nearly every major illness and aspect of care, we have concentrated on guidelines associated with primary care practice.

We thank Ursula A. Poehling, B. A. for her assistance with the literature search.

A DISCREPANCY BETWEEN GUIDELINES AND PRACTICE

Evidence of the discrepancy between guidelines and practice abounds in the literature. Two striking examples concern smoking cessation counseling and the diagnosis and treatment of depression. In the first example, physicians strongly agreed with the concept of taking an active role in helping their patients to quit smoking, yet fewer than two-thirds of the clinicians had ever offered any counseling to their patients about smoking cessation (Cohen et al., 1987). The second example concerns the detection and treatment of depression. The rate of failure to diagnose depression by primary care providers is quite high, with estimates ranging from 60% to 80%. However when clinicians do diagnose and treat depression, they tend to prescribe medication at lower doses and for less time than recommended by guidelines (Brown, Shye, McFarland, 1995; German et al., 1987; Katon, von Korff, Lin, Bush, & Ormel, 1992; Perez-Stabel, Miranda, Munoz, & Ying, 1990). In both of these examples serious discrepancies exist between suggested and delivered care.

Several reasons account for this gap between practice and clinical guidelines. These can be classified in three areas relating to physician, clinical practice, and clinical guidelines. Physician issues include time constraints, a lack of knowledge, and the difficulty of objectively judging performance. Clinical practice factors include local constraints, the nature of medical care, and systems that are inefficient to identify guideline discrepancies and address them. Clinical guidelines themselves also contribute to the gap between practice and guidelines. The number of clinical practice guidelines published and distributed to physicians continues to increase annually. In 1992, the American Medical Association identified at least 1,300 practice guidelines from more than 50 organizations, which was nearly double the number of guidelines available in 1990 (Kibbe, Kaluzny, & McLaughlin, 1994). Unfortunately, many of these newly developed guidelines have not been disseminated in such a way as to alter the practice patterns of physicians (Wise & Billi, 1995). Both the content and format of guidelines can impact implementation. For instance, a strong research literature orientation instead of a practical clinical decision orientation (yes or no) limits its appeal to practitioners (Wise & Billi, 1995). Further, the range of values in guidelines also limits their impact, since guidelines tend to identify the thresholds of appropriate patient care, within which physicians and patients must still make discrete medical care decisions (Wise & Billi, 1995). Guidelines often seem to ignore the practical issues faced by practitioners and the clinical milieu in which the use of guidelines is embedded (Basinski, 1995). Before physicians view guidelines as precise tools to use in the construction of optimal patient care, they must be convinced that guidelines contain clear, evidence-based recommendations, and that there is a distinct advantage to them in changing practice styles to follow guidelines.

Reasons for the discrepancy between guidelines and practice concern attitudinal, contextual, and guideline issues which conspire to make optimal practice difficult to achieve at best. Fortunately, the gap can be narrowed, because these are surmountable obstacles. Considerable research has identified methods to increase physician behaviors that contribute to desirable health outcomes and to eliminate medical practices with no benefit or potential harm. Theory-derived interventions have been used to increase guideline implementation.

THE TRANSTHEORETICAL MODEL (TTM) FOR BEHAVIOR CHANGE

The key to improving physician implementation of clinical practice guidelines is to view it as behavior change, and to examine the amount and complexity of the change that is sought. For the most part, implementing clinical guidelines requires complex changes. Further, the amount of change required is often significant, especially if the interventions disrupt a familiar, albeit inefficient, system of care. We refer the reader to the excellent chapter in this volume contributed by Prochaska, Johnson, and Lee (Chapter 3) for an in-depth discussion of the Transtheoretical Model for Behavior Change. We have used the model as a basis for several intervention studies because of the rigorous conceptual and scientific work done to identify and develop the key constructs of the model, and the applicability of these concepts to clinical practice.

TTM suggests that change requires movement through discrete motivational stages over time, the active use of different processes of change at different stages, and the modification of cognitions, affect, and behaviors (Prochaska, 1995; Prochaska, Redding, Harlow, Rossi, & Velicer, 1994; Rossi et al., 1994). The Transtheoretical Model has a strong track record in studies of behavior change, ranging from smoking cessation, weight control, substance abuse, high-fat diets, exercise acquisition, high-risk sexual behavior, condom use, delinquent behavior, sun exposure, radon testing, mammography screening, and physicians practicing preventive medicine with smokers (Prochaska, 1994; Prochaska et al., 1994).

Stages of Change

The model describes the stages of change as a developmental sequence: precontemplation, contemplation, preparation, action, maintenance. Unlike other stage theories, however, progression through the stages is not necessarily linear (Prochaska et al., 1994). Those in the precontemplation stage are not seriously considering change within the next 6 months (for example, changing their system for monitoring and managing patients on oral anticoagulation therapy). Adults in the contemplation stage are seriously thinking about changing some behavior (e.g., quit smoking) within the next 6 months. The preparation stage pertains to people who are ready for action and are seriously planning to change within the next month. In this stage, people have already taken some steps toward action. Action involves overt modification of the behavior in question. Action is the busiest, most demanding stage in the model. Maintenance is the period that begins after about 6 months of continuous successful behavior change. Maintenance is a time of continued process use and relapse prevention.

Processes of Change

Progress from stage to stage is mediated by processes of change, which are overt and covert strategies used to modify behaviors. The processes of change include consciousness-raising, environmental reevaluation, self-reevaluation, social liberation, dramatic relief, helping relationship, self-liberation, counterconditioning, reinforcement management, and stimulus control. Use of experiential processes appears to peak in the contemplation and preparation stages, while behavioral process use peaks in the action stage (Rossi et al., 1994). However, it is important to note that no one process of change alone is going to produce significant change. Behavior change involves a series of interventions, processes, or techniques that accumulate over time to have an impact (Prochaska, 1995; Prochaska & DiClemente, 1983).

IMPEDIMENTS TO CHANGE

Despite the ample evidence that behavior change is possible, significant barriers to change exist. These impediments can range from contextual to personal characteristics. Individual attributes of clinicians and patients can impede guideline implementation. In addition, medical care is delivered in contexts which can influence practice patterns. The next section discusses obstacles to the improvement of clinical practice guideline implementation related to physician, context, and patient issues.

Physician Issues Limiting Implementation

Impediments at the physician level may include a lack of familiarity with guidelines, not knowing how to reach the levels of recommended care, or not being convinced that the guideline recommendations are worth implementing in a hectic practice setting. Anything which discourages thinking, planning, or initiating a change that improves guideline implementation is a hurdle to overcome. The literature suggests that barriers to patient counseling by physicians include a lack of counseling skills and the perceived ineffectiveness and lack of confidence in counseling (Lewis, Wells, & Ware, 1986; Marcus et al., 1995; Orleans, George, Houpt, & Brodie, 1985). A lack of training and familiarity with recommended behaviors (e.g., skills, procedures) also blocks implementation. Further, the amount of information with which physicians must cope may limit their effectiveness (Cohen, Weinberger, Hui, Tierney, & McDonald, 1985). One-fifth to one-half of primary care practitioners in the United States were found to be unaware or to not use new evidence about six common preventive procedures (Williamson, German, Weiss, Skinner, & Bowes, 1989). Moreover, the sheer enormity of the amount of new information and research findings published each year make it difficult for physicians to stay up to date. Much of what graduates learn in medical school is judged to be out of date within 10 years (Sherman & Davis, 1995). The failure of clinicians to acquire new knowledge appears to be a serious concern (Day, Norcini, & Webster, 1988). For example, Haynes, Ramsden, McKibbon, Walker, & Johnston (1991) reported that even with unlimited no-charge access in clinical settings, practitioners searched MEDLINE only about once a week, and even less when fees where imposed. However, some argue that the lack of compliance with preventive guidelines in primary care practice may actually reflect the priorities of the physician and saturated workloads rather than a lack of information (Karuza et al., 1995). Further, preventive activity factors, such as costs, risks, inaccessibility, and false-positive results also impact physician performance of preventive services (McPhee, Bird, Fordham, Rodnick, & Osborn, 1991). Physician factors, such as forgetfulness, lack of time or training, and confusion about conflicting and complex clinical recommendations diminish the effectiveness of guidelines. Clearly, the time constraints faced by practitioners limit guideline implementation. For example, a large health maintenance organization simplified the Agency for Health Care Policy and Research (AHCPR)'s *Guideline for the Treatment of Depression in Primary Care*, because "Primary care physicians have about two minutes to solve questions about how to treat depressed patients with drugs" (Brown et al., 1995, p. 6).

The gap between desired and delivered care is widened by the likelihood of physicians to overestimate their compliance with clinical guidelines (Cohen et al., 1985). Chart audits and patient surveys frequently indicate lower rates of physician compliance with guidelines than do physicians' self-reports (Giles et al., 1993; Glanz & Gilboy, 1992; Marcus et al., 1995; Neighbor, Scott, Schaad, MacDonald, & Van, 1991). Thus, physicians may not be motivated to change current behavior if they do not recognize that a discrepancy exists between current and desired practice.

Medical Practice Issues Limiting Implementation

Hurdles to overcome at the practice level include organizational system, time, and practice "chaos" issues. For instance, practice barriers to counseling by physicians to increase physical activity include lack of organizational support, little or no reimbursement, and limited availability of materials to aid both the patient and physician (Marcus et al., 1995). Clinical anecdotes indicate that whenever a clinic gets busy, health maintenance matters get overlooked or deferred (Tape & Campbell, 1993). Callahan and colleagues (1994) accurately described the reality of primary care practice, where patient visits typically are limited to 10–15 minutes, visits are separated by months rather than weeks, and where nearly every older patient has comorbidity. Major changes in personnel or business arrangements often preclude preventive care by contributing to a chaotic atmosphere in practices (Dietrich, Woodruff, & Carney, 1994). Healthcare system factors such as lack of reimbursement for recommended procedures, inconvenience, and scheduling difficulties all contribute to the gap between prevention guidelines and practice. The very nature of primary care contributes to this gap because clinicians are trained to deal with presenting symptoms (i.e., the primary task for an outpatient visit) which leaves little time for preventive care activities (i.e., secondary tasks) (Litzelman, Dittus, Miller, & Tierney, 1993). Local values and interests influence the acceptance of guidelines. A lack of trained personnel or limited access to necessary diagnostic equipment are two local constraints that can make guideline implementation difficult. For example, the availability of a flexible sigmoidoscope dramatically increased the compliance rate with recommended colorectal cancer screening procedures (Rodney, Quan, Johnson, & Beaber, 1982). Inefficient patient care systems can result from several causes, such as the failure to adjust established practice patterns to current changes in patient flow, administrative disorganization, or staff turnover.

Patient Issues Limiting Implementation

A variety of patient factors have been found to interfere with recommended cancer prevention activities, such as apathy or noncompliance, acute illness, anxiety, discomfort, or refusal (McPhee et al., 1991). Many physicians believe that their patients are not motivated to take suggested actions. For example, a survey of family physicians found that 77% of respondents believed patients lacked the motivation necessary to reduce intake of saturated fats, and 57% believed female patients were not motivated to practice breast self-examination (Henry, Ogle, & Snellman, 1987). Traditionally, physicians are trained to respond to patients' complaints. Unfortunately, patients rarely complain about diseases they do not yet have. Patients are not taught to actively seek preventive care and are not apt to say, "I don't have the flu. Do you think we ought to do something so I continue to not have the flu?" If patients appropriately requested such services, perhaps they would be more likely to receive them (Cohen, Halvorson, & Gosselink, 1994). Patients through their informed demands could be a new and strong force for preventive care (Hiss, 1986). Hampered by a lack of understanding of the basis for most medical decisions, and handicapped by unrealistic expectations of medical care, patients are rarely prepared to maximize time spent with the physician (Greenfield, Kaplan, & Ware, 1985). Most patients are aware of the time constraints of primary care and often prefer to focus attention on acute problems at the expense of important prevention activities. In addition, patients may be unwilling or unable to pay for procedures that are not covered by insurance.

REVIEWING EFFECTIVE INTERVENTIONS

Those who design effective interventions recognize that impediments to optimal performance can arise at multiple levels, and tailor their interventions to overcome the specific obstacles. Behavior change is a complex process. An individual physician might be at different stages of readiness for different behaviors. For example, a physician may be prepared to increase ordering of screening mammograms for age-eligible patients, but not even contemplating changing screening for colorectal cancer. Further, interventions that are designed to last over time need to be flexible enough to accommodate progression through stages. The appropriate change strategy might be a multistage approach that would expose individuals to a variety of strategies. One of the challenges for interventionists is to determine the most effective techniques for helping precontemplators to process information more clearly (consciousness-raising), to increase their emotional awareness of the problem (dramatic relief), and to increase their understanding of how their self-image is affected by change (self-reevaluation). For those in later stages, techniques need to be tested for reinforcing small steps towards desired behaviors (reinforcement management) (Prochaska, 1995).

The evidence is clear and suggests that academic outreach visits and the use of practice-wide system approaches are superior methods in effecting changes in physician behavior (Davis, Thomson, Oxman, & Haynes, 1995). The reason for their success is that they are able to facilitate multiple processes of change. An example integrating the two approaches to intervention is our current study: Project GUIDE. This study determines the impact of AHCPR Urinary Incontinence Clinical Practice Guideline adoption on primary care physicians and older adult patients. The intervention begins with an orientation workshop to educate the practice team about the problem, provide feedback on their current performance, and highlight the benefits of change (consciousness-raising, dramatic relief, environmental and self-reevaluation, self-liberation). At the conclusion of the workshop, each primary care practice team works out a detailed plan to implement the urinary incontinence guidelines in their practice and specifies who will be responsible for each aspect of implementation. Follow-up is provided by clinical faculty members who serve as "academic detailers" during the intervention period. The academic detailers can motivate physicians and help move precontemplation—contemplation—preparation stage persons in a single follow-up visit. A subsequent follow-up appointment helps the physician and practice team to restructure the healthcare environment to support change (stimulus control, reinforcement management, counterconditioning) and provide social support (helping relationship). Both approaches (e.g., academic detailing and an office-systems approach) involve a longer period of intervention and support, which help to sustain change and prevent relapse. The key to success is to shepherd the persons involved along the continuum of change, working in harmony with how people change naturally (Prochaska, 1995).

Changing Motivation: Moving From Precontemplation to Preparation

Movement from precontemplation to preparation involves a restructuring of thought processes about behavior and beliefs in self-efficacy. Interventions designed to change a physician's motivation to implement clinical practice guidelines are effective for progress from the precontemplation stage to the contemplation stage (see Figure 12.1). One example is the use of opinion leaders to prompt colleagues to begin thinking about making changes in practice styles. Processes of change such as consciousness-raising, dramatic relief, environmental reevaluation, self-reevaluation, and self-liberation facilitate movement through these early stages of change. Educational materials, conferences, feedback, and the use of local consensus are educational interventions that have been used to modify physician behavior.

Educational Materials

Educational materials include the distribution of published or printed recommendations for clinical care, audiovisual materials, and electronic or computer-produced publications. Clearly, physicians do not adopt new or improved practices as a natural consequence of their exposure to information. In fact, the mere distribution of printed materials has been found to

PRECONTEMPLATION	CONTEMPLATION	PREPARATION	ACTION	MAINTENANCE
Restructure Thought Processes in Self-Efficacy		*Change Thoughts About Behavior and Beliefs*	*Restructure Environment, Provide Social Support and Reward Desired Behavior*	
Use Interventions Designed To:				
	Change Motivation		**Initiate And Support Behavior Change**	
Consciousness Raising *provide information*				
			Counterconditioning *substitute new behavior*	
	Self-Reevaluation *benefits to physician*			
		Self-Liberation *belief that change is possible*		
Dramatic Relief *move emotionally*				
			Helping Relationships *social support*	
			Reinforcement Management *rewards, punishment*	
Environmental Reevaluation *benefits to others of physician's change*				
			Stimulus Control *rearrange environment*	

FIGURE 12.1 The Stages and Processes of Change

Adapted from "Why Do We Behave the Way We Do?", by J. O. Prochaska, 1995. *Canadian Journal of Cardiology, 11,* (Supp. A).; and "Strong and Weak Principles for Progressing from Precontemplation to Action on the Basis of Twelve Problem Behaviors," by J. O. Prochaska, 1994. *Health Psychology, 13.*

have little or no impact on physician behavior, often because physicians do not review the educational materials that are mailed to them (Anderson et al., 1994; Rabin et al., 1994). There are no magic formulas which will cause knowledge to jump off the page and into practice (Greer, 1988). Previous controlled studies of prescribing behavior have generally failed to support the efficacy of printed educational materials when used alone to improve medical decision making (Soumerai & Avorn, 1984; Soumerai, McLaughlin & Avorn, 1989). Similarly, Lomas and colleagues (1989) found that the dissemination of consensus statements was not effective in reducing repeat cesarean section procedures. However, when used as an early step in the process of change, educational materials can contribute to the restructuring of thought processes and improving motivation. Cohen et al. (1985) found modest effects of reading educational materials on physicians' adherence to recommended standards of care.

Conferences

Conferences typically require participation of healthcare providers in lectures, workshops, teleconferences, or traineeships outside their practice settings. Levinson and Roter (1993) reported that participation in a 2½ day workshop improved physicians' communication skills. The workshops employed role-playing, a small group format, and allowed participants to specify their personal learning objectives. Educational conferences may be effectively used to change physicians' motivations and restructure thoughts about behavior related to guideline implementation, especially when participants have the chance to view effective role models, practice the new behavior, and get feedback on their performance.

Audit and Feedback

Audit and feedback include any summary of clinical performance of health care over a specified period, with or without recommendations for clinical action. The information may have been obtained from medical record reviews, computerized databases, patients, or by observation. The identification of a discrepancy between what the practice is doing vis-a-vis what it should be doing can be an effective step in the adoption of recommended prevention services (Kaluzny et al., 1991). Meyer, van Kooten, Marsh, & Prochaska (1991) found that a computerized medical record system increased healthcare maintenance recommendations. Szczepura, Wilmot, Davies, & Fletcher (1994) reported that feedback was just as effective in changing practice behavior as was feedback in combination with a facilitator. Intensive screening and feedback of patient-specific treatment recommendation increased the recognition and treatment of late-life depression. In that study a practice-enabling, physician-targeted intervention improved compliance with recommended standards of care for late-life depression in primary care (Callahan et al., 1994). Monthly feedback with peer comparison improved some aspects of cervical screening (Buntinx et al., 1993). Feedback has been effective, especially personalized feedback provided by an opinion leader or respected person. Buntinx et al. (1993) reported that feedback in the form of written quality assessments plus monthly overviews and peer comparison, had a positive influence on the identification of endocervical cells in the smears submitted. Feedback may be effective in changing motivation through providing information designed to raise consciousness and provide dramatic relief.

Local Consensus

A somewhat different approach involves the local consensus process, where providers are included in discussions to ensure agreement that the chosen clinical problem is important and the approach to managing it appropriate. Karuza et al. (1995) found that the small-group consensus process was found to increase physician rates of influenza vaccinations. Interventions based on group dynamics and sensitive to local practice contexts can be useful in facilitating adoption of guidelines by physicians. The interaction involved in this process can be quite useful in restructuring the thought process via consciousness-raising, dramatic relief, environmental and self-reevaluation. Such group-consensus processes might be well-suited to the trend toward group practices and managed care.

Initiating and Supporting Change: Moving From Preparation to Maintenance

Following a restructuring of thought processes and beliefs about self-efficacy, the task becomes to intervene in such a way as to initiate and support change. The environment must be restructured, social support provided, and desired behavior rewarded. The processes of change that help movement from preparation to action to maintenance include counterconditioning, helping relationships, reinforcement management, and stimulus control. Interventions such as outreach visits, local opinion leaders, and chart reminders have been effective in helping to initiate and support behavior change.

Outreach Visits

A very effective intervention has been the use of outreach visits by a trained person (e.g., physician, pharmacist, nurse, or other professional) who provides information and ongoing support to clinicians in their practice setting. The information may consist of feedback on the provider's performance or topic-specific information. Academic detailing is highly effective because it can facilitate several processes of change, which help to guide physicians along entire the continuum of change. Avorn & Soumerai (1983) found that drug therapy decisions were improved via outreach, while no change was observed among physicians who were mailed educational materials. Soumerai et al. (1993) demonstrated that brief focused educational outreach visits by transfusion specialists substantially improved the appropriateness and cost-effectiveness of blood product use in surgery. Similarly Dietrich et al. (1992) found that assistance from a facilitator in the development of an office system consisting of flow sheets, external identifiers for patient charts, health education charts and brochures, and patient-held diaries were used effectively to improve the provision of cancer screening and prevention services. The educational strategy of opinion leaders doing "detailing" based on the guideline in this study (delivery after previous cesarean section) produced a significant impact on the practice patterns of physicians at community hospitals (Lomas et al., 1991). Opinion leaders with educational support generated community-wide change and improved compliance with the cesarean guideline. Targeted, professionally based, face-to-face educational outreach efforts have reduced unnecessary repeat cesarean sections and the use of contraindicated or expensive drugs (Avorn & Soumerai, 1983; Lomas et al., 1991; Soumerai et al., 1989).

Opinion Leaders

Within any group of physicians there are a few physicians who have significant influence on the behavior of their colleagues through interaction in the informal communication network (Stross, Hiss, Watts, Davis, & MacDonald, 1984). Local opinion leaders generally are identified by their colleagues to be "educationally influential" clinicians. Through the informal provision of information, opinion leaders can have an impact on their colleagues' practice patterns. Depending on their role in an intervention, an opinion leader could inform, move emotionally, and support behavior change in physicians trying to improve guideline implementation. Lomas et al. (1991) found that the use of opinion leaders resulted in a reduction in the rate of cesarean section births, while the use of feedback and audit resulted in no change. Educational-influential clinicians were found to positively influence the behavior of other primary care providers (e.g., the use of IV administered fluids, antibiotics, single agent bronchodilators, and respiratory therapy services) (Stross et al., 1984). Clinical champions were used as advocates of a guideline for the cost-effective care of hypertension (Aucott et al., 1996). Aucott and colleagues reported that the prescribing behavior of clinicians was modified, resulting in the increased use of guideline medications and decreased use of nonguideline medications. Brown et al. (1995) described the process by which a large HMO used local opinion leaders to help adapt AHCPR's depression guideline so that local providers would increase the diagnosis and treatment of depression. They suggested that the translation of science-oriented national guidelines by local opinion leaders into user-oriented documents tailored to local audiences can add great value to the guideline development process without sacrificing science-derived integrity (Brown et al., 1995).

Reminders

Another successful intervention strategy involves the use of reminders. Reminders entail any intervention, manual or computerized, that prompts the healthcare provider to perform a clinical action. Examples include concurrent or intervisit reminders to professionals about desired actions such as screening or other preventive services, enhanced laboratory reports or administrative support (e.g., follow-up appointment systems or stickers on charts). Tape and Campbell (1993) found that a computerized medical record system increased healthcare maintenance recommendations. Similarly, McPhee et al., (1991) reported that computerized reminders significantly increased physicians' performance of cancer prevention activities in community-based practices. Analogous findings were reported by Litzelman et al. (1993) who found that requiring physicians to respond to computer-generated reminders improved compliance with preventive care protocols. Velicer, Prochaska, & Bellis (1993) suggested that an expert computer system approach can provide a cost-effective, viable means of intervening for smoking cessation. Further, medical residents using a computerized medical record that included healthcare maintenance reminders were more likely to recommend preventive measures for their patients (Tape & Campbell, 1993). Reminders given to physicians during scheduled patient visits improved compliance with preventive care guidelines (Barnett & Winickoff, 1990; Litzelman et al., 1993; Tierney, Hui, & McDonald, 1986). However, Cowan, Heckerling and Parker (1992) found that fact-sheet reminders alone, without an enabling system or facilitator, failed to improve performance of periodic health examinations.

Multifaceted Interventions

Multifaceted interventions use a combination of techniques to modify physician behavior. Oxman, Thomson, Davis, and Haynes (1995) reviewed 102 studies and concluded that there are no "magic bullets" for improving the quality of health care, but that there are a wide range of interventions available, that, if used appropriately, could lead to important improvements in professional practice and patient outcomes. In general, studies that use multiple methods to intervene (e.g., outreach visits, education materials, and reminders) are the most effective in improving physician performance. Multifaceted interventions can overcome multiple barriers (motivational or environmental) to recommended levels of care.

Two recent examples of randomized controlled trials used a multifaceted approach to improve clinical practice concern cancer prevention and the prevention of sexually transmitted diseases. The first example, the Partners for Cancer Prevention study, used multistage interventions including support from a medical liability carrier, a motivational videotape, a task-delineated office manual, chart flowsheets, patient activation forms, practice feedback reports, a designated prevention coordinator within each practice, and regular telephone calls and office visits by project staff (see Cohen et al., 1994). The intervention strategies were designed to trigger a number of processes of change (Figure 12.2). The feedback reports about discrepancies between recommended levels of care and actual care were intended to raise consciousness. Project staff visited the practices to provide follow-up (dramatic relief and helping relationship). The malpractice-incentive and patient-initiated discussion served to spur the physicians to reevaluate the benefits of their change on others (environmental reevaluation). Self-reevaluation was prompted by the peer discussions at a project orientation workshop. Participants returned a letter of intent to participate in the project indicating that they believed that change in practice patterns was possible (self-liberation). Stimulus control was provided by flowsheets and patient health checks which were often attached to patient charts. Counterconditioning was achieved through integrating the practice-based intervention information and materials (e.g., flow sheets, patient health checks, education materials, office coordinator, and the orientation workshop) into the practice environment. Through deploying interventions to address both motivational and environmental issues they were able to significantly enhance cancer prevention in the primary care settings.

The second example sought to determine whether office-based interventions increased primary care physicians' risk assessment of and counseling practices for patients regarding sexually transmitted disease (STD) and the Human Immunodeficiency Virus (HIV). Rabin and colleagues (1994) compared physicians who were mailed educational materials, those who received the materials coupled with a simulated patient instructor office visit, and a control group. The educational materials were very comprehensive and consisted of cover letters from the Director of the National Institute for Allergy and Infectious Diseases and from the project directors; a taped example of physician assessment of sexual risk and risk reduction counseling; a monograph containing the most recent information on risk assessment and coun-

PRECONTEMPLATION	CONTEMPLATION	PREPARATION	ACTION	MAINTENANCE
Restructure Thought Processes		*Change Thoughts About Behavior and Beliefs in Self-Efficacy*	*Restructure Environment, Provide Social Support and Reward Desired Behavior*	
Consciousness raising *(provide information)* Feedback reports on baseline medical record review and patient surveys	**Self-reevaluation** *(benefits to physician of behavior change)* Video tape and peer discussion at orientation		**Stimulus control** *(rearrange environment)* Flow sheet, patient health check Education materials Office coordinator, orientation	
Dramatic relief *(move emotionally)* Follow-up with project staff, influentials on video		**Self-liberation** *(belief that change is possible)* Letter of intent Agree to medical record review		
Environmental reevaluation *(benefits to others of behavior change)* Patient-initiated discussion via patient health check and health tips malpractice insurance incentive			**Counterconditioning** *(substitute new behavior)* Flow sheet, patient health check Chart reminders	
			Helping relationship *(social support)* Continued contact with project staff	

Figure 12.2 Partners for cancer prevention.

Adapted from "Changing Physician Behavior to Improve Disease Prevention," by S. J. Cohen, H. W. Halrorson, & C. A. Gosselink. 1994. *Preventive Medicine, 23.*

seling to prevent STD/HIV infection; sample patient education materials; guidelines from the U.S. Preventive Services Task Force; a resource directory; and a wall chart on diagnosing and treating sexually transmitted diseases produced by the Centers for Disease Control. The role-played assessment of risks and counseling about STDs and HIV infection with a simulated patient-instructor lasted about 15 minutes, and the instructor then provided the clinician with feedback on the interaction from a patient's perspective. A letter reiterating the main points was mailed to the physician within three weeks of the visit. Consciousness was raised through the cover letters, monograph, and other educational materials (see Figure 12.3). Similarly, the reevaluation processes (self- and environmental reevaluation) were facilitated through the cover letters, monograph, resource directory, and patient education materials. Self-liberation, or the belief that change is possible, was prompted through the examples of desired clinical behavior (audiotape, wall chart). The simulated patient visit and feedback on physician performance facilitated a number of processes of change: counterconditioning, helping relationship, and reinforcement management. They reported that the multifaceted approach significantly increased the frequency of physicians' risk assessment and risk reduction counseling for sexually transmitted diseases and HIV infection.

Despite the success of these and other examples, a 10-year review of the literature on CME indicated that the more effective methods, such as systemic practice-based interventions and outreach visits, are rarely used by CME providers (Davis et al., 1995).

Many interventions have modest or negligible practical effects in altering health professional performance when used alone. However, when coupled with other strategies, the effects may be cumulative and significant. There is a need in the area of health professional performance to include appropriate diagnostic strategies to determine reasons for suboptimal performance, to identify barriers to change, and to carefully select the interventions most likely to be effective in light of the diagnosed problem.

CONCLUSIONS

A result of the trend toward managed care and the growing desire to reduce the variability of care delivery is an increase in both the number and importance of clinical practice guidelines. In general, guidelines are useful tools that may be used to enhance patient care. Discrepancies between recommended levels of care and actual practice exist for a variety of reasons. Multifaceted interventions to narrow the gap between guidelines and practice are generally most effective, especially if the interventions consider the amount and complexity of change, and target all persons involved in the

PRECONTEMPLATION	CONTEMPLATION	PREPARATION	ACTION	MAINTENANCE
Restructure Thought Processes	Change Thoughts About Behavior and Beliefs in Self-Efficacy		Restructure Environment, Provide Social Support and Reward Desired Behavior	
Raise Consciousness *(Provide information)* Cover letter Monograph Educational materials	**Dramatic Relief** *(Move emotionally)* Simulated patient visit	**Self-Liberation** *(Belief that change is possible)* Audiotape CDC wall chart		
	Environmental Reevaluation *(Benefits to others of changed behavior)* Cover letter Monograph Educational materials		**Counterconditioning** *(Substitute new behavior)* Simulated patient visit and feedback	
	Self-Reevaluation *(Benefits to self of behavior change)* Cover letter Monograph Educational materials		**Helping Relationship** *(Social support)* Simulated patient visit and feedback	
			Reinforcement Management *(Rewards, punishment)* Verbal feedback on performance Written feedback on performance	

Figure 12.3 Sexually transmitted disease prevention practices.

Adapted from "Improving Office Based Physicians' Preventions Practices for Sexually Transmitted Disease," by D. J. Rabin, B. O. Bockeloo, E. S. Marx, M. A. Bowman, N. K. Russell, & A. Willis, 1994, *Annals of Internal Medicine, 121*.

delivery of care. However such interventions tend to be of a longer duration, more complex, and expensive than typical CME activities. Moreover, guidelines may continue to be ignored, or perceived as an irritant and threat to physician autonomy unless implementation strategies and benefits are clearly explicated (Kaluzny et al., 1995). In addition, if those who develop and publish guidelines are serious about elevating the standard of care, they must produce guidelines that are relevant to the real-life situations of busy physicians.

As our health care system continues to undergo change, guideline implementation may become more challenging and more promising. The trend toward evidence-based medicine should result in an expansion of guidelines. The availability of point-of-service computerized patient record systems will have the potential to provide important patient-tailored reminders, reduce drug-drug interactions, and readily link distant subspecialty expertise. The trend toward managed care and capitation may result in the availability of new resources, such as disease case managers who are directed to improving care without diminishing the role of the primary care provider. While the principles of behavior modification will not change, interventions to improve care will need to evolve and adapt to meet the challenges of the future.

REFERENCES

Anderson, F. A., Wheeler, H. B., Goldberg, R. J., Hosmer, D. W., Forcier, A., & Patwardhan, N. A. (1994). Changing clinical practice: Prospective study of the impact of continuing medical education and quality assurance programs on use of prophylaxis for venous thromboembolism. *Archives of Internal Medicine, 154*, 669–677.

Aucott, J. N., Pelecanos, E., Dombrowski, R., Fuehrer, S. M., Laich, J., & Aron, D. C. (1996). Implementation of local guidelines for cost-effective management of hypertension. *Journal of General Internal Medicine, 11*, 139–146.

Avorn, J., & Soumerai, S. B. (1983). Improving drug-therapy decisions through educational outreach: A randomized controlled trial of academically based "detailing". *The New England Journal of Medicine, 308*, 1457–1463.

Barnett, G. O., & Winickoff, R. N. (1990). Quality assurance and computer-based patient records. *American Journal of Public Health, 80*, 527–528.

Basinski, A. S. (1995). Evaluation of clinical practice guidelines. *Canadian Medical Association, 153*,1575–1581.

Brown, J. B., Shye, D., & McFarland, B. (1995). The paradox of guideline implementation: How AHCPR's depression guideline was adapted at Kaiser Permanente Northwest Region. *Journal on Quality Improvement, 21*, 5–21.

Buntinx, F., Knottnerus, J. A., Crebolder, H. F., Seeger, T., Essed, G. G., & Schouten, H. (1993). Does feedback improve the quality of cervical smears? A randomized controlled trial. *British Journal of General Practice, 43*, 194–198.

Callahan, C. M., Hendrie, H. C., Dittus, R. S., Brater, D. C., Hui, S. L., & Tierney,

W. M. (1994). Improving treatment of late life depression in primary care: A randomized clinical trial. *Journal of American Geriatric Society, 42*, 839–846.

Cohen, S. J., Christen, A. G., Katz, B. P., Drook, C. A., Davis, B. J., Smith, D. M., & Stookey, G. K. (1987). Counseling medical and dental patients about cigarette smoking: The impact of nicotine gum and chart reminders. *American Journal of Public Health, 77*, 313–316.

Cohen, S. J., Halvorson, H. W., & Gosselink, C. A. (1994). Changing physician behavior to improve disease prevention. *Preventive Medicine, 23*, 284–291.

Cohen, S. J., Weinberger, M., Hui, S. L., Tierney, W. M., & McDonald, C. J. (1985). The impact of reading on physicians' non-adherence to recommended standards of medical care. *Social Science Medicine, 21*, 909–914.

Cowan, J. A., Heckerling, P. S., & Parker, J. B. (1992). Effect of a fact sheet reminder on performance of the periodic health examination: A randomized controlled trial. *American Journal of Preventive Medicine, 8*, 104–109.

Davis, D. A., Thomson, M. A., Oxman, A. D., & Haynes, R. B. (1995). Changing physician performance: A systematic review of the effect of continuing medical education strategies. *Journal of the American Medical Association, 274*, 700–705.

Day, S. C., Norcini, J. J., & Webster, G. D. (1988). The effects of changes in medical knowledge on examination performance at the time of recertification. In D. S. Dabney (Ed.), *Proceedings of the Twenty-Seventh Annual Conference on Research in Medical Education*, (pp 139–144). Washington, DC: Association of American Medical Colleges.

Dietrich, A. J., Woodruff, C. B., & Carney, P. A. (1994). Changing office routines to enhance preventive care: The preventive GAPS approach. *Archives of Family Medicine, 3*, 176–183.

Dietrich, A. J., O'Connor, G. T., Keller, A., Carney, P. A., Levy, D., & Whaley, F. S. (1992). Cancer: Improving early detection and prevention. A community practice randomized trial. *British Medical Journal, 304*, 687–690.

Fantl, J. A., Newman, D. K., Colling, J., et al. *Urinary incontinence in adults: Acute and chronic management.* (Clinical Practice Guideline, No. 2, 1996 Update). (AHCPR Publication No. 96-0682). Rockville, MD: U.S. Department of Health and Human Services. Public Health Service, Agency for Health Care Policy and Research.

German, P. S., Shapiro, S., Skinner, E. A., Von Koff, M., Klein, L. E., Turner, R. W., Teitelbaum, M. L., Burke, J., & Burns, B. J. (1987). Detection and management of mental health problems of older patients by primary care providers. *Journal of the American Medical Association, 257*, 489–493.

Giles, W. H., Anda, R. F., Jones, D. H., Serdula, M. K., Merritt, R. K., & Destefano, F. (1993). Recent trends in identification and treatment of high blood cholesterol by physicians: Progress and missed opportunities. *Journal of the American Medical Association, 269*, 1133–1138.

Glanz, K., & Gilboy, M. B. (1992). Physicians, preventive care, and applied nutrition: Selected literature. *Academic Medicine, 67*, 776–781.

Greenfield, S., Kaplan, S., & Ware, J. E. (1985). Expanding patient involvement in care: Effects on patient outcomes. *Annals of Internal Medicine, 10*, 520–528.

Greer, A. (1988). The state of the are versus the state of the science. *International*

Journal of Technology Assessment in Health Care, 4, 5–26.

Haynes, R. B., Ramsden, M. F., McKibbon, K. A., Walker, C. J., & Johnston, M. (1991). Online access to MEDLINE in clinical settings: Impact of introducing user fees. *Bulletin of the Medical Library Association, 79*, 377–381.

Henry, R. C., Ogle, K. S., & Snellman, L. A. (1987). Preventive medicine: Physician practices, beliefs, and perceived barriers for implementation. *Family Medicine, 19*, 110–113.

Hiss, R. G. (1986). The activated patient: A force for change in diabetes health care and education. *The Diabetes Educator, 12*, 225–231.

Kaluzny, A. D., Harris, R. P., Strecher, V. J., Stearns, S., Qaquish, B., & Leininger, L. (1991). Prevention and early detection activities in primary care: New directions for implementation. *Cancer Detection and Prevention, 15*, 459–464.

Kaluzny, A. D., Konrad, T. R., & McLaughlin, C. P. (1995). Organizational strategies for implementing clinical guidelines. *Journal on Quality Improvement, 21*, 347–351.

Karuza, J., Calkins, E., Feather, J., Hershey, C. O., Katz, L., & Majeroni, B. (1995). Enhancing physician adoption of practice guidelines: Dissemination of influenza vaccination guideline using a small-group consensus process. *Archives of Internal Medicine, 155*, 625–632.

Katon, W., von Korff, M., Lin, E., Bush, T., & Ormel, J. (1992). Adequacy and duration of antidepressant treatment in primary care. *Medical Care, 30*, 67–76.

Kibbe, D. C., Kaluzny, A. D., & McLaughlin, C. P. (1994). Integrating guidelines with continuous quality improvement: Doing the right thing the right way to achieve the right goals. *Journal on Quality Improvement, 20*, 181–191.

Levinson, W., & Roter, D. (1993). The effects of two continuing medical education programs on communication skills of practicing primary care physicians. *Journal of General Internal Medicine, 8*, 318–324.

Lewis, C. E., Wells, K. B., & Ware J. (1986). A model for predicting the counseling practices of physicians. *Journal of General Internal Medicine, 1*, 14–19.

Litzelman, D. K., Dittus, R. S., Miller, M. E., & Tierney, W. M. (1993). Requiring physicians to respond to computerized reminders improves their compliance with preventive care protocols. *Journal of General Internal Medicine, 8*, 311–317.

Lomas, J., Anderson, G. M., Domnick-Pierre, K., Vayda, E., Enkin, M. W., & Hannah, W. J. (1989). Do practice guidelines guide practice? The effects of a consensus statement on the practice of physicians. *New England Journal of Medicine, 321*, 1306–1311.

Lomas, J., Enkin, M., Anderson, G. M., Hannah, W. J., Vayda, E., & Singer, J. (1991). Opinion leaders vs. audit and feedback, to implement practice guidelines. *Journal of the American Medical Association, 265*, 2202–2207.

Marcus, B. H., Pinto, B. M., Clark, M. M., DePue, J. D., Goldstein, M. G., & Silverman, L. S. (1995). Physician-delivered physical activity and nutrition interventions. *Medicine, Exercise, Nutrition, and Health, 4*, 325–334.

McPhee, S. J., Adair Bird, J., Fordham, D., Rodnick, J. E., &Osborn, E. H. (1991). Promoting cancer prevention activities by primary care physicians. *Journal of the American Medical Association, 266*, 539–544.

Meyer, T. J., Van Kooten, D., Marsh, S., & Prochaska, A. V. (1991). Reduction of polypharmacy by feedback to clinicians. *Journal of General Internal Medicine,*

6, 133–136.

Neighbor, W. J., Scott, C. S., Schaad, D. C., MacDonald, S. C., & Van, C. R. (1991). Assessment and counseling of coronary risk factors by family practice residents. *Journal of Family Practice, 32*, 273–281.

Orleans, C. T., George, L. K., Houpt, J. L., & Brodie, K. H. (1985). Health promotion in primary care: A survey of U.S. family practitioners. *Preventive Medicine, 14*, 636–647.

Oxman, A. D., Thomson, M. A., Davis, D. A., & Haynes, R. B. (1995). No magic bullets: A systematic review of 102 trials of interventions to improve professional practice. *Canadian Medical Association Journal, 153*, 1423–1431.

Perez-Stabel, E. J., Miranda, J. Munoz, R.F. & Ying, Y.W.. (1990). Depression in medical outpatients: Under-recognition and misdiagnosis. *Archives of Internal Medicine, 50*, 1083–1088.

Prochaska, J. O. (1994). Strong and weak principles for progressing from precontemplation to action on the basis of twelve problem behaviors. *Health Psychology, 13*, 47–51.

Prochaska, J. O. (1995). Why do we behave the way we do? *Canadian Journal of Cardiology, 11 (Supplement A)*, 20A–25A.

Prochaska, J. O., & DiClemente, C. C. (1983). Stages and processes of self-change of smoking: Toward an integrative model of change. *Journal of Consulting and Clinical Psychology, 51*, 390–395.

Prochaska, J. O., Johnson, S., & Lee, P. (1998). The transtheoretical model of behavior change. In S. A. Shumaker, E. Schron, J. Ockene, & W. L. McBee (Eds.), *The handbook of health behavior change*, (2nd ed.). New York: Springer Publishing Company.

Prochaska, J. O., Redding, C. A., Harlow, L. L., Rossi, J. S., & Velicer, W. F. (1994). The transtheoretical model of change and HIV prevention: A review. *Health Education Quarterly, 21*, 471–486.

Prochaska, J. O., Velicer, W. F., Rossi, J. S., Goldstein, M. G., Marcus, B. H., Rakowski, W., Fiore, C., Harlow, L. L., Redding, C. A., Rosenbloom, D., & Rossi, S. R. (1994). Stages of change and decisional balance for 12 problem behaviors. *Health Psychology, 13*, 39–46.

Rabin, D. L., Boekeloo, B. O., Marx, E. S., Bowman, M. A., Russell, N. K., & Willis, A. G. (1994). Improving office-based physicians' prevention practices for sexually transmitted diseases. *Annals of Internal Medicine, 121*, 513–519.

Rodney, W. M., Quan, M. A., Johnson, R. A., & Beaber, R. J. (1982). Impact of flexible sigmoidoscopy on physician compliance on colorectal cancer screening protocol. *Journal of Family Practice, 15*, 885–889.

Rossi, S. R., Rossi, J. S., Rossi-DelPrete, L. M., Prochaska, J. O., Banspach, S. W., & Carelton, R. A. (1994). A process of change model for weight control for participants in community-based weight loss programs. *The International Journal of Addictions, 29*, 161–177.

Sherman, C. D., & Davis, D. A. (1995). CME in oncology: From where we were to where we are going. *Journal of Cancer Education, 10*, 131–136.

Soumerai, S. B., & Avorn, J. L., (1984). Efficacy and cost-containment in hospital pharmacotherapy: State of the art and future. *Milbank Quarterly, 62*, 447–474.

Soumerai, S. B., McLaughlin, T. J., & Avorn, J. (1989). Improving drug prescribing in primary care: A critical analysis of the experimental literature. *Milbank Quarterly, 67*, 268–317.

Soumerai, S. B., Salem-Schatz, S., Avorn, J., Casteris, C. S., Ross-Degnan, D., & Popovsky, M. A. (1993). A controlled trial of educational outreach to improve blood transfusion practice. *Journal of the American Medical Association, 270*, 961–966.

Stross, J. K., Hiss, R. G., Watts, C. M., Davis, W. K., & MacDonald, R. (1984). Continuing education in pulmonary disease for primary-care physicians. *American Review of Respiratory Disease, 127*, 739–746.

Szczepura, A., Wilmot, J., Davies, C., & Fletcher, J. (1994). Effectiveness and cost of different strategies for information feedback in general practice. *British Journal of General Practice, 43*, 19–24.

Tape, T. G., & Campbell, J. R. (1993). Computerized medical records and preventive health care: Success depends on many factors. *The American Journal of Medicine, 94*, 619–625.

Tierney, W. M., Hui, S. L., & McDonald, C. J. (1986). Delayed feedback of physician performance versus immediate reminders to perform preventive care: Effects on physician compliance. *Medical Care, 24*, 659–666.

Velicer, W. F., Prochaska, J. O., & Bellis, J. M. (1993). An expert system intervention for smoking cessation. *Addictive Behavior, 18*, 269–290.

Williamson, J. W., German, P. S., Weiss, R., Skinner, E. A., & Bowes, F. (1989). Health science information management and continuing education of physicians: A survey of U. S. primary care practitioners and their opinion leaders. *American Internal Medicine, 110*, 151–160.

Wise, C. G, & Billi, J. E. (1995). A model for practice guideline adaptation and implementation: Empowerment of the physician. *Journal on Quality Improvement, 21*, 465–476.

13

Adolescent Tobacco Use and the Social Context

David G. Altman and Christine Jackson

INTRODUCTION

Since publication of the 1964 Surgeon General's Report on Smoking and Health, much has been learned about factors that influence the initiation, maintenance, and cessation of smoking. Thirty years after the landmark Surgeon General's Report (U.S. Public Health Service, 1964), there are numerous achievements to cite and pressing challenges yet to overcome. The overall downward trend in adult tobacco use rates in the United States from the 1960s to the 1990s is one of the most important public health accomplishments of this century, although this decrease has slowed in the last few years. Of great concern, however, is that about one-quarter of the U.S. population uses tobacco regularly. Among adolescents, the smoking rate remained flat through the decade of the 1980s, and began to increase in the 1990s. Moreover, tobacco companies remain highly profitable, allowing them to generously fund marketing campaigns to attract new tobacco users and to expand their reach into foreign countries.

The failure to prevent young people from using tobacco raises questions about the efficacy of our intervention approaches. Indeed, our primary response to the problem of adolescent tobacco use has been to deliver school-based prevention programs. Data from evaluations of the current programs suggest that their effects are generally modest in the short-term and uncertain in the long-term (Cleary, Hitchcock, Semmer, Flinchbaugh & Pinney, 1988; Flay, 1985; Glynn, 1989; Rooney & Murray, 1996; U.S. Department of Health and Human Services, 1994). A notable exception is a 6-year longitudinal evaluation of a school-based program in 56 schools that presented the first encouraging news about the long-term efficacy of a model school-based interevention. In this study, the investigators found that smoking rates were 15–25% lower in the intervention group (Botvin, Baker, Dusenbury, Botvin, & Diaz, 1995). Unfortunately, such high quality programs have limited national dissemination. More commonly, schools around the country implement untested or ineffective programs.

The discrepancies between pro-health concepts taught in school-based prevention programs and the pro-smoking messages that youth observe and experience first-hand in their communities contribute to the problem of adolescent tobacco use. For example, in a typical classroom-based program, students are taught how to resist social pressures to smoke. Yet, in the community, these messages in schools are strongly countered by pro-tobacco messages. Adolescents observe an abundant supply of tobacco, a willingness on the part of merchants to sell them tobacco, lack of enforcement of tobacco-related laws, little evidence that the community views teenage tobacco use as a problem, and pervasive tobacco marketing promising independence, romance, and recreation to those who use tobacco. Peer pressure to use tobacco can succeed only if the substances around which pressure is exerted (in this case, tobacco) are available, affordable, and perceived positively. Easy access to cigarettes by minors, low tax rates (and therefore relatively less expensive tobacco), and tobacco marketing may increase the opportunities and motives for young people to use tobacco, and may enhance their ability to serve as influences on others. Thus, preventing adolescent tobacco use is not simply a matter of equipping individuals with peer-pressure resistance skills. While imparting resistance skills is an important component to a comprehensive intervention, neglecting factors that influence peer pressure is a strategic error and is an example of focusing on a mediating rather than an antecedent cause of the problem.

AN ECOLOGICAL APPROACH TO TOBACCO CONTROL

Adolescent tobacco use is a complex behavior, rooted in biological, social, environmental, historical, and cultural contexts. To adequately understand it, one must account for how it is influenced at multiple levels of analyses. This chapter focuses on how environmental, policy, and interpersonal factors influence tobacco use and offers suggestions for preventing adolescent tobacco use. Although physiological factors in the initiation and maintenance of tobacco use are beyond the scope of this chapter, we subscribe to the perspective that nicotine addiction is an important factor in the development and maintenance of tobacco use (Food and Drug Administration, 1995; Lynch & Bonnie, 1994; U.S. Department of Health and Human Services, 1988; U.S. Department of Health and Human Services, 1989).

Our approach is influenced by ecological and systems theories. These theories view behavior as a function of the surrounding context. Articulation of an ecological approach has been provided by others writing in diverse disciplines (Binder, Stokols, & Catalano, 1975; Bronfenbrenner, 1977; Kelly, 1966, 1968, 1971, 1988; Lewin, 1951; McLeroy, Bibeau, Steckler, & Glanz, 1988; Mills & Kelly, 1972; Moos, 1979; Rappaport, 1977; Stokols, 1992; Trickett, Kelly, & Todd, 1972; Vincent & Trickett, 1983). At its most basic level, ecological theory posits that individuals and settings are mutually influential, that this influence occurs in subsystems at multiple levels of analysis, and that influence changes over time and settings. Ecological theory is thus guided by the principle that the whole is more than the sum of its parts and that behavior and environment are viewed as interdependent rather than independent. Furthermore, an ecological perspective considers different levels of analysis like the layers of an onion, each system nested within another, with each system constrained both by the system it surrounds and the system that surrounds it (Wicker, 1979). Central to this chapter are the implications of taking a social-ecological perspective in the design and implementation of health promotion interventions. Thus, an interventionist committed to the ecological model would search for points of leverage at multiple levels of analysis in the sociocultural context and would use multiple approaches to change.

Few studies of health behavior specify the sequence or causal linkages by which individuals influence, and are influenced by, the larger social context (Altman & King, 1986; Winett, King & Altman, 1989). The ultimate goal of all interventions directed at tobacco-related behavior, regardless of the level of analysis, is to improve the health status of individuals, since individuals, not systems or environments, experience illness and health. The focus of macrolevel interventions (e.g., increasing the tax on cigarettes) may also influence the actions that individuals take (e.g., not purchasing cigarettes). Similarly, a goal of many microlevel interventions (e.g., teaching worksite employees how to quit smoking) may influence actions taken at higher levels of analysis (e.g., implementation of a worksite smoking policy). There are interactional and synergistic connections among levels of analysis. The means by which individuals are reached and influenced, however, can vary as a function of the level at which one intervenes. In more cases than not, there is a reciprocity of influence between levels of analysis (Winett et al., 1989). Furthermore, individuals and systems are not "mutually exclusive or opposite ends of a political or theoretical continuum (Green, 1986, P. 29)." In the case of tobacco use, focusing on one level has concomitant costs and benefits. Curtailing and eventually eliminating smoking on school grounds may require changes in organizational policies that are agreeable to parents, teachers, administrators, and students; implementation of educational programs for students and parents; development of cessation programs for individuals attempting to quit smoking; and enforcement of age-of-sale laws in retail outlets near schools.

TOBACCO USE AMONG ADOLESCENTS

The use of tobacco by young people remains a substantial threat to the nation's health (Food and Drug Administration, 1995; Lynch & Bonnie, 1994; U.S. Department of Health and Human Services, 1989; U.S. Department of Health and Human Services, 1994). Over 3 million U.S. adolescents are current smokers and over 1 million adolescent males use smokeless tobacco (Cummings, Pechacek, & Shopland, 1994; U.S. Department of Health and Human Services, 1994). These children serve as the replacements for the 400,000 American smokers who die and the 1.3 million who quit using tobacco each year (Lynch & Bonnie, 1994). Every day, approximately 3,000 children and teenagers become regular tobacco users (Lynch & Bonnie, 1994). Tobacco use is a behavior that almost always starts in adolescence. Of adults who use tobacco regularly, 37% started by the age of 14, and 89% started by the age of 18 (Lynch & Bonnie, 1994). The mean age of initiation is 14.5 years and the the mean age of daily use is 17.7 years (U.S. Department of Health and Human Services, 1994).

Although more than 50 million Americans have quit smoking since the first Surgeon General's Report in 1964, monthly use of tobacco among high-school senior males has not changed much since 1980, while use among females has dropped only slightly (Giovino et al., 1994; Johnston, O'Malley & Bachman, 1993; U.S. Department of Health and Human Services, 1994). Unfortunately, we are far from the Year 2000 goal of a 15% youth initiation rate (McGinnis & Lee, 1995). Thus, despite ongoing efforts to prevent tobacco use among young people, by any standard these efforts are falling far short of stated goals. Our inability to prevent adolescent tobacco use, now a problem two decade old, requires us to critically examine our intervention strategies and tactics. We suggest here that progress can be made with more careful consideration of the environmental context of tobacco use and its interrelationship with peer and family influences.

THE ENVIRONMENTAL CONTEXT OF TOBACCO USE

Marketing

Expenditures

Tobacco companies use an array of advertising and promotion strategies to market their products. Advertising appears in newspaper and magazines and on outdoor or transportation signage (e.g., billboards, store windows, cash registers, buses, and subways). Promotions include offering coupons and retail value-added merchandising, promotional allowances for retailers participating in promotional programs, specialty item distribution, point-of-sale displays, sponsorship of public entertainment, sporting events, and movies, and distribution of tobacco samples.

Substantial resources support tobacco marketing campaigns. Except for automobile companies, tobacco companies spend more on marketing than any other consumer product industry. In 1993, the tobacco companies spent $6.2 billion on advertising and promotion expenditures for cigarettes, over 90% of which was spent on promotions (Federal Trade Commission, 1995a; Federal Trade Commission, 1995b). Marketing expenditures have increased rapidly in the past few decades, climbing from about $261 million in 1964, to $491 million in 1975, to their current level (1993) of over $6 billion. During the mid-1990s, expenditures increased by almost $1 billion each year. Similarly, for marketing of smokeless tobacco, the tobacco companies spent $119 million in 1993, up from $80 million spent in 1985 (Federal Trade Commission, 1995b).

Over the past two decades, a shift has occurred in the proportion of money expended on promotions versus advertising. Whereas advertising previously received about three-quarters of the total marketing budget, it now receives less than 10%. The primary forms of promotional marketing in 1993 included cents-off coupons and retail value added (42% of total expenditures), promotional allowances (26%), distribution of branded specialty items (12%), and point-of-sale displays (7%). Sponsorship is the fastest growing category of tobacco marketing. Consumer product companies generally use sponsorships as a springboard for other marketing efforts ("IEG's Complete Guide to Sponsorship," 1995).

Functions

There is consensus that tobacco marketing functions to maintain or increase brand share among current users, and to expand markets by persuading nonusers to initiate use (Food and Drug Administration, 1995; Warner et al., 1992). Warner articulated a set of direct and indirect mechanisms by which marketing might affect use (Warner, 1986; Warner et al., 1992). Direct mechanisms include:

1. Reducing the resolve of current users to quit or to reduce the amount consumed;
2. increasing relapse among users who have quit; and
3. increasing current users' consumption.

Indirect mechanisms include:

1. Suppressing media coverage of the health effects of tobacco;
2. contributing to an environment in which use is perceived as normative; and
3. decreasing opposition to tobacco company policy positions.

On balance, there is strong empirical evidence for the effect of indirect mechanisms, and moderately strong evidence for the effect of direct mechanisms.

Effects on Adolescents

As noted previously, adolescent tobacco use rates began to increase in the 1990s, after a 10-year period of being relative flat. Interestingly, the Joe Camel cartoon character was launched by the RJ Reynolds Tobacco Company in 1987, immediately preceding the increase in adolescent tobacco use. Before RJ Reynolds used this cartoon figure, about 4% of adolescents used Camel cigarettes. After just a few years of the Joe Camel cartoon campaign, the youth market share for the Camel brand had increased to about 13% (Barker, 1994; USDHHS, 1994). At about the same time as the Joe Camel campaign, Philip Morris spent substantial resources to promote its leading brand, Marlboro, as part of a campaign that solidified Marlboro's dominance among adolescents and adults. Lorillard's youth brand, Newport, bolstered by its "Alive with Pleasure" campaign showing youthful actors engaging in frolic and romance, also increased in popularity among youth during this period (from 8.2 to 12.7%).

One study found that from the early 1970s to the mid-1980s, adolescents received increasingly more explicit targeting by tobacco advertising in popular magazines. This study, a content analysis of almost 800 tobacco advertisements, found that the ratio of tobacco advertisements in youth magazines compared to advertisements in other popular magazines increased substantially over this timeframe (Albright, Altman, Slater, & Maccoby, 1988; Altman, Slater, Albright, & Maccoby, 1987; Basil et al., 1991).

A U.S. study of adolescents ages 12–17 found that over one-third had either collected tobacco coupons (e.g., Camel Cash, Marlboro Adventure Miles), had a promotional catalogue, or owned a promotional item; over 10% had owned a promotional item. Extrapolating these data, it was estimated that over 7 million U.S. teenagers had participated in a tobacco promotion campaign (Coeytaux, Altman, & Slade, 1995). A study in California of adolescent and adult smokers found that 15% of boys and 9% of girls owned tobacco promotion items. The gender effect found for adolescents was similar to that found for adults (men = 26% tobacco promotion ownership, women = 18%) (Pierce, Gilpin, Rosbrook, Davis, & Wright, 1995).

There is some evidence of an association between participation in promotional campaigns and susceptibility to tobacco use (Altman, Levine, Coeytaux, Slade, & Jaffe, 1996). Altman and colleagues found that when an adolescent was aware of tobacco promotions, the predicted odds of being a tobacco user or being susceptible tobacco use were two times greater as compared to an adolescent who was unaware of promotions. When an adolescent was aware of promotions, had an adolescent friend who owned a promotional item, had received tobacco, and had participated directly in a tobacco promotional campaign, the predicted odds increased to about 22 (Altman et al., 1996).

The association between the awareness of tobacco company marketing and perceptions of tobacco use is also evident among children (Food and Drug Administration, 1995; Lynch & Bonnie, 1994; USDHHS, 1994). For example, in a study of the cartoon character, Joe Camel, practically all 6-year-old children (over 90 percent) successfully matched the Camel logo to a photo of cigarettes. These six year old participants achieved about the same match rate with Mickey Mouse and the logo for the Disney Channel (Fischer, Schwartz, Richards, Goldstein, & Rojas, 1991).

Another study found that over 80% of 12- to 13-year-old never-smokers could identify benefits to tobacco use, nearly 60% named a favorite cigarette advertisement, and over 40% expressed a brand preference (Evans, Farkas, Gilpin, Berry, & Pierce, 1995). An Australian study of over 5,000 children 10 to 12 years of age found that children who expressed attitudinal approval of tobacco advertisements were over twice as likely to smoke 1 year later as compared to children who did not approve (Alexander et al., 1983).

After a thorough review of the evidence, the FDA concluded that there was substantial quantitative and qualitative evidence supporting a causal relationship between tobacco product marketing and adolescent tobacco use. Likewise, they suggested that there was strong evidence supporting the efficacy of antismoking media campaigns (Food and Drug Administration, 1995).

Brand Switching

Despite evidence to the contrary, the tobacco industry continues to maintain that their marketing is designed to influence current smokers to switch brands, rather than to attract nonsmokers. Examining the brand-switching argument of the tobacco industry raises questions about the actual intent of cigarette advertisers. Each year, about 1 million smokers die and another 1.5 million smokers quit smoking. The tobacco industry must recruit about 2.5 million new smokers each year just to maintain the current smoking prevalence rate (Warner, 1986). Since the majority of smokers begin smoking by the end of their teenage years (Johnston, O'Malley, & Bachman, 1994b), 5,000 children and teenagers would have to start smoking each day of the year for the tobacco industry to maintain the smoking prevalence rate. In addition:

1. Only 9% of smokers switch brands each year (Federal Trade Commission, 1985);
2. over two-thirds of existing cigarette brands are owned by Philip Morris and RJ Reynolds, and thus about 93% of brand switching occurs among brands owned by the same company (Tye, Warner, & Glantz, 1987);
3. assuming a brand-switching argument, in 1983 the tobacco industry would have spent about $346 for every smoker who switched brands at the same time that the after-tax profits generated by the average smoker was about $80.00, thereby resulting in significant monetary losses (Tye et al., 1987); and
4. expenditures for cigarette advertising in magazines with large young male and female readerships is high (Davis, 1987).

The 1971 Broadcast Ban on TV and Radio Cigarette Advertising

From July 1, 1967 to December 31, 1970, television and radio broadcasters were required under the FCC Fairness Doctrine to donate air time to antismoking media to balance advertising sponsored by the tobacco industry. The FCC ruled that the ratio of antismoking ads to smoking ads had to be no less than one to five (Abernethy & Teel, 1986). In 1975 dollars, this amounted to about $75 million per year of free commercial air time for antismoking messages (Food and Drug Administration, 1995). The effects of the resulting media antismoking campaign—a 7% decline in per capita cigarette consumption—suggested that it was effective in countering the effects of tobacco advertising (Food and Drug Administration, 1995; Hamilton, 1972; Teel, Teel, & Bearden, 1979; Warner, 1986; Warner et al., 1986). One analysis suggested that the antismoking messages reduced per capita consumption about 2 times as much as cigarette advertising increased it (Hamilton, 1972). Econometric studies suggest that the advertising ban reduced the teenage smoking prevalence rate by as much as 0.6% from 1970–1974 (Warner, 1986).

When legislation was passed in 1971 banning tobacco advertising on television and radio, public health advocates were hopeful that per capita consumption of cigarettes would fall sharply. Interestingly, however, overall per capita consumption did not start dropping until the mid-1970s. One explanation for this finding was the effectiveness of the antismoking campaign. That is, the banning of tobacco ads on television and radio, which eliminated any rights to equal broadcast time for health messages (except for public service announcements), produced a dramatic increase in tobacco advertising and promotion expenditures in other venues (e.g., outdoor, magazines, sponsorship of events), and may have contributed to an increase in the overall consumption of tobacco products (Teel et al., 1979). The ban, then, may not have accomplished what health advocates had hoped; indeed, a major effect was to reduce access of health advocates to public media (Teel et al., 1979). Moreover, because print media readerships are more loyal than television viewers, and because it is more cost-effective to deliver messages through print channels than through broadcast channels, the ban may actually have benefitted the tobacco industry (Teel et al., 1979). Indeed, the tobacco companies were ultimately supportive of the ban. Teel et al. (1979) suggest that by diverting tobacco advertising money to print media, the ban may be the primary explanation for the appearance, growth, and economic prosperity of special-interest magazines as well as newspapers. In addition, it may well have contributed to the increase in tobacco promotions.

Since the early 1960s, antismoking campaigns, events, and messages have occurred in several forums: broadcast media, narrowcast media, and community events. In an analysis of the effects of the overall antismoking campaign (beginning with the Surgeon General's Report in 1964), Warner illustrated that in the absence of this broadbased campaign, per capita consumption of cigarettes would have been 20 to 30% higher by 1975 and 40% higher by 1978 (Warner, 1977; Warner, 1981). Evaluations of the antismoking media campaign in California, funded by a 25 cent increase in the state excise tax on tobacco, has reduced tobacco consumption. One study estimated that the media campaign influenced, either directly or indirectly, 44% of the almost 500,000 Californians who quit smoking between 1990–1991 (Popham, 1993). Another study of the increase in the California excise tax compared the relative effects of the tax increase with the media campaign (Hu, Sung & Keeler, 1995). This study found that between 1990 and 1992, the tax increase reduced sales of cigarettes by 819 million packs while the media campaign reduced sales by 232 million packs (Hu et al., 1995).

Short of a total advertising and promotion ban in this country, other options include allowing only tombstone advertising (e.g., restricting ad content to pictures of cigarette packages or the brand name, and disallowing models, slogans, scenes, or colors); strict enforcement of an advertising and promotion code to remove false and misleading imagery; counteradvertising paid by the federal excise tax or tobacco company contributions; changes in tax laws to eliminate tax deductions for cigarette advertising and promotion expenditures; and banning ads in magazines and other outlets with large youth exposure (Food and Drug Administration, 1995; Warner, 1986). The regulations proposed by the Food and Drug Administration in 1995 (Food and Drug Administration, 1995) were the most far-reaching and comprehensive ever recommended by the federal government.

Media Practices Affecting Modeling of Smoking

The portrayal of tobacco use in the mass media may play a role in the way that adolescents perceive social norms about use. A content analysis of routine prime time television shows in the fall of 1984 (116 hours of programming) revealed the following: about one act of smoking took place during each hour of programming, almost two-thirds of the smokers were lead characters, males were three times more likely to be smoking than females; and 70% of smokers were in "strong or enduring roles" (as opposed to "bad or outside the law") (Cruz & Wallack, 1986). Moreover, there was only one instance in 116 hours of programming in which the potential desire to quit smoking was portrayed.

Similar positive portrayals of tobacco use in motion pictures have been documented. Evidence that consumer products advertised implicitly in movies results in increased sales is evident in the movie "ET," in which the promotion of Reese's Pieces candy resulted in an 85% increase in sales. In the movie "Superman II," Philip Morris paid to have Marlboro displayed prominently throughout the movie. In the Walt Disney movie "Baby," the lead character was a smoker ("R. J. Reynolds Reaches Kids," 1986). Along the same lines, smoking was associated with God in the adolescent movie "Two of a Kind," in which, for example, one of God's assistants drives a bus with a huge Camel cigarette advertisement on the side. The promotion of cigarettes in movies planned and strategic rather than coincidental.

Cost

The taxation of cigarettes is regulated by federal and state government. As of 1995, Virginia had the lowest tax rate per pack (2.5 cents) while Washington had the highest (81.5 cents). Worldwide, the U.S. has the lowest tobacco excise tax of all developed nations (USDHHS, 1995). The tax per pack is 46 cents in the U.S., $1.52 in France, and $4.07 in Denmark (USDHHS, 1995). Moreover, the tax burden on a pack of cigarettes sold in the U.S. has dropped from 48% in 1955 to 30% in 1993 (Lynch & Bonnie, 1994).

In 1993, approximately $12 billion in tobacco excise taxes was collected by local governments ($187 million), state governments ($6.2 billion), and the federal government ($5.5 billion) (Tobacco Institute, 1994). In the 1990s, several states considered raising state excise taxes on tobacco as a means of decreasing consumption and raising revenue; tax initiatives were passed in California, Massachusetts, and Arizona.

The tax rates on cigarettes and the impact on the retail price of a pack of cigarettes are related to smoking behavior. It has been estimated that an 8 cent decrease in the federal cigarette excise tax would encourage about 1 million young people ages 12–25 and several hundred thousand adults to become smokers (Warner et al., 1986). Conversely, an 8–16 cent increase in the tax would encourage 1–2 million young people and 800,000–1.5 million adults to either quit or not take up the habit. Sensitivity to cigarette prices is inversely related to age, due in part to the fact that young people generally are less addicted to nicotine and on average have less discretionary income than older adults (Warner et al., 1986). It has been estimated that the overall price elasticity of tobacco is -0.4, meaning that for every 10% increase in the price of tobacco, there is a 4 percent decrease in consumption (Lynch & Bonnie, 1994; National Cancer Institute, 1993). The price elasticity for adolescents and young adults has been estimated at about -1.4, meaning that for every 10% increase in the price of tobacco, there is a 14% decrease in use and smoking participation (Chaloupka & Wechsler, 1995).

One policy alternative is to set aside a few cents of the federal excise tax on tobacco for an antismoking media campaign. One cent per pack would generate about $250 million in annual revenue, enough for a sizeable public health campaign, to help pay for healthcare costs generated by smokers, or for assistance in tobacco farmer diversification efforts. If 5 cents were earmarked, $1.5 billion would be generated and each smoker would pay about $27 each year (Warner, 1986).

Access to Cigarettes by Minors

Access to cigarettes is a critical determinant of whether people (particularly children and adolescents), experiment with or maintain smoking behaviors. Since few smokers begin smoking after high school (Johnston, O'Malley & Bachman, 1994a) and one-third to two-thirds of adolescents who smoke two or more cigarettes become habitual smokers (Benowitz, 1988), efforts to prevent the adoption of smoking must focus on preventing children and adolescents from becoming addicted. Limiting access to tobacco can contribute to prevention. Indeed, three small, cross-sectional studies have reported reductions in tobacco use following decreases in tobacco accessibility

(J. R. DiFranza, Carlson, & Caisse, 1992; Hinds, 1992; Jason, Ji, Anes, & Birkhead, 1991).

Although most states have laws regulating tobacco sales to minors, these laws are rarely enforced (J. R. DiFranza, Norwood, Garner & Tye, 1987; DiFranza, 1995; Food and Drug Administration, 1995; U.S. Inspector General, 1995; U.S. Department of Health and Human Services, 1990; U.S. Department of Health and Human Services, 1994) and minors have little trouble obtaining tobacco. Estimates on the number of packs of cigarettes sold illegally to U.S. minors each year range from a low of 255 million to a high of 947 million (Cummings et al., 1994; DiFranza 1995; DiFranza & Tye, 1990). A national survey representative of students attending school found that over 76% of 8th-graders and 90% of 10th-graders believed that it would be "fairly easy" or "very easy" for them to obtain tobacco (Johnston, 1995).

Minors are typically able to purchase tobacco on 50–85% of attempts from over-the-counter sources (OTC) and on 80–100% of attempts from vending machines (Abernathy, 1994; Altman et al., 1992a; Altman et al., 1992b; Altman, Foster, Rasenick-Douss, & Tye, 1989; Altman, Rasenick-Douss, Foster, & Tye, 1991; Carruthers & McDonald, 1995; J. R. DiFranza & Brown, 1992; Forster, Hourigan, & McGovern, 1992; Keay, Woodruff, Wildey, & Kenney, 1993; Klonoff, Fritz, Landrine, Riddle, & Tully-Payne, 1994; Radecki & Zdunich, 1993; Wildey et al., 1995). There is also some evidence that shoplifting and "bumming" cigarettes are sources for minors, especially among early adolescents (Cismoski & Sheridan, 1994; J. R. DiFranza, Eddy, Brown & Ryan, 1995). A national study of adolescents ages 12–17 found that the percent of minors who reported buying their own cigarettes increased from 58 to 62% between 1989 and 1993 (Centers for Disease Control and Prevention [CDCP], 1996). This study also found that: (1) about half of minors who attempted to purchase tobacco were never asked to provide age identification; and (2) smokers ages 12–15 were about 44% more likely than smokers ages 16–17 to use vending machines to obtain tobacco.

Most health professionals agree that merchant and community education is an important component to a comprehensive, community-based program to reduce sales to minors (Altman et al., 1991, 1992b; Choi, Novotny, & Thimis, 1991; J. R. DiFranza, 1995; J. R. DiFranza et al., 1992; J. R. DiFranza et al., 1987; Feighery, Altman, & Shaffer, 1991; Gambescia & Corcoran, 1991; Jason et al., 1991; Kirn, 1987; USDHHS, 1990, 1994; Wildey et al., 1995). There is also agreement among health professionals that whenever possible, a licensing system and enforcement of age-of-sale laws are essential components of preventive intervention. Enforcement operations that involve youth must, however, carefully consider the protection of minors involved in such operations (Billows, Schnopp-Wyatt, & Jason,

1995). Also, some communities have not been able to enlist the support of local police, district attorneys, or other enforcement agents to actively enforce age-of-sale laws (Biglan et al., 1995; Carruthers & McDonald, 1995; Keay et al., 1993; Wildey et al., 1995).

In recent years, tobacco companies have undertaken efforts to alert retailers to the problem of illegal sales of tobacco to minors, although these programs have been shown to be ineffective (J. R. DiFranza & Brown, 1992; J. R. DiFranza, Savageau, & Aisquith, 1996). In surveys of the general public, there is strong public support for taking aggressive action to curtail illegal sales to minors (CDC, 1991; Forster, McBride, Jeffery, Schmid, & Pirie, 1991; Lynch & Bonnie, 1994; Strouse & Hall, 1994; USDHHS 1994; University of California at San Diego & California Department of Health Services, 1990). A 1994 national random digit dial survey of 2,345 U.S. adults found overwhelming support for policies that limit minors' access to tobacco (Strouse & Hall, 1994).

The greater the risk young people must take to obtain tobacco and the more community norms reject adolescent tobacco use, the lower the likelihood that adolescents will begin to use tobacco. Ultimately, preventing adolescent tobacco use is best accomplished through the delivery of a broad range of interventions, from education to legislation (Altman et al., 1992a; Glynn, Greenwald, Mills, & Manley, 1993). Easy access to tobacco undermines other tobacco control measures directed at adolescents, such as school-based interventions. Consistency between what adolescents see in the community and what they hear in school-based programs may help improve the effectiveness of school-based programs.

U.S. Tobacco Company Plan to Expand Smokeless Tobacco User Base

In the regulations on tobacco issued by the Food and Drug Administration (FDA) in 1995, the FDA reviewed and published internal tobacco company documents (Food and Drug Administration, 1995). One of these documents, obtained through discovery in a lawsuit against the U.S. Tobacco Company [UST] depicted UST's strategy to expand market share of their smokeless tobacco products. Many of the factors discussed in this chapter (e.g., advertising, sampling, promotions, peer influence, and cost) were used by UST in a coordinated plan to attract new users and to keep current users addicted. The UST smokeless tobacco product line (Bandits, Long Cut, Skoal, and Copenhagen [Cope]) includes low-nicotine brands (e.g., Bandits) and high-nicotine brands (e.g., Copenhagen). UST had an explicit "graduation" strategy of moving consumers from using the lower-profit and lower-nicotine-level brands such as Bandits to higher-addiction (and higher-profit) brands such as Copenhagen, this strategy was summarized in an internal industry document:

"Skoal Bandits, which is at the bottom of the previous graduation chart, 'will continue to fuel the new user base to assure graduation to our priority moist brands'" (FDA, 1995, p. 286).

Another company statement noted: "Sample Skoal Bandits often and intensively in and around the retail account to create new customers and feed the graduation process (FDA, p. 286)." UST's graduation strategy was built on using marketing tactics (e.g., sampling, advertisements, promotions) and peer influence to first build a customer base for lower-nicotine starter products with the long-term goal of encouraging a stepwise progression to higher-nicotine, premium, higher-cost products.

Public relations is another major strategy that tobacco companies use to control the way that tobacco issues are framed. One example of this strategy is money given by tobacco companies to Democratic and Republican National Committees. In 1995, for example, the Center for Responsive Politics found that Philip Morris ($1.2 million) and RJR Nabisco ($800,000) topped the list of corporate givers. Brown and Williamson ($265,000), the Tobacco Institute ($175,000), and U.S. Tobacco ($150,000) were ranked 17th, 37th, and 51st, respectively (Babcock, 1996). In sum, UST's strategy reflects the fact that to promote tobacco use (and, for our purposes, to prevent use), a multilevel, multifaceted strategy is required.

As a counterforce to tobacco industry efforts, various organizations have increased efforts to promote public health through tobacco control. In 1994, for example, the influential National Academy of Sciences convened a working group to review tobacco use among children and youths and to issue a report on their findings and recommendations (Lynch & Bonnie, 1994). Likewise, various health organizations have issued policy statements about tobacco over the past decade. For example, the American Heart Association has called for an increase in the federal excise tax, elimination or restriction of tobacco advertising and promotion, assurance of nonsmokers' rights, and identification of methods to assist tobacco farmers in the transition to farming other crops or to other professions (Warner et al., 1986). The Food and Drug Administration has issued proposed regulations on a wide variety of initiatives to protect children and youth (FDA, 1995). The American Medical Association, through its flagship journal, the *Journal of the American Medical Association*, has published at least yearly special issues on tobacco, and has issued strong policy positions on a range of tobacco issues. During the 1980s, tobacco policy research became a legitimate area of research inquiry and action (Davis, 1995).

Family Socialization Processes

Youth risk behaviors are also affected by factors in the immediate social environment. In particular, family socialization processes can affect the development of risk-taking behaviors. Socialization is a process through which children learn and internalize the normative beliefs, values, knowledge, skills and behaviors valued by members of their social groups (Baumrind, 1966; Clausen, 1968). Social norms are powerful determinants of behavior because approval by one's social groups is often linked to compliance with group norms, and because individuals generally try to avoid acting in ways that are inconsistent with their own internalized belief system (Maccoby, 1980; Moscovici, 1985; Smith, 1982).

Tobacco use by children and adolescents may be influenced by general socialization processes within the family. Parenting practices and their capacity to predispose some children to engage in risk-taking behaviors are particularly important to consider. "Parenting practices" is a general term referring to the childrearing practices of parents across a variety of parent-child interactions. Developmental theorists have identified parental demandingness and responsiveness (i.e., warmth/acceptance) as the key dimensions of parenting (Baumrind, 1966; Baumrind, 1978; Maccoby & Martin, 1983; Roberts, 1986; Steinberg, Elmen, & Mounts, 1989). Each dimension is a composite of specific parenting behaviors; for example, demandingness refers to setting and enforcing clear standards of behavior; actively monitoring and supervising a child's activities; maintaining structure and regimen in a child's life, and making maturity demands consistent with the developmental phase of a child. Parental responsiveness includes supporting a child's independence and individuality; relating to the actual child rather than to an idealized child; respecting a child's rights; and expecting a child to respect a parent's rights.

Research conducted over the last 30 years has established causal relationships between parenting practices and children's development of personal, academic, and social competencies (Baumrind, 1978; Coopersmith, 1981; Dornbusch, Ritter, Leiderman, Roberts, & Fraleigh, 1987; Grolnick & Ryan, 1989; Maccoby & Martin, 1983; Steinberg et al., 1989). This body of research strongly indicates that children of parents who balance high demandingness with high responsiveness and warmth (authoritative parents) are more likely to develop strong personal and social competencies, and are more likely to maintain a close relationship with their parents, than children whose parents are demanding but not responsive (authoritarian parents), are responsive but not demanding (lax parents), or are low on both dimensions (uninvolved parents) (Baumrind, 1966; Baumrind, 1978; Clausen, 1968; Dodge, Pettit, McClaskey, & Brown, 1986; Maccoby & Martin, 1983). It is noteworthy that the primary aim of current school-based smoking prevention programs is to engender the very competencies which parenting has been shown to influence.

Relatively few studies have been conducted to test a direct relationship between parenting practices and tobacco use. Most of the relevant findings come from studies of drug use by adolescents. Kandel and colleagues (Kandel,

Yamaguchi, & Chen, 1992) found that closeness to parents and extent of control exercised by parents were the two strongest (inverse) predictors of adolescents' initiation of use of alcohol and other drugs. In a 12-year longitudinal study, Pulkkinen (1982) found that children of authoritative or child-oriented families were less likely as adolescents to use tobacco, alcohol or other drugs than those whose parents were authoritarian or uninvolved. Simons and Robertson found that parent rejection, defined as the adolescent's perceptions of lack of parent support, concern, and interest, was negatively associated with adolescent self-esteem, and positively associated with multiple substance use (Simons & Robertson, 1989). Thus, in addition to the direct effect of parent modeling of tobacco use (discussed below), these studies suggest that general parenting also influences adolescents' substance use behaviors. Research is needed to investigate causal links between parenting practices and children's development of risk-taking behaviors, including tobacco use.

A parent's role in tobacco-specific socialization can take several forms. Parents' own use is an important predictor of child use of tobacco (Murray, Kiryluk, & Swan, 1985; Nolte, Smith & O'Rourke, 1983). However, socializing activities go well beyond modeling of actual use to include modeling of the consequences of use, and modeling of avoiding use, as when a parent requests nonsmoking sections in restaurants. Communicating about tobacco use, setting household rules that prohibit indoor smoking, and setting clear expectations about the negative consequences of trying smoking are other examples of tobacco-specific socialization variables. Through these and other socializing mechanisms, parents influence their children's perceptions of the prevalence, social acceptability, and personal and social consequences of tobacco use.

Another type of antismoking socialization activity includes parent involvement in countering pro-smoking influences in the surrounding environment. Parents may, for example, counter the positive images of smoking presented in cigarette advertisements and promotions, and they may use smoking models on television programs as cues to discuss the negative consequences of smoking. Parents may also make salient the public regulations that restrict sale of tobacco to minors, and that restrict or ban smoking in public spaces (as when a parent tells a child why smokers stand outside buildings to smoke).

Parents may also assume an advocacy role to enhance antismoking socialization for their children. Parental support of organized efforts to increase tobacco taxes, ban vending machines, or ban free distribution of cigarettes at public events sends a strong antismoking message to children. In sum, parents may act not only to modify smoking socialization processes within the home; they also may act to modify higher-level community and regulatory factors which have implications for smoking initiation by children.

While some parents may be proactive in socializing their children against tobacco use, it is likely that the majority view tobacco use as a problem of adolescence, and so remain passive during the childhood years. Importantly, a passive orientation is not devoid of a socializing effect. Baumrind, for example, posits that children often interpret parent passivity as tacit approval or lack of disapproval (Baumrind & Moselle, 1985). Thus, parents who do not actively challenge the many pro-smoking influences to which their children are exposed may effectively allow these other social influences to take effect.

At present, little is known about the prevalence, timing, or content of naturally occurring family socialization regarding tobacco use. Research is needed that identifies barriers to preventive socialization, examines variation in socialization across population subgroups, and tests for a relationship between antismoking socialization and tobacco use by children.

SUMMARY

The costs of tobacco use are staggering. Each year tobacco-related illnesses cost the U.S. about $50 billion in healthcare costs alone (USDHHS, 1995). The fact that the U.S. public underestimates the risk of tobacco use relative to other risks (e.g., in a national survey 36% thought AIDS was the most serious health risk, while only 9% mentioned smoking) (USDHHS, 1995) suggests that more knowledge about tobacco prevention and cessation is needed. In this chapter, we outlined some of the environmental, policy, and interpersonal factors that may affect tobacco-related behavior, and suggested that attention to such contextual factors may advance efforts to prevent tobacco use, especially among adolescents.

A theme of this chapter was that tobacco-related behavior, and the settings in which such behavior occurs, are interdependent. It can be difficult, however, to discriminate the relative contributions of multiple levels of influence on specific tobacco-related knowledge, attitudes, and behaviors. Similarly, assessing the interrelationships and potential synergistic effects between levels is difficult. The critical issue is how behavior is influenced by, and influences, multiple levels of analysis in a complex web of place and time.

The ideas in this chapter suggest a number of future research issues. First, the field of health psychology and the specific issues of health behavior change discussed throughout this book would benefit from incorporating a multilevel, social-context perspective into research. In addition to simply cataloging and measuring contextual variables, it is important to study how variables at different levels interact or link.

Second, methodological advances are needed. While the tools to measure the social context of health phenomena are perhaps less developed than the tools to measure intrapsychic constructs, their development is essential to an adequate understanding of health-related behaviors.

Third, health-behavior researchers should collaborate with other social and health scientists for complementary theories, concepts, and methodologies. In particular, researchers and practitioners interested in behavior change would benefit enormously from examining and using theories and concepts beyond the personal and interpersonal levels of analysis (Winett et al., 1989).

Fourth, the societal impact of health-related issues needs to be more salient. For example, although the focus in this chapter was on youth tobacco use in the U.S., it is important to recognize that whatever progress is made in this country is offset by soaring tobacco use rates overseas. U.S. tobacco companies have aggressively expanded their presence in overseas markets, particularly new markets in the former Eastern Bloc and Asia. They have done this by building overseas manufacturing facilities; engaging in joint ventures with, or buying outright, foreign-owned tobacco companies; providing money, technology, and technical assistance to foreign growers; establishing public relations enterprises; countering efforts to educate people about the relationship between smoking and ill health; and interfering with governmental efforts to pass public health policies (Chapman & Wong, 1990; Mackay, 1994; Naett, 1994).

Much has been accomplished to slow the epidemic of tobacco-related disease, and there is reason to maintain optimism about future progress. The rate at which progress is made in reducing tobacco use and in understanding other health behaviors is, however, critically dependent upon attending to the influences of the larger social context and upon changing the policy environment.

REFERENCES

Abernathy, T. J. (1994). A community-based tobacco prevention project. *Canadian Journal of Public Health, 85*, 82–84.

Abernethy, A. M., & Teel, J. E. (1986). Advertising regulation's effect upon demand for cigarettes. *Journal of Advertising, 15*, 51–55.

Albright, C. L., Altman, D. G., Slater, M. D., & Maccoby, N. (1988). Cigarette advertisements in magazines: Evidence for a differential focus on women's and youth magazines. *Health Education Quarterly, 15*, 225–233.

Alexander, H. M., Callcott, R., Dobson, A. J., Hardes, G. R., Lloyd, D. M., O'Connel, D. L., & Leeder, S. R. (1983). Cigarette smoking and drug use in school children: IV. Factors associated with changes in smoking behavior. *International Journal of Epidemiology, 12*, 59–66.

Altman, D., Carol, J., Chalkley, C., Cherner, J., DiFranza, J., Feighery, E., Forster, J., Gupta, S., Records, J., Slade, J., Talbot, B., & Tye, J. (1992a). Report of the tobacco policy research study group on access to tobacco products in the United

States. *Tobacco Control, 1*(supplement), S45–S51.

Altman, D. G., Feighery, E., Records, J., Kropp, R., Erikson, J., & Allard, A. (1992b). *Tobacco-free youth: How to reduce sales to minors in your community*. Palo Alto, CA: Stanford Health Promotion Resource Center.

Altman, D. G., Foster, V., Rasenick-Douss, L., & Tye, J. B. (1989). Reducing the illegal sale of cigarettes to minors. *JAMA, 261*, 80–83.

Altman, D. G., & King, A. C. (1986). Approaches to compliance in primary prevention. *The Journal of Compliance in Health Care, 1*, 55–73.

Altman, D. G., Levine, D. W., Coeytaux, R., Slade, J., & Jaffe, R. (1996). Tobacco promotion and susceptibility to tobacco use among adolescents aged 12 through 17 years in a nationally representative sample. *American Journal of Public Health, 86*, 1590–1593.

Altman, D. G., Rasenick-Douss, L., Foster, V., & Tye, J. B. (1991). Sustained effects of an education program to reduce sales of cigarettes to minors. *American Journal of Public Health, 81*, 891–893.

Altman, D. G., Slater, M. D., Albright, C. L., & Maccoby, N. (1987). How an unhealthy product is sold: Cigarette advertising in magazines, 1960–1985. *Journal of Communication, 37*, 95–106.

Babcock, C. R. (1996, March 11). Parties raised nearly $60 million in "soft" 1995 donations. *Washington Post*, p. A17.

Barker, D. (1994). Changes in the cigarette brand preferences of adolescent smokers: United States, 1989–1993. *Morbidity and Mortality Weekly Report, 43*, 577–581.

Basil, M. D., Schooler, C., Altman, D. G., Slater, M. D., Albright, C. L., & Maccoby, N. (1991). How cigarettes are sold in magazines: Special messages for special markets. *Health Communication, 3*, 75–91.

Baumrind, D. (1966). Effects of authoritative parental control on child behavior. *Child Development, 37*, 887–907.

Baumrind, D. (1978). Parental disciplinary patterns and social competence in children. *Youth & Society, 9*, 239–275.

Baumrind, D., & Moselle, K. A. (1985). A developmental perspective on adolescent drug abuse. *Advances in Alcohol and Substance Abuse, 4*, 41–67.

Benowitz, N. L. (1988). Pharmacologic aspects of cigarette smoking and nicotine addiction. *New England Journal of Medicine, 319*, 1318–1330.

Biglan, A., Henderson, J., Humphrey, D., Yasui, M., Whisman, R., Black, C., & James, L. (1995). Mobilising positive reinforcement to reduce youth access to tobacco. *Tobacco Control, 4f*, 42–48.

Billows, W. D., Schnopp-Wyatt, D., & Jason, L. A. (1995). Reducing the risk to minors participating in an urban intervention program. *Tobacco Control, 4*, 92.

Binder, A., Stokols, D., & Catalano, R. (1975). Social ecology: An emerging multidiscipline. *The Journal of Environmental Education, 7*, 32–43.

Botvin, G. J., Baker, E., Dusenbury, L., Botvin, E. M., & Diaz, T. (1995). Long-term follow-up results of a randomized drug abuse prevention trial in a white middle-class population. *Journal of the American Medical Association, 273*, 1106–1112.

Bronfenbrenner, U. (1977). Toward an experimental ecology of human development. *American Psychologist, 32*, 513–531.

Carruthers, S., & McDonald, C. (1995). The availability of cigarettes to minors in Perth, Western Australia. *Tobacco Control, 4*, 49–52.

Center for Disease Control. (1991). Public attitudes regarding limits on public smoking and regulation of tobacco sales and advertising - 10 U.S. Communities, 1989. *MMWR, 40*, 344–353.

Centers for Disease Control and Prevention. (1996). Accessibility of tobacco products to youths aged 12–17 years: United States, 1989 and 1993. *Morbidity and Mortality Weekly Report, 45*, 125.

Chaloupka, F. J., & Wechsler, H. (1995). *Price, tobacco control policies and smoking among young adults* (Working paper No. 5012). Chicago: National Bureau of Economic Research.

Chapman, S., & Wong, W. L. (1990). *Tobacco control in the Third World*, Penang: International Organisation of Consumers.

Choi, W. S., Novotny, T. E., & Thimis, A. T. (1991). Restricting minors' access to tobacco: A review of state legislation. *American Journal of Preventive Medicine, 8*, 19–22.

Cismoski, J., & Sheridan, M. (1994). Tobacco acquisition practices of adolescents in two Wisconsin communities. *Wisconsin Medical Journal, 93*, 585–591.

Clausen, J. A. (1968). Perspectives on childhood socialization. In J. A. Clausen (Ed.), *Socialization and Society* (pp. 131–181). Boston: Little, Brown and Co.

Cleary, P. D., Hitchcock, J. L., Semmer, N., Flinchbaugh, L. J., & Pinney, J. M. (1988). Adolescent smoking: Research and health policy. *Milbank Quarterly, 66*, 137–171.

Coeytaux, R. R., Altman, D. G., & Slade, J. (1995). Tobacco promotions in the hands of youth. *Tobacco Control: An International Journal, 4*, 253–257.

Coopersmith, S. (1981). *The antecedents of self-esteem.* Palo Alto, CA: Consulting Psychologists Press.

Cruz, J., & Wallack, L. (1986). Trends in tobacco use on television. *American Journal of Public Health, 76*, 698–699.

Cummings, K. M., Pechacek, T., & Shopland, D. (1994). The illegal sale of cigarettes to US minors: Estimates by state. *American Journal of Public Health, 84*, 300–302.

Davis, R. M. (1987). Current trends in cigarette advertising and marketing. *New England Journal of Medicine, 316*, 725–732.

Davis, R. M. (1995). Tobacco policy research comes of age. *Tobacco Control, 4*, 6–9.

DiFranza, J. R., & Tye, J. B. (1990). Who profits from tobacco sales to children? *JAMA, 263*, 2784–2787.

DiFranza, J. R. (1995). Active enforcement of minors' access laws: A moral and ethical imperative. *Tobacco Control, 5, 5.*

DiFranza, J. R., & Brown, L. J. (1992). The tobacco institute's "It's the Law" campaign: Has it halted illegal sales of tobacco to children? *American Journal of Public Health, 82*, 1271–1272.

DiFranza, J. R., Carlson, R. R., & Caisse, R. E. (1992). Reducing youth access to tobacco. *Tobacco Control, 1*, 57–8.

DiFranza, J. R., Eddy, J. J., Brown, L. F., & Ryan, J. L. (1995). Tobacco acquisition and cigarette brand selection among youth. *Tobacco Control, 3*, 334–338.

DiFranza, J. R., Norwood, B. D., Garner, D. W., & Tye, J. B. (1987). Legislative efforts to protect children from tobacco. *Journal of the American Medical Association, 257*, 3387–3389.

DiFranza, J. R., Savageau, J. A., & Aisquith, B. F. (1996). Youth access to tobacco: The effects of age, gender, vending machine locks, and "It's the Law" programs. *American Journal of Public Health, 86*, 221–224.

Dodge, K. A., Pettit, G. S., McClaskey, C. L., & Brown, M. M. (1986). Social competence in children. *Monographs of the Society for Research in Child Development, 51*(2).

Dornbusch, S. M., Ritter, P. L., Leiderman, P. H., Roberts, D. F., & Fraleigh, M. J. (1987). The relation of parenting style to adolescent school performance. *Child Development, 58*, 1244–1257.

Evans, N., Farkas, A., Gilpin, E., Berry, C., & Pierce, J. P. (1995). Influence of tobacco marketing and exposure to smokers on adolescent susceptibility to smoking. *Journal of the National Cancer Institute, 87*, 1538–1545.

Federal Trade Commission. (1985). *Report to Congress: Pursuant to the Federal Cigarette Labeling and Advertising Act 1984*, Washington, DC: U.S. Government Printing Office.

Federal Trade Commission. (1995a). *Report to Congress: Pursuant to the Federal Cigarette Labeling and Advertising Act.* . Washington, DC: Federal Trade Commission.

Federal Trade Commission. (1995b). *Report to Congress: pursuant to the Comprehensive Smokeless Tobacco Health Education Act of 1986*. Washington, DC: Federal Trade Commission.

Feighery, E., Altman, D. G., & Shaffer, G. (1991). The effects of combining education and enforcement to reduce tobacco sales to minors. *JAMA, 266*, 3168–71.

Fischer, P. M., Schwartz, M. P., Richards, J. W., Goldstein, A. O., & Rojas, T. H. (1991). Brand logo recognition by children aged 3 to 6 years: Mickey Mouse and Old Joe the Camel. *Journal of the American Medical Association, 266*, 3145–3148.

Flay, B. R. (1985). Psychosocial approaches to smoking prevention: A review of findings. *Health Psychology, 4*, 449–488.

Food and Drug Administration. (1995). Regulations restricting the sale and distribution of cigarettes and smokeless tobacco products to protect children and adolescents: Proposed rule analysis regarding FDA's jurisdiction over nicotine-containing cigarettes and smokeless tobacco products. *Federal Register, 60*, No. 155.

Forster, J. L., Hourigan, M., & McGovern, P. (1992). Availability of cigarettes to underage youth in three communities. *Preventive Medicine, 21*, 320–328.

Forster, J. L., McBride, C., Jeffery, R., Schmid, T. L., & Pirie, P. L. (1991). Support for restrictive tobacco policies among residents of selected Minnesota communities. *American Journal of Health Promotion, 6*, 99–104.

Gambescia, S. F., & Corcoran, R. D. (1991). Youth access to tobacco: Future promise after decades of neglect. *Future Choices, 3*, 37–43.

Giovino, G. A., Schooley, M. W., Zhu, B. P., Chrismon, J. H., Peddicord, J. P., Merritt, R. K., Husten, C. G., & Erikson, M. P. (1994). Surveillance for selected tobacco-use behaviors: United States: 1900–1994. Morbidity and Mortality Weekly Report, 43*(SS-3), 1–43.*

Glynn, T. J. (1989). Essential elements of school-based smoking prevention programs. *Journal of School Health, 59,* 181–188.

Glynn, T. J., Greenwald, P., Mills, S. M., & Manley, M. W. (1993). Youth tobacco use in the United States: Problem, progress, goals, and potential solutions. *Preventive Medicine, 22,* 568–575.

Green, L. W. (1986, September). Individuals vs. systems: An artificial classification that divides and distorts. *HealthLink,* 29–30.

Grolnick, W. S., & Ryan, R. M. (1989). Parent styles associated with children's self-regulation and competence in school. *Journal of Educational Psychology, 81,* 143–154.

Hamilton, J. L. (1972). The demand for cigarettes: Advertising, the health scare, and the cigarette advertising ban. *Review of Economic Statistics, 54,* 401–411.

Hinds, M. W. (1992). Impact of a local ordinance banning tobacco sales to minors. *Public Health Reports, 107,* 355–358.

Hu, T. W., Sung, H. Y., & Keeler, T. E. (1995). Reducing cigarette consumption in California: Tobacco taxes vs. an anti-smoking media campaign. *American Journal of Public Health, 85,* 1218–1222.

IEG's complete guide to sponsorship: Everything you need to know about sports, arts, event, entertainment and cause marketing. (1995). Chicago, IL: IEG.

Jason, L. A., Ji, P. Y., Anes, M. D., & Birkhead, S. H. (1991). Active enforcement of cigarette control laws in the prevention of cigarette sales to minors. *JAMA, 266,* 3159–61.

Johnston, L. D. (1995). *Smoking rates climb among American teen-agers, who find smoking increasingly acceptable and seriously underestimate the risks.* Ann Arbor, MI: The University of Michigan News and Information Service.

Johnston, L. D., O'Malley, P. M., & Bachman, J. G. (1993). *National trends in drug use and related factors among American high school students and young adults, 1975–1992.* Rockville, MD: U.S. Department of Health and Human Services.

Johnston, L. D., O'Malley, P. M., & Bachman, J. G. (1994a). *National survey results on drug use from the Monitoring the Future Study, 1975–1992: Volume 1. Secondary school students.* Rockville, MD: National Institute on Drug Abuse.

Johnston, L. D., O'Malley, P. M., & Bachman, J. G. (1994b). *National trends in drug use and related factors among American high school students and young adults, 1975–1993.* Rockville, MD: U.S. Department of Health and Human Services.

Kandel, D. B., Yamaguchi, K., & Chen, K. (1992). Stages of progression in drug involvement from adolescence to adulthood: Further evidence for the gateway theory. *Journal of Studies on Alcohol, 20,* 447–457.

Keay, K. D., Woodruff, S. I., Wildey, M. B., & Kenney, E. M. (1993). Effect of a retailer intervention on cigarette sales to minors in San Diego County, California. *Tobacco Control, 2,* 145–151.

Kelly, J. G. (1966). Ecological constraints on mental health services. *American Psychologist, 21,* 535–539.

Kelly, J. G. (1968). Toward an ecological conception of preventive interventions. In J. W. J. Carter (Ed.), *Research contributions from psychology to community mental health* (pp. 75–99). New York: Behavioral Publications.

Kelly, J. G. (1971). Qualities for the community psychologist. *American Psychologist, 26,* 897–903.

Kelly, J. G. (1988). *A guide to conducting prevention research in the community.* New York: Haworth.

Kirn, T. F. (1987). Laws ban minors' tobacco purchases but enforcement is another matter. *Journal of the American Medical Association, 257*, 3323–3324.

Klonoff, E. A., Fritz, J. M., Landrine, H., Riddle, R. W., & Tully-Payne, L. (1994). The problem and sociocultural context of single-cigarette sales. *Journal of the American Medical Association, 271*, 618–620.

Lewin, K. (1951). *Field theory in social science.* New York: Harper/Torch.

Lynch, B. S., & Bonnie, R. J. (1994). *Growing up tobacco free: Preventing nicotine addiction in children and youths.* Washington, DC: National Academy Press.

Maccoby, E. E. (1980). *Social development.* New York: Harcourt Brace Jovanovich.

Maccoby, E. E., & Martin, J. A. (1983). Socialization in the context of the family: Parent-child interaction. In E. M. Hetherington (Ed.), *Socialization, personality, and social development* (Vol. 4, pp. 1–101). New York: John Wiley.

Mackay, J. (1994). The fight against tobacco in developing countries. *Tubercle and Lung Disease, 75*, 8–24.

McGinnis, J. M., & Lee, P. R. (1995). Healthy people 2000 at mid decade. *Journal of the American Medical Association, 273*, 1123–1129.

McLeroy, K. R., Bibeau, D., Steckler, A., & Glanz, K. (1988). An ecological perspective on health promotion programs. *Health Education Quarterly, 15*, 351–377.

Mills, R. C., & Kelly, J. G. (1972). Cultural adaptation and ecological analogies: Analysis of three Mexican villages. In S. E. Golannn & C. Eisdorfer (Eds.), *Handbook of community mental health*, . New York: Appleton-Century-Crofts.

Moos, R. H. (1979). Social ecological perspectives on health. In G. C. Stone, F. Cohen, & N. E. Adler (Eds.), *Health psychology: A handbook* (pp. 523–547). San Francisco: Jossey-Bass.

Moscovici, S. (1985). Social influence and conformity. In G. Lindzey & F. Aronson (Eds.), *Handbook of social psychology* (pp. 347–412). New York: Random House.

Murray, M., Kiryluk, S., & Swan, A. V. (1985). Relation between parents' and children's smoking behaviour and attitudes. *Journal of Epidemiology and Community Health, 39*, 169–174.

Naett, C. (1994). The tobacco industry and Eastern Europe: International Trade Fair and Symposium, Moscow, 21–24 September 1993. *Tobacco Control, 3*, 163–165.

National Cancer Institute. (1993). *The impact of cigarette excise taxes on smoking among children and adults: Summary report of a National Cancer Institute expert panel.* Bethesda, MD: National Cancer Institute.

Nolte, A. E., Smith, B. J., & O'Rourke, T. (1983). The relative importance of parental attitudes and behavior upon youth smoking behavior. *Journal of School Health, 53*, 264–271.

Pierce, J. P., Gilpin, E. A., Rosbrook, B., Davis, B., & Wright, W. (1995). *Who is receptive to current tobacco industry marketing practices?* Manuscript submitted for publication.

Popham, W. J. et al. (1993). Do anti-smoking media campaigns help smokers quit? *Public Health Reports, 108*, 510–513.

Pulkkinen, L. (1982). Self-control and continuity from childhood to late adolescence. In P. B. Baltes & O. G. Brian (Eds.), *Life-span development and behavior* (Vol. 4, pp. 63–104). New York: Academic Press.

Radecki, T. E., & Zdunich, C. D. (1993). Tobacco sales to minors in 97 US and Canadian communities. *Tobacco Control, 2*, 300–305.

Rappaport, J. (1977). *Community psychology: Values, research, and action.* New York: Holt, Rinehart, and Winston.

R. J. Reynolds reaches kids with "Moviegoer". (1986). *Tobacco and Youth Reporter, 1*, 13–14.

Roberts, W. L. (1986). Nonlinear models of development: An example from the socialization of competence. *Child Development, 57*, 1166–1178.

Rooney, B. L., & Murray, D. M. (1996). A meta-analysis of smoking prevention programs after adjustment for errors in the unit of analysis. *Health Education Quarterly, 23*, 48–64.

Simons, R. L., & Robertson, J. F. (1989). The impact of parenting factors, deviant peers, and coping style upon adolescent drug use. *Family Relations, 38*, 273–281.

Smith, M. J. (1982). *Persuasion and human action: A review and critique of social influence theories.* Belmont, CA: Wadsworth.

Steinberg, L., Elmen, J. D., & Mounts, N. S. (1989). Authoritative parenting, psychosocial maturity, and academic success among adolescents. *Child Development, 60*, 1424–1436.

Stokols, D. (1992). Establishing and maintaining healthy environments: Toward a social ecology of health promotion. *American Psychologist, 47*, 6–22.

Strouse, R., & Hall, J. (1994). *Robert Wood Johnson Foundation Youth Access Survey: Results of a national household survey to assess public attitudes about policy alternatives for limiting minors' access to tobacco products* (Report #26023). Princeton, NJ: Mathematica Policy Research, Inc.

Teel, S. J., Teel, J. E., & Bearden, W. O. (1979). Lessons learned from the broadcast cigarette advertising ban. *Journal of Marketing, 43*, 45–50.

Tobacco Institute. (1994). *The tax burden of tobacco. Volume 29.* Washington, DC: Tobacco Institute.

Trickett, E. J., Kelly, J. G., & Todd, D. M. (1972). The social environment of the high school: Guidelines for individual change and organizational redevelopment. In S. E. Golann & C. Eisdorfer (Eds.), *Handbook of community mental health* (pp. 331–406). New York: Appleton-Century-Crofts.

Tye, J. B., Warner, K. E., & Glantz, S. A. (1987). Tobacco advertising and consumption: evidence of a causal relationship. *Journal of Public Health Policy, 8*, 492–508.

U.S. Department of Health and Human Services. (1988). *The health consequences of smoking: Nicotine addiction. A report of the Surgeon General* (DHHS Publication No. PHS88–8406). Rockville, MD: U.S. Department of Health and Human Services.

U.S. Department of Health and Human Services. (1989). *Reducing the health consequences of smoking: 25 years of progress: A report of the Surgeon General* (DHHS Publication No. CDC89–8411). Rockville, MD: U.S. Department of Health and Human Services.

U.S. Department of Health and Human Services. (1990). *Smoking and health, a national status report: A report to Congress/Department of Health and Human*

Services (2nd ed.). (DHHS (CDC) 87–8396). Rockville, MD: U.S. Department of Health and Human Services.

U.S. Department of Health and Human Services. (1994). *Preventing tobacco use among young people: A report of the Surgeon General.* Atlanta, GA: Centers for Disease Control.

U.S. Department of Health and Human Services. (1995). *Tobacco-control activities in the United States, 1992–1993: Biennial report to Congress.* Atlanta, GA: Centers for Disease Control

University of California at San Diego & California Department of Health Services. (1990). *Tobacco use in California, 1990: A preliminary report documenting the decline of tobacco use.* Sacramento, CA: California Department of Health Services.

United States Department of Health and Human Services. (1990). *Youth access to cigarettes* (OEI-02-90-02310). Washington, DC: Health and Human Services, Office of the Inspector General, Office of Evaluation and Inspections.

United States Department of Health and Human Services. (1994). *Preventing tobacco use among young : A Report of the Surgeon General.* Atlanta, GA: Centers for Disease Control.

U.S. Inspector General. (1995). State oversight of tobacco sales to minors. Washington, DC: Author.

U.S. Public Health Service. (1964). *Smoking and Health. Report of the Advisory Committee to the Surgeon General of the Public Health Service.* U.S. Department of Health, Education, and Welfare, Public Health Service, Center for Disease Control. PHS Publication No. 1103.

Vincent, T. A., & Trickett, E. J. (1983). Preventive interventions and the human context: Ecological approaches to environmental assessment and change, *Preventive psychology: Theory, research and practice* (pp. 67–86). New York: Pergamon.

Warner, K. E. (1977). The effects of the anti-smoking campaign on cigarette consumption. *American Journal of Public Health,* 67(7), 645–50.

Warner, K. E. (1981). Cigarette smoking in the 1970s: The impact of the antismoking campaign on consumption. *Science, 211*, 729–731.

Warner, K. E. (1986). *Selling smoke: Cigarette advertising and public health.* Washington, DC: American Public Health Association.

Warner, K. E., Butler, J., Cummings, K. M., D'Onofrio, C., Davis, R. M., Flay, B., McKinney, M., Myers, M. L., Pertschuk, M., Robinson, R. G., Ryden, L., Schudson, M., Tye, J., & Wilkenfeld, J. (1992). Report of the Tobacco Policy Research Study Group on tobacco marketing and promotion. *Tobacco Control, 1*(supplement), S19–S23.

Warner, K. E., Ernster, V. L., Holbrook, J. H., Lewit, E. M., Pertschuk, M., Steinfeld, J. L., Tye, J. B., & Whelan, E. M. (1986). Promotion of tobacco products: Issues and policy options. *Journal of Health Politics, Policy and Law, 11*, 367–392.

Wicker, A. W. (1979). *An introduction to ecological psychology.* Monterey, CA: Brooks-Cole.

Wildey, M. B., Woodruff, S. I., Agro, A., Keay, K. D., Kenney, E. M., & Conway, T. L. (1995). Sustained effects of educating retailers to reduce cigarette sales to minors. *Public Health Reports, 110*, 625–629.

Winett, R. A., King, A. C., & Altman, D. G. (1989). *Health psychology and public health.* New York: Pergamon.

SECTION IV
Lifestyle Change and Adherence Issues Within Specific Populations

Sally A. Shumaker, Editor

There are many factors that influence lifestyle changes and adherence which are common across groups. However, there are also factors that are specific within groups. Such population strata variables as economic status, education, gender, ethnicity and race, rural/urban, access to care, and age, each contain characteristics that differentially explain the group's receptiveness and ability to initiate healthy lifestyle changes, as well as the group's ability to maintain new behaviors. In order to maximize the effectiveness of strategies designed to initiate and maintain healthy behaviors, it is important for behavioral scientists and healthcare providers to be sensitive to both within- and between-group differences. In Section IV, three chapters examine the role of age in furthering our understanding of lifestyles and adherence.

In Chapter 14, Orlandi and Dalton consider the importance of *establishing* healthy behaviors and avoiding unhealthy behaviors early in life. Given that lifestyle choices account for most premature deaths in the United States, and that most of these "choices" (e.g., food preferences, activity levels, smoking) are established in our youth, the importance of preventing the adoption of risky behaviors in our youth is clear. Further, even after an unhealthy behavior has been adopted, the longer the behavior persists, the more resistant it is to change. Thus, targeting youth for both prevention and intervention is critical. Orlandi and Dalton provide a review of the factors that influence health-related behaviors among youth, the intervention opportunities that exist for youth, and the barriers for youth adopting new health behaviors or discarding unhealthy old behaviors. Taking a levels of analysis approach to the issue, these authors consider factors from the intrapersonal to environmental/societal level that impact on the health behaviors of youths, and the various "channels" ranging from individual to societal, to reach youth. Orlandi and Dalton then provide a critical review of some of the most promising youth-based intervention programs, and end their chapter with a look toward the future: what we have learned from prior research and where we need to go from here in order to maximize the efficacy of youth-based health promotion.

In Chapter 15, Murdaugh draws our attention to the other end of the age spectrum: older adults. The elderly represent the fasting growing portion of the population of the United States. For many older adults, the targets for changes necessitated to improve health represent lifelong habits that are well-established and resistant to change. Further exacerbating this situation is the fact that chronic illnesses increase with age, and often older adults are faced with multiple comorbidities that require complex behavioral and pharmacological treatments. In this chapter, Murdaugh provides an in-depth review of the complex nature of nonadherence among older adults and the multiple factors that influence nonadherence among the elderly (e.g., ability, desire, physical and emotional health, the social environment, and pharmokinetics). Recognizing the heterogeneity of the elderly population, Murdaugh goes on to consider methods to assess an elder's capacity to adhere. She concludes the chapter with a critical analysis of potential strategies for enhancing optimal adherence among the elderly.

Adolescents are particularly vulnerable to adopting risky health behaviors. At a time when authority and adult norms are constantly questioned, peer pressure is strong, and one feels immortal, risky behaviors (e.g., reckless driving, unprotected sex, substance abuse) can be very seductive. Coupling this turbulent life stage with an already compromised health state presents a major challenge to the healthcare providers and behavioral scientists who work with adolescents with chronic diseases such as diabetes, asthma, or arthritis. Not surprisingly, adolescents with chronic diseases have been found to be at greater risk for nonadherence to treatment regimens than any other age group. In Chapter 16, Rapoff considers the challenge of adherence among adolescents with a chronic condition. He provides a review of the prevalence and consequences of adherence problems among adolescents. He then carefully reviews the factors that correlate with and predict nonadherence, including: the patients and their families, the conditions or diseases, and the treatment regimens. Rapoff discusses methods for improving adherence among adolescents with chronic conditions, and in the final section of the chapter, he considers the clinical implications of strategies designed to maximize healthy behaviors and adherence among this vulnerable group.

14

Lifestyle Interventions for the Young

Mario A. Orlandi and Lesa T. Dalton

INTRODUCTION

Children and youth represent our future; maintaining their health should be one of highest priorities. Because poor health takes a tremendous toll on a nation's resources—both directly, through the cost of treating disease, and indirectly, through lowered productivity and reduced social well-being—steps taken to enhance the health of our youth today can reap significant economic and social rewards in the future. The basic premise of this chapter is that health status can be influenced by interventions designed to promote a healthy lifestyle, and that such interventions are most cost-efficient when delivered early in life and early in the natural history of a health problem's development.

The chapter begins by providing a rationale and logic for youth-focused lifestyle interventions as a critical component of broader public health initiatives. A framework for planning and implementing health-promotion interventions for the young is then described. Opportunities for promoting health among the young are contrasted with anticipated barriers and examples of prototypical programs are described. Concluding comments focus upon the need for integrated, rather than piecemeal, solutions and strategic planning, rather than crisis management, as we approach the new millennium.

THE LOGIC OF LIFESTYLE INTERVENTIONS FOR YOUTH

Lifestyle interventions are planned initiatives designed to promote health-enhancing behavior and to inhibit health-compromising behavior. In order to appreciate the particular value of lifestyle interventions for children and youth, it is important to understand (1) the relationship between behavior and health and the extent to which a health problem or illness can potentially be influenced or avoided through behavior change; (2) the particular value of lifestyle interventions delivered early in the lifespan; and (3) the determinants of behavior which are appropriate targets for youth interventions.

THE ROLE OF LIFESTYLE IN DETERMINING HEALTH

The U.S. Public Health Service has identified four major factors which contribute to avoidable illness or premature death (United States Department of Health, Education, and Welfare [USDHEW], 1979). Their epidemiological data showed for the first time that, in developed countries such as the United States, 20% of avoidable illness was caused primarily by heredity factors, 20% by environment, 10% by inadequacies of the health-care delivery system, and 50% by lifestyle or behavioral choices. These data demonstrate that, to a large extent, individuals can control their health and longevity by the type of lifestyle they choose to lead. The influence of these data on medical care systems and public health planning has been enormous. To appreciate this fully, it is useful to look at some of these issues historically.

It is now understood that lifestyle choices can be influenced and shaped by psychological, sociological, and environmental interventions collectively grouped under the heading of "health promotion." This is, however, a relatively new term which had its origins in a generalized epidemiological model first proposed by Leavell and Clark (1965), who defined "health promotion" as a prepathogenic level of intervention designed to enhance the general health and well-being of an individual. This approach was consistent with a subsequent formulation by the World Health Organization [WHO] (1977) which redefined health as a "state of complete physical, mental, and social well-being; not merely the absence of disease or infirmity." While Leavell and Clark viewed health promotion as related conceptually to primary prevention, they clearly distinguished it from traditional notions of disease prevention in that, rather than merely reducing disease risk, the goal was seen as improving performance in all aspects of human functioning. The definition for health promotion commonly used today was developed by

Green (1979) and groups under the rubric of health promotion "any combination of health education and related organizational, political, and economic interventions designed to facilitate behavioral and environmental adaptations that will improve or protect health." (p. 161)

As a result of efforts to define health promotion, a new way evolved of conceptualizing the determinants of health; the locus of responsibility for an individual's health; and the steps that could be taken to enhance health status. By elevating personal health behavior to the status of a primary health determinant, individuals were made to bear a portion of the responsibility for their own health, and interventions designed to influence lifestyle choices were provided with a logical and scientifically justified rationale.

The Advantages of Early Intervention

While the potential clearly exists to influence the health status of all individuals through interventions designed to modify lifestyle decisions, there are distinct advantages to intervening when individuals are younger. Many of the most significant health problems of adulthood have their origins in risk factors established during childhood. The most extensively studied of these risks are those related to chronic health disorders such as heart disease and cancer. The major risk factors for these diseases originate during childhood when tobacco use is initiated, dietary patterns are established, and exercise habits are learned (Stone, Perry, & Luepker, 1989).

The longer such behaviors remain an integral part of an individual's lifestyle repertoire, the more difficult it is to modify them (United States Department of Health and Human Services [USDHS], 1991). Similarly, individuals who exhibit one or more unhealthy lifestyle behaviors are more likely to develop others (Centers for Disease Control [CDC], 1991). It has also been conclusively shown that some of the physiological processes that lead to chronic disease in adults begin in childhood. For example, autopsy studies have demonstrated that early indicators of atherosclerosis, including plaque formation, are already evident in children (Newman, Wattigney, & Berenson, 1991), and that these indicators are correlated with elevated blood cholesterol levels in the young (PDAY Research Group, 1990). These factors, combined with the difficulty and cost associated with interventions like smoking cessation and weight reduction among adults, argue persuasively for the need for interventions early in life.

It is clear that significant segments of our youth are already at risk for a variety of preventable health and social problems. For example, 72% of all deaths among school-age youth and young adults ages 5–24 result from only four causes: motor vehicle crashes (30%); other unintentional injuries (12%); homicide (19%); and suicide (11%). In addition, approximately 1 million pregnancies occur among adolescents and more than 10 million cases of sexually transmitted diseases (STDs) are documented in the youngest age group (ages 15–29) for which data are recorded (Kann et al., 1995).

When this information is combined with the epidemiological data related to chronic diseases, it becomes clear that the following six categories of behaviors which are the leading causes of morbidity and mortality affecting the nation today are established during youth:

1. Behaviors that contribute to unintentional and intentional injury;
2. tobacco use;
3. alcohol and other drug use;
4. sexual behaviors that contribute to unintended pregnancy and STDs, including HIV infection;
5. unhealthy dietary patterns; and
6. physical inactivity.

Interventions which have the potential to influence such behaviors and lifestyle choices at an early age are both justified and needed.

Determinants of Health-Related Behavior Among Youth

Lifestyle interventions that have the potential to be effective among youth include those designed to promote health-enhancing behaviors and those designed to inhibit health-compromising behaviors. In order for such interventions to be efficacious, they must take into account and attempt to influence factors that are determinants of youth behavior—particularly those behaviors related to known risks for health problems and disease.

Most of what we know today regarding the determinants of health behavior among youth was derived from intervention development research. When this research began in earnest over three decades ago, our knowledge of what determined behavior and how to influence it was limited. A primary focus of these studies was the prevention of tobacco use because of this risk factor's preeminent status as the most significant cause of avoidable death and disease yet identified—a distinction which it maintains to this day (USDHHS, 1989). Early efforts tested the theory that providing youth with information about the risks of unhealthy behavior and the benefits of leading a healthy life would shape their lifestyle decisions. It was soon determined, however, that knowledge about health and disease does not have a significant effect on health-related behaviors (Goodstadt, 1978). Such approaches ignored a host of interpersonal, psychological, and environmental factors that influence behaviors.

Analogous to the informational approaches were affective interventions. Thses were based on the assumption that changes in attitudinal variables such as self-esteem and self-efficacy would influence health-related behavioral choices. However, when adolescents were taught skills such as stress management or decisionmaking to enhance their sense of self-efficacy, significant effects on behaviors were not achieved (Tobler, 1986).

The results of each study testing a theory which focused on a single factor or category of factors as determinants of health-related behaviors underscored the need to consider multiple factors. Gradually there evolved a number of theories which were based on the realization that health-related behaviors are either learned through social interaction or have social contingencies which provide positive or negative reinforcements. Evans (1983) referred to this as the Social Influences Model, through which he attempted to provide adolescents with resistance against the influences that promote poor health (e.g., mass media, product advertising, peer pressure). Kendall and Hollon (1979) developed a cognitive behavioral approach which assumed the importance of both social and psychological factors, and that behaviors such as tobacco use are learned as a method for meeting social needs. This approach adopted the basic social influences approach and added role-playing, behavioral rehearsal, and reinforcement of pressure-resistance skills. Results from the evaluations of these approaches to smoking prevention have been promising, though they are subject to a number of methodological limitations (Flay, 1985).

The Life-Skills Training Model combines the elements of both the social influences and social cognitive approaches, and incorporates methods to develop greater autonomy, self-esteem, and self-confidence from the affective approaches. This approach, which has been shown to be highly effective, also provides considerable training to help adolescents cope with a broad range of social challenges (Botvin & Eng, 1982).

The social influences, cognitive-behavioral, and life-skills approaches are each examples of interventions that are grounded in Bandura's social learning theory (Bandura, 1986). An underlying assumption of social learning theory is that behavior is dynamic and depends on environmental, intrapsychic, and interpersonal constructs that influence each other simultaneously. Adherence to this model has led intervention developers to incorporate various components in a variety of combinations, delivered through multiple channels, in order to reach youth with positive health messages in a style that is more consistent with the dynamic, integrated manner in which competing, negative health messages are delivered. What has been learned about the determinants of youth behavior can be used to guide the development of new and innovative interventions.

IDENTIFYING INTERVENTION OPPORTUNITIES AND ANTICIPATING BARRIERS

Children today grow up in an environment that increasingly encourages risk-taking behaviors and lifestyles that are not conducive to good health. In order to intervene in ways that effectively discourage and overcome these influences, it is necessary to consider the domains defined by social learning theory and the variety of channels through which the intervention can be delivered. These different domains and delivery channels may be used to define a framework for planning lifestyle interventions for youth. Social learning theory, for example, identifies three domains which can be considered in planning a lifestyle intervention for youth: the intrapsychic, the interpersonal, and the broader environmental domain. Some of the various channels for delivering interventions include the school, the home, the community, and the mass media. Each of these channels will be discussed separately and then considered collectively as part of the intervention planning process.

Intrapsychic Factors

This domain includes each of the many psychological processes that an individual goes through as situations and sets of stimuli are synthesized, analyzed, and then translated into behavior. Broadly speaking, these processes include cognitive factors (e.g., awareness, knowledge); affective factors (e.g., attitudes, beliefs, values, perceptions of self, behavioral intentions); and skills. Successful interventions typically incorporate various combinations of these factors to inform, motivate, and train individuals to adopt healthy lifestyles.

Interpersonal Factors

A critical element of social learning theory is the degree to which other people provide an individual with either positive or negative forms of social reinforcement for performing certain behaviors. These people may be family members, relatives, friends, peers, or others. The motivation to gain social acceptance or to avoid social disapprobation is very powerful, and operates differently at different points during the passage from childhood through adolescence to adulthood.

Environmental Factors

The broader societal environment is saturated with negative health influences. These include powerful images on television, in books, magazines, and movies, and other forms of mass media that are used to shape young people's impressions of who and what are acceptable. Since such images are typically selected to sell particular products or services, they are seldom consistent with messages designed to promote positive health habits. When the products being sold are themselves vehicles of poor health (e.g., tobacco or alcohol products), the influence which must be overcome is even more powerful.

The School as an Intervention Delivery Channel

Nearly 48 million students, or about 20% of the American population, are enrolled in public and private schools nationwide (O'Rourke, 1995). Schools provide excellent access for reaching children and youth. The majority of youth lifestyle interventions which have been developed and tested have been designed for implementation through the schools. Despite the obvious opportunities which schools provide for intervening with youth, a number of barriers should be noted. Many school systems do not recognize lifestyle interventions as appropriate subject matter for their curricula. Under considerable pressure to achieve high standards in traditional subjects like reading, science, and mathematics, some school systems view lifestyle-intervention programs as unnecessary. Similarly, most school systems do not have the resources to adopt and implement such programs.

The Home as an Intervention Delivery Channel

Parents and other family members can have a significant influence on the development of a young person's health-related attitudes and practices. Children often develop risk factors that are similar to those of their parents and siblings, though comparable patterns of healthy behavior can be promoted as well (Perry et al., 1988). When a home environment is unhealthy, it tends to invalidate other health-promotion messages which children and youth receive in school or through other channels (Winett et al., 1992). Interventions designed for delivery through the home are, however, more difficult to deliver systematically (i.e., in a particular scope and sequence) than are school-based programs, and implementation fidelity tends to be more of a problem with home delivery than with teacher-led classroom programs.

The Community as an Intervention Delivery Channel

Some initiatives are intended for delivery through other community organizations (such as Boy's or Girl's Clubs) or throughout the general community. The advantage of targeting interventions through these additional community channels is that they provide more opportunities for reaching youth in settings that are not typically thought of as delivery points for lifestyle interventions. Such settings have particular applicability for youth that are frequently absent from schools or who are less likely to receive interventions through other channels. In addition, students who have received interventions via other channels have an opportunity to validate and support those positive health messages. Barriers to community-based interventions include: difficulty in delivering in any particular scope and sequence, and the challenge of consistent implementation (Pentz, Dwyer, et al., 1989).

The Mass Media as an Intervention Delivery Channel

Lifestyle interventions may be delivered through mass media, such as radio, television, movies, magazines, and other communication vehicles typically used for product advertising. Since these types of communications are often delivered periodically, it is possible to achieve an approximation of desired scope and sequence, though implementation fidelity is difficult to control. A typical use of such media is to support interventions delivered through other channels and to provide messages that compete with the advertising of unhealthy products such as tobacco (Flay et al., 1988).

Program Planning

The behavioral determinants and delivery channels described above provide a useful framework for planning lifestyle interventions for youth. Successful programs often attempt to deliver a series of intervention messages over a specified time period that address particular health-related behaviors in a variety of ways. By identifying both the social-learning or behavioral focus and the delivery channel for any particular intervention message, appropriate objectives for that intervention can be identified and the program's success more reliably evaluated.

INNOVATIVE INTERVENTION PROGRAMS

A wide variety of programs have been developed that can be defined in terms of the social learning factors and delivery channels described above. Several are reviewed here which represent unique approaches or innovations that can serve as prototypes to program planners working in comparable settings.

The Minnesota Home Team

The Home Team was developed to educate youth about cancer risk factors through a home-based intervention involving parents (Perry et al., 1988).

The intervention targeted third-graders and their parents in Minnesota and North Dakota; a study was conducted to compare the efficacy of parental involvement in cancer risk reduction for youth with a more traditional, school-based approach. Four conditions were established to test the efficacy of this nutrition-focused program. Using schools as the unit of sampling, 31 schools were blocked by state and randomly assigned to one of four conditions: the school based Hearty Heart program (HH); the home-based Home Team program (HT); both programs in sequence (HH, HT); or a no-treatment control group (C).

The Hearty Heart program, an established third grade curriculum, was implemented by teachers over a 5-week period. The Home Team, also a 5-week program, was a correspondence course sent in packets to parents on a weekly basis. The packets were designed as a family game using a baseball motif. Similar to the school-based curriculum, the Home Team emphasized skills to modify the diet, participation in recipe planning and food selection, and setting goals for behavior change.

Data included pre- and post-test surveys conducted either in school (HH) or in the home (HT) by trained personnel; observations, both in class and in the home; a 24-hour dietary recall, and a urine sample from a subset of students. The Home Team approach had a positive influence on behavior for both children and their families. Fat intake, percentage of calories from saturated fat, and percentage of calories from monounsaturated fat were all significantly lower for children in Home Team groups, independent of participation in the Hearty Heart School curriculum (Crockett, Mullis, Perry, & Luepker, 1989).

The Texas A Su Salud Project

An intervention designed for Hispanic populations called "A Su Salud," (To Your Health), targeted Mexicans in two southern Texas cities (Eagle Pass and Del Rio) and Piedras Negras, a border city in Mexico. Initially, this was a 5-year longitudinal, community-based study aimed at smoking prevention and cessation. As part of the larger study, an additional community intervention project was introduced in Eagle Pass to reduce general health risks and promote health behavior change.

The A Su Salud intervention distinguished itself from other mass media health promotion programs through its use of role models as part of the message design (Ramirez & McAlister, 1988). In addition, the project recruited community volunteers to serve as program spokespersons. Using physicians, local residents who had recently initiated a lifestyle change to improve their health, and nonsmoking youth, television programs were developed to address local health concerns. Fifteen different programs were developed using a news format through which physicians discussed health information (See Amezcua, McAlister, Ramirez, & Espinoza, 1990 for more information).

Though the overall program attempted to reach both adults and children, a number of the intervention activities were designed specifically for children. For example, through programs delivered at the elementary, junior-high, and high-school levels, children were encouraged to advocate for nonsmoking and to help their parents quit. Also, student behavior was targeted for other lifestyle interventions, specifically in the area of substance abuse prevention. At the elementary level, school librarians were given teachers' manuals and a video cassette describing role-play activities. The content focused on preventing the onset of tobacco and other drug use and resisting peer pressure to smoke.

Since the youth intervention was only a component of the larger community program, there were no data reported regarding the effectiveness of the youth activities. However, results from other school-based smoking prevention programs suggest that parents are pressured to quit smoking by their children, and there is a consistent correlation between parent and youth smoking, indicating that influencing smoking among youth has the potential to influence adult smokers (Bowen, Dalton, Walker, Crystal, & Orlandi, 1995).

Life Skills Training

The Life Skills Training program is a school-based, substance abuse prevention program utilizing a competency enhancement approach; it has been evaluated through a series of more than eight intervention field trials since the early 1980s. The program, which has been tested among youth populations from a variety of socioeconomic and racial/ethnic backgrounds, stresses self-improvement by focusing on the development of important personal and social skills.

The LST program is designed to be introduced in the 7th grade and consists of 12 units which are presented over the course of 15–20 class sessions. Booster sessions in the 8th and 9th grade are designed to reinforce material covered in the first year of the program. There are 10 booster sessions in the second year and 5 booster sessions in the third year (Dusenbury & Botvin, 1992). Program providers must be good role models who do not engage in substance abuse and who exemplify the skills being taught. Teachers, peer role models, and health professionals have been successfully trained to deliver the LST program. The extent of training has been based on the providers' experience and background.

Thousands of youth have participated in this program which has demonstrated effectiveness in preventing substance use. Problem drinking and the use of marijuana and cigarettes have all been reduced, with behavioral changes lasting up to 3 years. However, the developers have noted that disadvantaged youth need positive life options in their environment to increase the program's ability to effect change.

The Midwestern Prevention Project

The Midwestern Prevention Project was a 6-year longitudinal school-based substance abuse prevention intervention supported by a wide variety of community-based components. It was implemented in 107 schools in Kansas City and Indianapolis. The intervention schools employed mass media, parent, community organizations, and health policy programming to reduce the prevalence of gateway drug use among adolescents (Pentz et al., 1989).

The intervention's school component consisted of a 10-session program for resisting and counteracting drug influences. This program incorporated a set of prevention practice activities to be carried out by the students with their parents. The school intervention was supported by mass media events and programs, parent education activities promoting effective parent-child communication and interaction, and school health-policy initiatives. Extensive media coverage of program messages and goals including commercials, news clips, press conferences, and talk shows helped to promote the various intervention efforts. A smaller panel study of 16 schools tested the effects of this prevention program as it related to individual risk factors for drug abuse. Researchers tracked students from grade 6 to grade 10 in schools where communities had either been exposed to the entire intervention or, in the case of control schools, were exposed to mass media and community-organization efforts.

The results from the smaller study indicated that the community-based prevention program was effective in reducing the prevalence of monthly cigarettes smoked and marijuana use at the 9th and 10th grade levels. This occurred 3 years after delivery of the school-based component, suggesting that the intervention, reinforced by other community components, had sustained effects. Assignment of schools in this study were random, overcoming a limitation of previous reports from the larger study, and contributing greatly to the interpretability of the findings. The smaller study design did not permit assessment of the effects of mass media and community-organization efforts to condition. It is apparent, however, that the mass media program and community-organization efforts alone had a relatively modest impact on primary outcomes as compared to the comprehensive program (Johnson et al., 1990).

Violence Prevention Project

The Violence Prevention Project of Boston, Massachusetts, was an effort to combine mass media with a curriculum designed to effect behavior change

(Hausman, Spivak, Prothrow-Stith, & Roeber, 1992). A unique aspect of this study is that it sought to involve various sectors of the community in the delivery of a violence-prevention intervention, with the intention of the community taking ownership of the project in the process.

Youth between the ages of 10 and 19 from two Boston neighborhoods with high violent crime rates and low socioeconomic status were targeted for intervention. Other neighborhoods served as control sites. The project trained community service providers from a variety of agencies to deliver an established violence-prevention curriculum that was tailored to their particular setting. Promotional materials such as posters and T-shirts were distributed throughout the intervention neighborhoods to support the curriculum and promote the mass media campaign.

Local public television stations aired two television programs which the project team designed for the mass media campaign, and which were supported by a local advertising club. The campaign was designed to (1) raise public awareness of the issue of adolescent violence; (2) provide a visual message to youth about the consequences of their behavior; and (3) reinforce the message of violence prevention that was promulgated throughout the community. The slogan for the campaign was "Friends for life, don't let friends fight".

Youth participation in project activities was tracked through various agencies involved in the project. Approximately 46% of the agencies implemented some form of continuous violence education activities, and 42% reported implementing at least one related activity. A follow-up survey indicated that approximately 56% of the youth sampled reported some exposure to violence-prevention activities. Although this study had several limitations, the authors noted that participating community agencies continued to implement the violence prevention activities a year after the study had concluded.

San Diego Family Health Project

The San Diego Family Health Project provides another view of family interventions in action. Using elementary schools both as the sampling unit and for recruitment purposes, 206 Mexican and Anglo-American families with at least one child in either fifth or sixth grade participated in this cardiovascular risk-reduction project (Nader et al., 1989). An intensive recruitment process to improve cohort maintenance was carried out, this included take-home surveys, two to three informational meetings, and take-home measurement activities. Subsequently, baseline data were collected on the remaining participants. Families were given financial incentives after baseline and were contacted repeatedly throughout the intervention phase to maximize involvement. Participation rates remained high throughout the course of the 24-month study.

Intervention families received 3 months of intensive weekly interventions, followed by 9 months of monthly or bimonthly maintenance sessions. Families were grouped for ethnic homogeneity. The four-part program began with a family aerobic exercise session. Parents and children were then separated into groups for educational sessions. Games were used in the children's group to facilitate the educational process. Families then reconvened into one group setting to assess progress, engage in group problem-solving, set behavior change and support goals, and mutually encourage progress in health habit changes. Finally, a social time, often with music, was held. Families took turns bringing a healthy snack (often a new recipe) for others to try.

Data included physiological measures such as blood pressure and serum cholesterol, dietary recall assessments, direct observations, and health-knowledge scales. Overall, the results indicated that both populations in the treatment group attained more knowledge of behavior modification skills related to CVD risk reduction than did the control group. In addition, researchers noted that there were more changes among the Anglo-American intervention participants than their Mexican-American counterparts, and that intervention subjects changed dietary behavior more than their physical activity.

Home-Based HIV/AIDS Prevention Project

Another innovative approach to reducing risk factors in youth involved an HIV/AIDS prevention intervention based on a video program targeting children aged 12–14 (Winett et al., 1992). This project was carried out in Roanoke, Virginia and was a home-based program involving parents and family recruitment by their physicians.

The 49 families recruited for the initial study were randomly assigned to either an experimental or control group. All families received an in-home baseline assessment and then experimental families received the video program and were instructed by family interviewers in its use. Parents were advised to view the entire program first and then to watch it again with their children.

The four-part program totals 120 minutes. The first tape includes: (1) an introduction describing the rationale for the program; (2) facts about HIV transmission; (3) identification of youth risk factors associated with HIV; and (4) a description of various preventive measures. Tape 2 presents a short drama of a typical family with one older and two younger teenagers. The story line follows the family through several small crisis situations demonstrating that, although the family members like one another and communicate well, the family as a unit and each family member individually would be helped with problem-solving and assertiveness.

The third tape fosters skill-building by showing a family using the skills they have acquired to address the family issues depicted in Tape 2. Though the authors reported that the evaluation indicated that the video program needed modification, they were encouraged by the potential to provide a HIV/AIDS prevention intervention to large numbers of families through this relatively cost-efficient and innovative format. In addition, there was evidence that the home-based video program was effective in increasing knowledge related to HIV/AIDS prevention and problem-solving.

The Boy and Woman Bear Program

The Boy and Woman Bear Program is a computer software innovation addressing cancer risk reduction in Native American adolescents (Schinke, Moncher, & Singer, 1994). Based on the Seneca Nation legend known as The Boy Who Lived with Bears, the researchers developed an adaptation of the story entitled the "Boy and the Woman Bear." The story focuses on translating food choices and eating habits into native customs and traditions in ways that make use of successful intervention approaches employed previously for a Native American youth intervention on tobacco use. In that intervention, the use of tobacco for traditional and ceremonial purposes is distinguished from nontraditional habitual smoking, highlighting its harmful effects.

Study participants were randomly assigned to either the treatment or control condition. A pre-test was given through an interactive computer program that prompted them to respond to multiple-choice questions. Control students answered the same questions via paper and pencil. After completing the pre-test, intervention participants viewed the computer program which consists of 77 separate visual screens that pictorially present the "Boy and the Woman Bear" story. Control students viewed a 30-minute videotape in school which told a story about a youth taught by his mentor how to make everyday decisions and resolve problems. Upon completion of both stories, the post-test was administered to each group.

The results of this pilot indicated that when compared to control students, the intervention students had increased their knowledge of nutritional information related to risk reduction, and had developed a positive attitude towards initiating behaviors related to good health. The outcome data also suggest that the personal computer holds potential as an effective method for delivering cancer-prevention interventions.

The Television, School, and Family Project

While many lifestyle intervention programs for youth consider mass media and school-based components separately, the Television, School, and Family Project (TVSFP) sought to determine both the combined and the independent effects of using mass media to enhance school-based tobacco control curricula (Flay et al., 1988). The TVSFP curriculum contains seven key elements: (1) correction of norms (particularly misperceptions of the prevalence of tobacco use among adolescents and in the general population); (2) awareness of peer influences to smoke; (3) development of peer resistance skills; (4) awareness of family influences to use tobacco; (5) development of media influence resistance skills; (6) instruction on the social and physiological consequences of smoking; and (7) development of decision-making skills.

An evaluation of this intervention involved 7th-grade students and their families in Southern California attending 47 public schools in Los Angeles and San Diego. These schools were randomly assigned to 5 conditions. The study was designed to determine the relative efficacy of three approaches to the delivery of a smoking and drug-abuse prevention curriculum: (1) a social resistance classroom curriculum plus mass broadcast TV segments (CR & TV); (2) classroom-only (CR-Only); and (3) mass broadcast TV segments with only classroom encouragement to view (TV-only). A health information attention control curriculum group and a measurement-only group were established as the two controls.

Outcomes measuring youth tobacco use, intent to smoke, knowledge and attitudes towards tobacco and health, and parent smoking prevalence and cessation were among some of the dependent variables analyzed. Although researchers admit that the television program was poorly implemented and the classroom component was delivered inconsistently, there were indications that the combined use of mass media and classroom components can enhance the effectiveness of either component provided alone. It was also apparent that the combined format was widely accepted by students, parents, and teachers.

The Know Your Body Program

The Know Your Body (KYB) Program is a comprehensive, skills-based health promotion program targeting elementary schools (Resnicow, Cross & Wynder, 1993). It is designed to empower children—from kindergarten through grade 6—with the knowledge, attitude, skills, and experience necessary to practice positive health behaviors and control risk factors related to factors such as nutrition; alcohol, tobacco, and other drug use; exercise; dental care; disease prevention; injury prevention; self-management; growth and development; healthy relationships; consumer advocacy; and environmental health.

The KYB program consists of five components: a skills-based health education curriculum, teacher/coordinator training, a biomedical screening, extracurricular activities, and program evaluation. Extracurricular activities constitute one optional component of KYB. Each module contains a list of activities and projects that are incorporated into daily instruction. These include recycling drives, fitness walks, peer leadership programs, and heart-healthy food-tasting parties. These activities are designed to creatively involve children, parents, teachers, administrators, health professionals, and community members. Schools have the option of modifying the program to accommodate their needs, goals, philosophy, and capacity. The program was developed as a tool for integrating health activities with other subject areas, such as math, science, social studies, language arts, dramatic arts, and communication arts. Each teacher's guide utilizes a variety of teaching methods such as small-group activities, cooperative teaming, role-playing and simulations, brainstorming, and whole-group processing.

The impact of the KYB program has been evaluated in a number of randomized field trials. These studies have shown that after a 3-year follow-up, consistent positive intervention effects persisted for a number of outcome measures including systolic blood pressure, diastolic blood pressure, smoking, HDL cholesterol, and health knowledge. Results for other outcomes were mixed.

Summary: Strengths and Weaknesses

The intervention programs described have approached the challenge of promoting health among youth in a wide variety of ways. There are several perspectives from which these programs can be summarized and compared: first, according to the risk factors or health factors that are targeted; second, according to the delivery channels employed; and, third, according to the extent to which evaluation has played an integral role in the program's development. Table 14.1 compares the programs reviewed in this chapter along these dimensions.

As Table 14.1 shows, the majority of the programs reviewed are designed to address a single risk factor or related group of factors. Narrowly focused programs of this sort are, in fact, much more common than multiple risk-factor or comprehensive programs. This is partially due to the fact that comprehensive programs are more expensive and more difficult to administrate. It is also due to the fact that the National Institutes of Health, which are organized around specific diseases, have for decades promoted disease-specific and single risk-factor interventions in an attempt to further the goals of the individual institutes. For this reason, program planners who want to address a range of health problems are often confronted with the challenge of trying to implement and coordinate a large number of separate programs simultaneously. More often than not, they decide instead to take a selective approach and ignore some health problems for the sake of others they consider more critical.

Table 14.1 also notes that the programs reviewed have been designed for implementation through various delivery channels including, for example,

TABLE 14.1 Comparison of Intervention Programs

Program Name	*Risk Factor or Health Factor*	*Delivery Channel*	*Evaluation Focus*
The Minnesota Home Team Program	cancer risk reduction	family	high
A Su Salud Program	tobacco use control	community organizations, mass media	low
Life Skills Training Program	drug use prevention	school	high
Midwestern Prevention Project	drug use prevention	school, family, mass media	high
Violence Prevention Project	violence prevention mass media	community organizations, low	
San Diego Family Health Project	cardiovascular disease prevention	family	medium
Home Based HIV/AIDS Prevention Project	HIV / AIDS prevention	family	medium
Boy and Woman Bear Program	cancer risk reduction	personal computer	medium
Television, School, and Family Project	tobacco use control	school, family, mass media	high
Know Your Body Program	comprehensive	school, family	high

the school, the home or family, and mass media. Though a decade ago lifestyle interventions for youth were restricted primarily to school-based programs, significant advances have been made in the development of out-of-school approaches. It is important to note that recent development has emphasized the role of home-based and mass media approaches both as adjuncts to school-based programs and as stand-alone interventions. Little effort has been made, however, to coordinate these various approaches, or to maximize their collective effects on the youth who participate in them.

Finally, Table 14.1 also notes considerable variation in the priority which each program gives to evaluation as an integral aspect of development. Program developers who place a high priority on evaluation have carried out formative research to improve the intervention's appropriateness for its target group; they have tested the intervention in a true experimental design; they have assessed multiple indicators, including knowledge, attitude, behavior, and physiological validation when appropriate; and they have used longitudinal designs to determine whether changes observed in the short term are maintained over the long term. Unfortunately, many programs are either poorly evaluated or not evaluated at all. When this occurs it is difficult, if not impossible, to determine whether they have been effective.

PREPARING FOR THE FUTURE

This chapter has described lifestyle interventions for youth from a variety of perspectives. A case was made for the planning and implementation of early preventive interventions as effective strategies for controlling avoidable disease and death, as well as a variety of other social and economic problems known to be correlated with poor health.

In conclusion, this final section addresses the need as we approach the new millennium for integrated, rather than piecemeal, solutions to the planning of lifestyle interventions for the young. Needed improvement is identified in three areas.

First, there is a need for a greater emphasis on program evaluation. Unfortunately, the programs which are more likely to incorporate evaluation into their developmental planning are those which have been created through research grants. From this perspective, evaluation is more of a funding agency requirement rather than a planning tool. Since evaluation requires resources, perhaps it should be advocated that all agencies which fund larger research initiatives should also set aside funds to promote evaluation among those program developers who do not usually have sufficient resources to consider this option. Adequate training would clearly be a prerequisite, as would the creation of a mechanism for administering such evaluation funds that would operate separately from the routine research grant process. If youth health programs that hold great potential are never adequately evaluated, they can make very little contribution to the common enterprise of public health promotion—and this represents a tremendous and unfortunate loss that is entirely avoidable.

Second, there is a great need for youth health promotion programs and initiatives that strive to exert their influence at levels beyond the home, the school, or even the realm of individual television programs. Despite the influence that the types of programs reviewed in this chapter may have on youth in the short term, those effects tend to fade over time. One reason for this may be that the broader social context within which our youth are growing up is both powerful and equivocal with respect to many health values. Movies, music videos, books, magazines, advertisements, the Internet and other media tend to work in concert to establish the social normative structure that youth reference when they choose healthy or unhealthy lifestyles. From this perspective, it is unfortunate that unhealthy lifestyles, including violence, drug use and unprotected sex, are promoted through these channels. No government or private organization has yet made a concerted effort to broadly promote a healthy lifestyle as a social norm—something that youth would in fact expect of themselves and others.

Third, there is a need for greater coordination of youth health programs. While the wide range of innovative interventions described is certainly a tribute to their developers, they represent, to a great extent, an admixture of approaches that benefit very little from their efforts in common, and that fail to achieve any significant economies of scale. Unfortunately, some of these initiatives are even redundant, due primarily to the lack of any central coordination or integration of these impressive efforts. Despite the central role that schools can play in promoting health among children and adolescents, the majority of our nation's states have yet to mandate comprehensive health education for the young. Such legislation is desperately needed, as are efforts to coordinate and share information about interventions designed to control avoidable morbidity and mortality through early intervention. If strategic planning for the future health of our children replaces the mindset of crisis management, all succeeding generations will be the beneficiaries.

REFERENCES

Amezcua, C., McAlister, A., Ramirez, A., & Espinoza, R. (1990). *A Su Salud*: Health promotion in a Mexican-American border community. In N. Bracht (Ed.), *Health promotion at the community level.* (pp. 257–277). Newbury Park, CA: Sage.

Bandura, A. (1986). *Social foundations of thought and action.* Englewood Cliffs, NJ: Prentice-Hall.

Botvin, G. J., & Eng, A. (1982). The efficacy of a multicomponent approach to the prevention of cigarette smoking. *Preventive Medicine, 11*, 199–211.

Bowen, D., Dalton, L., Walker, R., Crystal, S., & Orlandi, M. A. (1995). Promoting community-wide tobacco control activities by involving schools. In B. Thompson, D. Burns, & W. Lynn (Eds.), *Community-based interventions for smokers: The COMMIT field experience* (Smoking and Tobacco Control Monograph No. 6) (pp. 209–224). Bethesda, MD: National Cancer Institute.

Centers for Disease Control. Selected tobacco use and dietary patterns among high school students in the United States (1992). *Morbidity and Mortality Weekly Report, 41*, 417–421.

Crockett, S. J., Mullis, R., Perry, C. L., & Luepker, R. V. (1989). Parent education in youth-directed nutrition interventions. *Preventive Medicine, 18*, 471–491.

Dusenbury, L., & Botvin, G. J. (1992). Substance abuse prevention: Competence enhancement and the development of positive life options. *Journal of Addictive Diseases, 11*, 29–45.

Evans, R. I. (1983). Deterring smoking in adolescents: Evolution of a research program in applied social psychology. *International Review of Applied Psychology, 32*, 71–83.

Flay, B. R. (1985). Psychological approaches to smoking prevention: A review of findings. *Health Psychology, 4*, 449–488.

Flay, B. R., Phil, D., Branno, B. R., Johnson, C. A., Hansen, W. B., Ulene, A. L., Whitney-Saltiel, D. A., Gleason, L. R., Sussman, S., Gavin, M. D., Glowacz, K. M., Sobol, D. F., & Spiegel, D. C. (1988). The Television, School and Family Smoking Prevention and Cessation Project: I. Theoretical basis and program development. *Preventive Medicine, 17*, 585–607.

Flay, B. R., Phil, D., Miller, T. Q., Hedeker, D., Siddiqui, O., Britton, C. F., Brannon, B. R., Johnson, C. A., Hansen, W. B., Sussman, S., & Dent, C. (1995). The Television, School, and Family Smoking Prevention and Cessation Project: VIII. Student outcome and mediating variables. *Preventive Medicine, 24*, 29–40.

Goodstadt, M. S. (1978). Alcohol and drug education: Models and outcomes. *Health Education Monographs, 6*, 263–279.

Green, L. (1979). National policy in the promotion of health. *International Journal of Health Education, 12*, 161–168.

Hausman, A. J., Spivak, H., Prothrow-Stith, D., & Roeber, J. (1992). Patterns of teen exposure to a community-based violence prevention project. *Journal of Adolescent Health, 13*, 668–675.

Johnson, C. A., Pentz, M. A., Weber, M. D., Dwyer, J. H., Baer, N., MacKinnon, R., & Hansen, W. B. (1990). Relative effectiveness of comprehensive community programming for drug abuse prevention with high-risk and low-risk adolescents. *Journal of Consulting and Clinical Psychology, 58*, 447–456.

Kann, L., Warren, C. W., Harris, W. A., Collins, J. L., Douglas, K. A., Collins, M. E., Williams, B. I., Ross, J. G., & Kolbe, L. J. (1995). Youth risk behavior surveillance: United States. *Journal of School Health, 65*, 163–171.

Kendall, P. C., & Hollon, S. D. (1979). *Cognitive-behavioral interventions: Theory, research, and practice*. New York: Academic.

Leavell, H. R., & Clark, E. G. (1965). *Preventive medicine for the doctor in his community* (3rd Ed.). Toronto: McGraw-Hill.

McAlister, A. L., Ramirez, A. G., Amezcua, C., Pulley, L., Stern, M. P., & Mercado, S. (1992). Smoking cessation in Texas-Mexico border communities: A quasi-experimental panel study. *American Journal of Health Promotion, 6*, 274–279.

Nader, P. R., Saltis, I. F., Patterson, T. L., Abramson, I. S., Rupp, J. W., Senn, K. L., Atkins, C. J., Roppe, B. E., Morris, J. A., Wallace, J. P., & Vega, W. A. (1989). A family approach to cardiovascular risk reductions: Results from the San Diego Family Health Project. *Health Education Quarterly, 16*, 229—224.

Newman, W. P., III, Wattigney, W., & Berenson, G. S. (1991). Autopsy studies in United States children and adolescents: Relationship of risk factors to atherosclerotic lesions. *Annals of the New York Academy of Science, 623*, 16–25.

O'Rourke, T. W. (1995). Creating capacity: A research agenda for school health education. *Journal of School Health, 65*, 33–37.

PDAY Research Group. (1990). Relationship of atherosclerosis in young men to serum lipoprotein cholesterol concentrations and smoking: A preliminary report from the PDAY (Pathobiological Determinants of Atherosclerosis in Youth) Research Group. *Journal of the American Medical Association, 264*, 3018–3024.

Pentz, M. A., Dwyer, J. H., MacKinnon, D. P., Flay, B. R., Phil, D., Hansen, W. B., Wang, E. Y., & Johnson, C. A. (1989). A multicommunity trial for primary prevention of adolescent drug abuse. *Prevention of Drug Abuse, 261*, 3259–3267.

Pentz, M. A., MacKinnon, D. P., Dwyer, J. H., Wang, E. Y., Hansen, W. B., Flay, B. R., & Johnson, C. A. (1989). Longitudinal effects of the Midwestern prevention projects on regular and experimental smoking in adolescents. *Preventive Medicine, 18*, 304–321.

Perry, C. L., Luepker, R. V., Murray, D. M., Kurth, C., Mullis, R., Crockett, S., & Jacobs, D. R. Jr. (1988). Parent involvement with children's health promotion: The Minnesota Home Team. *American Journal of Public Health, 78*, 1156–1160.

Ramirez, A. G., & McAlister, A. L. (1988). Mass media campaign: *A Su Salud. Preventive Medicine, 17*, 608–621.

Resnicow, K., Cross, D., & Wynder, E. (1993) The Know Your Body Program: A review of evaluation studies. *Bulletin of the New York Academy of Medicine, 70*, 188–207.

Schinke, S. P., Moncher, M. S., & Singer, B. R. (1994). Native American youths and cancer risk reduction: Effects of software intervention. *Society for Adolescent Medicine, 15*, 105–110.

Stone, E. J., Perry, C. L., & Luepker, R. V. (1989). Synthesis of cardiovascular behavioral research for youth health promotion. *Health Education Quarterly, 16*, 155–169.

Tobler, N. S. (1986). Meta-analysis of 143 adolescent drug prevention programs: Quantitative outcome results of program participants compared to a control or comparison group. *Journal of Drug Issues, 16*, 537–567.

United States Department of Health, Education, and Welfare. (1979). *Healthy people: The U.S. Surgeon General's Report on health promotion and disease prevention.* Washington, DC: U.S. Government Printing Office.

United States Department of Health and Human Services. (1989). *Reducing the health consequences of smoking: 25 years of progress: A Report of the Surgeon General, 1989.* (DHHS Publication No. (CDC) 89–8411). Atlanta, GA: Centers for Disease Control.

United States Department of Health and Human Services. (1991). *Healthy people 2000: National health promotion and disease prevention objectives*. (Publ. No. (PHS) 91–50212). Washington, DC: U.S. Government Printing Office.

Winett, R. A., Anderson, E. S., Moore, J. F., Sikkema, K. J., Hook, R. J., Webster, D. A., Taylor, C. D., Dalton, J. E., Ollendick, T. H., & Eisler, R. M. (1992). Family/media approach to HIV prevention: Results with a home-based, parent-teen video program. *Health Psychology, 11*, 203–206.

World Health Organization. (1977). *Health needs of adolescents* (WHO Technical Report Series, No. 609). Geneva: Author.

15

Problems With Adherence in the Elderly

Carolyn L. Murdaugh

INTRODUCTION

The "graying of America" is widely recognized (White, Cartwright, Cornoni-Huntley, & Brock, 1986). In 1990 persons over the age of 65 constituted 12.5% of the population as compared to only 3% in the late 1800s, and this number is expected to increase to approximately 30% by the year 2020 (American Association of Retired Persons (AARP), 1992; U.S. Bureau of Census, 1990). Persons aged 85 years and older are the most rapidly growing segment of the population and will continue to increase significantly as the population in the United States proceeds to age into the next century. Increased prevalence of chronic diseases in persons aged 65 and older implies increased healthcare utilization with resultant higher healthcare costs. Elderly spend twice as much time in the hospital as younger persons and account for two times as many hospitalizations and over 40% more physician office visits than persons under age 65 (AARP, 1992). Physician visits and over-the-counter and prescription drug use increase with age. Persons over age 65 average eight physician visits annually, compared to five visits per year for persons under the age of 65. Medication consumption is higher in the elderly than in other age groups (Stewart, Moore, May, Marks, & Hale, 1991). Prescription drugs are only surpassed by nursing home care costs in out-of-pocket expenses incurred by the elderly (Waldo, 1987). These trends are not expected to change, as further technological advances will facilitate the treatment of chronic diseases, and new pharmacologic agents will continue to enter the healthcare market (Burke, Jolson, Goetsch, & Ahronheim, 1992).

Although the elderly are the largest consumers of healthcare services, older persons prefer to be cared for at home. Thus adherence will persist as a major healthcare issue for all healthcare professionals, as older persons will need to learn to use what are often complex treatment and pharmacologic regimens for multiple chronic illnesses.

This chapter discusses the multiple factors that contribute to nonadherence to medical regimens in the elderly. Forms of nonadherence in medication therapy, a major problem in older persons, and possible reasons for medication nonadherence are described. Factors which influence one's ability or desire to adhere, such as one's physical and emotional health, the social environment, and drug-age pharmokinetic factors, are summarized. Methods to assess an elder's capacity to adhere are examined, and the chapter concludes with a review of potential strategies to increase adherence in the elderly.

TYPES AND CAUSES OF NONADHERENCE TO MEDICATION REGIMENS

The elderly are the largest consumers of pharmaceutical agents. Although elderly comprise only 12% of the population, they use over 25% of all prescription medications and approximately 40% of nonprescription drugs (Rowe & Ahronheim, 1992). An average of 11 prescriptions are filled each year by elderly persons living in the community. The most common classes of prescribed medications are cardiovascular agents, diuretics, analgesics, gastrointestinal agents, diabetic agents, and potassium supplements (Jones-Grizzle & Draugalis, 1993). The elderly also purchase and consume seven times more over-the-counter medications than younger persons (Waldo, 1987). The commonly used over-the-counter drugs are analgesics, laxatives, antihistamines, and sympathomimetics (Yee & Williams, 1996). As previously mentioned, medication costs are second only to nursing home costs in out-of-pocket expenses in this age group. It is estimated that the elderly pay 54% of all prescription drug costs each year. Healthcare costs are also incurred because of the large number of hospitalizations for drug-related illnesses. More than 200,00 elderly are admitted to hospitals annually because of adverse drug reactions or experience an adverse drug reaction during hospitalization (Esposito, 1995).

The number of prescriptions and the purchase of over-the-counter medications does not reflect high adherence rates. Medication adherence in the elderly has been estimated to be as low as 40% to as high as 75% (Ostrum, et al.,

1988). Medication nonadherence places an elderly person at risk for debilitating health, increased hospitalization, and death. Approximately 40% of hospitalizations in persons over the age of 65 have been attributed to medication nonadherence (Col, Fanale, & Kronholm 1990). The increased physician outpatient and emergency room visits, hospitalizations, and nursing home admissions place the cost of nonadherence at $13 to 22 billion per year (Bond & Hussar, 1991). Thus, the remainder of the chapter focuses on medication nonadherence due to the magnitude of this problem in the elderly.

Overuse and Underuse

Intentional and nonintentional overuse and underuse are two forms of nonadherence to medication regimens in the elderly (Salzman, 1995). Intentional overuse is usually attributed to the belief that the prescribed dose is ineffective or that "more is better" to relieve symptoms or promote recovery. Forgetfulness may result in unintentional overuse. Patients may not remember taking a medication and take a second dose. Forgetfulness is also the most common reason for unintentional under use of medications. Intentional underuse also occurs when the patient does not believe the medication is needed or does not want to be overmedicated. Intentional underuse also occurs when elders deny the diagnosis of an illness. Medication "hoarding", or saving medication for a future problem, is another example of intentional under use and is often related to the high costs of drugs. Some prescriptions are never filled, another method of intentional under use. Lack of financial resources to pay for prescriptions also results in intentional under use. Nonadherence is more common in the elderly who do not have insurance to cover medications. Uncomfortable side effects of medications may also result in intentional underuse or even termination of the medication. The response cost or incompatibility of the medication regimen with the elder's daily activities also results in intentional underuse (Luciano & Herruro, 1992). For example, doses may be skipped or eliminated if they interfere with social or lifestyle activities. Last, the inability to perform simple tasks which depend on adequate functional performance, such as the ability to open a medication bottle or cut pills, results in unintentional underuse.

Common explanations for nonadherence to medications, in addition to the factors associated with aging discussed in the first section of this chapter, include the complexity and duration of drug regimens, adverse side effects of medications, and lack of information and poor instruction about the drugs.

Complexity of Drug Regimen

The presence of more than one chronic illness in many elderly results in the administration of a large number of medications. More than one specialist may be consulted for elderly persons with chronic illnesses, resulting in multiple prescribers and prescriptions. Thus polypharmacy, or the indiscriminate prescribing of multiple concurrent drugs, is commonplace. Excessive and often inappropriate prescribing behaviors of physicians are not uncommon. Reasons have been documented and include the failure to make an adequate diagnosis due to inadequate clinical assessment before initially prescribing; the influence of the pharmaceutical industry, which promotes prescribing; overenergetic treatment, which leads to incremental prescribing; patient or family demands; failure to conduct careful medication histories; inadequate review of patient records, resulting in a failure to discontinue drugs; and a lack of continuity of care between acute and outpatient facilities (Walley & Scott, 1995). Adherence has been reported to be inversely related to the number of medications prescribed (Gilbert, Luszcz, & Owen, 1993). Three or more drugs have been associated with greater nonadherence. The increased number of drugs are associated with a more complex administration schedule, which is also a deterrent to adherence. Multiple dosing schedules, as compared to single or twice-daily doses, may interfere with leisure activities or sleep and are more likely to be forgotten by the elderly. In addition, the consumption of multiple drugs may result in unpleasant drug-drug interactions, in which one drug may either interfere with or enhance the action of another, or one drug may change the manner in which the body handles another drug (Yee & Williams, 1996). Changes in drug regimens or switching from brand names to generic drugs are confusing to the elderly and may also result in nonadherence (Walley & Scott, 1995).

Adverse Side Effects

Several factors increase the risk of side effects of medications in the elderly. As previously described, older persons react differently to medications because of age-related changes which may alter drug distribution and transport, metabolism, and excretion. These factors increase an older person's susceptibility to side effects of drugs at therapeutic doses. The complexity of the regimen, including the number and dosage of drugs and the duration of the regimen, increase the likelihood of drug incompatibility and drug interactions. Often, more than one physician may be treating the elder, and no one physician coordinates the drug regimen. Multiple chronic illnesses which may alter drug metabolism and excretion, such as cardiovascular, liver, and renal diseases, may also increase the risk of negative side effects. The elderly are at a increased risk for these side effects because many of the side effects they experience, such as confusion, forgetfulness, or weakness, are misattributed to aging or a disease process, instead of to a drug reaction.

Adverse side effects increase the risk of nonadherence, as they are often more troublesome than the disease itself, as in the case of hypertension, which is usually asymptomatic. In addition, many side effects make it difficult for an elder to continue the treatment regimen, annoying symptoms may include confusion, sedation, dizziness, diuresis, appetite and mood changes, constipation, sleep disturbances, and problems with gait instability and physical performance. Antihypertensive agents, the most commonly prescribed medication in the elderly, may cause psychiatric symptoms (Callahan, 1992). Any of these side effects may cause a deterioration in both physical health and quality of life. Many elderly become nonadherers because they do not consider the side effects to be abnormal and do not report them, or they may not know what to do if side effects occur. In addition, they may be embarrassed to report symptoms such as forgetfulness or confusion, because they believe they will be labeled "demented."

Lack of Information and Inadequate Instructions

Knowledge of medications and their side effects is a major factor in adherence. The problem of lack of knowledge is twofold; physicians and other health care professionals often do not provide adequate information, and many elderly are hesitant to ask for information. Health care provider-patient communication is an ongoing problem and is considered a major factor to take into account in patient adherence. Many older persons believe they do not receive adequate information about their prescriptions from their healthcare providers (Williams et al., 1992). It is estimated that as many as 50% of patients leave physicians' offices without an understanding of their medical regimens. When explanations are provided, they are couched in medical terminology that is foreign to most people, including elderly patients. Persons are less likely to follow a prescribed regimen when the instructions are not clear and supportive. Elderly patients are often too inhibited or inarticulate to ask needed questions; or they do not want to be viewed as what they perceive to be a "problem patient", so they do not acknowledge their lack of understanding (Dimatto, 1994). Aging changes, including hearing and visual difficulties as well as increased forgetfulness and decreased attention span, also interfere with an elder's ability to understand and remember instructions. Persons adhere to regimens they understand and believe in and have the ability to follow. Therefore, provision of adequate information and instructions is key to promoting medication adherence.

FACTORS THAT PROMOTE NONADHERENCE IN THE ELDERLY

Multiple factors contribute to the problem of nonadherence in elderly persons. Physical changes that occur with aging, such as declining functional performance and visual, hearing, and cognitive alterations, influence an elderly person's ability to remain independent and follow a medical regimen. In addition, emotional health, specifically depression, is considered a potential factor in nonadherence in the elderly. The social environment, which includes social networks and support, companionship, friendships, living arrangements and financial resources, also plays a role in the promotion of adherence. All of these health status changes and social environmental factors are described in more detail below to provide an understanding of their potential function in the problem of nonadherence in the elderly.

Physical Changes: Functional Performance

Functional performance declines in the elderly (Lafata, Koch, & Weissert, 1994). Functional decline is related to loss of muscle strength and joint flexibility as well as balance and gait changes. More than poor posture results from decreases in strength and flexibility. Loss of strength and flexibility compounds problems in walking or performing activities of daily living (Lewis, 1996). However, decreases in strength may go unnoticed for long periods because normal daily activities do not require great strength (Rice 1989). Strength, flexibility, and balance insure adequate gait or mobility. Bilateral standing balance is necessary to free the upper extremeties for activities, while unilateral balance is essential for stepping over obstacles and climbing stairs. Changes in gait that occur in aging include slowed walking speed, flexion in the thoracic spinal area, a loss of the lordic curve in the lumbar spine, a forward head position, short shuffling steps, and a loss of normal arm movement (Leiper & Craik, 1991). Functional performance is essential for the accomplishment of everyday activities such as bathing, dressing, toileting, shopping, preparing meals, using transportation, performing simple psychomotor skills, and taking medications. Changes which result in a deterioration in mobility and the capacity to maintain independence affect one's ability to perform activities necessary to adhere to certain treatment regimens.

Physical Changes: Visual

Visual changes occur with aging; reduced vision is the most common sensory problem in the aged, and at least 90% of persons over age 60 need correction of vision (Heath, 1992b). The major visual impairment in the elderly, presbyopia, is caused by a loss of elasticity and increased density of the lens. The ciliary muscles which hold the lens also lose their ability to accommodate rapidly, resulting in the need for bifocal lenses. Age-related ocular changes include altered depth perception, increased light threshold, arcus senility, increased eyelid laxity, and decreased tear production. Cataracts are the most common ocular disease in the elderly. Two other major ocular diseases affecting the elderly are glaucoma and macular degeneration (Maguire, 1996). All three of these diseases result in visual impairments, and glaucoma and macular degeneration can result in blindness. In addition, chronic diseases that increase with age, such as diabetes mellitus, cause eye changes that may result in blindness.

Visual problems often go undetected until late in the disease process because health professionals may associate these changes with aging and overlook them (Faye, 1984). Poor vision interferes with an elder person's capability to adhere to medical regimens due to the inability to see in order to perform household tasks, drive, and read.

Physical Changes: Hearing

Hearing loss, or presbycusis, is the most underreported and unrecognized sensory impairment in geriatric medicine (Heath, 1992a). Elderly persons with hearing problems may wait 5 years or more before seeking medical assistance (Hull, 1985). Hearing loss results in a decreased perception of higher frequency tones as well as auditory signal distortion which may result in inappropriate responses. Such responses are often misinterpreted, and elderly who experience this problem may withdraw due to frustration in communication. Signs such as withdrawal from conversations, inappropriate responses, inattentiveness, and difficulty in following directions are often interpreted as confusion or cognitive decline in the elderly instead of a correctable hearing problem (Gennis, Garry, Haaland, Yeo, & Goodwin, 1991). Because hearing loss is usually not diagnosed and managed appropriately, elderly who do not hear or misinterpret medical information, or who are reluctant to ask questions because they are concerned they will not hear the response may be more likely to not adhere to medical regimens.

Physical Changes: Cognitive Function

Declines in cognitive function occur with age. Increased age is associated with changes in recent memory, psychomotor speed, concept formation, visual spacial praxis, and visual perceptual function (Flicker, Ferris, & Reisberg, 1993). It is estimated that cognitive impairment is present in as many as 11% of persons over age 65, and for persons over the age of 85 the prevalence increases to as high as 20% (Livingston, Hawkins, Graham, Blizard, & Mann, 1990). Alzheimer's-related dementia is the most common cause of cognitive impairment. Silent or unrecognized dementia has been reported to be as high as 52% among persons with early cognitive deterioration (Ross et al., in press). Early signs of cognitive impairment are often diagnosed as "normal" aging, hearing loss, or depression, leading to undetected cases until advanced stages (Canadian Task Force, 1991).

Although memory impairment is considered the hallmark of dementia, it is also a useful gauge of physical and psychological functioning in older persons without dementia. Memory includes the processes related to the acquisition, storage and retrieval of verbal, visual and motor information (Zarit & VanderBos, 1990). Cognitive resources are considered to be the most important resource for maintaining everyday functioning (Poon et al., 1992). Thus cognitive changes, namely memory loss, become issues when an elder is unable to recall and use information necessary to perform everyday activities, including the ability to remember information needed to plan and follow treatment and pharmacologic regimens (Conn, Taylor, & Miller, 1994).

Emotional Health: Depression

Depression may range from the expression of a sad mood to a mental state characterized by dejection, loss of hope, and absence of cheerfulness (Teri & Wagner, 1992). Almost half of the population over 60 years of age report symptoms of depression (Blazer, Hughes, & George, 1987). Losses associated with aging, such as death of a spouse or friends, moving from one's home, and termination of a career, are thought to contribute to depression in the elderly. Depression may produce physical, psychological, and cognitive symptoms (Cummings, 1994; Teri & Wagner, 1992). Physical symptoms include sleep disturbances, appetite or weight changes, fatigue, and loss of libido. Emotional aspects include a pervasive dysphoric mood, feelings of worthlessness, suicidal thoughts, and loss of self-esteem. Cognitive symptoms may include difficulty with memory, concentration, and confusion.

Physician and patient factors have been attributed to the underdiagnosis and treatment of depression. As with other changes in the elderly, depressive symptoms are often considered predictable complaints of chronic illnesses and are ignored (Callahan, 1992). A relationship between depression and morbidity and mortality has been reported (Carney, Freedland, Eisen, Rich, & Jaffe, 1995). Depression is also associated with more functional complaints, greater numbers of physician office visits and hospitalizations, and poor adherence. One proposed explanation is that depression is also associated with poor social support, functional impairment, and cognitive deficits —all factors which are associated with nonadherence.

Social Environment: Social Network and Social Support

Social networks and supports have been positively linked to the health and well-being of older persons (Antonucci, 1990; Felton & Berry, 1992; House, Landis, & Umberson, 1988). Social networks are predictive of access to support and other needed resources. The major types of social support are emotional, informational, and instrumental or tangible support. Supportive contacts and relationships may positively affect health through earlier recognition of symptoms and a greater likelihood of seeking medical care, which decreases the need for hospitalization or nursing home admissions, and provision of assistance to sustain treatment regimens. Social isolation, the lack of social and community relationships, has been associated with poor health (Berkman, 1983; Dean, Kalody, & Wood, 1989). Estimates are that between 25 and 35% of persons over age 65 live alone. Elderly who live alone, especially elderly women, are also more likely to have a low income (Commonwealth Fund, Commission, 1988). Both of these factors contribute to the difficulties encountered by elderly persons in adhering to a treatment regimen.

Social Environment: Financial Resources

The advent of the Social Security system and government programs for medical care, such as Medicare and Medicaid, have improved the economic status of persons over age 65. Fewer persons over age 65 now live below the poverty line. However, these statistics mask differences by age and race (Hess, 1990). The median income for White married couples in 1989 was $21,000. However, for women living alone, annual income dropped to $8,000, and $5,000 was reported for African Americans (United States Bureau of the Census, 1989). Since women live longer than men, are three and a half times more likely to be widowed, and earn lower salaries in their lifetime, women are at increased risk for nonadherence due to limited financial resources.

The high costs of prescriptions and medical supplies, and inadequate Medicare reimbursement, pose additional barriers to adherence for persons with low incomes as well as for persons with fixed incomes. Many elderly cannot afford to pay for all of the medications prescribed, and make their own decisions about which ones to omit. Many are not covered by any insurance other than government programs, which do not reimburse outpatient medication expenses. Since multiple drugs are usually prescribed, annual costs have estimated to range from $600 to as high as $3,000 (Stuart & Lago, 1989). Most of these costs are out-of-pocket expenses for the elderly. Persons on fixed incomes usually have limited funds available after paying for food, housing, and other medical care, resulting in unfilled drug prescriptions or intentional dose-skipping or drug-hoarding.

Drug-Age Pharmokinetics

Older persons respond differently to medications than younger people because of age-related changes that occur in the body. Pharmokinetic alterations include changes in absorption, distribution, metabolism, and elimination (Ives, 1992; Yee & Williams, 1996). Absorption of drugs by passive diffusion is not affected by aging. However, alterations in gastric motility and blood flow can influence drug absorption. Distribution or transportation of drugs throughout the body may be altered by age-related changes, including a decreased lean body mass, increased body fat, and decreased total body water. Thus dosages of water-soluble drugs, including digoxin, propranolol, and cimetidine need to be altered, as well as drugs that are distributed into adipose tissue. In addition, fat-soluble drugs such as barbiturates and phenothiazines produce prolonged actions or adverse effects due to the large amounts that may be stored in fat.

The major site for drug metabolism is in the liver. Hepatic mass and hepatic blood flow decrease with age. This decreased blood flow means a decreased extraction (first pass) of the drug by the liver which produces an increase in serum drug levels and clinical effects of certain drugs, such as propanalol, verapamil, and some opiates.

The kidney is the major organ of drug excretion. Renal blood flow and perfusion decreases with age. Therefore, dosages must be reduced for drugs that are dependent on renal blood for excretion, such as digoxin, lithium, and penicillin. In addition to the effects of aging on the four parameters of pharmokinetics, common chronic illnesses, such as congestive heart failure, cirrhosis, nutritional deficiencies, hypertension, and kidney diseases, may impair absorption, metabolism, and excretion. Significant adverse side effects and toxicity may occur if the physician does not understand these age-related changes in pharmokinetics when prescribing pharmacologic therapies and prescribes incorrect doses. Deleterious effects or perceived lack of benefits result in nonadherence as well as increased health care costs, due to hospitalizations and physician office visits.

In summary, aging affects the physiological, psychological, and social aspects of a person's life (Birren & Fisher, 1991). Functional, visual, hearing and cognitive changes that occur with aging determine a person's ability to make lifestyle changes or follow treatment and medication regimens. Social isolation, the converse of social support, often results from deaths of spouses and close friends. Socially isolated and depressed elders are less likely to adhere to treatments or make necessary lifestyle changes. Finally, greater attention is needed to address pharmokinetic changes to prevent needless healthcare utilization as well as nonadherence. All of these factors, which may not be controllable by the elder, must be considered when assessing potential adherence problems and designing programs to increase adherence.

ASSESSMENT OF THE CAPACITY TO ADHERE

The first step to facilitate adherence in the elderly is assessment of the capacity to follow a regimen, as physical, cognitive, and social environmental barriers place these persons at risk for nonadherence. Assessment of adherence needs to occur before a medication or treatment regimen begins, not after a program has been implemented. This case is made by Fitten, Coleman, Siembieda, Ye, Ganzell, (1995) who advocate assessment of cognitive and functional performance to evaluate understanding as well as capacity to institute a treatment program for persons potentially at risk for nonadherence. Comprehension is a key component in decisionmaking, as elders must understand information in order to make appropriate decisions on which to act (Salthouse, 1996). In one study, persons in their 60s and 70s had error rates ranging from 16 to 21% when asked to prepare a medication schedule with the prescription in front of them, evidence that adherence is not likely if persons do not comprehend instructions (Morrell, Park, & Poon, 1990). A more recent study found that judgement and memory impairment produced the most errors when elders were presented with difficult medication regimen scenarios (Fitten et al., 1995). Since impaired mental status is a major risk factor for nonadherence, assessment of cognitive functioning is essential.

Physical measures as well as social environmental measures also need to be taken into account when assessing the capacity of elders to adhere. The healthcare provider must be knowledgeable of any physical impairments that may influence adherence. For example, the performance of self- care and instrumental activities of daily living indicate one's ability to care for self and to manage one's property (Willis 1996). Hearing and visual difficulties may interfere with comprehension of the treatment regimen. Social environmental assessment provides information about the elder's living arrangements and available assistance from a spouse, family member, or friend, as well as the ability to pay for medications and equipment or obtain transportation for medical appointments.

Assessment of cognitive functioning as well as physical and social support and financial resources prior to initiating a regimen is achieved through ongoing communication by a healthcare professional. The time allotted to an initial detailed assessment for adherence will pay off over time. Short, reliable, and valid questionnaires that are easy to administer are available to assess cognitive functioning and both self-care and instrumental activities of daily living. It must be kept in mind that many factors influence compliance other than the ability to initiate and follow a regimen. However, an initial thorough assessment provides a major step in reducing potential barriers to adherence.

STRATEGIES TO INCREASE ADHERENCE IN THE ELDERLY

Understanding of and adherence to the current medication regimen should be evaluated following assessment of the elderly person's capacity to follow the prescribed therapy. A detailed medication history is necessary prior to implementing an educational program so that strategies to increase adherence can be tailored to individual needs. The medication regimen itself also deserves scrutiny as changes in dosing, timing, etc. may increase adherence. Communication between the elder and the healthcare professional is a major factor in improving adherence (Salzman, 1995). Therefore, the healthcare provider must be knowledgeable of the elements of effective communication that promote adherence. Since forgetting is a major problem in adherence in the elderly, educational and behavioral strategies that promote adherence should be initiated. Last, a multidiscliplinary approach is central to promoting adherence in the elderly.

MEDICATION HISTORY ASSESSMENT

Initially, a detailed medication history should be taken to obtain information about current prescription and over-the-counter medications, prior prescription and over-the-counter medications, and home remedies. Social drug use, including alcohol, tobacco, and caffeine, should also be ascertained, as these may interfere with or alter prescribed drugs. One successful strategy is to request that the elder bring in all prescription, over-the-counter, borrowed, and outdated medications in the home at the initial visit. This "paper bag test" will provide a picture of the person's medication habits (Ham, 1992). Next the elder should be queried about the medications. Questions need to be asked to obtain information about medication dosages and schedules, side effects and other problems when taking the medications, and knowledge about the drugs and disease being treated. Questions should be open-ended and nonthreatening and asked in a supportive, nonpunitive manner. A supportive atmosphere will facilitate honest answers about adherence issues without fear of reprisal.

Medication Regimen Analysis

Potential adherence issues may be addressed through an ongoing review of the medication regimen, while focusing on the patient as well as the disease. First, prescription instructions need to be detailed, avoiding directions such as "Take as directed" or "Take as needed," as they may not be understood (Ives, 1992). Easily administered dosage forms should be prescribed that consider such problems as difficulty in swallowing pills. A careful review is needed to keep the regimen as simple as possible, as the elderly should take as few drugs as necessary. Drugs that can be administered in a single or twice-daily dose should be prescribed whenever possible. Dosage timing should be adjusted so that the schedule does not interfere with the elder's daily activities. Therapeutic endpoints for prescribed drugs should be established and medications that are no longer needed should be discontinued as soon as possible, as prolonged regimens increase the potential for nonadherence. Last, safety caps should not be dispensed, as many elderly are unable to open medications with these caps. Ongoing attention to all aspects of the medication regimen decreases the potential for adverse side effects and increases the likelihood of adherence. Strategies which will improve adherence include changing the education of physicians and healthcare providers who prescribe, in addition to educating the elderly (Wally & Scott, 1995).

Effective Communication

Elements of effective communication between physicians and elderly persons have been reviewed in the literature (McCormick & Inui, 1992). Timing of communication episodes, quality of the encounter, and importance of involvement of the significant other are applicable in promoting constructive communication between healthcare professionals and elderly persons to increase adherence with treatment programs. Effective communication enables healthcare providers to furnish essential information in a meaningful manner as well as elicit the elder's concerns and questions about the medication regimen.

Timing

Scheduled, ongoing contacts with a consistent healthcare provider, rather than "as-needed" visits, are necessary to prevent or reduce side effects and polypharmacy and to monitor cognitive and physical changes which may interfere with adherence (McCormick & Inui 1992; Wally & Scott 1995). Follow-up visits are critical after a hospital or other health care facility discharge, the death of a spouse, a change in living arrangements, or a decline in cognitive or physical functioning, as any transition increases the elder's risk for nonadherence as well as other potentially debilitating consequences.

Quality of Encounter

The quality of the patient-healthcare provider relationship has a significant bearing on satisfaction with care, which in turn influences an elder's motivation to adhere with a prescribed regimen (Sherbourne, Hays, Ordway, DiMatto, Kravitz, 1992). It may be the most important ingredient in whether behavior change occurs. Empathetic listening and genuine interest in the elder convey respect, instill trust, and decrease communication barriers. Sensitivity to cognitive, physical, and social environmental barriers enable the healthcare provider to plan and implement realistic regimens which provide the types of supports essential for success. The quality of the encounter is enriched when sufficient time is spent with the elder to provide individualized information, assess response to current medications, answer questions, address concerns, and provide encouragement and support (Beisecker & Beisecker, 1990; Dimatto et al., 1993).

Significant Other Involvement

Inclusion of the spouse, a family member, or friend is a major factor in the management of the elder's chronic illness treatment regimen, especially if there is declining cognitive or physical functioning. Household members can contribute information about elders and their living environments that is crucial to understanding potential adherence issues. The significant other may also administer the medications or insure that the elder is taking the medication. Illness is a family affair, as everyone in the household is affected. Therefore, active participation by a spouse, son, or daughter facilitates adherence to medication and other treatments that may be prescribed. In addition, side effects or other problems are likely to be observed and reported earlier, decreasing the need for hospitalization. Significant others or caregivers need to be present during provider-patient communications about the medication regimens and during all educational activities.

Educational Strategies

Educational strategies have traditionally been the mainstay to improve adherence with medication and other treatment regimens, with varying levels of success for persons of all ages (Eposito, 1995; Morris & Schultz, 1992). Educational strategies are based on the premise that provision of information about the disease and its treatment is a necessary first step. In other words, elders must first understand their illness and its consequences and comprehend the benefits of the prescribed regimen before they are able to make lifestyle adjustments needed to implement a regimen. Multiple educational strategies are more effective than a single strategy. For example, verbal communication as well as written information is more beneficial than written information alone. Multiple strategies which take into account verbal, visual, and auditory channels are particularly effective to reinforce information in the elderly. Medical and technical terminology should be avoided when possible, and care must be taken to avoid presenting too much information in one session, as a reduced attention span may result in remembering only some or none of the information. A stepwise approach, in which information is presented in small increments, enables the elder to believe that adherence is both beneficial and possible (Herrier & Boyce, 1993). Individualized one-to-one educational sessions that are flexible are more effective than structured group approaches. Flexibility in the educational process is critical to adjust for varying levels of involvement, difficulties with comprehension, and changes in beliefs and attitudes.

Other educational strategies include active involvement of the elder as much as possible in the teaching-learning process. Active involvement enables the healthcare provider to evaluate understanding of information as well as to provide opportunities to ask questions and practice new skills, such as insulin injections or urine checks. The "show-and-tell" technique has been effectively implemented by pharmacists in the Indian Health Service to confirm understanding of the medication regimen (Herrier & Boyce, 1993). First, the medication is shown to the patient. The patient is then asked what the medication is for, how is it to be taken, and what types of problems, if any, are experienced. Design and packaging information which takes into account visual problems and educational levels also demands attention.

Behavioral Strategies

Behavioral strategies are defined as the application of various mechanisms or aids to increase adherence, rather than the traditional definition, which is rooted in classical or operant conditioning (Goldfried & Goldfried, 1980). Behavioral strategies are effective, as they address the problem of declining cognitive and physical functioning in the elderly. For example, aids which remind elders to take their medications have been shown to improve adherence (Wong & Norman, 1987). Reminders may be as simple as a chart, special medication containers such as a daily dispenser or weekly medication tray, or a special calendar or mealtime dispensing pack. Color-coded bottles have also been used. Special packaging simplifies the medication regimen by organizing the medications. The packaging can also serve as a mechanism to monitor adherence. Telephone or mail prompts to refill prescriptions are also helpful in promoting adherence.

Additional strategies which address declining memory have been implemented with varying levels of success. Cues within the environment are frequently used as reminders (Wallsten et al., 1995). For example, the elderly can be taught to take medications when drinking their morning coffee or juice, at mealtimes, or during certain television programs, or they may devise their own cues. Reminders from significant others are valuable complements to environmental cues.

Multidisciplinary Approach

A team approach which incorporates the expertise of multiple healthcare providers, namely physicians, pharmacists, and registered nurses, enhances adherence. Each provider contributes a special expertise that is complementary, rather than competitive. For example, physicians are responsible for diagnosing and prescribing medications. Physicians also monitor patients for adverse side effects and provide education. Pharmacists fill prescriptions and review drugs for potential drug-drug interactions. They conduct drug reviews to reduce the cost of medications as well as reduce the number of medicines prescribed. In addition, pharmacists dispense educational materials and may provide education as well. The responsibilities of registered nurses vary with their role. For example, nurse practitioners may prescribe medications. Nurses in acute care, nursing home, and other institutional settings administer medications and monitor patients for effectiveness as well as adverse side effects. In addition, nurses provide information about the medication regimen and teach skills that may be needed to administer medications such as insulin injections. In the community setting nurses make home visits to monitor the elderly for side effects and other issues that may influence adherence to the medication regimen. Ongoing communication among the three healthcare providers is essential to optimize care and promote adherence.

SUMMARY

The number of persons over the age of 65 is increasing faster than any other segment of the population. This group also is the largest consumer of healthcare services. The increase in chronic illnesses in the elderly necessitates lifelong, complex medication and treatment programs that may produce unpleasant and uncomfortable side effects. Problems with adherence result from these adverse side effects as well as cognitive and physical decline and a lack of social support and financial resources. Thus, adherence in the elderly is a complicated issue. The health care provider should begin with an assessment of factors beyond the control of the patient, such as cognitive decline and change in vision, hearing, or physical performance. These factors enable the provider to determine the elder's capacity to adhere before prescribing a complex drug regimen.

Potential causes of nonadherence, including the complexity of the regimen, adverse side effects, and lack of understanding, should supplement the information obtained about the elders to facilitate the choice of strategies to increase adherence. Effective communication between the elder and healthcare providers is paramount. While educational and behavioral strategies may promote adherence, no one strategy is completely effective. Ongoing gerontological research is critical, as the problem of nonadherence in the elderly is expected to continue and even increase as the elderly population expands into the next century.

REFERENCES

American Association of Retired Persons. (1992). *A profile of older Americans*. Long Beach, CA: Author.

Antonucci. T. C. (1990). Social supports and social relationships. In *R. H. Binstock & L. K. George (Eds.), Handbook of aging and the social sciences* (3rd ed.). (pp. 205–226) San Diego: Academic Press.

Beisecker, A. E., & Beisecker, T. D. (1990). Patient information seeking behavior when communicating with doctors. *Medical Care, 28*, 19–28.

Berkman, L. F. (1983). The assessment of social networks and social support in the elderly. *Journal of the American Geriatrics Society, 31*, 743–762.

Birren, J. E., & Fisher, L. M. (1991). Aging and slowing of behavior: Consequences for cognition and survival. *Nebraska Symposium on Motivation, 39*, 1–37.

Blazer, D. G., Hughes, D. C., & George, L. K. (1987). The epidemiology of depression in elderly community populations. *Gerontologist, 27*, 281–287.

Bond, W. S., & Hussar, D. A. (1991). Detection methods and strategies for improving medication compliance. *American Journal of Hospital Pharmacy, 48*, 1978–1988.

Burke, L. B., Jolson, H. M., Goetsch, R. A., & Ahronheim, J. C. (1992). Geriatric drug use and adverse drug event reporting in 1990: A descriptive analysis of two national data bases. In J. W. Rowe & J. C. Ahronheim (Eds.), *Annual Review of Gerontology and Geriatrics*, Vol. 12, (pp. 1–28). New York: Springer Publishing Co.

Callahan, C. M. (1992). Psychiatric symptoms in elderly patients due to medications. In J. W. Rowe & J. C. Ahronheim (Eds.), *Annual Review of Gerontology and Geriatrics*, New York: Springer Publishing Company.

Canadian Task Force on the Periodic Health Examination. (1991). Periodic health examination, 1991 update: 1. Screening for cognitive impairment in the elderly. *Canadian Medical Association Journal, 144*, 425–431.

Carney, R. M., Freedland, K. E., Eisen, S. A., Rich, M. W., & Jaffe, A. S. (1995). Major depression and medication adherence in elderly persons with coronary artery disease. *Health Psychology, 14*, 88–90.

Col, N., Fanale, J. E., & Kronholm, P. (1990). The role of medication noncompliance and adverse drug reactions in hospitalization of the elderly. *Archives of Internal Medicine, 150*, 841– 845.

Commonwealth Fund Commission on Elderly Persons Living Alone. (1988). *Aging alone*. Washington, DC: U.S. Government Printing Office.

Conn, V., Taylor, S., & Miller, R. (1994). Cognitive impairment and medication adherence. *Journal of Gerontological Nursing*, 41–47.

Cummings, J. L. (1994). Depression in neurologic diseases. *Psychiatric Annals, 24*, 525–531.

Dean, A., Kalody, B., & Wood, P. (1989). The effects and types of support from adult children on depression in elderly persons. *Journal of Community Psychology, 17*, 341–355.

DiMatto, M. R. (1994). Enhancing patient adherence to medical recommendations. *Journal of the American Medical Association, 271*, 79, 83.

DiMatto, M. R., Sherbourne, C. D., Hays, R. D., Ordway, L., Kravitz, R. L.,

McGlynn, E. A., Kaplan, S., & Rogers, W. H. (1993). Physician's characteristics influence patients' adherence to medical treatment: Results from the Medical Outcomes Study. *Health Psychology, 12*, 93– 102.

Esposito, L. (1995). The effects of medication education on adherence to medication regimens in an elderly population. *Journal of Advance Nursing, 21*, 935–943.

Faye, E. E. (1984). Maintaining visual functioning in the elderly. *Bulletin of the New York Academy of Medicine, 60*, 987.

Felton, B. J., & Berry, C. A. (1992). Do the sources of the urban elderly's social support determine its psychological consequences? *Psychology and Aging, 7*, 89–97.

Fitten, I. J., Coleman, L., Siembieda, D. W., Ye, M., & Ganzell, S. (1995). Assessment of capacity to comply with medication regimens in older patients. *Journal of the American Geriatric Society, 43*, 361–367.

Flicker, C., Ferris, S. H., & Reisberg, B. (1993). A two-year longitudinal study of cognitive functioning normal aging and Alzheimer's Disease. *Journal of Geriatric psychiatry and Neurology, 6*, 84–96.

Gennis, V., Garry, P. J., Haaland, K. Y., Yeo, R. A., & Goodwin, J. S. (1991). Hearing and cognition in the elderly. *Archives of Internal Medicine, 151*, 2259–2264.

Gilbert, A., Luszcz, M., & Owen, N. (1993). Medication use and its correlates among the elderly. *Australian Journal of Public Health, 17*, 18–22.

Goldfried, M. R., & Goldfried, A. P. (1980). Cognitive change methods. In F. H. Kanfer & A. P. Goldstein (Eds.), *Helping people change* (2nd ed.). (pp. 97–130). New York: Pergamon.

Ham, R. J. (1992). Assessment. In R. J. Ham & P. D. Sloane (Eds.). *Primary care geriatrics*, (2nd ed.). (pp. 64–94). St. Louis: Mosby-Year Book.

Heath, J. M. (1992a). Hearing. In R. J. Ham & P. D. Sloane (Eds.), *Primary care geriatrics* (2nd ed.) (pp. 490–497). St. Louis: Mosby-Year Book.

Heath, J. M. (1992b). Vision. In R. J. Ham & P. D. Sloane (Eds.). *Primary care geriatrics* (2nd ed.), pp. 482–489. St. Louis: Mosby-Year Book.

Herrier, R. N. & Boyce, R. W. (1993). Compliance with prescribed drug regimens. In R. Bressler & M. D. Katz (Eds.), *Geriatric pharmacology* (pp. 63–78). New York: McGraw-Hill.

Hess, B. B. (1990). The demographic parameters. *Generations, 14*(3), 12–14.

House, J. S., Landis, K. R. & Umberson, D. (1988). Social relationships and health. *Science, 241*, 540–545.

Hull, R. H. (1985). Hearing aids for the older adult: Considerations for fitting and dispensing. *Seminars in Hearing, 6*, 181–195.

Ives, T. J. (1992). Pharmacotherapeutics. In R. J. Ham & P. D. Sloane (Eds.), *Primary care geriatrics* (2nd ed., pp. 194–208). St. Louis: Mosby-Year Book.

Jones-Grizzle, A. J., & Draugalis, J. R. (1993). Demographics. In J. W. Rowe & J. C. Ahronheim (Eds.), *Annual Review of Gerontology and Geriatrics* (pp. 1–8). New York: Springer Publishing Company.

Lafata, J. E., Koch, G. G., & Weissert, W. (1994). Estimating activity limitation in the noninstitutionalized population: A method for small areas. *American Journal of Public health, 84*, 1813–1817.

Leiper, C. I., & Craik, R. L. (1991). Relationship between physical activity and temporal-distance characteristics of walking in elderly women. *Physical Therapy, 11*, 791–803.

Lewis, C. B. (1996). Musculoskeletal changes with age: Clinical implications. In C. B. Lewis (Ed.), *Aging The Health Care Challenge* (3rd ed.), (pp. 147–176). Philadelphia: F. A. Davis.

Livingston, G., Hawkins, A. R., Graham, N. D., Blizard, B. A., & Mann, A. (1990). The Gospel Oak study: Prevalence rates of dementia, depression and activity limitation among elderly residents in inner London. *Psychological Medicine, 20*, 137–146.

Luciano, M. C., & Herruzo, J. (1992). Some relevant components of adherence behavior. *Journal of Behavioral Therapy and Experimental Psychiatry, 23*, 117–124.

Maguire, G. H. (1996). The changing realm of the senses. In C. B. Lewis (Ed.), *Aging: The health care challenge* (3rd ed.) (pp. 126–146). Philadelphia: F. A. Davis.

McCormick. W. C., & Inui, T. S. (1992). Geriatric preventive care: Counseling techniques in practice settings. *Clinics in Geriatric Medicine, 8*, 215–228.

Morrell, R. W., Park, D. C., & Poon, L. W. (1990). Effects of labeling techniques on memory and comprehension of prescription information in young and old adults. *Journal of Gerontology, 45*, 166–172.

Morris, L. S., & Schulz, R. M. (1992). Patient compliance: An overview. *Journal of Clinical Pharmacy and Therapeutics, 17*, 283–295.

Ostrum, F. E., Hammarlund, E. R., Christensen, D. B., Plein, J. B., Kethley, A. J. (1985) Medication usage in an elderly population. *Medical Care, 23*, 157–170.

Poon, L. W., Martin, P., Clayton, G. M., Messner, S., Noble, C. A., & Johnson, M. A. (1992). The influence of cognitive resources on adaptation and old age. *International Journal of Aging and Human Development, 34*, 31–46.

Rice, C. L. (1989). Strength in an elderly population. *Archives of Physical Medicine and Rehabilitation, 70*, 391–397.

Ross, G. W., Abbot, R., Petrovich, H., Masaki, K., Murdaugh, C., Trockman, C., & White, L. (1997). Silent dementia: Frequency and characteristics in elderly Japanese-American men: The Honolulu-Asia aging study. *Journal of the American Medical Association, 277*(10), 800–805.

Rowe, J. W., & Ahronheim, J. C. (1992). Geriatric medication use: Translating knowledge into practice. In J. W. Rowe, & J. C. Ahronheim (Eds.), *Annual Review of Gerontology and Geriatrics*, (pp. vii–viii). New York: Springer.

Salthouse, T. A. (1996). Commentary: A cognitive psychologist's perspective on the assessment of cognitive competency. In M. Smyer, K. W. Schaie & M. B. Kapp (Eds.), *Older adult's decision-making and the law* (pp. 29–39). New York: Springer.

Salzman, C. (1995). Medication compliance in the elderly. *Journal of Clinical Psychiatry, 56* (suppl 1), 18–23.

Sherbourne, C. D., Hays, R. D., Ordway, L., DiMatto, M. R., & Kravitz, R. L. (1992). Antecedents of adherence to medical recommendations: Results from the Medical Outcomes Study. *Journal of Behavioral Medicine, 15*, 447–468.

Stuart, B., & Lago, D. (1989). Prescription drug coverage and medical indigence among the elderly. *Journal of Aging and Health, 1*, 451–469.

Stewart, R., Moore, M., May, F., Marks, R., & Hale, W. (1991). Changing patterns of therapeutic agents in the elderly. *Age and Ageing, 20*, 182–188.

Teri, L., & Wagner, A. (1992). Alzheimer's disease and depression. *Journal of Consulting and Clinical Psychology, 60*, 379–391.

U.S. Bureau of the Census. (1989). Poverty in the United States. *Current Population Reports* (Series P-60, No. 163). Washington DC: Government Printing Office.

U.S. Bureau of the Census. (1990). Population Division. Washington DC: Author.

Waldo, D. R. (1987). Outpatient prescription drug spending by the Medicare population. *Health Care Financing Review, 9*, 83–89.

Wallsten, S. M., Sullivan, R. J., Hanlon, J. T., Blazer, D. G., Tyrey, M. J., & Westlund, R. (1995). Medication taking behaviors: 1. the high-and low-functioning elderly: McArthur field studies of successful aging. *The Annals of Pharmacotherapy, 29*, 359–364.

Walley, T., & Scott, A. K. (1995). Prescribing in the elderly. *Postgraduate Medical Journal, 71*, 466–471.

White, L. R., Cartwright, W. S., Cornoni-Huntley, J., & Brock, D. B. (1986). Geriatric epidemiology. In C. Eisdorfer (Ed.), *Annual Review of Gerontology and Geriatrics* (Vol. 6), 251–311.

Williams, B. R., Nichol, M. B., Lowe, B. F., McCombs, J. S., Yoon, P. S., & Lipson, L. G. (1992). Pharmacist interventions in residential care facilities. In J. W. Rowe & J. C. Ahronheim (Eds.) *Annual Review of Gerontology and Geriatrics* (pp. 150–162). New York: Springer.

Willis. S. L. (1996). Assessing everyday competence in the cognitively challenged. In M. Smyer, K. W. Schaie & M. B. Kapp (Eds.), *Older adult's decision-making and the law* (pp. 29–39). New York: Springer.

Wong, B. S., & Norman, D. C. (1987). Evaluation of a novel medication aid, the calendar blister-pak, and its effect on drug compliance in a geriatric outpatient clinic. *Journal of the American Geriatrics Society, 35*, 21–26.

Yee, B. W. K., & Williams, B. J. (1996). Medication management and appropriate substance use in the elderly. In C. B. Lewis (Ed.), *Aging: The Health Care Challenge* (3rd ed.), (pp. 325–363). Philadelphia: F. A. Davis.

Zarit, S. H., & VanderBos, G. R. (1990). Effective evaluation of memory in older persons. *Hospital and Community Psychiatry, 41*, 9–10, 16.

16

Adherence Issues Among Adolescents With Chronic Disease

Michael A. Rapoff

INTRODUCTION

WARNING: ADOLESCENCE MAY BE HAZARDOUS TO YOUR HEALTH. Although relatively healthy from a traditional epidemiologic perspective, adolescents are particularly vulnerable to health risks which result from high-risk behaviors such as substance abuse, unprotected sex, reckless vehicle use, and self- or other-inflicted violence (Blum, 1987; Elliott, 1993; Elster & Kuznets, 1994). There is also some evidence for covariation among high-risk behaviors; that is, adolescents who engage in one type of risky behavior (e.g., alcohol abuse) tend to engage in other risky behaviors (e.g., unprotected sex) (Elliot, 1993; Millstein & Igra, 1995). From a primary prevention perspective, these lifestyle-related health threats need to be addressed by health-promotion efforts in the home, school, and community as discussed in other chapters in this volume. This chapter will focus on secondary or tertiary prevention for adolescents who already experience compromised

Preparation of this manuscript was supported, in part, by grant MCJ–200617 from the Maternal and Child Health Bureau (Title V, Social Security Act), Health Resources and Services Administration, Department of Health and Human Services.

health from contracting a chronic disease such as asthma, cancer, diabetes, or juvenile rheumatoid arthritis (JRA). The goal of health promotion for these young people is to minimize the physical and psychosocial morbidity associated with these diseases and thereby extend the length and quality of life (Blum, 1992).

Although chronic physical illnesses affect a relatively small proportion of adolescents (Newacheck, 1989; Newacheck & Taylor, 1992), they carry the potential for causing significant medical and psychosocial morbidity and even increased mortality, while consuming a disproportiante amount of health care resources (Holden & Nitz, 1995). Nonadherence to medical treatment is considered a major contributor to increased morbidity, mortality, and health care utilization and costs (Jay, Litt, & Durant, 1984; Rapoff & Barnard, 1991). Adolescents with chronic diseases have been found to be at greater risk for nonadherence to regimens for cancer (Smith, Rosen, Trueworthy, & Lowman, 1979; Tebbi et al., 1986); cystic fibrosis (Gudas, Koocher, & Wypij, 1991; Patterson, 1985); diabetes (Anderson, Auslander, Jung, Miller, & Santiago, 1990; Bond et al., 1992; Jacobson et al., 1987; Jacobson et al., 1990; Johnson et al., 1992; Kovacs, Goldston, Obrosky, & Iyengar, 1992; La Greca, Follansbee, & Skyler, 1990), and renal disease (Beck et al., 1980; Brownbridge & Fielding, 1994).

In addition to negotiating the normal developmental challenges, adolescents with chronic diseases have to cope with pain, fatigue, limitations in their daily activities, and demanding medical regimens. These regimens can be time-consuming, intrusive, and of little immediate benefit (Rapoff & Barnard, 1991). This chapter reviews the prevalence, consequences, and correlates and predictors of adherence problems for adolescents with chronic diseases, as well as strategies for improving adherence.

PREVALENCE OF ADHERENCE PROBLEMS

The average nonadherence rate to medical regimens for chronic pediatric diseases is often cited to be about 50% (Jay et al., 1984; Rapoff & Barnard, 1991). However, nonadherence rates vary across different diseases, types of regimens, and methods of defining and measuring adherence. There is also variability in adherence across persons, across age groupings, and within the same persons over time.

Table 16.1 summarizes nonadherence rates to various chronic disease regimens from 25 studies that included or exclusively reported on adolescents with chronic diseases. Several conclusions can be drawn from reviewing these studies:

1. There is wide variability in nonadherence rates across different diseases and types of regimens, with a tendency toward lower adherence to more complex and intrusive regimen components;
2. adherence to regimens for diabetes has been studied most frequently (36% of studies), followed by medications for cancer (20% of studies) and relatively few (2 or 3) for the remaining chronic diseases;
3. the majority of these studies (52%) assessed adherence with medications;
4. many of these studies (40%) relied on less objective methods of assessing adherence, such as patient, parent, or health care provider ratings; and
5. varied and relatively arbitrary criteria have been used to classify patients in a dichotomous fashion (adherent or nonadherent) based on cross-sectional and single assessments of adherence.

NONADHERENCE CONSEQUENCES

Potentially serious health consequences can result from adherence failures (Rapoff & Barnard, 1991; Varni & Wallander, 1984). Incomplete adherence to immunosuppressive drugs has been linked to heart, kidney, and liver transplant failures (Stuber, 1993). In one study (Ettenger et al., 1991), 64% (30/47) of adolescents were found to be nonadherent, with 15% rejecting their allografts and 26% experiencing graft dysfunction attributed to nonadherence. These adherence-related transplant failures are particularly tragic, given that approximately 19% of heart, 12% of liver, and 1% of kidney potential adolescent recipients die while on organ transplant waiting lists (Stuber, 1993). Adherence failures have also been implicated in the rise in mortality due to asthma in children and adolescents (Sly, 1988) and the reemergence of drug-resistant infectious diseases such as tuberculosis (Bloom & Murray, 1992; Gibbons, 1992). Drug-resistant microbes evolve when bacteria exposed to different and incomplete doses of antimicrobials develop a defense against these drugs. The potential for drug-resistant microbes could be especially threatening to young people with compromised immunity, such as those with cancer and cystic fibrosis, who are prone to opportunistic infections.

The cost-effectiveness of medical care can be adversely affected by nonadherence (Rapoff & Barnard, 1991; Smith, 1985). Money may be wasted on unused medications or other therapies which are not followed. Physician visits and hospitalizations may also be increased for nonadherent patients (Sly, 1988). For example, the costs associated with treating drug-resistant infectious diseases has been estimated to be between $100 million and $200 million a year in the United States alone (Gibbons, 1992).

TABLE 16.1 Nonadherence Rates for Selected Chronic Disease Regimens (Studies Which Include or Exclusively Report on Adolescents).

Reference	Sample	Disease & Regimen	Adherence Measure	Results
Eney & Goldstein, 1976	N=43 3-16yrs	Asthma Theophylline	Serum assay (therapeutic range=10-20ug/ml or higher)	88% of sample had sub-therapeutic levels. Median level=2.65ug/ml: range= 0-15.4)
Radius et al., 1978	N=80 9mos.-17yrs (M=7.7yrs)	Asthma Theophylline	Serum assay	34% had negative values
Smith et al., 1979	N=52 8mos-17yrs	Cancer Prednisone	Urine Assay (<18.7kgs/cr defined as subtherapeutic)	33% had subtherapeutic levels
Lansky et al., 1983	N=31 2.1-14.3yrs (M=7.2yrs	Cancer Prednisone	Urine Assay (<18.7kgs/cr defined as subtherapeutic)	42% had subtherapeutic levels (M=19.88; range=4.95-40.05)
Tebbi et al., 1986	N=46 2.5-23yrs. (M=6.85yrs)	Cancer Prednisone	Patient and parent report (corroborated by serum assay). Nonadherence defined as any missed dose during preceeding month.	Nonadherence rates, post-diagnoses, at 2wks=18.8%; at 20wks=39.5%; & at 50wks=35%
Phipps & DeCuir-Whalley, 1990	N=54 1mos.-20yrs (M=9yrs)	Cancer Antibiotics as part of bone marrow transplant	Review of patient chart and notes from psychosocial team meetings	"Significant" adherence difficulties identified in 52% of sample

TABLE 16.1 *(continued)*

Festa, Tamaroff, Chasalow, & Lanzkowsky, 1992	*N*=50 (2 samples with M=15.6yrs and M=19.1yrs.)	Cancer Prednisone (N=21) for ALL. Penicillin (N=29) for postsplenectomy prophylaxis.	Serum assay for prednisone Urine assay for penicillin	52% nonadherent to prednisone 48% nonadherent to penicillin
Passero et al., 1981	*N*=58 (no specific ages given)	Cystic Fibrosis Antibiotics, Vitamins, Chest physiotherapy, & Diet	Patient report	Incomplete adherence for: antibiotics=7%; vitamins=10%; chest physiotherapy=60%; & diet=80%.
Czajkowski & Koocher, 1986	*N*=40 13-23 yrs	Cystic Fibrosis Chest physiotherapy, Diet, Medications, Recording daily input and output, & cooperation with medical tests (on inpatient unit).	Medical and nursing notes used to rate degree of adherence (rater not specified)	35% of sample identified as being nonadherent

(continued)

TABLE 16.1 *(continued)*

Reference	Sample	Disease & Regimen	Adherence Measure	Results
Lorenz et al., 1985	N=90 9-15yrs (M=12.8yrs)	Diabetes Diet	Observations (unobtrusively done in camp setting) Error rate calculated by summing additions & deletions to meal plan divided by the total number of exchanges	Mean error rate=.35 (standard deviation=.19)
Wing et al., 1985	N=282 (M=13.2yrs) N=209 completed adherence measure	Diabetes Blood glucose monitoring	Patient report (frequency of monitoring in the past month)	12% not monitoring 25% monitoring <1 once/day 37% monitoring 1-2/day 26% monitoring 3 or >/day
Wilson & Endres, 1986	N=18 12-18yrs	Diabetes Blood glucose monitoring	Meters with memory (patients and parents unaware of memory capabilities)	30% of blood tests not performed over 6wks. Mean=40% of blood tests recorded by patient but not registered by meter. Mean=18% of blood tests not recorded by patients were registered by meter

TABLE 16.1 *(continued)*

Wing et al., 1986	N=62 (M=13.5yrs)	Diabetes Blood glucose monitoring	Observation of blood glucose monitoring technique by trained observers in clinic	48% estimated blood glucose within 20% of actual value Sterile technique poor; only 10% worked on a tissue or paper towel and none washed hands 40% incorrectly timed test 21% did not adequately wipe blood from testing strip
Jacobson et al., 1987 cents	N=57 9-15yrs (M=12.8yrs)	Diabetes Diet Insulin usage Blood glucose monitoring	Health Care Provider Ratings on a 4-point scale (4=excellent, 3=good, 2=fair, 1=poor) for each regimen component and a composite index	First 9-mos interval mean adherence ratings by regimen: diet=3.2; insulin usage=3.3; blood glucose monitoring=2.8 & composite index=3 Second 9-mos interval mean adherence ratings by regimen: diet=2.9; insulin usage=3; blood glucose monitoring=2.5 & composite index=2.7 (second 9-mos interval significantly lower than first) Adolescents vs. preadoles- had significantly lower adherence on diet, blood glucose monitoring, & the composite index

(continued)

TABLE 16.1 *(continued)*

Reference	Sample	Disease & Regimen	Adherence Measure	Results
Jacobson et al., 1990	N=61 9-16yrs	Diabetes Diet Insulin usage Blood glucose monitoring	Health Care Provider Ratings on a 4-point scale (4=excellent, 3=good, 2=fair, 1=poor) Composite index derived from regimen components	Mean adherence ratings by year: Yr. 1=3.07; Yr. 2=2.83; Yr. 3=2.63; & Yr. 4=2.43
Hentinen & Kyngas, 1992	N=47 15-17yrs	Diabetes Insulin Diet Glucose monitoring	Patient report (questionnaire) with patient responses used to categorize adherence as high, average, or low	Percent of patients categorized as having low adherence by regimen component: insulin=3%; diet=34%; glucose monitoring=38%
Kovacs et al., 1992	N=95 8-13yrs. (M=11.1yrs)	Diabetes Insulin use Glucose monitoring Diet	Diagnosis of medical nonadherence by clinicians based on structured interviews with patients and parents	29.5% of sample were nonadherent Nonadherence emerged an average of 3.5yrs after disease onset
Schmidt et al., 1992	N=69 4-18yrs (M=14.2yrs)	Diabetes Diet	Patient dietary records over a 3-day period Registered dietitian tallied the number of food exchanges that deviated from prescribed meal plans	Mean daily deviation from prescribed food exchanges=23.8% (patients added or deleted, on average, about one of four exchanges)

TABLE 16.1 *(continued)*

Litt & Cuskey, 1981	N=82 (M=12yrs)	Juvenile Rheumatoid Arthritis Salicylates	Serum Assay (<$20mg/dl defined nonadherence)	45% of patients nonadherent Mean serum level=21.3mg/dl
Litt et al., 1982	N=38 (M=14yrs)	Juvenile Rheumatoid Arthritis Salicylates	Serum assay (<$20mg/dl defined nonadherence)	45% of patients nonadherent Mean serum level=20.79mg/dl
Beck et al., 1980	N=21 3-20yrs	Renal disease immunospressive drugs, post-transplant	Pill counts	43% of patients were nonadherent (all were adolescents)
Ettenger et al., 1991	N=165 (M=13.5yrs) Adherence analyzed for subset of 70 patient	Renal disease immunospressive drugs, post-transplant	Patient report & serum assay (patients classified as nonadherent if they reported missing any medications for 3 or more days in 1 week or if serum level was "abnormally low"	50% (35 of 70) were nonadherent Nonadherence rate higher for adolescents (64%)

(continued)

TABLE 16.1 *(continued)*

Reference	Sample	Disease & Regimen	Adherence Measure	Results
Kurtin et al., 1994	N=23 10-19yrs (M=16yrs)	Renal disease Medications Diet	Nurse rated adherence on a 5-point scale ("very often" to "never") Nonadherence defined as those patients rated as "sometimes", "almost never", or "never" adherent	59% of patients rated as nonadherent
Friedman et al., 1986	N=25 9-17yrs	Seizures Phenobarbital	Saliva assay (<3.0 ug/ml defined nonadherence)	21% of patients nonadherent Mean saliva level=5.11 ug/ml
Hazzard et al., 1990	N=35 9-16yrs	Seizures Anticonvulsant medications	Serum assay (nonadherence defined as subtherapeutic levels for 3 separate assays obtained an average of 2.52 months apart)	56% of patients nonadherent

These serious health and economic consequences of nonadherence illustrate the importance of identifying correlates of adherence, particularly those which can be modified to improve adherence to therapeutic regimens. These efforts have the potential of increasing treatment efficacy, reducing disease-related morbidity and mortality, reducing unnecessary health care costs, and improving the yield from clinical drug trials.

CORRELATES AND PREDICTORS OF NONADHERENCE

There are few extant theoretical models which have been proposed and tested that are relevant to the pediatric medical adherence literature, with the exception of variations on the Health Belief Model (HBM) (Rapoff, 1996). Most studies examine correlates or predictors of adherence through correlational or regression analyses, or classify patients as adherent or nonadherent and test for significant between-group differences along factorial dimensions. Patient, family, disease, and regimen factors have been commonly studied as correlates or predictors of adherence. These types of studies can be helpful in identifying risk factors for adherence problems, even if a particular variable (e.g., age) can not be altered to improve adherence. These empirically derived factors can also assist researchers in formulating adherence theories which can then be tested and refined through experimentation (Rapoff & Barnard, 1991).

Patient/Family Factors

Demographics

A number of patient and family-related demographic variables have been associated with adherence. As mentioned, adolescents are at higher risk for nonadherence to regimens for cancer, cystic fibrosis, diabetes, and renal disease. The few studies that examined patient gender effects are less clear than those examining patient age. Males have been found to be less adherent to regimens for cystic fibrosis (Patterson, 1985) and diabetes (Lorenz, Christensen, & Pichert, 1985). However, one study found that males were more adherent than females to insulin-injection and exercise regimens for diabetes (Johnson, Freund, Silverstein, Hansen, & Malone, 1990).

Parental and family demographics have also been studied as correlates of adherence. Lower SES, in general, and lower parental educational levels, specifically, have been associated with nonadherence to regimens for asthma (Radius et al., 1978), cystic fibrosis (Patterson, 1985), diabetes (Bobrow, AvRuskin, & Siller, 1985), and renal disease (Brownbridge & Fielding, 1994). Adolescents whose parents are separated or divorced are less likely to be adherent to regimens for asthma (Radius et al., 1978) and renal disease (Brownbridge & Fielding, 1994). In addition, patients in larger families and patients whose mothers work outside the home are less likely to be adherent to regimens for cystic fibrosis (Patterson, 1985).

Knowledge/Health Beliefs

Patients who are less knowledgeable about their disease and treatment tend to be less adherent to regimens for cancer (Tebbi et al., 1986), cystic fibrosis (Gudas et al., 1991), and diabetes (La Greca et al., 1990). However, patient knowledge in one study was not associated with adherence to medications for renal disease (Beck et al., 1980). A different picture emerges with parental knowledge about their child's disease and treatment. In one study, maternal knowledge of diabetes was unrelated to adherence for adolescents but significantly correlated for preadolescents (La Greca et al., 1990).

Factors related to the Health Belief Model (HBM) have been examined in several studies from parents' and patients' perspectives. The HBM posits four sets of variables that predict or explain adherence:

1. *perceived susceptibility*, which is the perceived risk of contracting a particular condition;
2. *perceived severity*, which is a subjective evaluation of the seriousness of contracting or of not receiving treatment for an illness;
3. *perceived benefits*, which refers to beliefs about the effectiveness of treatment options; and
4. *perceived barriers*, which is a type of cost-benefit analysis wherein the person compares the potential costs (including feasibility and potential side effects) of following a particular regimen versus its potential benefits (Janz & Becker, 1984).

In addition, the HBM emphasizes the importance of internal or external cues to action to prompt adherence.

Higher susceptibility or vulnerability and severity, as rated by mothers, has been associated with better adherence to medications for asthma (Radius et al., 1978) and, as rated by patients, for cancer (Tamaroff, Festa, Adesman, & Walco, 1992). In contrast, higher perceived threat or severity by adolescents has been associated with lower adherence to regimens for diabetes (Bond et al., 1992), and to lower adherence to chest physiotherapy for cystic fibrosis (Gudas et al., 1991). Higher levels of perceived benefits, as assessed by mothers, has been associated with better adherence to asthma medications (Radius et al., 1978) and (as assessed by patients) with diabetes regimens (Bobrow et al., 1985; Bond et al., 1992; McCaul et al., 1987). Ratings by parents and adolescents of higher perceived barriers has been uniformly related to poorer adherence to regimens for asthma (Radius et al., 1978) and diabetes (Glasgow, McCaul, & Schafer, 1986; McCaul et al., 1987). The presence of relevant cues to action as assessed by adolescents has been associated with better adherence to diabetes regimens (Bond et al., 1992).

Adjustment and Coping

Adolescent adjustment and coping variables have been frequently examined as correlates of adherence with fairly consistent results. Higher self-esteem has been associated with better adherence to diabetes (Jacobson et al., 1987), JRA (Litt, Cuskey, & Rosenberg, 1982), and seizure (Friedman et al., 1986) regimens. Greater autonomy and personal independence has been related to higher adherence to regimens for JRA (Litt et al., 1982) and seizures (Friedman et al.,1986). Higher social functioning, better disease-specific adjustment, and an internal locus of control have all been associated with higher adherence to diabetes regimens (Jacobson et al., 1987). A sense of optimism has been associated with better adherence to regimens for cystic fibrosis (Gudas et al., 1991), and greater problem-solving skills predicted higher adherence to diabetes regimens (McCaul et al., 1987). Patient and parental satisfaction with care has been associated with better adherence to seizure medications (Hazzard, Hutchinson, & Krawiecki, 1990).

On the negative side of the ledger, adolescents with more behavior problems (Jacobson et al., 1987) and who have a psychiatric disorder (Kovacs et al., 1992) are less likely to be adherent to diabetes regimens. Increased anxiety and depression have also been related to poor adherence to regimens for renal disease (Brownbridge & Fielding, 1994) and the use of denial has been associated with poor adherence to cancer medications (Tamaroff et al., 1992).

Several studies have examined family and parental adjustment and coping as correlates of adherence, with "family environment" variables studied most frequently. Greater family support, expressiveness, harmony, integration, cohesion, and organization have been associated with higher adherence to regimens for cystic fibrosis (Patterson, 1985), diabetes (Hauser et al., 1990; La Greca et al., 1995; McCaul et al., 1987), renal disease (Kurtin, Landgraf, & Abetz, 1994), and seizures (Friedman et al., 1986). In addition, mother-daughter interactions characterized by clear communication, empathy, and positive conflict resolution have been associated with higher adherence to diabetes regimens (Bobrow et al., 1985). Somewhat surprisingly, paternal "nagging" has been associated with better adherence to diabetes regimens (Burroughs, Pontious, & Santiago, 1993).

On the negative side, higher marital satisfaction has been related to lower adherence to cystic fibrosis regimens (Geiss, Hobbs, Hammersley-Maercklein, Kramer, & Henley, 1992). Parental coping difficulties have been associated with poor adherence to JRA (Wynn & Eckel, 1986) and renal (Brownbridge & Fielding, 1994) regimens. Increased parental depression has been related to poor adherence to renal disease regimens (Brownbridge & Fielding, 1994) and greater parental anxiety has been related to lower adherence to seizure medications (Hazzard et al., 1990). Also, those parents who placed more behavioral restrictions on their children tended to have children who were less adherent to their seizure medications (Hazzard et al., 1990).

Parental Monitoring

The lack of parental monitoring of their adolescents' adherence to treatment-related activities has been implicated as a contributor to nonadherence. Family situations where there is ambiguity about who assumes primary responsibility for regimen tasks, or where parental monitoring and supervision is low, have been associated with lower adherence to regimens for cancer (Tebbi, Richards, Cummings, Zevon, & Mallon, 1988), diabetes (Anderson et al., 1990; Bobrow et al., 1985; Ingersoll, Orr, Herrold, & Golden, 1986), and renal disease (Beck et al., 1980). In a sample of 12- to 21-year-olds with diabetes, parental supervision virtually ceased by the time children were 15 years of age (Ingersoll et al., 1986). This relative lack of parental involvement in monitoring adolescents' adherence to treatment regimens may explain why parental knowledge of diabetes is unrelated to adherence for adolescents but significantly correlated with adherence for preadolescents (La Greca et al., 1990), and why parental ratings of adherence for older adolescents is a poor predictor of metabolic control but a significant predictor for younger adolescents (Burroughs et al., 1993).

Disease Factors

Duration

Longer disease duration has been associated with poorer adherence to regimens for diabetes (Bond et al., 1992), JRA (Litt & Cuskey, 1981), and renal disease (Brownbridge & Fielding, 1994). Also, longitudinal studies have found significant deterioration in adherence over time to diabetes regimens, with nonadherence emerging an average of 3.5 years after diabetes onset (Jacobson et al., 1990; Kovacs et al., 1992).

Symptoms

One might expect that increased symptomatology would be related to greater adherence, but this has not been the case with the few studies investigating this variable. Greater numbers of health problems and hospitalizations has been associated with lower adherence to renal disease regimens (Brownbridge & Fielding, 1994). Also, higher numbers of parent-reported seizures have been associated with lower adherence to anticonvulsant medications (Hazzard et al., 1990).

Perceived Severity

As mentioned in the previous section, patient's and parent's perceptions of severity have contrasting relationships with adherence. Patient's perception of higher severity has been related to lower adherence (Gudas et al., 1991) while parent's perception of higher severity relates to higher adherence (Radius et al., 1978). However, patient's and parent's ratings of severity seem be more useful in predicting adherence than do healthcare provider severity ratings (Rapoff & Barnard, 1991).

Regimen Factors

Type and Complexity

Adherence tends to be lower with complex regimens such as chest physiotherapy for cystic fibrosis (Passero, Remor, & Salomon, 1981), dietary regimens for diabetes (Glasgow et al., 1986), and exercise regimens for JRA (Rapoff, Lindsley, & Christophersen, 1985) in contrast to less complex medication regimens.

Costs

Treatment costs can be prohibitive for some families and result in nonadherence (Rapoff & Barnard, 1991). A telephone survey of 138 patients with rheumatic diseases revealed that of those who had a physician visit and purchase of medication in the month before the survey, 40.7% of the parents reported difficulty paying physician-related charges and 25.3% had problems paying medication-related expenses (McCormick, Stemmler, & Athreya, 1986). Further studies are needed to specifically relate treatment costs and adherence to determine if costs influence or are influenced by adherence or if costs are primarily related to disease severity.

Side Effects

Chronic disease treatments can have unpleasant side effects, such as stomach pain from anti-inflammatory medications and joint pain from exercising affected joints in the treatment of JRA (Rapoff, 1989). However, few studies have examined this factor. One of the few located showed that bad-tasting medications related to lower adherence to asthma medications (Radius et al., 1978).

Efficacy

As previously noted, regimens which are perceived by parents and patients as more efficacious are better adhered to (Bobrow et al., 1985; Bond et al., 1992; McCaul et al., 1987; Radius et al., 1978). However, regimen efficacy (in terms of treatment outcome) is usually assumed to be partially determined by adherence. There is support for this connection, as higher adherence has been related to better metabolic control of diabetes (Burroughs et al., 1993; Johnson et al., 1992; Kovacs et al., 1992; Kuttner, Delamater, & Santiago, 1990). Most likely, the relationship between efficacy and adherence is bidirectional. A related issue is delayed benefits of treatments even when patients are highly adherent (Rapoff & Barnard, 1991). For example, an adequate trial of nonsteroidal anti-inflammatory medications in the treatment of JRA is considered to be at least 8 weeks (Lovell, Giannini, & Brewer, 1984).

Summary and Implications

A "risk profile" can be developed for adolescents with chronic diseases who are likely to be nonadherent to their medical regimens. These adolescents tend to come from families that are preoccupied with dysfunctional interaction patterns or, by contrast, with positive social and recreational activities outside the home, that consume time, energy, and resources that could be directed to supervising and managing treatment regimens. Their families are also likely to be larger or in the lower socioeconomic strata, with only one parent living in the home. Their parents tend to be less educated, in general, or specifically about their disease and treatment. Also, their parents are prone to adjustment and coping difficulties and may place undue restrictions on their children's activities.

The adolescents are likely to have adjustment and coping difficulties and be less knowledgeable about their disease and treatment. They are also likely to have primary responsibility for carrying out regimen tasks with little or no direct supervision by their parents. Both the parents and the adolescents tend to hold beliefs that undermine adherence efforts, such as perceiving more costs than benefits from adhering to treatment regimens. These adolescents have also had to cope with their disease and treatment over a period of years, with fluctuations in the type and severity of symptoms associated with their disease. They have also been prescribed regimens that are often complex, intrusive, costly, produce negative side effects, and are not immediately efficacious.

The flip side of this discussion is that "resource" factors can also be gleaned from these studies which point to specific ways patients can be helped to achieve better adherence. It is clear that a positive family environment is critical to supporting adolescent adherence to chronic disease regimens. Most adolescents report being close to their parents, respect them, and rely on them for support (Coleman & Hendry, 1990; Crockett & Petersen, 1993). Part of this support by parents involves shared responsibility for treatment regimen tasks and monitoring. Developing autonomy from parents is an important developmental task for adolescents, and close supervision by parents is not as feasible or in, some cases, desirable (Coleman & Hendry, 1990; Crockett & Petersen, 1993). For some adolescents, this decrease in parental supervision increases the likelihood of engaging in misconduct and health-risking behaviors (Crockett & Petersen, 1993). Thus, parents have to balance their adolescents' needs for autonomy, with supervision.

ADHERENCE IMPROVEMENT

Adherence improvement strategies can be broadly classified as educational, organizational, and behavioral (Dunbar, Marshall, & Hovell, 1979). Educational strategies primarily rely on verbal and written instructions designed to inform patients and their parents about the illness, regimen tasks, the importance of adherence, and strategies for improving adherence.

Organizational strategies target changes in the healthcare delivery system, such as increasing assessibility to healthcare services, simplifying regimens, and providing more intense supervision of patients by healthcare providers. Behavioral strategies refer to behavior change procedures, such as patient or parental monitoring, contracting, and token economy programs, designed to alter specific adherence behaviors. Most studies utilize these strategies in combination.

Table 16.2 provides details on adherence improvement studies, primarily conducted with chronically ill adolescents. Overall, there are strikingly few intervention studies. Six of the 10 studies located were concerned with improving adherence to diabetes regimens, no studies were located relevant to regimens for cancer, cystic fibrosis, renal disease, or seizures. However, several conclusions can be drawn from these studies.

Educational strategies are rarely attempted in isolation, but are usually combined with behavioral strategies (e.g., Pieper, Rapoff, Purviance, & Lindsley, 1989). This may occur because educational strategies have limited utility in improving adherence, in part, due to ceiling effects. That is, those patients selected for intervention studies were probably exposed to extensive educational efforts that had their impact on adherence prior to study entry

TABLE 16.2 Adherence Intervention Studies Involving Adolsecents With Chronic Diseases

Reference	Sample/Disease	Regimen/Measure	Procedures	Outcome
Eney & Goldstein, 1976	N=90 (3-16yrs) Asthma	Theophylline Serum/salivary assays	Random selection but not assignment to 2 groups: Gr 1 had no specific intervention. Gr 2 patients Informed that drug ingestion was being monitored and physicians were more "directive" in discussing adherence.	11% of patients in Gr 1 had therapeutic drug levels vs. 42% in Gr 2.
Tinkelman et al., 1980	N=20 (11-18yrs) Asthma	Theophylline Serum assay & pill counts	Random assignment to short-acting (q 6 hr) or sustained-release (q 12hrs) theophylline. Dosing instructions given for both preparations.	Signficantly higher adherence with sustained-release vs. short-acting theophylline by pill counts. No significant difference in serum levels.
Epstein et al., 1981	N=17 (6-16yrs) Diabetes	Urine glucose testing Direct observation	Random assignment to practice condition (patients tested 20 prepared samples but not informed of results) or feedback condition (patients tested samples and given feedback about accuracy).	Mean number of correct urine glucose estimations were significantly higher for feedback (7.2) vs. practice (3.8) conditions post-training.

TABLE 16.2 *(continued)*

Schafer et al., 1982	N=3 (16-18yrs) Diabetes	Urine glucose testing, Insulin use, Exercise, Wearing diabetic information bracelet, and blood glucose testing assessed by patient self-monitoring records.	Multiple baseline across-behaviors design with baseline followed by goal setting and (if needed) contingency contracting conditions.	Goal setting alone effective in improving adherence to wearing info, exercise, & urine testing for subject 1 and for urine testing & exercise for subject 2; goal setting plus contracting improved adherence to insulin use for subject 2; nothing effective for subject 3 who was experiencing severe family problems.
Carney et al., 1983	N=3 (10-14yrs) Diabetes	Blood glucose testing Patient records and used testing strips. Ghb levels	Multiple baseline across subjects with baseline followed by point system exchanged for money and special activities.	All 3 patients showed improvement in % of tests performed with 2 patients improving from <5% in baseline to 87% and 93% after treatment. Gains were maintained at 4-mos follow-up. Ghb levels improved from baseline (10.1%, 15.2%, & 9.1%) to follow-up (9.4%, 11.7%, & 6.0%).

(continued)

TABLE 16.2 *(continued)*

Reference	Sample/Disease	Regimen/Measure	Procedures	Outcome
Snyder, 1987	N=1 (14yrs) Diabetes	Insulin use Urine glucose testing Diet Patient self-monitoring records with independent checks by mother and school nurse	Quasi-experimental single-subject design. Following self-monitoring baseline, patient exposed to self-monitoring plus monetary incentives and then to an additional condition involving hospitalization contingent on hypo- or hyperglycemic episodes for 36 hrs in a private room with no TV, visitors, books, and minimal staff interaction. Behavioral contacting and communication/conflict resolution training was also implemented for antisocial behavior and mother-child conflict.	Mean number of diabetes self-care activities performed was 5.6 during self-monitoring baseline, 6.3 during self-monitoring + reinforcement, and 8.5 during self-monitoring + reinforcement + punishment; 1-mo. follow-up showed maintenance of gains. Also, decreases in antisocial behavior and conflicts and increases in school attendance noted. However, anecdotal reports at 6-mos. post-treatment indicated deterioration of gains with patient hospitalized for drug abuse.
Satin et al., 1989	N=32 (mean age=14.6yrs). Diabetes	Insulin use Urine glucose testing Diet Exercise Parental ratings of self-care (1=very	Random assignment to one of three groups: Gr 1-patients and parents met for 6 weekly sessions to discuss diabetes and management; Gr 2-identical to Gr 1 plus	No significant differences between groups in self-care ratings. Significant decrease in Ghb levels at 6-wk post-intervention for Gr 2 vs. Gr 3. Significant difference in attitudes towards teenager with diabetes (more

TABLE 16.2 *(continued)*

		careful to 5=careless). Ghb levels Attitudes towards teenage with diabetes scales. Family Environment Scale	included a parent simulation of diabetes regimen; or Gr 3-control group.	positive) for Gr's 1 & 2.
Wysocki et al., 1989	*N*=42 (mean age=14yrs) Diabetes	Blood glucose testing Insulin use Diet Exercise Automated recording of blood glucose (reflectance meters). 24-hr recall patient and parent interviews. Ghb levels. Attitudes towards diabetes and diabetes adjustment scales	30 patients randomly assigned to meter-alone (MA) or meter-plus-contract (MC) groups. Remaining 12 patients in conventional-therapy (CT) control group. MA gr patients earned money for bringing meters to clinic. MC gr patients earned money contingent on glucose testing frequency.	By 8th week, MC gr had significantly higher frequency of glucose testing. No differences in overall adherence, Ghb levels, or patient/parent attitudes and adjustment to diabetes.

(continued)

TABLE 16.2 *(continued)*

Reference	Sample/Disease	Regimen/Measure	Procedures	Outcome
Rapoff et al., 1988	*N*=1 (14yrs) JRA	Medications Pill counts Disease activity measures	Single-subject withdrawal design. Following baseline, regimen simplified (q.i.d to t.i.d); token system in the home for 10wks, then withdrawn for 7 wks, reinstated for 7 wks, and then maintenance phase for 8 wks (where token system reintroduced if adherence was <80% for 2consecutive wks. Token system then completely withdrawn.	Mean adherence levels by condition were: baseline=44%; simplified regimen=59%; token system=100%; withdrawal of token system=77%; token system reinstated=99%; maintenance phase=92%; and 9-mos follow-up=97%. Less disease activity evident during simplified regimen and token system phases.
Pieper et al., 1989	*N*=3 (11–18 yrs) Rheumatic diseases	Medications Pill counts	Multiple baseline across-subjects. Following baseline, patients and parents given instructionsin clinic about medications, adherence, and monitoring/ reinforcement strategies.	Because over- as well as underdosing occurred, patients classified as adherent if pill counts indicated 80–120% of doses were taken. The mean % of pill counts in acceptable range were: baseline =38%, 7%, & 33%; intervention=89%, 67%, & 88%; 6-mos. follow-up=100% for all patients; and 12-mos. follow-up=67% for 2 patients.

(Rapoff & Barnard, 1991). Also, knowing about something (declarative knowledge) is quite different than knowing how to do something (procedural knowledge) or performing in accordance with expectations (Glaser & Bassok, 1989; Reese, 1989).

The primary organizational strategies used have been physician monitoring and simplifying regimens. Increased physician monitoring has improved adherence to asthma medications (Eney & Goldstein, 1976). Simplifying regimens, by reducing the number of medication doses, has improved adherence to medications for asthma (Tinkelman, Vanderpool, Carroll, Page, & Spangler, 1980) and JRA (Rapoff, Purviance, & Lindsley, 1988).

By far the most frequently tested and effective strategies have been behaviorally based, including explicit training and feedback (Epstein, Figueroa, Farkas, & Beck, 1981), goal-setting and contracting (Schafer, Glasgow, & McCaul, 1982), and reinforcement programs (Carney, Schechter, & Davis, 1983; Rapoff et al., 1988; Wysocki, Green, & Huxtable, 1989). Sometimes punishment procedures have been added when reinforcement contingencies have not been sufficient (Snyder, 1987). However, most of these studies have included small samples and have used fairly complicated interventions that are not likely to be feasible for routine use in subspecialty settings.

The most intriguing study reviewed in Table 16.2 is one reported by Satin, La Greca, Zigo, and Skyler (1989), who employed a parent simulation component whereby parents simulated their children's diabetes regimens. This simulation, coupled with weekly support and educational sessions, resulted in improvements in metabolic control of patients' diabetes.

CLINICAL IMPLICATIONS

Based on this and other reviews (Friedman & Litt, 1987; Jay et al., 1984; Meichenbaum & Turk, 1987; Rapoff & Barnard, 1991; Rapoff & Christophersen, 1982; Varni & Wallander, 1984), several clinical implications can be drawn.

Cooperative Alliance

Patients and their families are not satisfied with a passive role in their health care. Most want a greater role in making decisions regarding their health (Cassell, 1991). Chronic disease care needs to be a collaborative effort between adolescents, their parents, and providers. A first step in this approach is to set explicit and mutually agreed-upon treatment goals. Patients and their families may be less inclined to follow treatment plans that fail to address their goals, which are usually related to functional concerns such as relating to peers, academic success, and engaging in recreational and social activities.

Greater involvement of adolescents in this clinical alliance also recognizes their need for autonomy and their increased cognitive sophistication (Coleman & Hendry, 1990; Crockett & Petersen, 1993).

Developmental Sensitivity

Providers who treat adolescents need to be sensitive to their developmental needs, challenges, and capacities. Among these are physical, cognitive, self-identity and esteem, and autonomy issues (see Crockett & Petersen, 1993, for an excellent review of individual and social factors impacting health promotion with adolescents). For example, we expect adolescents, in their transition to adulthood, to be more self-governed and responsible for their behavior. However, there needs to be a balance between giving adolescents opportunities to exercise their autonomy while minimizing risks to their health and well-being.

Parental Monitoring and Support

Clearly, parental involvement, in the form of appropriate monitoring, shared responsibility, and articulation and enforcement of reasonable limits is critical to enhancing adherence to medical regimens and the competencies of adolescents, in general (Crockett & Petersen, 1993). An "authoritative" parenting style seems to be the most useful approach. This style has been characterized as "a constellation of parent attributes that includes emotional support, high standards, appropriate autonomy granting, and clear, bidirectional communication" (Darling & Steinberg, 1993, p. 487). This type of parenting approach has been associated with better adherence to medical regimens for adolescents.

Education

Educational strategies are necessary, but not sufficient, to maintain adherence to regimens for chronic diseases (Rapoff & Christophersen, 1982). The content needs to be expanded to include not only disease and treatment information but specific instructions on how to maintain adherence and why consistent adherence is important (Rapoff & Barnard, 1991). Educational methods also need to be expanded beyond verbal and written information-giving, to include modeling, behavioral rehearsal, and contingent performance feedback (e.g., Epstein et al., 1981). Educational content and methods need to capitalize on the developing ability of adolescents to engage in abstract thinking (Crockett & Petersen, 1993). In addition, education needs to be viewed as an ongoing process for patients and families. When patients are first diagnosed, they and their parents may be too anxious to adequately attend to and retain complex information required to master multicomponent chronic disease regimens. Also, regimens are periodically altered, which necessitates educational updates or booster sessions.

Healthcare Delivery

There is a tendency for providers to "blame" patients and their families for adherence problems while ignoring how they themselves interact with patients and families to deliver healthcare (Dunbar-Jacob, 1993; Rapoff & Barnard, 1991). Generally, "consumer-friendly" clinical settings need to be developed in order to enhance satisfaction with medical care and thereby promote adherence. This includes pleasant physical surroundings, prompt and accessible care, and a consistent provider (Rapoff & Barnard, 1991). Also, providers need to take care how they prescribe regimens. Patients and their families have a finite amount of time, energy, and resources to devote to medical regimens, if they are to maintain some semblance of a normal family life (Patterson, 1985). Providers need to minimize the complexity, costs, and negative side effects of regimens. It is also incumbent on providers to prescribe regimens that are efficacious. Patients and families want their provider to be sensitive and caring but not at the expense of competency.

Adherence Incentives

Ideally, patients are prescribed treatments which rapidly and pervasively control their disease symptoms. Thus, the "natural" reinforcer for adherence is that patients get and feel better. However, this rarely happens in treating complex chronic diseases. This situation creates the necessity of using "contrived" reinforcers, such as token systems, to improve and maintain adherence until disease symptoms abate or remit. This review and others (Friedman & Litt, 1987; Jay et al., 1984; Meichenbaum & Turk, 1987; Rapoff & Barnard, 1991; Rapoff & Christophersen, 1982; Varni & Wallander, 1984) clearly show the effectiveness of behavioral procedures in improving adherence to chronic disease regimens. But positive reinforcement may not be sufficient in some cases (e.g., Snyder, 1987). Parents may need assistance in the use of appropriate discipline strategies such as token fines (Rapoff, 1994). This may be particularly difficult for parents of chronically ill patients as evidenced by studies which show that these parents (relative to parents of healthy children) are more likely to excuse their children's misbehavior and fail to set limits (Ievers, Drotar, Dahms, Doershuk, & Stern, 1994; Walker, Garber, & Van Slyke, 1995). The importance of setting and enforcing reasonable limits can be explained to parents as vital to fostering self-discipline in their children. This is particularly important for children with chronic diseases, who need a higher level of self-discipline than healthy children, given the increased demands and challenges of living with a chronic illness.

At-Risk Patients and Families

In some cases, medical nonadherence can be symptomatic of, or exist concurrently with, patient or family dysfunction. For some adolescents, this may be part of a broader pattern of externalizing (e.g., oppositional and defiant disorder) or internalizing disorders (e.g., depression). There may also be parental or family problems. These types of problems may need to be addressed before or concurrent with efforts to manage medical nonadherence, and are better addressed by mental health professionals who have extensive experience with adolescents in medical settings (Rapoff & Barnard, 1991).

Inflated Importance of Adherence

This is a paradoxical way to conclude a chapter that has emphasized the importance of adherence in improving the health of adolescents with chronic diseases. Adherence and treatment outcome parameters may be influenced by factors unrelated to patient behavior. For example, subtherapeutic assay levels may reflect inadequate dosing, pharmacokinetic variations in metabolism, and interactions with other drugs (Backes & Schentag, 1991). Also, unless medications (such as theophylline and insulin) are adjusted in response to pubertal growth spurts, poor treatment outcomes among adolescents may be misattributed to nonadherence (Barnard, 1986; Cary, Hein, & Dell, 1991). However, when confronted with less than adequate outcomes in the treatment of chronic diseases for adolescents, a reasonable first step is to investigate the contribution of patient adherence.

REFERENCES

Anderson, B. J., Auslander, W. F., Jung, K. C., Miller, J. P., & Santiago, J. V. (1990). Assessing family sharing of diabetes responsibilities. *Journal of Pediatric Psychology, 15*, 477–492.

Backes, J. M., & Schentag, J. J. (1991). Partial compliance as a source of variance in pharmacokinetics and therapeutic drug monitoring. In J. A. Cramer & B. Spilker (Eds.), *Patient compliance in medical practice and clinical trials* (pp. 27–36). New York: Raven.

Barnard, M. U. (1986). Care of the child with Type I diabetes. In *Pediatrics: Nursing update*, (Vol. 1) (pp. 1–8). Princeton, NJ: Continuing Professional Education Center.

Beck, D. E., Fennell, R. S., Yost, R. L., Robinson, J. D., Geary, D., & Richards, G. A. (1980). Evaluation of an educational program on compliance with medication regimens in pediatric patients with renal transplants. *Journal of Pediatrics, 96*, 1094–1097.

Bloom, B. R., & Murray, C. J. L. (1992). Tuberculosis: Commentary on a reemergent killer. *Science, 257*, 1055–1064.

Blum, R. W. (1987). Contemporary threats to adolescent health in the United States. *Journal of the American Medical Association, 257*, 3390–3395.

Blum, R. W. (1992). Chronic illness and disability in adolescence. *Journal of Adolescent Health, 13*, 364–368.

Bobrow, E. S., AvRuskin, T. W., & Siller, J. (1985). Mother-daughter interaction and adherence to diabetes regimens. *Diabetes Care, 8*, 146–151.

Bond, G. G., Aiken, L. S., & Somerville, S. C. (1992). The health belief model and adolescents with insulin-dependent diabetes mellitus. *Health Psychology, 11*, 190–198.

Brownbridge, G., & Fielding, D. M. (1994). Psychosocial adjustment and adherence to dialysis treatment regimes. *Pediatric Nephrology, 8*, 744–749.

Burroughs, T. E., Pontious, S. L., & Santiago, J. V. (1993). The relationship among six psychosocial domains: Age, health care adherence, and metabolic control in adolescents with IDDM. *The Diabetes Educator, 19*, 396–402.

Carney, R. M., Schechter, K., & Davis, T. (1983). Improving adherence to blood glucose testing in insulin-dependent diabetic children. *Behavior Therapy, 14*, 247–254.

Cary, J., Hein, K., & Dell, R. (1991). Theophylline disposition in adolescents with asthma. *Therapeutic Drug Monitoring, 13*, 309–313.

Cassell, E. J. (1991). *The nature of suffering*. New York: Oxford University Press.

Coleman, J. C., & Hendry, L. (1990). *The nature of adolescence* (2nd ed). New York: Routledge.

Crockett, L. J., & Petersen, A. C. (1993). Adolescent development: Health risks and opportunities for health promotion. In S. G. Millstein, A. C. Petersen, & E. O. Nightingale (Eds.), *Promoting the health of adolescents: New directions for the twenty-first century* (pp. 13–37). New York: Oxford Press.

Czajkowski, D. R., & Koocher, G. P. (1986). Predicting medical compliance among adolescents with cystic fibrosis. *Health Psychology, 5*, 297–305.

Darling, N., & Steinberg, L. (1993). Parenting style as context: An integrative model. *Psychological Bulletin, 113*, 487–496.

Dunbar, J. M., Marshall, G. D., & Hovell, M. F. (1979). Behavioral strategies for improving compliance. In R. B.Haynes, D. W. Taylor, & D. L. Sackett (Eds.), *Compliance in health care* (pp.174–190). Baltimore: The Johns Hopkins University Press.

Dunbar-Jacob, J. (1993). Contributions to patient adherence: Is it time to share the blame? *Health Psychology, 12*, 91–92.

Elliott, D. S. (1993). Health-enhancing and health-compromising lifestyles. In S. G. Millstein, A. C. Petersen, & E. O. Nightingale (Eds.), *Promoting the health of adolescents: New directions for the twenty-first century* (pp. 119–145). New York: Oxford Press.

Elster, A. B., & Kuznets, N. J. (1994). *AMA Guidelines for Adolescent Preventive Services (GAPS): Recommendations and rationale*. Chicago, IL.: American Medical Association

Eney, R. D., & Goldstein, E. O. (1976). Compliance of chronic asthmatics with oral administration of theophylline as measured by serum and salivary levels. *Pediatrics, 57*, 513–517.

Epstein, L. H., Figueroa, J., Farkas, G. M., & Beck, S. (1981). The short-term effects of feedback on accuracy of urine glucose determinations in insulin dependent diabetic children. *Behavior Therapy, 12*, 560–564.

Ettenger, R. B., Rosenthal, J. T., Marik, J. L., Malekzadeh, M., Forsythe, S. B., Kamil, E. S., Salusky, I. B., & Fine, R. N. (1991). Improved cadaveric renal transplant outcome in children. *Pediatric Nephrology, 5*, 137–142.

Festa, R. S., Tamaroff, M. H., Chasalow, F., & Lanzkowsky, P. (1992). Therapeutic adherence to oral medication regimens by adolescents with cancer: 2. Laboratory assessment. *Journal of Pediatrics, 120*, 807–811.

Friedman, I. M., & Litt, I. F. (1987). Adolescents' compliance with therapeutic regimens. *Journal of Adolescent Health Care, 8*, 52–67.

Friedman, I. M., Litt, I. F., King, D. R., Henson, R., Holtzman, D., Halverson, D., & Kraemer, H. C. (1986). Compliance with anticonvulsant therapy by epileptic youth. *Journal of Adolescent Health Care, 7*, 12–17.

Geiss, S. K., Hobbs, S. A., Hammersley-Maercklein, F., Kramer, J. C., & Henley, M. (1992). Psychosocial factors related to perceived compliance with cystic fibrosis treatment. *Journal of Clinical Psychology, 48*, 99–103.

Gibbons, A. (1992). Exploring new strategies to fight drug-resistant microbes. *Science, 257*, 1036–1038.

Glaser, R., & Bassok, M. (1989). Learning theory and the study of instructions. *Annual Review of Psychology, 40*, 631–666.

Glasgow, R. E., McCaul, K. D., & Schafer, L. C. (1986). Barriers to regimen adherence among persons with insulin-dependent diabetes. *Journal of Behavioral Medicine, 9*, 65–77.

Gudas, L. J., Koocher, G. P., & Wypij, D. (1991). Perceptions of medical compliance in children and adolescents with cystic fibrosis. *Journal of Developmental and Behavioral Pediatrics, 12*, 236–242.

Hauser, S. T., Jacobson, A. M., Lavori, P., Wolfsdorf, J. I., Herskowitz, R. D., Milley, J. E., Bliss, R. (1990). Adherence among children and adolescents with insulin-dependent diabetes mellitus over a four-year longitudinal follow-up: II. Immediate and long-term linkages with the family milieu. *Journal of Pediatric Psychology, 15*, 527–541.

Hazzard, A., Hutchinson, S. J., & Krawiecki, N. (1990). Factors related to adherence to medication regimens in pediatric seizure patients. *Journal of Pediatric Psychology, 15*, 543–555.

Hentinen, M., & Kyngas, II. (1992). Compliance of young diabetics with health regimens. *Journal of Advanced Nursing*, 17, 530–536.

Holden, E. W., & Nitz, K. (1995). Epidemiology of adolescent health disorders. In J. L. Wallander & L. J. Siegel (Eds.), *Adolescent health problems: Behavioral perspectives* (pp. 7–21). New York: Guilford.

Ievers, C. E., Drotar, D., Dahms, W. T., Doershuk, C. F., & Stern, R. S. (1994). Maternal child-rearing behavior in three groups: Cystic fibrosis, insulin-dependent diabetes mellitus, and healthy children. *Journal of Pediatric Psychology, 19*, 681–687.

Ingersoll, G. M., Orr, D. P., Herrold, A. J., & Golden, M. P. (1986). Cognitive maturity and self-management among adolescents with insulin-dependent diabetes mellitus. *Journal of Pediatrics, 108*, 620–623.

Jacobson, A. M., Hauser, S. T., Lavori, P., Willett, J. B., Cole, C. F., Wolfsdorf, J. I., Dumont, R. H., & Wertlieb, D. (1994). Family environment and glycemic control: A four-year prospective study of children and adolescents with insulin-dependent diabetes mellitus. *Psychosomatic Medicine, 56*, 401–409.

Jacobson, A. M., Hauser, S. T., Lavori, P., Wolfsdorf, J. I., Herskowitz, R. D., Milley, J. E., Bliss, R., & Gelfand, E. (1990). Adherence among children and adolescents with insulin-dependent diabetes mellitus over a four-year longitudinal follow-up: I. The influence of patient coping and adjustment. *Journal of Pediatric Psychology, 15*, 511–526.

Jacobson, A. M., Hauser, S. T., Wolfsdorf, J. I., Houlihan, J., Milley, J. E., Herskowitz, R. D., Wertlieb, D., & Watt, E. (1987). Psychologic predictors of compliance in children with recent onset of diabetes mellitus. *Journal of Pediatrics, 110*, 805–811.

Janz, N. K., & Becker, M. H. (1984). The health belief model: A decade later. *Health Education Quarterly, 11*, 1–47.

Jay, S., Litt, I. F., & Durant, R. H. (1984). Compliance with therapeutic regimens. *Journal of Adolescent Health Care, 5*, 124–136.

Johnson, S. B., Freund, A., Silverstein, J., Hansen, C. A., & Malone, J. (1990). Adherence-health status relationships in childhood diabetes. *Health Psychology, 9*, 606–631.

Johnson, S. B., Kelly, M., Henretta, J. C., Cunningham, W. R., Tomer, A., & Silverstein, J. H. (1992). A longitudinal analysis of adherence and health status in childhood diabetes. *Journal of Pediatric Psychology, 17*, 537–553.

Kovacs, M., Goldston, D., Obrosky, S., & Iyengar, S. (1992). Prevalence and predictors of pervasive noncompliance with medical treatment among youths with insulin-dependent diabetes mellitus. *Journal of the American Academy of Child and Adolescent Psychiatry, 31*, 1112–1119.

Kurtin, P. S., Landgraf, J. M., & Abetz, L. (1994). Patient-based health status measurements in pediatric dialysis: Expanding the assessment of outcome. *American Journal of Kidney Diseases, 24*, 376–382.

Kuttner, M. J., Delamater, A. M., & Santiago, J. V. (1990). Learned helplessness in diabetic youths. *Journal of Pediatric Psychology, 15*, 581–594.

La Greca, A. M., Auslander, W. F., Greco, P., Spetter, D., Fisher, E. B., & Santiago, J. V. (1995). I get by with a little help from my family and friends: Adolescents' support for diabetes care. *Journal of Pediatric Psychology, 20*, 449–476.

La Greca, A. M., Follansbee, D., & Skyler, J. S. (1990). Developmental and behavioral aspects of diabetes management in youngsters. *Children's Health Care, 19*, 132–139.

Lansky, S. B., Smith, S. D., Cairns, N. V., & Cairns, G. F., Jr. (1988). Psychological correlates of compliance. *The American Journal of Pediatric Hematology/Oncology, 5*(1), 87–92.

Litt, I. F., & Cuskey, W. R. (1981). Compliance with salicylate therapy in adolescents with juvenile rheumatoid arthritis. *American Journal of Diseases of Children, 135*, 434–436.

Litt, I. F., Cuskey, W. R., & Rosenberg, B. A. (1982). Role of self-esteem and autonomy in determining medication compliance among adolescents with juvenile rheumatoid arthritis. *Pediatrics, 69*, 15–17.

Lorenz, R. A., Christensen, N. K., & Pichert, J. W. (1985). Diet-related knowledge, skill, and adherence among children with insulin-dependent diabetes mellitus. *Pediatrics, 75*, 872–876.

Lovell, D. J., Giannini, E. H., & Brewer, E. J. (1984). Time course of response to nonsteroidal anti-inflammatory drugs in juvenile rheumatoid arthritis. *Arthritis and Rheumatism, 27*, 1433–1437.

McCaul, K. D., Glasgow, R. E., & Schafer, L. C. (1987). Diabetes regimen behaviors: Predicting adherence. *Medical Care, 25*, 868–881.

McCormick, M. C., Stemmler, M. M., & Athreya, B. H. (1986). The impact of childhood rheumatic diseases on the family. *Arthritis and Rheumatism, 29*, 872–879.

Meichenbaum, D., & Turk, D. C. (1987). *Facilitating treatment adherence: A practitioner's guidebook*. New York: Plenum Press.

Millstein, S. G., & Igra, V. (1995). Theoretical models of adolescent risk-taking behavior. In J. L. Wallander & L. J. Siegel (Eds.), *Adolescent health problems: Behavioral perspectives* (pp. 52–71). New York: Guilford.

Newacheck, P. W. (1989). Adolescents with special health needs: Prevalence, severity, and access to health services. *Pediatrics, 85*, 872–881.

Newacheck, P. W., & Taylor, W. R. (1992). Childhood chronic illness: Prevalence, severity, and impact. *American Journal of Public Health, 82*, 364–371.

Passero, M. A., Remor, B., & Salomon, J. (1981), Patient-reported compliance with cystic fibrosis therapy, *Clinical Pediatrics, 20*, 264–268.

Patterson, J. M. (1985). Critical factors affecting family compliance with home treatment for children with cystic fibrosis. *Family Relations, 34*, 79–89.

Phipps, S., & DcCuir-Whalley, S. (1990). Adherence issues in pediatric bone marrow transplantation. *Journal of Pediatric Psychology, 15*, 459–475.

Pieper, K. B., Rapoff, M. A., Purviance, M. R., & Lindsley, C. B. (1989). Improving compliance with prednisone therapy in pediatric patients with rheumatic disease. *Arthritis Care and Research, 2*, 132–135.

Radius, S. M., Becker, M. H., Rosenstock, I. M., Drachman, R. H., Schuberth, K. C., & Teets, K. C. (1978). Factors influencing mother's compliance with a medication regimen for asthmatic children. *Journal of Asthma Research, 15*, 133–149.

Rapoff, M. A. (1989). Compliance with treatment regimens for pediatric rheumatic diseases. *Arthritis Care and Research, 2*, S40–S47.

Rapoff, M. A. (1996, Summer). Why comply? Theories in pediatric medical adherence research. *Progress Notes: Newsletter of the Society of Pediatric Psychology, 20*, 2–3, 6.

Rapoff, M. A. (1994). *Helping children follow their medical treatment program: Guidelines for parents of children with rheumatic diseases*. (Available from Michael Rapoff, PhD., University of Kansas Medical Center, Department of Pediatrics, 3901 Rainbow Blvd., Kansas City, KS. 66160–7330).

Rapoff, M. A., & Barnard, M. U. (1991). Compliance with pediatric medical regimens. In J. A. Cramer & B. Spilker (Eds.), *Patient compliance in medical practice and clinical trials* (pp. 73–98). New York: Raven.

Rapoff, M. A., & Christophersen, E. R. (1982). Compliance of pediatric patients with medical regimens: A review and evaluation. In R. B. Stuart (Ed.), *Adherence, compliance and generalization in behavioral medicine* (pp. 79–124). New York: Brunner/Mazel.

Rapoff, M. A., Lindsley, C. B., & Christophersen, E. R. (1985). Parent perceptions of problems experienced by their children in complying with treatments for juvenile rheumatoid arthritis. *Archives of Physical Medicine and Rehabilitation, 66*, 427–429.

Rapoff, M. A., Purviance, M. R., & Lindsley, C. B. (1988). Improving medication compliance for juvenile rheumatoid arthritis and its effect on clinical outcome: A single subject analysis. *Arthritis Care and Research, 1*, 1–5.

Reese, H. W. (1989). Rules and rule-governance: Cognitive and behavioristic views. In S. C. Hayes (Ed). *Rule-governed behavior: Cognition, contingencies, and instructional control* (pp. 3–84). New York: Plenum.

Satin, W., La Greca, A. M., Zigo, M. A., & Skyler, J. S. (1989). Diabetes in adolescence: Effects of a multifamily group intervention and parent simulation of diabetes. *Journal of Pediatric Psychology, 14*, 259–275.

Schafer, L. C., Glasgow, R. E., & McCaul, K. D. (1982). Increasing the adherence of diabetic adolescents. *Journal of Behavioral Medicine, 5*, 353–362.

Schmidt, L. E., Klover, R. V., Arfken, A. C. L., Delamater, A. M., & Hobson, D. (1992). Compliance with dietary and prescriptions in children and adolescents with insulin-dependent diabetes mellitus. *Journal of the American Dietetic Association, 92*, 567–570.

Sly, R. M. (1988). Mortality from asthma in children 1979–1984. *Annals of Allergy, 60*, 433–443.

Smith, M. (1985). The cost of noncompliance and the capacity of improved compliance to reduce health care expenditures. In *Improving medication compliance: Proceedings of a symposium*. Washington, DC: National Pharmaceutical Council.

Smith, S. D., Rosen, D., Trueworthy, R. C., & Lowman, J. T. (1979). A reliable method for evaluation drug compliance in children with cancer, *Cancer, 43*, 169–173.

Snyder, J. (1987). Behavioral anlysis and treatment of poor diabetic self-care and antisocial behavior: A single-subject experimental study. *Behavior Therapy, 18*, 251–263.

Stuber, M. (1993). Psychiatric aspects of organ transplantation in children and adolescents. *Organ Transplantation in Children and Adolescents, 34*, 379–387.

Tamaroff, M. H., Festa, R. S., Adesman, A. R., & Walco, G. A. (1992). Therapeutic adherence to oral medication regimens by adolescents with cancer. II. Clinical and psychologic correlates, *Journal of Pediatrics, 120*, 812–817.

Tebbi, C. K., Cummings, K. M., Zevon, M., Smith, L., Richards, J., & Mallon, J. (1986). Compliance of pediatric and adolescent cancer patients. *Cancer, 58*, 1179–1184.

Tebbi, C. K., Richards, M. E., Cummings, K. M., Zevon, M. A., & Mallon, J. (1988). The role of parent-adolescent concordance in compliance with cancer chemotherapy. *Adolescence, 23*, 599–611.

Tinkelman, D. G., Vanderpool, G. E., Carroll, M. S., Page, E. G., & Spangler, D. L.

(1980). Compliance differences following adminstration of theophylline at six- and twelve-hour intervals. *Annals of Allergy, 44*, 283–286.

Varni, J. W., & Wallander, J. L. (1984). Adherence to health-related regimens in pediatric chronic disorders. *Clinical Psychology Review, 4*, 585–596.

Walker, L. S., Garber, J., & Van Slyke, D. A. (1995). Do parents excuse the misbehavior of children with physical or emotional symptoms? An investigation of the pediatric sick role. *Journal of Pediatric Psychology, 20*, 329–345.

Wilson, D. P., & Endres, R. K. (1986). Compliance with blood glucose monitoring in children with type I diatetes mellitus. *The Journal of Pediatrics, 108*, 1022–1024.

Wing, R. R., Koeske, R., New, A., Lamparski, D., & Becker, D. (1986). Behavioral skills in self-monitoring of blood glucose: relationship to accuracy. *Diabetes Care, 9*, 330–333.

Wing, R. R., Lamparski, D. M., Zaslow, S., Betschart, J., Simmens, L., & Becker, D. (1985). Frequency and accuracy of self-monitoring of blood glucose in children: relationship to glycemic control. *Diabetes Care, 8*, 214–218.

Wynn, K. S., & Eckel, E. M. (1986). Juvenile rheumatoid arthritis and home physical therapy program compliance. *Physical & Occupational Therapy in Pediatrics, 6*, 55–63.

Wysocki, T., Green, L., & Huxtable, K. (1989). Blood glucose monitoring by diabetic adolescents: Compliance and metabolic control. *Health Psychology, 8*, 267–284.

SECTION V

Lifestyle Change and Adherence Issues Among Patients With Chronic Disease

Wendy L. McBee, Editor

Adaptation to living with a chronic health condition often requires challenging lifestyle changes and maintenance of healthier behaviors. This section focuses on the implementation and integration of lifestyle interventions and self-management issues among older adults with chronic obstructive pulmonary disease (COPD), adolescent and adult diabetics, and patients with cancer.

In Chapter 17, Kaplan et al. describe co-management behaviors that may enhance the quality of life of COPD patients, though these interventions may not necessarily directly affect pulmonary functioning. Comprehensive pulmonary rehabilitation programs, which may contain components such as exercise, education, psychosocial support, and chest physiotherapy, have demonstrated multiple short-term benefits in health status. The long-term effects of these programs are currently being investigated. Although it is not likely possible to change the course of the disease in this patient population, investigators are optimistic that behavior change, in the form of co-management, may help these patients live fuller lives.

In Chapter 18, Glasgow and Eakin emphasize the complexities of diabetes self-management and introduce a conceptual model that integrates the multiple influences of a diabetes self-management regimen. Review of the diabetes control regimen, including self-management of smoking, diet, foot care, blood glucose monitoring, physical activity, and depression, indicates improper management and education in several areas. The importance of the patient-provider interaction is discussed, and the results of an impressive randomized clinical trial that utilized the services of a highly skilled multidisciplinary team of medical and behavioral scientists are described. A model that integrates interventions across all societal levels and allows for appropriate patient participation in interactions with providers may be the most beneficial in terms of overall quality of life for the diabetic patient.

In Chapter 19, Peterman and Cella discuss the role of adherence in treating cancer patients of all ages. As with many diseases, the extent of behaviors requested of cancer patients is broad, and adherence rates vary widely depending upon the behavior being examined. Very few interventions to improve adherence among cancer patients have been proposed to date, but given the life-threatening consequences for patients who do not adhere to some portion of their treatment regimen, the need for such a comprehensive program is emphasized.

17

Co-Management of Chronic Obstructive Pulmonary Disease

Robert M. Kaplan, Elizabeth G. Eakin, Andrew L. Ries, Michelle Toshima, and Catherine J. Atkins

Chronic obstructive pulmonary disease (COPD) is a major cause of disability in most western countries. Behavior and COPD are inseparably intertwined. Extensive evidence over the past 30 years suggests that smoking behavior is the major risk factor for the development of emphysema and chronic bronchitis (American Thoracic Society, 1995). In addition, several epidemiologic studies have shown that the rate of decline in pulmonary function for affected patients decreases with cessation of smoking behavior (American Thoracic Society, 1995; Anthonisen et al., 1994; Austin, 1976). Thus, individual behavior is a major risk factor for the development and maintenance of COPD, and behavioral management strategies are important in the care of COPD patients.

Once diagnosed, patients with COPD are asked to follow a complex regimen that may include monitoring and managing symptoms with multiple medications, respiratory care techniques, regular exercise, proper nutrition/hydration, pacing and relaxation. These are referred to as co-management or self-care behaviors to acknowledge that it is the patient, under medical guidance, who is largely responsible for managing their disease on a day-to-day basis. Previously we, as well as many others, used the terms "compliance" and "adherence" when discussing patients' regimen-related behaviors. We have moved away from these terms because they often imply that following or not following the COPD regimen is a dichotomous phenomenon; that is, that the patient either "complies with" or "adheres to" the entire regimen, or is labeled as noncompliant. As will be discussed in later sections, recent studies have shown that the various COPD co-management behaviors are not highly correlated. Thus, knowing that a patient is taking medications as prescribed tells you little about whether she is engaging in other aspects of the COPD regimen. COPD co-management involves a complex number of behaviors, each of which may have multiple determinants.

In this chapter, we focus on behavioral programs for patients with COPD. As the review will suggest, the contemporary literature contains few descriptions of systematically evaluated programs. Before considering the behavioral interventions, it will be worthwhile to review the definition of COPD and its etiology, prevalence, and medical management.

THE CHRONIC OBSTRUCTIVE PULMONARY DISEASES

American Thoracic Society defines COPD as "a disease state characterized by the presence of airflow obstruction due to chronic bronchitis or emphysema. The airflow obstruction is generally progressive, may be accompanied by airway hyper-reactivity and may be partially reversible," (American Thoracic Society, 1995, p. 577). Chronic bronchitis, emphysema, and asthma are the three diseases most commonly associated with COPD. The common denominator of these disorders is expiratory flow obstruction due to airway narrowing, although the cause of airflow obstruction is different in each. Also, in many patients airflow obstruction may be attributed to more than one specific condition.

Emphysema

Emphysema is characterized by abnormal permanent enlargement of the air spaces resulting from destruction of the walls of the alveoli. Alveoli are clusters of air spaces at the ends of the airways in the lung. As the alveolar walls break down, individual alveoli coalesce, and the lung gradually loses its elasticity. This loss of lung elasticity means that the airways are not held open during expiration and tend to collapse. Air gets trapped in these damaged areas, and the lungs become inflated and enlarged (American Thoracic Society, 1995; Snider, Faling, & Rennard, 1994).

Chronic Bronchitis

Chronic bronchitis is defined as the presence of chronic productive cough for 3 months in each of 2 successive years in a patient in whom other causes of chronic cough have been excluded. It is the result of chronic inflammation of the cells lining the breathing passages (bronchi). The inflammation causes the cells to swell and produce excess quantities of mucus. The swelling and excess mucus result in narrowing of the bronchi, which, in turn, obstructs the airflow and produces chronic cough (American Thoracic Society, 1995).

Asthma

Asthma is a disease characterized by reversible airway narrowing and increased responsiveness to various stimuli such as infection, allergy, cold air, or cigarette smoke. The airway narrowing is caused by smooth muscle spasm, inflammation, and/or oversecretion of mucus. Chronic asthma may develop when the condition persists and does not reverse.

The common feature shared in emphysema, chronic bronchitis, and chronic asthma is difficulty in expelling air from the lungs during expiration. In practice, the clinical signs and symptoms of these conditions are often very similar. In fact, many patients with COPD have varying combinations of emphysema, chronic bronchitis, and asthma. However, asthma differs from chronic bronchitis and emphysema in that at least a component of the obstruction can be reversed by the administration of a bronchodilator medication.

ETIOLOGY

Cigarette smoking is the major risk factor and accounts for nearly 90% of COPD. Compared to nonsmokers, current smokers have approximately 10 times the relative risk of developing COPD. The risk is equal for men and women. Previously, COPD was more common in men due to higher smoking rates. In recent years, the increased smoking rate for women is reflected in increased COPD rates.

There is marked individual variation in susceptibility, and host factors play an important role. Only about 10% to 15% of smokers develop significant obstructive lung disease. In susceptible individuals, smoking is associated with an accelerated decline in lung function over many years that is dose-related to the amount of smoking.

Exposure of nonsmokers to the smoke of others in an indoor environment (secondhand smoke) is associated with an increase in respiratory infections and lung disease in children and to modest changes in lung function in adults. However, it has not been clearly established that passive smoke exposure alone leads to clinically significant obstructive lung disease.

There is some evidence that environmental exposures, such as air pollution and occupational dusts and fumes, are harmful for persons with underlying lung disease and may increase the risk for developing COPD. However, it is not clear whether these effects are independent of smoking. There is also growing evidence that a history of childhood respiratory infections increases the risk for developing COPD in later life (American Thoracic Society, 1995; Snider et al., 1994).

EPIDEMIOLOGY

COPD has become an important public health problem for at least four reasons: (1) it is a major cause of death; (2) it affects a large number of persons; (3) incidence is increasing; and (4) it has a major impact upon activities of daily living (Crystal, 1987). Because COPD is insidious, with a long latency period before clinical recognition, official statistics underestimate morbidity and mortality.

As of 1990, COPD had moved up to the fourth leading cause of death in the United States (Higgins, 1989; Sherill, Lebowitz, & Burrows, 1990). COPD was listed as the underlying cause of more than 90,000 deaths in 1991, accounting for approximately 4% of all deaths. In addition, it was a contributing cause for an additional 5%. In persons 55 to 74 years of age, COPD ranks third among men and fourth among women. In contrast to other major diseases, death rates from COPD have increased considerably in recent years, nearly 38% between 1979 and 1991 (National Center for Health Statistics, 1994).

In the United States, the overall prevalence is approximately 4% to 6% in men and 1% to 3% in women; COPD is recognized in approximately 10% to 15% of adults over age 55 (Feinleib et al., 1989; Higgins & Thom, 1989). The 1989 National Health Interview Survey estimated that 12 million adults had chronic bronchitis and 2 million had emphysema. From 1979 through 1985, the prevalence rates for COPD peaked at 65 to 74 years of age: 136/1,000 in men and 118/1,000 in women. Recent trends indicate prevalence rates that are stable to decreasing in men but increasing among women. Death rates, however, are still higher in men (male:female ratio of 1.7 in 1991) (Snider et al., 1994).

The impact of COPD on morbidity is even greater than on mortality. In the National Health Interview Survey in 1985, COPD accounted for 5% of doctors' office visits and more than 13% of all hospitalizations (Feinleib et al., 1989). COPD is an enormous cause of disability and reduced function among affected individuals.

Epidemiological studies of Burrows and coworkers have identified two main syndromes with different risk factors and natural histories. The "usual" emphysematous form is associated closely with cigarette smoking.

Such individuals develop airflow obstruction insidiously over many years with minimal symptoms, followed by clinical disease in later years with progressive symptoms and high morbidity and mortality. The second form of COPD, chronic asthmatic bronchitis, is associated with risk factors of atropy, high serum IgE, and bronchial hyperreactivity. These individuals develop chronic airflow obstruction independent of smoking, although smoking may provide added risk. Asthmatic bronchitis is more amenable to medical therapy and has better prognosis and survival than the emphysematous type (Burrows, 1991).

Due to the long latency period between smoking exposure and clinical disease, morbidity and mortality from COPD continue to increase, despite decreasing smoking rates. Lower smoking rates will, ultimately, reduce the burden of COPD, but not for many years. With increased overall life expectancy and lower death rates from other major diseases, the impact of COPD will be magnified in our aging population.

PHARMACOLOGICAL INTERVENTIONS

Despite major advances in diagnosis and medical therapeutics, many patients do not receive optimal benefit from standard medical care. While some aspects of COPD are treatable, the medical regimen is extremely complex. Traditional medical management of COPD consists primarily of various medications. However, treatment may also include respiratory chest physiotherapy techniques, exercise, and advice to quit smoking. Most patients are confronted with complex combinations of antibiotics, bronchodilators, anti-inflammatory drugs, and, in some cases, supplemental oxygen.

For this review, all papers since 1980 on co-management of or compliance with the COPD regimen, as well as literature reviews published prior to 1980 (Atkins, 1981; Haynes, Taylor, & Sackett, 1979), were examined. The results of the search, summarized in Table 17.1, revealed few studies that have directly addressed the issue of co-management of COPD, especially regarding traditional medical regimens. The studies considered different treatments in diverse samples and employed various definitions of and measurements for self-care. Unfortunately, few conclusions, if any, can be drawn from the current literature.

Published studies have considered co-management with regard to a variety of different regimens. Adherence with oxygen therapy in Scotland was reported by Morrison, Skwarski, and MacNee (1995). Among COPD patients who were prescribed 24-hour oxygen, only 14% were in full adherence. The average use was 14.9 hours per day, and 44% used their oxygen less than 15 hours per day. These patients also had poor adherence with other aspects of the regimen. Although all patients were requested to have

TABLE 17.1 Summary of Studies on Compliance in COPD

Citation	Regimen	Sample	Measure	Definition	Compliance
Taylor, Kinney, & McDevitt (1984)	Theophyline	63 patients in General Practice clinics (Northern Ireland)	Plasma throphyline levels before and after treatment	Δ Plasma level <5.8 µg/ml at 350 mg dose/day and <9.6 µg/ml at 700 mg/day	60% of patients
			Tablet counting	Taking >80% of prescribed medications	
Chryssidis et al. (1981)	Aerosol therapy (Salbutamol and Beclomethasone diproprionate)	84 outpatients and 30 recently discharged patients (South Australia)	Estimation of compliance by weight of canisters at 1 and 2 months	Compliance score = #doses used divided by #doses prescribed	Mean compliance scores at 1 month = 98.5%, at 3 months = 110.8%
James et al. (1981)	Prescribed drug therapy	185 patients in chest/asthma/allergy clinics (London)	Self-report of drug taking patterns by questionnaire	Maintenance therapy—patients who took prescribed medication regularly	49% of patients
				Full compliance—patients who took prescribed m edication regularly + adjusted therapy according to symptom exacerbation	30% of patients

TABLE 17.1 *(continued)*

IPPB Group Trial (1983)	Intermittent Positive Pressure Breathing therapy	500 patients in multicenter trial	Number of minutes on therapy as measured by recording device	Did assigned therapy >25 minutes/day	50% of patients
	Compressor Nebulizer therapy	485 patients in multicenter trial	attached to the machines		
Kaplan, Atkins, & Reinsch (1984)	Exercise prescription	76 patients randomized into 1 of 5 experimental groups	Self-report of time spent walking (walking logs)	Mean cumulative time spent walking in minutes	Cognitive/Behavioral modification group had greatest compliance
Costello et al. (1995)	Low flow oxygen	99 hospitalized patients	Delivery of oxygen	Number of nasal cannulae displaced during night	49% dislodged oxygen delivery device during night. Dislodging was more common for V enturi face masks than for nasal cannulae
Morrison et al. (1995)	Long-term oxygen therapy	519 COPD patients (Scotland). Approximately equal numbers of males and females, mean age 85 years	Hours of therapy per day	Use of oxygen > 15 hours/day	56% met definition of compliance, study had high mortality rate

(continued)

TABLE 17.1 *(continued)*

Citation	Regimen	Sample	Measure	Definition	Compliance
Simmons et al. (1996)	Metered-dose inhaler	231 participants in Lung Health Study	Nebulizer Chronolog that records the date and time of each medication dose	Matching of dose to prescription	Compliance variable. Typically compliance was highest prior to a follow-up visit and declines following the visit
O'Hara et al. (1993)	Aerosolized inhalers (either placebo or active	3,923 male and female participants in the Lung Health Study	Self-reports and canister weights	Reduced weight of aerosol canister	81% by self-report and 66% by canister weight
Rand et al. (1995)	Metered-dose inhaler	3,923 male and female participantsin the Lung Health Study	Self-reports and canister weights	Reduced weight of aerosol canister	After 2 years self-reported compliance was 70%, with 48% confirmed by canister weight

acute arterial blood gas measurements within 12 months, only about half obtained the tests. In another study from the UK, patients who were prescribed oxygen for less than 24 hours (in this case 15 hours/day) obtained high levels of adherence (Restrick et al., 1993).

Long-term adherence with inhaled medications was evaluated in the Lung Health Study (Rand, Nides, Cowles, Wise, & Connett, 1995). This was one of the first trials to evaluate inhaled bronchodilator medication used regularly over time. The Lung Health Study was a large clinical trial ($N = 3{,}923$) of smoking intervention and bronchodilator therapy for the early stages of COPD. Early in the trial, self-report data suggested that nearly 70% of the patients adhered to the regimen. This rate dropped only slightly over the next 18 months. In addition to self-reports, the investigators weighed the canisters containing the medications. Self-reports confirmed by canister weights showed that 48% of the patients had good adherence at 1 year. Nonadherence rates involved overuse of medication. Further analysis demonstrated that those who overuse medication are also likely to inaccurately report their smoking status.

Personality measures tend not to be good predictors of co-management. A scale designed to assess medication adherence in COPD has been developed by Powell (1994), but the scale's clinical value remains unknown. A variety of studies have investigated demographic characteristics associated with COPD self-care behaviors. For example, the Lung Health Study suggested that participants who were better self-managers tended to be married, older, White, and to have more severe disease. These participants also had less shortness of breath and were hospitalized or confined to bed less often (Rand et al., 1995). Studies of adherence with nebulizer therapy from the Intermittent Positive Pressure Breathing Study showed that about half of the patients were adherent and half were nonadherent. Those who adhered tended to be Caucasian, married, abstain from alcohol and cigarette use, and have more severe shortness of breath. Further, those patients with more severe disease were also more likely to adhere (Turner, Wright, Mendella, & Anthonisen, 1995).

Some variables thought to predict co-management often fail to do so. For example, it is commonly assumed that heavy drinkers will be less likely to follow the regimen than those who drink less. In the Lung Health Study, alcohol consumption was used as a predictor of the ability to quit smoking. The results revealed that heavy alcohol use (greater than 25 drinks per week) was not a significant predictor of relapse in smoking cessation. However, binge drinking (defined as eight or more drinks per occasion once a month or more) was associated with greater smoking cessation relapse (Murray, Istvar, Voelker, Rigdon, & Wallace, 1995).

Estimated or measured adherence values do not appear to converge on a specific rate or even a specific pattern. James et al. (1985) reported that only half of their patients took their medicine regularly. The Intermittent Positive Pressure Breathing (IPPB) clinical trial, which used objective assessments of actual time on oxygen therapy, found only half of the patients using oxygen at least 25 minutes per day, the minimal level for clinical efficacy. However, a noteworthy similarity among studies investigating pharmacological therapy was the mention of overcompliant patients, referring to those individuals who regularly took more than their prescribed amount of medication. Chryssidis, Frewin, Frith, and Dawes (198l), for example, reported that the use of high doses of aerosol therapy often exceeded prescription rates. The mean percentage of prescribed dose actually used was 98.5% at l-month follow-up and 110.86% at 2-month follow-up. Since there was variability for each of these estimates, it appears that some portion of the patients took considerably more medications than was prescribed. It is not surprising that patients suffering from COPD, a highly symptomatic disorder, would overuse a medication that provides rapid symptomatic relief.

Electronic medication monitors may be valuable methods for improving adherence among patients with COPD. One study evaluated 251 COPD patients participating in a multi-site clinical trial of nebulizer therapy. The patients were divided into an intervention and a control group. Using an electronic medication monitor known as the Nebulizer Chronolog, the intervention group received feedback on the accuracy of their medication use. Patients receiving feedback were significantly more likely to adhere to the regimen and use medications correctly than those in the control group (Nides et al., 1993).

The traditional view of compliance/noncompliance, in which the patient either strictly follows or fails to follow a treatment recommendation, may no longer be the optimal direction of co-management research. The degree of adherence required for the desired outcome, be it adherence to a prescribed regimen or maximizing quality or life, varies from treatment to treatment, and should be considered. To date, few studies have systematically evaluated co-management with regard to the COPD regimen, and in these few cases, the focus has been on drug and oxygen therapy. Further, only a few studies evaluating interventions to improve COPD patients' ability to manage their disease have been reported. Several commentaries have offered strategies for enhancing co-management; however, none of these have been systematically studied.

MEDICAL MANAGEMENT

Since COPD is generally recognized at an advanced stage, medical management requires close supervision and attention from physicians and other allied health professionals. The primary goals of management should be directed toward preventive health strategies to slow progression, maintain function, and reduce complications. Treatments may include a variety of modalities (Snider et al., 1994). It is most important to encourage patients to stop smoking to slow the progression of disease. Because the diseases may be largely irreversible when recognized, however, smoking cessation may not result in significant return of lost lung function. However, smoking cessation will slow the accelerated rate of decline in function seen in current smokers. Chest physiotherapy techniques may be very helpful in controlling chronic cough and sputum. General health measures, including regular exercise, may promote improved health and fitness.

A variety of medications may also be used. Bronchodilator medications are used to treat any reversible component of the airway obstruction and should generally be tried in all patients. Inhaled beta-2 selective sympathomimetic and anticholinergic drugs are the mainstays of bronchodilator therapy. Both types of medicines result in relaxation of bronchial smooth muscle, but because they act by different mechanisms, their effects may be additive. Sympathomimetic drugs may be given either orally or by inhalation. Newer sympathomimetic (beta-2) medications act more selectively on bronchial smooth muscle and have a lower incidence of side effects from action at other sites. Inhaled medicines generally have the advantage of fewer systemic side effects than oral preparations.

Recently, anticholinergics have gained in prominence in the treatment of COPD. Although their bronchodilating effects have been known for many years, the selectivity and minimum of side effects for new agents such as ipratropium bromide have increased their usefulness. The drugs are reported to be more effective in larger airways, making them particularly useful for patients with COPD.

Theophylline preparations have been used in treating patients with COPD for many years. However, their use has decreased because of frequent problems with toxicity, the need for regular monitoring of blood levels, and the advent of newer, more selective bronchodilating agents. The mechanism of bronchodilation from theophylline is still not clearly defined. Theophylline has other potentially beneficial effects such as improved diaphragmatic function, reduced dyspnea, increased mucociliary clearance, and stimulation of respiratory drive. Older patients are particularly susceptible to toxicity. In addition, many patients may be tried and managed on corticosteriods, both oral and inhaled, to control inflammation and to treat reversible airway obstruction. Antibiotics are used to control infections and acute exacerbations of bronchitis. Other types of medications may also be indicated for individual patients.

Some patients with significant hypoxemia (low blood oxygen levels) may be treated with supplemental oxygen. Two important clinical trials demonstrated the benefits of long-term oxygen therapy. In the NIH-sponsored multicenter Nocturnal Oxygen Therapy Trial (NOTT), hypoxemic patients with COPD were randomly assigned to receive oxygen therapy for either 12 or 24 hours (Nocturnal Oxygen Therapy Trial Group, 1980). In the British Medical Research Council study, hypoxemic COPD patients received either no oxygen or 15 hours of therapy (Petty & Cherniak, 1981). Both studies demonstrated a significant reduction in mortality associated with the use of oxygen. Patients receiving continuous oxygen therapy had significantly reduced mortality compared with patients receiving intermittent oxygen (12 or 15 hours). The highest mortality rate was seen in patients who received no oxygen. In addition, the 24-hour oxygen group experienced higher scores on general quality of life measures (McSweeney, Grant, Heaton, Adams, & Timms, 1982) and, after 1 year, on selected tests of cognitive function (Heaton, Grant, McSweeny, Adams, & Petty, 1983). Although oxygen is expensive and inconvenient for patients to use, there are now several types of oxygen therapy systems available, including portable units for ambulation, that allow for continuous therapy (Tiep, 1990). Therefore, with the use of oxygen, hypoxemic patients with COPD can remain active and engage in a variety of physical activities and beneficial exercises.

BEHAVIORAL AND REHABILITATION PROGRAMS IN COPD

In addition to drug interventions, behavioral changes, especially in the areas of smoking and physical activity, are usually recommended for patients with COPD. Because of the well-documented association between smoking and COPD, successful smoking-prevention programs are expected to reduce the incidence of these diseases. Smoking-cessation programs are also valuable. However, by the time patients become function-limited, substantial numbers of them have stopped smoking on their own. There is considerable interest in the effects of smoking cessation for smokers with mild airway obstruction who may be at risk for COPD.

In the NIH Lung Health Study, participants in the two smoking intervention groups showed significantly smaller declines in Force Expiratory Volume in One Second ($FEV_{1.0}$) than did those in the control group. Most of this difference occurred during the first year following entry into the study and was attributable to smoking cessation, with those who achieved sustained smoking cessation experiencing the largest benefit.

Although patients with COPD can benefit greatly from exercise (Bell & Jensen, 1977), adherence to a physical regimen is often poor because activity can cause shortness of breath and fatigue. The more severely disabled patients open complain that their situation is hopeless and one over which they have little control (Fix, Daughton, & Kass, 1981). Long-term maintenance of physical exercise is difficult even when patients are initially motivated, and it may be an even more serious problem for the chronically ill (National Institutes of Health, 1981).

There is no medical cure for COPD. Because of the insidious origin of the disease and the large pulmonary reserve, COPD is generally not recognized until late in its course. Although standard medical treatment provides some relief for patients with COPD, the disease is largely irreversible and patients are disabled with symptoms (e.g., breathlessness) that limit their daily activities significantly.

Comprehensive pulmonary rehabilitation programs have been developed to provide a multidisciplinary therapeutic program tailored to the needs of the individual patient (American Association of Cardiovascular and Pulmonary Rehabilitation, 1993; Casaburi & Petty, 1993; Hodgkin, Connors, & Bell, 1993; Lertzman & Cherniak, 1976; Ries, 1990). Such programs may include several components, including individual assessment, education, instruction in respiratory and chest physiotherapy techniques, psychosocial support, and supervised exercise training (American Association of Cardiovascular and Pulmonary Rehabilitation, 1993; Ries et al., 1995). The primary goal of pulmonary rehabilitation is to restore the patient to the highest possible level of independent function. Successful programs can help patients to become better educated and more involved in their own care. In addition, patients will have reduced symptoms, improved exercise tolerance, fewer hospitalizations and physician visits, and more gainful employment (American Thoracic Society, 1981, 1995; Ries, 1990). Pulmonary rehabilitation programs have expanded substantially in recent years and are now an accepted form of comprehensive therapy for many COPD patients (American Thoracic Society, 1981, 1995; Ries, 1990).

An important component of most pulmonary rehabilitation programs has been the establishment of a regular exercise regimen. Specific physical conditioning exercises, such as walking, can be undertaken by the patient to help maintain lung function and improve the remainder of the oxygen delivery system (Ries, 1994). In several published studies, the improvements in patients with COPD following rehabilitation training have been striking (Ries, 1990). Specifically, appropriate physical conditioning exercises can improve maximum oxygen consumption and endurance, reduce heart rate, improve ventilator efficiency, and increase tolerance for exercise.

There have been few controlled studies evaluating pulmonary rehabilitation programs or their components. Reports from nonrandomized studies typically suggest that the objectives can be achieved (Ries, 1990). A few controlled trials documented the benefits of exercise programs for patients with COPD. Cockroft (1981) randomly assigned 39 patients to a 6-week exercise program or to a no-treatment control group. In comparison to the control group, patients in the exercise group experienced subjective benefits and increased the amount of distance they could walk in 12 minutes. However, the length of follow-up was only 2 months. McGavin and colleagues (1977) randomly allocated 24 COPD patients to a 3-month unsupervised stair-climbing home exercise program or to a nonexercise control group. The 12 patients in the exercise group noted subjective improvements and an increased sense of well-being and decreased breathlessness. They also reported an objective increase in the 12-minute walk distance and maximal level of exercise on a cycle ergometer. These changes did not occur in the control group. However, the length of follow-up was limited to 3 months. Ambrosino and coworkers (1981) randomly assigned 23 patients to a 1-month medical and rehabilitative therapy group and 28 patients to medical therapy alone (without exercise training). The experimental group improved in exercise tolerance and respiratory pattern (as evidenced by decrease in respiratory rate and increase in tidal volume). Again, these changes were not present in the control group.

Atkins, Kaplan, Timms, Reinsch, and Lofback (1984) reported the results of an experimental trial designed to evaluate behavioral and cognitive-behavioral programs for increasing exercise among patients with COPD. The patients underwent exercise testing on a treadmill and were given an exercise prescription. They were then randomly assigned to one of five experimental or control groups. The experimental groups were designed to increase participation in regular exercise. They included Behavior Modification, Cognitive-Behavioral Modification, and a Cognitive Modification Condition.

The Behavior Modification treatment included goal-setting, functional analysis of reinforcers, mediating walking, a behavioral contract, contingency management, and two sessions of relaxation training. In the Cognitive treatment, subjects experienced didactic interactions in which they learned to identify negative self-statements and to replace them with positive thoughts, to identify specific cues for promoting positive self-talk, and other similar strategies. The experimenter attempted to challenge irrational beliefs about walking whenever possible. The Cognitive-Behavioral group experienced many of the same positive self-talk exercises. However, they also received training in contingency management and two relaxation sessions. The attention control group received attention, but did not have training specifically directed toward increasing compliance. During six sessions, they completed a variety of questionnaires, including the MMPI, a life stress questionnaire, and the Trailmaker test from the Halstead-Reitan Battery (Reitan, 1971). The results of these tests and their relationship to lung disease were discussed during the sessions. A more detailed description of the treatments is given in Atkins et al. (1984). The first four sessions were held weekly during the month following the initial interview. Sessions were held biweekly the second month. Three months following the initial assessment, patients were reevaluated on all measures in the clinic. Outcome measures included a general Quality of Life Index, Pulmonary Function tasks, Exercise Tolerance tasks, and measures of Self-Efficacy.

Analysis of the data suggested that those in the Cognitive Behavior Modification Group increased their walking more than those in the other experimental or control groups. Patients in the three treatment groups walked more than those in the two control groups (Atkins et al., 1984). These changes were reflected as changes in exercise tolerance measured 1 month after the treatment. However, there were no significant changes in spirometric parameters. Several analyses were performed using a General Health Index (Kaplan, 1985) and a General Health Policy Model. Over the course of 18 months, the experimental and control groups showed significant differences on a quality-of-life index. These differences were used to calculate quality-adjusted life years and perform cost-effectiveness studies. There is considerable debate about the value of insurance reimbursement for behavioral and rehabilitation programs. The cost/effectiveness analyses suggested that behavioral and rehabilitation programs for COPD patients produce an equivalent of a well-year for approximately $23,000. This is comparable to other widely advocated healthcare programs (Toevs, Kaplan, & Atkins, 1984).

These same patients were studied again 3 years after the beginning of the program. At this time, observed differences between the experimental and control groups remained for the Quality of Well-Being measure (Atkins, Hayes, & Kaplan, 1984); yet substantial increases in variability precluded statistically significant effects. Analysis of the data using concepts derived from social learning theory (Bandura, 1977) suggested that perceived self-efficacy mediated changes in behavior and function (Kaplan, Atkins, & Reinsch, 1984).

Although comprehensive rehabilitation is believed to improve functional and psychosocial outcomes in patients with COPD, studies have not typically followed patients longer than 6 months. This has been problematic, because the effects of behavioral intervention are often short-lived. A treatment effect that lasts only 1 year, for example, may be of limited value because behavior modification does not cure the condition. Instead, continuing behavior change must be present.

In one of our recent studies, 119 patients with COPD were randomly assigned to either comprehensive pulmonary rehabilitation or to an education control group. Pulmonary rehabilitation consisted of 12 four-hour sessions distributed over an 8-week period (Ries et al., 1995). The content of the sessions was education, physical and respiratory care, psychosocial support, and supervised exercise. The education control group attended four 2-hour sessions that were scheduled twice per month, but did not include any individual instruction or exercise training. Topics included medical aspects of COPD, pharmacy use, breathing techniques and a variety of interviews about smoking, life events, and social support. Lectures covered pulmonary medicine, pharmacology, respiratory therapy, and nutrition. Outcome measures included lung function, maximum and endurance exercise tolerance, of perceived breathlessness, perceived fatigue, self-efficacy for walking, Centers for Epidemiologic Studies Depression (CES-D), and the Quality of Well-Being Scale (QWB).

In comparison to the educational group, the pulmonary rehabilitation group showed greater improvements on measures of exercise performance of both maximum level and endurance. In addition, the rehabilitation groups showed greater improvements for symptoms of breathlessness and self-efficacy. There were no differences between groups for measures of lung function, depression, or general quality of life. However, both groups experienced reductions in quality of life. For exercise variables, benefits tended to relapse toward baseline after 18 months of follow-up (Ries et al., 1995).

The lack of effects on pulmonary function was not unanticipated. Nearly all previous studies have also failed to show significant changes in lung function (Ries, 1990). Our failure to demonstrate benefits of pulmonary rehabilitation for measures of quality of life and depression was somewhat unexpected. Long-term benefits beyond 12 months were observed only for measures of exercise endurance and perceived breathlessness.

There are several potential explanations for the failure to demonstrate long-term benefits from comprehensive pulmonary rehabilitation. One explanation is that behavioral interventions, without long-term follow-up or maintenance sessions, such as rehabilitation, are inadequate to produce long-term change. Long-term maintenance of behavior change has also been difficult to demonstrate in research on smoking cessation (Fisher, Lichtenstein, Haire-Joshu, Morgan, & Rehberg, 1993), weight-loss (Brownell & Cohen, 1995), and exercise adherence (Blair et al., 1993). The finding that patients experience behavior change during treatment that is not maintained is consistent across a variety of different behavioral interventions (Kaplan & Simon, 1990).

The failure to obtain significant differences on quality-of-life outcomes may be explained by the insensitivity of these measures to small changes in general health status from interventions of this type. However, the QWB measure has been used in a variety of outcomes studies, and has shown significant associations with clinical measures for patients with lung diseases (Kaplan, Atkins, & Timms, 1984; Kaplan, Eakin, & Ries, 1993; Toeves et al., 1984). It is possible that questionnaires that are more specific to lung diseases may offer a more sensitive assessment.

Two other recently published randomized trials reported short-term benefits favoring pulmonary rehabilitation over conventional treatment. Goldstein, Gort, Avendano, and Guyatt (1994) reported significant improvement in exercise tolerance, dyspnea, and quality of life after 6 months in 45 patients receiving 8 weeks of in-patient pulmonary rehabilitation followed by 16 weeks of supervised out-patient care compared to 44 patients who received conventional care from their own physicians. Wijkstra, Van Altena, & Kraan (1994) reported significant improvement in exercise tolerance and quality of life in 28 patients who were randomly allocated to a home pulmonary rehabilitation program for 12 weeks compared to 15 patients who received no rehabilitation.

Sassi-Dambron, Eakin, Ries, & Kaplan (1995) conducted a randomized clinical trial to evaluate the effects of a modified pulmonary rehabilitation program on coping strategies for shortness of breath, but without exercise training. Eighty-nine patients with COPD were randomly assigned to the 6-week treatment or to a 6-week general health education control group. The treatment consisted of instruction and practice in techniques of progressive muscle relaxation, breathing retraining, pacing, self-talk, and panic control. Outcomes included the 6-minute walk test, quality of well-being, depression and anxiety scales, and six commonly used dyspnea (shortness of breath) measures. There were no significant differences between the treatment and control groups at the end of treatment or at 6-month follow-ups. The authors conclude that while dyspnea management strategies are an important component of COPD management, they should be taught in combination with other aspects of comprehensive pulmonary rehabilitation, namely structured exercise training.

MEASUREMENT OF OUTCOMES

Both behavioral and biomedical interventions should be evaluated in terms of their potential to improve health status and the quality of life. No behavioral or medical intervention can repair damaged lung tissue and restore pulmonary function (Unger, Moser, & Hansen, 1980). The objective of the interventions is to improve function and the quality of life. Several studies have demonstrated that function can improve in the absence of changes in measures of pulmonary function (Atkins et al., 1984; Kaplan & Ries, 1996a; Ries, Kaplan et al., 1995). Capturing these benefits requires a technology for measuring functioning and the quality of life.

It has been suggested that diseases and disabilities may have at least three important effects on health status: They may affect current functioning (quality of life); they may affect future functioning; or they may affect life expectancy (Kaplan et al., 1993). A variety of measures reviewed by Kaplan and Ries (1996b) are designed to measure these effects.

At least three different approaches have been used to evaluate patients with COPD. The Sickness Impact Profile (SIP) has been employed in a variety of major clinical trials. The SIP includes 136 items, which are divided into 12 categories. These categories are further clustered into three groups: Independent Categories, Physical, and Psychosocial (Bergner, Bobbitt, Carter, & Gilson, 1981). In the Nocturnal Oxygen Therapy Trial, the SIP was used to demonstrate that patients with COPD experienced severely curtailed quality of life in comparison to age-matched controls (McSweeney et al., 1982). The second approach is a questionnaire developed for the Rand Health Insurance Study. The Rand instruments include specific measures of physiologic health, physical health, mental health, and social health. In one study, it was demonstrated that the physical health measures correlated substantially with FEV1.0 (Allen, 1985). In addition, a recent study by Guyatt and colleagues (1985) demonstrated that the Rand instrument was highly correlated with performance on a walking test. A laboratory bicycle ergometer test was not as strongly correlated with other indices of disease severity.

We have proposed that a General Health Policy, and in particular a subcomponent known as the Quality of Well-Being Scale, has validity as an outcome measure for evaluating interventions for patients with COPD (Ries, Kaplan, et al., 1995). In medical research, program or treatment effectiveness is often measured using single indicators. In chronic lung disease, those indicators may be physiologic parameters such as pulmonary function, exercise performance, and pulmonary hemodynamics. These measures are essential for monitoring the course of a specific disease. Yet disease-specific indicators often fail to capture the total impact of a treatment, because they may allow side effects of treatment to be overlooked (Jette, 1980). Steroid drugs can modify many symptoms for patients with COPD, but they may also be associated with decreased immunity and increased susceptibility to many problems in the long run. A measure focusing only on pulmonary function may miss the overall impact of the treatment upon function and symptoms.

This approach expresses the benefits of medical care, behavioral intervention, or preventive programs in terms of well-years. These well-years integrate mortality and morbidity to express health status in terms of equivalence of well-years of life. Morbidity effects can be assessed through years of life lost. For example, a patient with COPD with a life expectancy of 73 years would have lost 13 years if he died at age 60. If 100 patients with COPD died at age 60 (and had a 73-year life expectancy), they collectively would have lost $100 \times 13 = 1{,}300$ life years.

Although COPD may result in early death, it is also a major cause of disability. Patients with decreased lung function experience reduced quality of life over an extended period of time. Our system allows the integration of quality-of-life information with mortality. For example, if the quality of life for the patient with COPD is reduced by one half, we say that the disease takes away 0.5 Quality Adjusted Life Years (QALYs) over the course of 1 year. If the disease affects two people, it will take away 1.0 QALYs (= 2×0.5) over a 1 year period. Our previous work has suggested that behavioral programs can improve the quality of life by as much as .073 units of well-being for 1 year. Thus, for each 100 patients receiving this benefit, 7.33 QALYs would be produced (Toevs et al., 1984).

FUTURE DIRECTIONS

Given the importance of COPD in terms of death, disability, and medical expense, it is surprising that so little attention has been devoted to systematic behavioral studies in this area. In contrast to nearly every other major medical condition, there are few published intervention studies evaluating the benefits of behavioral interventions to improve patients' ability to manage COPD. In addition, there are no population-based studies on co-management, and the extent to which adherence to various regimen components is a problem is not known. Also, the extent to which problems such as overcompliance affect detrimental outcomes for patients with COPD is unknown.

The Task Force on Lung Diseases for the NHLBI Workshop Adoption and Maintenance of Behaviors for Optimal Health suggested five directions for future research.

The regimen for patients with COPD requires many different behaviors. These might include the use of several different medications, exercise, respiratory therapy, and other aspects of self-care. In other chronic illnesses, for example, hypertension, adherence with one aspect of the regimen is often not correlated with adherence to other components. There is preliminary evidence for the same problem in COPD. In one study, self-reported participation in a variety of COPD co-management activities, including medication-taking, physical activity, diet, relaxation, breathing techniques, and respiratory care techniques (e.g., controlled coughing, bronchial drainage) was evaluated in 65 patients with COPD. Correlations between the co-management activities were conducted to evaluate the interrelationships among these activities. The correlations were generally small and nonsignificant, indicating that there is little relationship among COPD co-management activities. Stated differently, knowing that a patient is compliant with one aspect of the COPD regimen does not provide information about their participation in other aspects of the regimen. We need to move away from categorizing patients as "good" or "bad" compliers, and recognize the need to assess and address co-management behaviors individually (Eakin & Glasgow, 1996). More research is necessary to define the interrelationships between behaviors relevant to the management of COPD.

A second issue identified in this literature review is that overcompliance with aspects of the COPD regimen may be a problem. This is a particular concern for inhaled medications that provide symptomatic relief. More research is necessary in order to document overcompliance and evaluate effects upon health outcomes.

Further research is also needed to establish the links between co-management and attainment of health benefits. At present, little is known about how to improve self-care for patients with COPD. There are no published studies on increasing adherence to prescribed medications. Only a few studies consider improving adherence to behavioral regimens. The problem of smoking cessation among the elderly has also received insufficient study. These problems require further systematic investigation.

Finally, there is very little research on rehabilitation programs for patients with COPD. Though these programs are common, little is known about their effectiveness. Our recent clinical trial of rehabilitation in COPD suggested some short-term benefits. However, these benefits were attenuated over time (Ries, Kaplan, et al., 1995). We believe that the failure to find long-term effects is explained by poor long-term co-management. We are currently conducting a second trial in which all patients are assigned to rehabilitation. After completing the program, patients are randomly assigned to a program designed to enhance long-term self-care or to a control group. The study is designed to determine whether post-rehabilitation behavioral intervention can improve long-term self-management.

Rehabilitation programs for patients with COPD include many different components. For example, comprehensive programs often include exercise, education, chest physiotherapy, and psychosocial support. If the programs are shown to be effective, it is not clear what aspects of the program caused the benefits. Further studies are needed to identify the essential components of a successful program. Research on mechanisms of delivery and reimbursement for rehabilitation programs is also needed.

In summary, COPD is an important health problem that requires further systematic investigation. There has been very little behavioral research relevant to COPD. Yet behavior change, in the form of co-management, may be essential for obtaining optimal patient outcomes. Further research relevant to the clinical management of COPD should be encouraged.

REFERENCES

Allen, H. (1985, August). *Validity of measures in the Rand health insurance study.* Paper presented at the meeting of the American Psychological Association, Los Angeles, CA.

Ambrosino, N., Paggiaro, P. L., Macchi, M., Felieri, M., Toma, G., Lombard, F. A., DeiCesta. F., Parlanti, A., Loi, A., & Baschieri, L. (1981). A short-term effect of rehabilitative therapy in chronic obstructive pulmonary disease. *Respiration, 41,* 40–44.

American Association of Cardiovascular and Pulmonary Rehabilitation. (1993). Guidelines for pulmonary rehabilitation programs. Champaign, IL: Human Kinetics.

American Thoracic Society. (1981). Pulmonary rehabilitation. *American Review of Respiratory Diseases, 124*, 683–686.

American Thoracic Society. (1995). Standards for the diagnosis and care of patients with chronic obstructive pulmonary disease (COPD) and asthma. *American Review of Respiratory Diseases, 152*, S77–S120.

Anthonisen, N. R., Connett, J. E., Kiley, J. P., Altose, M. D., Bailey, W. C., Buist, A. S., Conway, W. A. J., Enright, P. L., Kanner, R. E., & O'Hara, P. (1994). Effects of smoking intervention and the use of an inhaled anticholinergic bronchodilator on the rate of decline of FEV1: The Lung Health Study [see comments]. *Journal of the American Medical Association, 272*, 1497–1505.

Atkins, C. J. (1981). *A randomized clinical trial comparing cognitive and behavioral strategies for exercise compliance among chronic obstructive pulmonary disease patients*. Unpublished doctoral dissertation, University of California, Riverside.

Atkins, C. J., Hayes, J., & Kaplan, R. M. (1984, June). *Four-year follow-up of behavioral programs in COPD*. Paper presented at the University of California Health Psychology Conference, Lake Arrowhead, CA.

Atkins, C. J., Kaplan, R. M., Timms, R. M., Reinsch, S., & Lofback, K. (1984). Behavioral programs for exercise compliance in COPD. *Journal of Consulting and Clinical Psychology, 52*, 591–603.

Austin, T. W. (1976). Cigarette smoking and chronic bronchitis. *British Medical Journal, 2*, 1261.

Bandura, A. (1977). Self-efficacy: Toward a unifying theory of behavior change. *Psychological Review, 84*, 191–215.

Bell, C. W., & Jensen, R. H. (1977). Exercise and stress testing in physical conditioning. In R. H. Jensen & I. Kass (Eds.), *Pulmonary rehabilitation medical manual* (pps. 50–91). Omaha, NE: University of Nebraska Medical Center.

Bergner, M., Bobbitt, R. A., Carter, W. B., & Gilson, B. S. (1981). The sickness impact profile: Development and final revision of a health status measure. *Medical Care, 19*, 787–806.

Blair, S. N., Powell, K. E., Bazzarre, T. L., Early, J. L., Epstein, L. H., Green, L.W., Harris, S. S., Haskell, W. L., King, A. C., Koplan, J. Marcus, B., Pafferbarger, R. S., & yeager, K. K. (1993). Physical inactivity: Workshop V. AHA Prevention Conference III: Behavior change and compliance: Keys to improving cardiovascular health. *Circulation, 88*, 1402–1405.

Brownell, K. D., & Cohen, L. R. (1995). Adherence to dietary regimens: 1. An overview of research. *Behavioral Medicine, 20*, 149–154.

Burrows, B. (1991). Epidemiologic evidence for different types of chronic airflow obstruction. *American Review of Respiratory Diseases, 143*, 1452–1455.

Casaburi, R., & Petty, T. (1993). *Principles and practice of pulmonary rehabilitation.* Philadelphia: Saunders.

Chryssidis, E., Frewin, D. B., Frith, P. A., & Dawes, E. R. (1981). Compliance with aerosol therapy in chronic obstructive lung disease. *New Zealand Medical Journal, 94*, 375–377.

Cockroft, A. E. (1981). Randomized controls trial of rehabilitation in chronic respiratory disease. *Thorax, 36*, 200.

Costello, R. W., Liston, R., & McNicholas, W. T. (1995). Compliance at right with low flow oxygen therapy: A comparison of nasal cannulae and venturi face masks. *Thorax, 50*, 405–406.

Crystal, R. G. (1987). Chronic obstructive pulmonary disease. In *Forty years of achievement in heart, lung, and blood research: A collection of essays in selected papers of biomedical research accomplishment*. Bethesda, MD: National Institutes of Health.

Eaking, E. G., & Glasgow, R. E. (1996). The physician's role in diabetes self-management: Helping patients to help themselves. *The Endocrinologist, 6*, 1–10.

Feinleib, M., Rosenberg, H. M., Collins, J. G., Delozier, J. E., Pokras, R., & Chevarley, F. M. (1989). Trends in COPD morbidity and mortality in the United States. *American Review of Respiratory Diseases, 140*, S9–S18.

Fisher E. B., Jr, Lichtenstein E., Haire-Joshu D., Morgan G. D., & Rehberg H. R. (1993). Methods, successes, and failures of smoking cessation programs. *Annual Review of Medicine, 44*, 481–513.

Fix, A. J., Daughton, D., & Kass, I. (1981). Behavioral sciences in pulmonary rehabilitation. *Applied Techniques in Behavioral Medicine, 1*, 263–294.

Goldstein, R., Gort, E., Avendano, M., & Guyatt, G. (1994). Randomised controlled trial of respiratory rehabilitation. *Lancet, 344*, 1394–1397.

Guyatt, G. H., Thompson, P. J., Berman, L B., Sullivan, M. J., Townsend, M., Jones, N. L., & Pugsly, S. O. (1985). How should we measure function in patients with chronic heart and lung disease? *Journal of Chronic Diseases, 38*, 517–524.

Haynes, R. B., Taylor, D. W., & Sackett, D. L. (1979). *Compliance in health care.* Baltimore: Johns Hopkins University Press.

Heaton, R. K., Grant, I., McSweeny, A. J., Adams, K. M., & Petty, T. L. (1983). Psychological effects of continuous and nocturnal oxygen therapy in hypoxemic chronic obstructive pulmonary disease. *Archives of lnternal Medicine, 143*, 1941–1947.

Higgins, M., & Thom, T. (1989). Trends is coronary heart disease in the United States. *International Journal of Epidemiology, 18*, S58–S66.

Hodgkin, J. E., Connors, G. L., & Bell, C. W. (1993). *Pulmonary rehabilitation guidelines to success* (2nd ed.). Philadelphia: Lippincott.

Intermittent Positive Pressure Breathing Trial Group. (1983). Intermittent positive pressure breathing therapy of chronic obstructive pulmonary disease. *Annals of Internal Medicine, 99*, 612–620.

James, P. N. E., Anderson, J. B., Priar, J. G., White, J. P., Henry, J. A., & Cochrane, G. M. (1985). Patterns of drug taking in patients with chronic airflow obstruction. *Postgraduate Medical Journal, 61*, 7–10.

Jette, A. M. (1980). Health status indicators: Their utility in chronic disease evaluation research. *Journal of Chronic Diseases, 33*, 567–579.

Kaplan, R. M. (1985). Quantification of health outcomes for policy studies in behavioral epidemiology. In R. M. Kaplan & M. H. Criqui (Eds.), *Behavioral epidemiology and disease prevention* (pp. 31–54). New York: Plenum.

Kaplan, R. M., Atkins, C. J., & Reinsch, S. (1984). Specific efficacy expectations mediate exercise compliance in patients with COPD. *Health Psychology, 3*, 223–242.

Kaplan, R. M., Atkins, C. J., & Timms, R. M. (1984). Validity of a quality of well-being scale as an outcome measure in chronic obstructive pulmonary disease. *Journal of Chronic Diseases, 37*, 85–95.

Kaplan, R. M., Eakin, E. G., & Ries, A. L. (1993). Psychosocial issues in the rehabilitation of patients with Chronic Obstructive Pulmonary Disease. In R. Casaburi & T. L. Petty (Eds.), *Principles and Practice of Pulmonary Rehabilitation*, (pp. 351–365). Philadelphia: Saunders.

Kaplan, R. M., & Ries, A. L. (1996a). Cognitive-behavioral interventions and the quality of life of patients with chronic obstructive pulmonary disease. In J. Bach (Ed.), *Pulmonary fehabilitation: The obstructive and paralytic conditions*, (pp. 133–144). Philadelphia: Hanley & Delfus.

Kaplan, R. M., & Ries, A. L. (1996b). Cost-effectiveness of pulmonary rehabilitation. In A. Fishman (Ed.), *Pulmonary rehabilitation* (pp. 379–398). New York: Marcel Dekker.

Kaplan, R. M., & Simon, H. J. (1990). Compliance in medical care: Reconsideration of self-predictions. *Annals of Behavioral Medicine, 12*(2), 66–71.

Lertzman, M. M., & Cherniack, R. M. (1976). Rehabilitation of patients with chronic obstructive pulmonary disease. *American Review of Respiratory Diseases, 114*, 1145–1165.

McGavin, C. R., Gupta, S. P., Lloyd, E. L., & McHardy, J. R. (1977). Physical rehabilitation of chronic bronchitis: Results of a controlled trial of exercises in the home. *Thorax, 32*, 307–311.

McSweeny, A. J., Grant, I., Heaton, R. K., Adams, K. M., & Timms, R. M. (1982). Life quality of patients with chronic obstructive pulmonary disease. *Archives of International Medicine, 142*, 473–478.

Morrison, D., Skwarski, K., & MacNee, W. (1995). Review of the prescription of domiciliary long term oxygen therapy in Scotland. *Thorax, 50*, 1103–1105.

Murray, R. P., Istvan, J. A., Voelker, H. T., Rigdon, M. A., & Wallace, M. D. (1995). Level of involvement with alcohol and success at smoking cessation in the lung health study. *Journal of Studies of Alcohol, 56*, 74–82.

National Center for Health Statistics, Centers for Disease Control (1994) Mortality Patterns—United States, 1992. *Morbidity and Mortality Weekly Report, 43*, 916–921.

National Institutes of Health. (1981). *Chronic obstructive pulmonary disease* (NIH Publication No. 81–2020). Bethesda, MD: U.S. Department of Health and Human Services.

Nides, M. A., Tashkin, D. P., Simmons, M. S., Wise, R. A., Li, V. C., & Rand, C. S. (1993). Improving inhaler adherence in a clinical trial through the use of the nebulizer chronolog [see comments]. *Chest, 104*, 501–507.

Nocturnal Oxygen Therapy Trial Group. (1980). Continuous or nocturnal oxygen therapy in hypoxemic chronic obstructive lung disease: A clinical trial. *Annals of Internal Medicine, 93*, 391–398.

O'Hara, P., Grill, J., Rigdon, M. A., Connett, J. E., Lauger, G. A., & Johnston, J. J. (1993). Design and results of the initial intervention program for the Lung Health Study: The Lung Health Study Research Group. *Preventive Medicine, 22*, 304–315.

Petty, T. L., & Cherniak, R. M. (1981). Comprehensive care of COPD. *Clinical Notes on Respiratory Diseases, 91, 653–659.*

Powell, S. G. (1994). Medication compliance of patients with COPD. *Home Healthcare Nurse, 12*, 44–50.

Rand, C. S., Nides, M., Cowles, M. K., Wise, R. A., & Connett, J. (1995). Long-term metered-dose inhaler adherence in a clinical trial. The Lung Health Study

Research Group. *American Journal of Respiratory and Critical Care Medicine, 152*, 580–588.

Reitan, R. M. (1971). Trial making test results for normal and brain damaged children. *Perceptual and Motor Skills, 33*, 575–581.

Restrick, L. J., Paul, E. A., Braid, G. M., Cullinan, P., Moore-Gillon, J., & Wedzicha, J. A. (1993). Assessment and follow-up of patients prescribed long term oxygen treatment. *Thorax, 48*, 708–713.

Ries, A. L. (1990). Position paper of the American Association of Cardiovascular and Pulmonary Rehabilitation: Scientific basis of pulmonary rehabilitation. *Journal of Cardiopulmonary Rehabilition, 10*, 418–441.

Ries, A. L. (1994). The importance of exercise in pulmonary rehabilitation. *Clinics in Chest Medicine, 15*, 327–337.

Ries, A. L., Kaplan, R. M., Limberg, T. M., & Prewitt, L. M. (1995). Effects of pulmonary rehabilitation on physiologic and psychosocial outcomes in patients with chronic obstructive pulmonary disease. *Annals of Internal Medicine, 122*, 823–832.

Ries, A. L., Moser, K. M., Sassi-Dambron, D. E., Bullock, P. J., Limberg, T. M., & Sheldon, J. B. (1995). *Shortness of breath: A guide to better living and breathing* (5th ed.) St. Louis: Mosby-Year Book.

Sassi-Dambron, D. E., Eakin, E. G., Ries, A. L., & Kaplan, R. M. (1995). Treatment of dyspnea in chronic obstructive pulmonary disease: A controlled clinical trial of dyspnea managementstrategies. *Chest, 107*, 724–729.

Sherrill, D. L., Lebowitz, M. D., & Burrows, B. (1990). Epidemiology of chronic obstructive pulmonary disease. *Clinics in Chest Medicine, 11*(3):375–387.

Simmons, M. S., Nides, M. A., Rand, C. S., Wise, R. A., & Tashkin, D. P. (1996). Trends in compliance with bronchodilator inhaler use between follow-up visits in a clinical trial. *Chest, 109*(4):963–968.

Snider, G. L., Faling, L. J., & Rennard, S. I. (1994). Chronic bronchitis and emphysema. In J. F. Murray and J. A. Nadel, (Eds). *Textbook of respiratory medicine* (2nd ed.) (pp. 1331–1397). Philadelphia: Saunders.

Taylor, D. R., Kinney, C. D., & McDevitt, D. G. (1984). Patient compliance with oral theophylline therapy. *British Journal of Clinical Pharmacology, 17*, 15–20.

Tiep, B. L. (1990). Long-term home oxygen therapy. *Clinics in Chest Medicine, 11*, 505–521.

Toevs, C. T., Kaplan, R. M., & Atkins, C. J. (1984). The costs and effects of behavioral programs in chronic obstructive pulmonary disease. *Medical Care, 22*, 1088–1100.

Turner, J., Wright, E., Mendella, L., & Anthonisen, N. (1995). Predictors of patient adherence to long-term home nebulizer therapy for COPD. The IPPB Study Group. Intermittent Positive Pressure Breathing. *Chest, 108*, 394–400.

Unger, K., Moser, K., & Hansen, P. (1980). Selection of an exercise program for patients with chronic obstructive pulmonary disease. *Heart and Lungs, 9*, 68–76.

Wijkstra, P. J., Van Altena, R., & Kraan, J. (1994). Quality of life in patients with chronic obstructive pulmonary disease improves after rehabilitation at home. *European Respiratory Journal, 7*, 269–273.

18

Issues in Diabetes Self-Management

Russell E. Glasgow and Elizabeth G. Eakin

"Diabetes" refers to a number of chronic diseases that have in common disruptions in glucose metabolism that result in hyperglycemia. Living with and managing diabetes presents a complex series of challenges with which patients must deal on a daily basis for the rest of their lives. Because of the complexity of these demands and the attendant psychosocial, family, emotional, developmental, health care, economic, and social issues involved in diabetes, it is increasingly being seen as a prototype for chronic disease management (N. M. Clark, Becker, Lorig, Rakowski, & Anderson, 1991; Von Korff, Gruman, Schaefer, Curry, & Wagner, 1997).

There are two primary types of diabetes. Type I diabetes is associated with childhood onset and results from an inability of the pancreas to produce the hormone insulin. Because insulin is necessary for life, individuals with Type I diabetes must inject insulin.[1] To adequately control their glucose levels, many persons must do so several times per day, and in appropriate

[1] A number of persons with Type II diabetes also inject insulin to better control their diabetes, and over a number of years Type II diabetes can gradually become Type I diabetes. The general distinction, however, is that patients with Type II diabetes do not require insulin to survive.

combination and sequence with other activities such as fingerstick glucose testing, regular meal timing and content, regular physical activity, and several other "safety-related procedures" (e.g., carrying sources of glucose, wearing diabetes ID and monitoring for signs of hyper- and hypo-glycemia). Because Type I diabetes occurs in childhood/adolescence, a time that is often demanding and conflictual for family members, and because the immediate consequences of poor management can be severe, dramatic, and potentially even fatal, it has resulted in a fair amount of research (Cox & Gonder-Frederick, 1992; Johnson, 1993).

Type II diabetes is by far the most prevalent type, accounting for 90–98% of all diabetes (Brownson, Remington, & Davis, 1993; Harris, Eastman, & Siebert, 1994; National Institute of Health [NIH], 1995). It is associated with adult onset and occurs far more frequently in obese, older adults (some studies estimate that as many as 20% of persons over age 65 may have diabetes). In Type II diabetes, there is endogenous insulin production, but the regulation of insulin and glucose is impaired through one of several mechanisms.

Type II is often co-occuring with other chronic diseases (e.g., hypertension, arthritis), further compounding the disease management requirements. It is also more common among Native Americans, Mexican-Americans, and African Americans than among Caucasians. The prevalence of Type II diabetes has been estimated to be as high as 50% among adult members of certain Indian tribes such as the Pima (NIH, 1995). Originally thought to be a milder form of diabetes, Type II diabetes has been found to result in the same long-term complications as Type I diabetes. Both diseases place persons at greater risk of heart disease (especially women), stroke, and a host of microvascular complications, including blindness or visual impairment from retinopathy, renal disease, amputations, and neuropathy.

Complexity of Diabetes Self-Management

Diabetes self-management refers to the various tasks in which patients must engage on a regular basis to manage their diabetes. The term "self-management" is used, rather than "compliance," to denote that (1) the diabetes regimen involves a changing and complex set of behaviors and is not a static or "all or none" phenomenon and (2) the patient has the primary role in carrying out the regimen, that is, 90–98% of diabetes management is conducted by the patient (R. M. Anderson et al., 1994; Coonrod, Betschart, & Harris, 1994; Etzwiler, 1994). Self-management activities include self-monitoring of blood glucose, proper use and adjustment of medications, engaging in regular exercise, following an appropriate eating plan, not smiling, and examining one's feet at regular intervals. Any of these behaviors may be difficult to incorporate into one's daily life. Taken together, and when done in an integrated sequence, they represent a complex set of multiply determined behaviors that is particularly challenging.

Frustration with patients who don't follow their diabetes regimens often leads to a label of being "noncompliant." However, one of the key findings from the literature on diabetes self-management is that adherence to one part of the regimen is not strongly related to adherence to other parts of the regimen (Orme & Binik, 1989; Peyrot & Rubin, 1994). In other words, the fact that a patient has difficulty following a prescribed eating plan does not mean that she is failing to adhere to blood glucose testing or foot-care recommendations.

A number of studies have evaluated patients' "barriers" to self-management (Glasgow, McCaul, & Schafer, 1986; Irvine, Saunders, Blank, & Carter, 1990; Schlundt, Pichert, Gregory, & Davis, 1996). Rather than labeling the patient as noncompliant, an attempt has been made to understand the factors that interfere with various aspects of the diabetes regimen. Commonly reported barriers include lack of family support, stress, being busy, being away from home, lack of insurance reimbursement (e.g., for glucose-testing strips), and lack of convenient, safe, low-cost places to exercise. In one such study, Glasgow et al. (1986) found that patients reported the highest frequency of barriers to dietary and exercise adherence and the fewest to medication-taking, and further, that patients' self-reported barriers to adherence were prospectively predictive of their level of diabetes self-care. Stated differently, patients with a greater number of barriers to a given regimen area tend to engage in that self-care activity less often. These findings suggest that helping patients to identify barriers to self-management and develop strategies to overcome these barriers should increase the frequency of their diabetes self-management activities.

Diabetes self-management training often occurs in the context of formal diabetes education programs for which standards have been published (American Diabetes Association (ADA) Task Force to Revise the National Standards, 1995). A recent review of diabetes self-management education programs found that there is substantial evidence supporting their efficacy and recommended that they become an integral part of diabetes treatment (Clement, 1995). The review concludes with three recommendations:

1. Interventions with the goal of helping people make and maintain behavior changes should make extensive use of behavior change strategies (and not rely solely on informational approaches);
2. Interventions should take into account the needs, preferences and abilities of the patient; and
3. Healthcare providers involved in helping patients manage their diabetes must work with the patients as an integrated team.

To these important points, we would add a fourth:

4. To produce lasting behavior change, the patient's social environment must be taken into account, and plans made for ongoing support of self-management behaviors.

Determination of Self-Management

Most diabetes research has approached diabetes self-management as if it were solely a function of interpersonal factors, such as knowledge and health beliefs. As illustrated in Figure 18.1, however, there are several levels of influence on self-management. Unfortunately, neither patients, healthcare providers, nor diabetes researchers have devoted much attention to these other factors, especially those toward the bottom of the pyramid, which

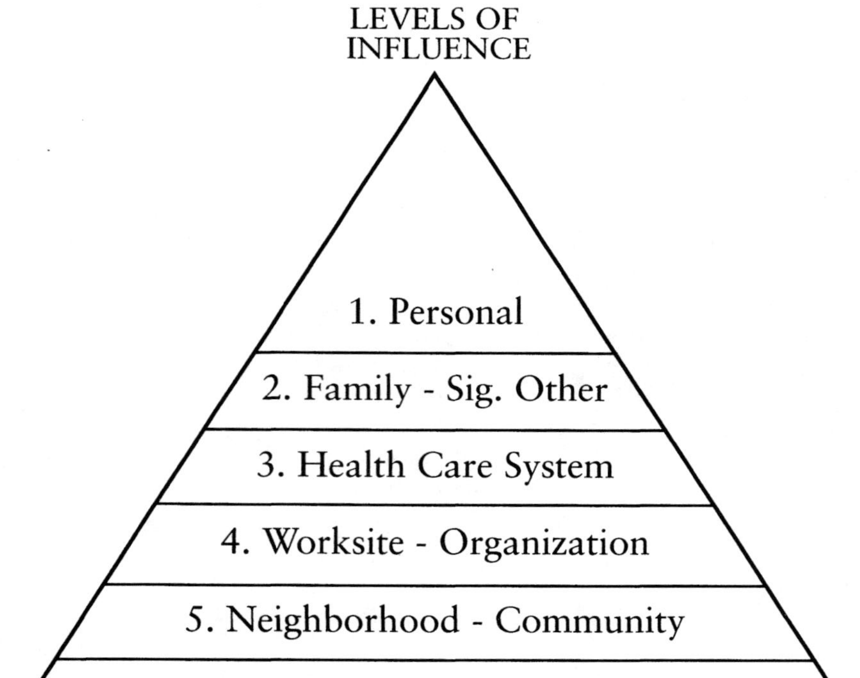
LEVELS OF INFLUENCE
1. Personal
2. Family - Sig. Other
3. Health Care System
4. Worksite - Organization
5. Neighborhood - Community
6. Media - Policy - Culture

Figure 18.1 Pyramid of influences.

impact far larger numbers of persons. As one moves toward the base of the pyramid, the factors also tend to become more complex and more difficult to change. This does not mean, however, that these factors are any less important or less influential (Green & Kreuter, 1991; Stokols, 1996).

Below and in Table 18.1 we briefly discuss key factors that act to either support or serve as barriers to self-management at each of the six levels of the pyramid.

At the *Personal* level, it appears that the most powerful influences on self-management behaviors are self-efficacy and the related concepts of empowerment (R. M. Anderson et al., 1995; Kingery & Glasgow, 1989) and problem-solving or coping skills (Toobert & Glasgow, 1991). There has also been a considerable literature on health beliefs or "personal models of diabetes" (e.g., Bond, Aiken, & Somerville, 1992; M. Z. Cohen, Tripp-Reimer, Smith, Sorofman, & Lively, 1994; Hampson, Glasgow, & Foster, 1995) demonstrating that patient perceptions of the seriousness of one's diabetes and especially the perceived effectiveness of diabetes treatment recommendations are related to self-management and/or glycemic control. However, with the exception of Hampson et al.'s research, such beliefs have generally not been shown to prospectively predict self-management or to remain significant after controlling for other factors. Knowledge of diabetes has generally *not* been found to be significantly related to self-management (Dunn, 1990; Glasgow & Osteen, 1992).

At the *Family/Significant Other* level, there have been many studies investigating the role of social support, or conversely the lack of support, on regimen adherence or glycemic control. The majority of studies have been with children or adolescents, and have been concurrent in nature. It appears that for both children and adults, social support aids diabetes self-management. Issues currently being investigated include finding ways to cost-effectively modify ongoing social support patterns, and determining how well-intended social support becomes transformed into "miscarried helping" (B. J. Anderson, 1996). In adolescents, the balance between adult and adolescent responsibility for self-management, and the developmental appropriateness of this balance, appears important to address (B. J. Anderson, 1996; Wysocki, Hough, Ward, & Green, 1992).

The *Healthcare Team and System* is another potent influence on chronic disease self-management. Across a number of health-related behaviors, patients rate advice from their doctors as one of the most important influences on their health-protective behaviors (e.g., smoking cessation, mammography screening). Of concern are unintended communications from health care providers that may imply that diabetes is not serious (e.g., "You just have a touch of diabetes") or that lifestyle components of the self-management regimen are not important ("If it was important for me to exercise, my doctor would have told me"). Another key issue is consistency of messages

TABLE 18.1 Factors Supporting and Interfering with Diabetes Self-Management at Each Level of Influence

Influence Level	Supportive Factors	Inhibitory Factors
1. Personal	Empowerment; High self-efficacy; Good problem-solving skills.	Lack of knowledge; Low self-efficacy.
2. Family/Significant Other	Social support; Shared exercise and eating patterns.	Miscarried helping (nagging); Poor role models.
3. Health Care Provider/System	Patient-centered perspectives; Integrated, systems approaches; Collaborative goal-setting; Follow-up support.	Lack of reimbursement or insurance coverage; Inconsistency among different team members.
4. Worksite/School/ Organization	Smoking policies; Availability of nutritious foods; Flexible schedules; Physical activity resources and opportunities.	Lack of control over schedules; Embarrassment; Lack of privacy.
5. Neighborhood/ Community	Awareness and use of nutrition, physical activity resources; support groups; strong library and volunteer programs.	Lack of nutrition education or self-management resources; Lack of safe, convenient exercise locations.
6. Regulatory, Policy and Incentive	Taxes and subsidies on tobacco and food products; Labeling information on food; Topics that media covers.	Auto-oriented society; Media that does not consider diabetes serious; Lack of support for diabetes education and self-management supplies.

across healthcare personnel. If the nurse emphasizes glucose testing, the physician encourages medication adjustment, and the dietician recommends low-fat eating, the patient can leave feeling overwhelmed and confused (Eakin & Glasgow, 1996; Glasgow & Eakin, 1996). Two factors receiving substantial empirical verification are the importance of follow-up support between office visits (Kirkman et al., 1994; Wasson et al., 1992) and the need to provide personalized, tailored interventions for patients rather than "one-size-fits-all prescriptions." Finally, health insurance reimbursement policies for health education and diabetes supplies are an obvious and important influence on self-management.

Worksites and School Environments are important for adults and adolescents, respectively, because of the number of hours per week spent in these settings. In particular, the policies of these institutions (and other organizations such as churches, fraternal organizations, etc.) toward health promotion generally, and diabetes self-management related tasks specifically, can have a profound influence on self-management (Padgett, Nord, Heins, & Arfken, 1996). The strongest evidence to date concerns the effects of workplace smoking policies and worksite and school cafeteria food choices and nutrition labeling on employee/student health behaviors (R. M. Davis, 1995; Glanz & Rimer, 1995). Another relevant factor is the scheduling and flexibility of work and schoolwork, which can facilitate or impede self-management. Finally, work and school policies, resources, and support/incentives for physical activity are important in establishing and maintaining regular exercise patterns (King et al., 1995; Sallis & Owen, 1996).

Neighborhood and Community Influences on self-management are potentially very important, but they have not been well researched. It is hypothesized that one's awareness of, access to, and participation in neighborhood and community activities that support healthy living are important determinants of level of self-management. For example, an individual who lives in a neighborhood with pleasant walking trails or by a shopping mall that sponsors a walking program will be more likely to engage in regular physical activity than one who does not (King et al., 1995). Peer support groups, buddy systems, and other strategies to involve lay volunteers have been popular and successful with other chronic diseases (Lorig, Mazonson, & Holman, 1993) and may also be with diabetes. In brief, the social environment in which one lives produces opportunities and support for self-management tasks, as well as challenges and barriers.

Finally, in the last row of Table 18.1 are listed *Societal Level Influences*, such as regulatory actions, policies, and incentives that act to promote or inhibit diabetes self-management. This is probably most clear regarding the lifestyle aspects of the regimen, where diabetes patients are repeatedly subjected to media messages that promote eating convenient high-fat foods, using tobacco to be young and sexy, and using numerous labor-saving devices to remain virtually sedentary. The tremendous and under-recognized influence of media, advertising, and regulatory policies (or lack of such) on health behaviors is only recently being recognized (Stauber & Rampton, 1995; Stokols, 1996).

Summary

Behavioral scientists have been prolific in developing, and to some extent testing, health-behavior models of diabetes and chronic disease self-management (e.g., Ewart, 1991; Glanz & Rimer, 1995; Glasgow, 1995; Green & Kreuter, 1991; Ruggiero & Prochaska, 1993; Wing, Epstein, Nowalk, & Lamparski, 1986). Unfortunately, these models have had less than the intended impact on diabetes practice. This is due at least partially to the fact that, with few exceptions, these models are complex and not easily understood by nontheoreticians or health professionals other than psychologists. Although we plead partially guilty to this tendency ourselves, we and others have recently tried to distill the key implications of our conceptual models into straightforward, practical principles that practitioners can apply in everyday encounters (B. J. Anderson & Rubin, 1996; Glasgow, 1995; Von Korff et al., 1997).

Opportunities for Behavioral Contributions to Diabetes Care

To date, behavioral research has had only modest impact on the clinical practice of diabetes care. There are several reasons for this, which include historical, professional training and turf issues, reimbursement policies, and the fact that mental health professionals have only recently become real members of the healthcare team. Tremendous opportunities for behavioral science contributions exist, however, given the complexity of the biopsychosocial issues in diabetes, the frequency of contact with diabetes patients, and the relatively low level of adherence to recommended guidelines (ADA, 1995; Diabetes Guidelines Advisory Group, 1996) by both patients or providers (Harris et al., 1994; Marrero, 1994).

To impact diabetes management, behavioral and psychological assessments, interventions, and models should be practical and efficient, be readily understood by nonpsychologists, and address issues that diabetes patients and providers (rather than psychologists) perceive as important needs (B. J. Anderson & Rubin, 1996; McCulloch, Glasgow, Hampson, & Wagner, 1994). Given the multiple demands and time pressures in most primary care clinical settings, a key guideline to keep in mind is that an assessment or intervention innovation must take little or no additional time—or alternatively, save time in other ways—if it is to be adopted widely. The use of computer technology that collects and immediately scores key behavioral assessment information addresses this issue. Other ways to achieve this goal may involve transferring management responsibilities to nonphysician (and likely non-mental health professional) members of the healthcare team, such as nurses, dieticians, and/or diabetes educators.

More time-consuming and expensive interventions (e.g., consultations with psychologists) may be justified for high-risk patients or for those for whom an initial standard level of self-management counseling and assistance proves insufficient (Fisher et al., 1997; Glasgow, 1995; Mazze, 1994). Such a "stepped-care model" is familiar to medical practitioners and has been advocated for other lifestyle factors such as smoking cessation and obesity.

Review of Self-Management Regimen Areas and Key Studies

Although space does not permit a comprehensive review of the diabetes self-management literature, we discuss key studies in each of several regimen areas (e.g., nutrition, physical activity, foot care, etc.), concluding with studies of multiple, integrated self-management activities. We have focused on intervention rather than correlational studies, and have emphasized a "best evidence" synthesis (Glasgow & Anderson, 1995; Slavin, 1986), relying to the extent possible on studies that are randomized or well-controlled; have relatively large and representative samples; and are sound methodologically.

Dietary Self-Management

Dietary issues have consistently been found to be the most difficult aspects of the diabetes regimen (Ary, Toobert, Wilson, & Glasgow, 1986; Fisher et al., 1997; Schlundt et al., 1996). This is partially due to the inherent difficulties and challenges in weight regulation (Wing, 1996), partly to interactions with other aspects of the diabetes regimen, such as taking insulin, which is associated with weight gain; and also to the pervasive and inescapable social and advertising cues to eat high-fat, low-fiber, processed foods. Many persons with Type II diabetes have a long history of attempting unsuccessfully to lose weight, often exacerbated by vague instructions from well meaning healthcare providers to "lose weight—it will help your glucose level" or from standard diet tearsheets not tailored to an individual's culture, dietary history, or food preferences.

Meta-analyses have found the effect sizes for dietary outcomes to be generally lower than those for other classes of diabetes outcome variables (Brown, 1990; Padgett, Mumford, Hynes, & Carter, 1988). Wing (1996) and colleagues have conducted the most systematic research in the diet area, focusing primarily on intensive, structured behavioral group and individual programs to produce weight loss. They have found that long-term interventions (e.g., regular meetings over periods as long as 2 years) may be required to produce stable weight loss, and that very low-calorie diets seem to increase weight loss, but require careful supervision. On a less optimistic note, they have also found that participants with diabetes tend to lose less weight than spouses participating in the same program (Wing, 1996), and that African Americans seem to lose less weight than Caucasians participating in their program (Wing & Anglin, 1996).

In contrast to the sobering conclusions above, recent findings from relatively brief public health-focused interventions that attempt to produce smaller changes in dietary fat intake in a high percentage of the population have been more optimistic. For example, Glasgow, Toobert, and Hampson (1996) have found that a brief computer-assisted dietary intervention conducted during regular outpatient office visits produced sustained changes at both 3-month and 12-month follow-ups in several measures of dietary behavior (percent of calories from fat, eating patterns), serum cholesterol levels, and patient satisfaction with the office visit compared to similar patients randomized to a usual care-plus-computer-assessment condition.

Tools that make it practical for busy practitioners to efficiently assess eating behaviors and design interventions based upon these assessments, have become available in recent years. Both Schlundt, Rea, Kline, and Pichert (1994) and Glasgow, Toobert, Hampson, and Noell (1995) have developed measures of common barriers to dietary self-management for persons with diabetes that can be used to tailor problem solving-based interventions. Also, the American Diabetes Association has issued revised dietary guidelines that, in contrast to previous dietary recommendations which recommended a standardized diet approach, now stress more behaviorally sophisticated guidelines for medical nutrition therapy, then include individualized assessment, negotiated goal setting, problem-solving, and ongoing evaluation (ADA, 1996).

Smoking

It is disturbing that the smoking prevalence rates among diabetes patients are approximately as high as those among the general population (Fisher et al., 1997; Haire-Joshu, 1991). This is of concern given the increased risk of diabetes patients to develop and die of heart disease (Brownson et al., 1993). It is not likely that providers intend to convey that stopping smoking is not important for patients having diabetes, but this is unfortunately the conclusion that patients sometimes reach because "My doctor did not mention anything about smoking."

By far the most consistent work on smoking cessation among persons with diabetes has been by Haire-Joshu, Fisher, and colleagues. Based upon their clinical experience and outcomes of medical office-based smoking cessation research in other settings, Fisher, Ziff, and Haire-Joshu (1996) have presented a succinct summary of key issue for healthcare team members to consider and implement. Possibly more important than any single action is the concept that the entire medical office and healthcare system needs to consider smoking status a vital sign (Fiore, 1991) and consistently approach it at each contact.

Foot Care

Despite the fact that a significant proportion of diabetes-related amputations are preventable (United States Department of Health and Human Services [USDHHS], 1992), studies have shown that most patients with diabetes do not engage in simple foot-care assessments, nor do physicians regularly examine the feet of their diabetes patients (Litzelman et al., 1993). In one of the best-controlled, most thorough studies of a diabetes self-management intervention, Litzelman and colleagues evaluated the effects of a multilevel intervention to increase patient and provider adherence to foot-care recommendations during the course of regular office visits. Patients in this study received education on foot care from a nurse, and then negotiated behavioral contracts regarding self-foot care. This was followed by a phone call 2 weeks later and postcard reminders about foot care at 1 and 3 months. Healthcare providers were given practice guidelines regarding foot care, and patients' folders contained prompts to providers to ask patients to remove their footwear, perform foot exams, and provide education on foot care. At the end of the 12-month randomized trial, intervention patients had significantly fewer foot lesions than usual care patients, and were more likely to perform self-foot care, to receive foot exams during office visits, and to receive foot-care education from their health care provider.

This study replicated one of the simplest and most impactful demonstrations of stimulus control strategies (S. J. Cohen, 1983), namely, that having patients remove their shoes and socks in the exam room dramatically increases the probability that a foot exam will be conducted by the provider. This also suggests the possibility of increasing provider adherence to other recommended guidelines by using patients as change agents (Kaplan, Greenfield, & Ware, 1989). Future studies would do well to apply this type of approach to other diabetes self-management areas, such as eye care, diet, exercise, and smoking cessation.

Blood Glucose Monitoring

In a series of studies over the past decade, Cox and colleagues have developed and evaluated a patient education program designed to teach Type I diabetes patients to better estimate their blood-glucose levels (e.g., Cox, Gonder-Frederick, & Clarke, 1996; Cox et al., 1989; Cox et al., 1995). Their program, called blood glucose awareness training (BGAT), involves teaching patients how to identify symptoms of both hypo- and hyperglycemia. Hypoglycemic, or low blood glucose, episodes can be disruptive and fear-provoking in their mild form. Severe hypoglycemia can cause marked neurologic dysfunction, increasing the risk of accidents, and can progress to loss of consciousness, coma, and even death. BGAT is taught in a series of seven weekly classes and makes use of a training manual and homework exercises that focus on estimation of blood glucose as well as the impact of insulin, food, and exercise on blood glucose levels. Results of a number of studies demonstrate that, in the short term, BGAT improves estimation of blood glucose levels and glycosylated hemoglobin (e.g., Cox et al., 1989, 1996). An evaluation of the long-term effects of BGAT (mean follow-up of 4.9 years) found that BGAT and BGAT booster sessions reduced the number of severe hypoglycemic episodes and automobile accidents (Cox, Gonder-Frederick, Julian, & Clarke, 1994). Finally, a recent multicenter trial (Cox et al., 1995) confirmed the efficacy of an enhanced version of BGAT in improving overall blood-glucose estimation accuracy.

Physical Activity

While regular, moderate physical activity is an important component of the diabetes regimen, it is also one of the more difficult self-care behaviors for patients to initiate and maintain (Ary et al., 1986). A review of the PsychLit and Medline literature from 1989 to 1996 revealed over 320 citations corresponding to the phrase "diabetes and physical activity." However, not one of these citations involved a study of an intervention to increase physical activity in patients with diabetes. The majority of studies were descriptive reports of the physical activity levels of patients with diabetes and factors related to physical activity, or laboratory studies of the acute effects of exercise on metabolism.

Exercise has been evaluated as an adjunct to diet in Type II diabetes (e.g., Wing et al., 1988). A review of the literature on the role of diet and exercise in weight control concludes that the most successful approach to long-term weight control involves programs that combine diet, exercise, and behavior modification (Wing, 1996).

Multiple Self-Management Outcomes

Interventions focused on multiple self-management outcomes (e.g., diet, exercise, SMBG) are commonly referred to as diabetes self-management education programs. The reader is referred to Brown (1990), Clement (1995),

Glasgow & Osteen (1992), Padgett et al., (1988), and Rubin and Peyrot (1992) for more comprehensive and meta-analytic reviews of the outcomes of such programs. Until recently, the majority of diabetes-education studies reported on diabetes knowledge and glycosylated hemoglobin as the primary outcomes. More recent studies have shifted their focus to include the measurement of patient self-care behaviors and quality of life as key outcomes (Glasgow & Osteen, 1992; R. M. Kaplan, 1990). Below, we describe a few of the key intervention studies in this area. These studies were chosen to represent a variety of approaches and levels of intervention intensity that have been effective in impacting multiple self-care outcomes.

R. M. Anderson et al. (1994) evaluated the impact of a diabetes education newsletter that was mailed to patients monthly over a 2-year period. Each newsletter was one page long, focused on a single topic, and recommended specific actions regarding diabetes self-care. Patients who found the newsletters to be most helpful were older, had more complications, lower income, less understanding of diabetes, and reported being in poorer overall health. While few patients reported having changed their behavior as a result of any single newsletter, when asked at follow-up whether they had made any changes in diabetes self-management, 54% of those who had read most or all of the newsletters reported making at least one behavior change.

Greenfield, Kaplan, Ware, Yano, and Frank (1988) evaluated an intervention to increase the participation of patients with Type I and Type II diabetes in their medical care. In this randomized trial, patients in the experimental group met for 20 minutes with a research staff person in the clinic while waiting for their physician visit. Patients were helped to better understand diabetes-related information in their medical charts, to identify medical issues likely to arise during the visit, and were encouraged to negotiate treatment decisions regarding these issues with the physician during the visit. Results of audiotaped patient-physician interactions indicated that experimental patients were significantly more effective in eliciting information from the physician. They also had significantly lower HbA_{1c} levels at follow-up, and reported decreased functional limitations as compared to the Usual Care control group, which met for 20 minutes with a research assistant to review standardized diabetes education materials.

Glasgow and colleagues (1992) evaluated an intervention designed to improve multiple self-care outcomes among older patients (age 60 and over) with Type II diabetes. This group-based intervention took place during 10 sessions over a 3-month period and focused on the development of individualized plans to aid participants in overcoming barriers to diet, exercise, and blood-glucose monitoring. The intervention was based on a problem-solving paradigm in which participants identified barriers to each of the self-management areas, worked with staff on coping strategies for each barrier, and were encouraged to try out and reevaluate the strategies. Using a randomized, wait-list control design, Glasgow and colleagues reported that the intervention resulted in significantly greater improvements in caloric intake, calories from fat, weight, and frequency of glucose testing.

Section Summary

This section has summarized some of the key issues and important studies that have been conducted in several different diabetes self-management areas. Using the "pyramid of influences" framework introduced in Figure 18.1, Table 18.2 summarizes what behavioral science has accomplished and issues that still need to be addressed. The following sections discuss two of the most currently active and controversial areas of diabetes research: patient-provider interactions and the implications of the DCCT.

Patient-Provider Interactions

A growing literature exists on the importance of patient-provider interactions and involving patients in medical decisionmaking, both across various patient groups (see L. A. Anderson & Sharpe, 1991, for a review) and in diabetes specifically (L. A. Anderson, 1990; R. M. Anderson & Funnell, 1990; Golin, DiMatteo & Gelberg, 1996). A variety of complex issues have been addressed, from evaluations of patients' desire for participation in the medical encounter to content analysis of patient-provider interactions (e.g., which party speaks more, who initiates conversation, and what topics are covered), and assessment of the impact of such interactions on patient self-management.

R. M. Anderson and colleagues have advocated a "patient empowerment" approach to diabetes care that recognizes the unique responsibility that patients with diabetes have for managing their disease (R. M. Anderson et al., 1995). This approach involves a collaborative relationship between patient and provider in which the physician acts as a consultant and assists the patient in making decisions about the daily management of diabetes.

It is important to be cognizant of the current context of medical care when discussing patient involvement in medical care. Over 75% of diabetes patients and an even higher percentage of adults with Type II diabetes receive their diabetes care from primary care providers. Primary care in the current era of health care reform/chaos is faced with an ever-increasing number of responsibilities and guidelines, with a simultaneous restriction in the resources and reimbursement for delivering these services (Vogt, 1993). For example, if a busy provider was to follow all of the consensus guidelines for care recommended by the U.S. Preventive Services Task Force ([USPSTF], 1996), she would need to complete 27 preventive activities, as well as deal with presenting complaints, prescriptions, and other issues, within the typi-

Table 18.2 Current Status Within Each Level of Influence

Level Of Influence	What We Do Well	What We Need More Of
1. Personal	Attend to self-efficacy; Individualizing Tx	Tailor recommendations based on patient 'models'; Problem-solving
2. Family-Significant Other	Assess social support; Demonstrate correlational relations	Practical ways to increase social support
3. Health Care System	High-tech tertiary care; Treat acute symptoms	Systems approaches; Prevention; Guidelines-based continuous care
4. Worksite-Organizational	Employee involvement; Group programs for motivated employees.	Reach small worksites; Increase participation rates; Worksite policy interventions.
5. Neighborhood-Community	Attempts to change whole community	Assess neighborhood/ environmental factors; Use existing community resources
6. Media, Policy, Legislation, and Incentives	Some documentation of impact of policies	Media advocacy; Use policy and media events as intervention opportunities; Behavioral economics
7. All Levels	Reasonable progress at individual levels	Awareness and use of resources at other levels

cal 10–15 minute visit. Thus, it is not surprising that behavioral, psychosocial, and emotional issues are often overlooked.

Another reason that behavioral and lifestyle issues are not usually addressed during primary care visits has to do with the training of physicians. Most medical training has followed an acute-illness paradigm in which doctors provide diagnosis and treatment on a reactive basis to alleviate and *cure* symptomatic complaints (R. M. Anderson et al., 1995; Greenlick, 1992). This paradigm works reasonably well for acute illnesses, but is much less effective in *managing* chronic illnesses such as diabetes. The implications of approaching diabetes as a chronic, public health disorder—instead of as acute illness—have received scant attention (Glasgow, Wagner et al., 1996; Lasker, 1993; McCulloch et al., 1994; Rubin & Peyrot, 1994; Vinicor, 1994).

We conclude this section with a concrete example of how behavioral diabetes self-management issues might be incorporated by healthcare teams during routine office visits. The flow chart in Figure 18.2 emphasizes three points:

1. The use of low-cost reminders to patients regarding self-management, both before the visit and via brief assessment of self-management activities while the patient waits to be seen;
2. A clear message from the physician regarding the importance of patient self-management activities; and
3. Referral to and use of allied health professionals (e.g., nurses, dieticians, and diabetes educators) to assist the patient in developing and following through with a personalized self-management plan.

The DCCT and Its Implications

The Diabetes Control and Complications Trial (DCCT, Research Group, 1993) was one of the most impressive multicenter randomized clinical trials ever conducted. The DCCT was an efficacy trial conducted with 1,441 adolescent and adult Type I diabetes patients who were randomized to either intensive intervention or usual care and followed for 6–8 years. Intensive therapy consisted of either multiple daily insulin injections or an insulin pump, glucose monitoring at least 4 times per day, state-of-the-art dietary and exercise management, insulin adjustment, support and attention of an expert healthcare team to address issues of motivation and emotional reactions, and an unprecedented level of patient contact. The purpose of the DCCT was to experimentally test the hypothesis that better control of blood glucose levels would result in reduced incidence of microvascular complications of diabetes. The trial was unequivocally successful in answering this question. The intensive intervention produced large effects: 76% reduction in risk for developing diabetic eye disease, 54% lower risk of developing kidney disease, and 60% lower risk for developing clinical neuropathy (DCCT, Research Group, 1993).

From a behavioral perspective, the most unusual and impressive feature of the DCCT was the amount, duration, integration, and availability of support provided to participants in the intensive intervention condition (Fisher

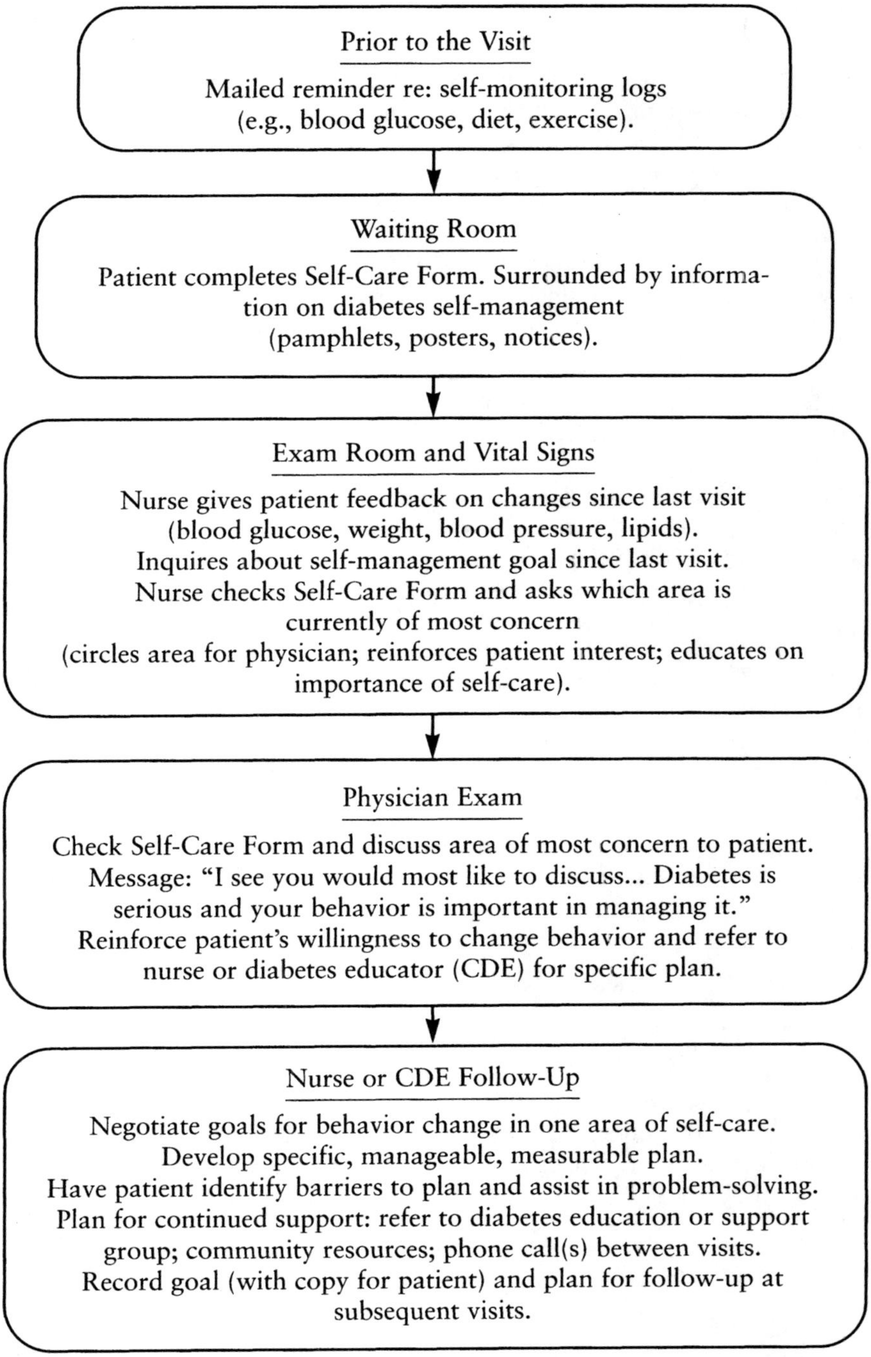

Figure 18.2 Flow of brief office-based diabetes self-management intervention.

et al., 1994; Lorenz et al., 1996). These services were provided by a highly skilled multidisciplinary team of endocrinologists, dieticians, nurses, diabetes educators, and behavioral scientists who were available to the participants 24 hours a day for 6–8 years. The DCCT was a powerful demonstration that an integrated team approach to intensive collaborative management of diabetes produces beneficial outcomes.

Despite the clearcut results, the implications of the DCCT have been controversial (e.g., Clark & Vinicor, 1996; Harris et al., 1994; McCulloch et al., 1994; Vinicor, 1994). Lively debates have revolved around three issues:

1. Is it practical, given our current health care system and cost constraints, to deliver the level of support tested in the DCCT? Most diabetes care occurs in the context of primary care provider offices that have far less expertise and resources than did the DCCT;
2. Do the results also apply to older Type II diabetes patients? Questions surround the pros and cons of intensive insulin therapy for Type II (Clark & Vinicor, 1996), which carries with it increased risk of hypoglycemic attacks, weight gain, and the possibility of increased cardiac disease (the major cause of morbidity among persons with Type II diabetes) from hyperinsulinemia;
3. Given that the relationship between level of glycemic control and probability of complications was almost linear, can we expect that population-based or wide-scale interventions of a less intensive nature (which would be more feasible but likely less effective) would reduce the overall level of the population risk, and thereby reduce the prevalence of diabetes complications?

Vigorous debate has served to bring issues of diabetes control, and the related discussion of behavioral and psychosocial issues in diabetes, to the national forefront (Fisher et al., 1994, 1996; Rubin & Peyrot, 1994).

Summary and Emerging Issues

Considerable progress has been made over the past decade in addressing behavioral aspects of diabetes (e.g., Clement, 1995; Cox & Gonder-Frederick, 1992; Fisher et al., 1997). Healthcare systems, providers, and diabetes patients are increasingly recognizing the importance and challenges of psychosocial issues in diabetes care. However, many challenges remains. This section briefly discusses issues in need of additional research.

Personalization

The 1990s patient-focused intervention, self-efficacy, and empowerment perspectives have been established. There is almost universal agreement that the patient should be the central member of the diabetes team, and that diabetes management plans and goals should be individualized to fit patient values, preferences, readiness to change, and situations (ADA, 1996; Clement, 1995; Ruggiero & Prochaska, 1993). However, research is needed to determine the most effective, practical, and efficient ways to deliver these services. In particular, new information technologies, including electronic patient records, touchscreen and hand-held computers, interactive multimedia systems, modem-based communications, and the Internet, have potential to enhance tailored patient care.

There is a need to increase our conceptual understanding of change processes and patient empowerment issues. The idea of tailoring interventions based upon psychological factors has intuitive appeal. However, to be defensible from a cost-effectiveness perspective, such tailoring applications should be demonstrated to be 1) significantly better than nontailored intervention, and 2) to be more effective (given the increased costs) than simply providing patients with a menu of intervention options and allowing them to tailor their own program.

Comorbidity

Most adult patients with diabetes have one or more other chronic disease (e.g., hypertension, arthritis, heart disease, back pain), as well as various levels of diabetes complications. Many patients also experience psychiatric comorbidities, including depression in particular (Lustman, Griffith, & Clouse, 1996). These disorders and their functional implications form an important part of the environment in which diabetes management occurs. Unfortunately, little attention has been given to these issues. In fact, many major studies, including the DCCT, have excluded persons with complications or comorbidities so that efficacy questions may be answered more "clearly." This situation needs to change, because diabetes and diabetes care do not occur in a vacuum, but rather in the context of other medical and social situations.

Quality of Life and Underserved Diabetes Populations

Possibly most central to the mission of the ADA, and two of the least researched areas, are (a) patient quality of life, and (b) ways to reach underserved segments of the diabetes population that usually do not receive patient education. These high-prevalence, underserved groups include Native Americans, Hispanic-Americans, African Americans, older adults, those living in rural areas, and the poor. The mission of the ADA (1995) is to "prevent and cure diabetes and to improve the lives of all people affected by diabetes . . . to make an every day difference in the quality of life for all people with diabetes." As Kaplan (1990) has argued, patient functioning and behavioral adjustment should be the primary outcomes on which we focus. Physiologic indices are useful to the extent that they predict behavioral functioning, impairment, and premature mortality (Davis, Hess, & Hiss, 1988).

Culturally diverse groups will constitute an increasingly larger proportion of the population, are more likely to develop diabetes, and are more likely to develop complications of diabetes (as well as other diseases). Yet, paradoxically, these groups are less likely to have sufficient access to or receive state-of-the-art diabetes management. These inequities, and their functional impacts, must be addressed. The challenges implied in reaching these populations are starting to be addressed (e.g., R. M. Anderson et al., 1996), but deserve even greater emphasis.

Methodological Issues

Given the current status of the literature, what is most needed are demonstrations that behavioral and psychoeducational assessments and interventions make a difference in the quality of life and outcomes of persons with diabetes. The field needs empirical documentation that psychological assessment and intervention procedures are practical, broadly applicable, cost-effective, and produce meaningful long-term results if they are to be adopted widely or accepted into clinical practice.

Much excellent psychological, psychometric, and intervention development work has been done, but many of these procedures are too extensive, time-consuming, or poorly understood (that is, not high in face validity to other disciplines) to be widely disseminated. As implied by Figures 18.1's Level 6, concerning cultural issues and policies, we should work to change existing reimbursement and healthcare policies that underemphasize or penalize prevention and psychosocial/behavioral procedures (Glasgow, 1996; Vogt, 1993). But the current reality is that for the next few years, this will be the environment and sociopolitical-financial context for diabetes care.

Psychosocial procedures—and other healthcare procedures—must do a better job of reaching a broad and representative segment of the population having diabetes and at risk of developing diabetes. Many individuals receive little or no diabetes education or services (Coonrod et al., 1994). This also raises complex social justice issues, since these underserved individuals tend to be poor, older, live in rural areas, and be persons of color.

A priority for future research should be studies that comprehensively address the complex relationships among patient characteristics, self-management behaviors, glycemic control, and other physiologic/risk factor outcomes. There is abundant evidence that these relationships are complex, multifactorial, and often not strong—possibly because they are moderated by medications, disease severity, comorbidities, and other factors (Glasgow,

McCaul, & Schafer, 1987; Johnson, 1994). Cardiovascular risk factors are important outcomes that have been relatively neglected by diabetes education research (Brown, 1990; Glasgow & Osteen, 1992). Smoking status, serum lipids, and physical activity have been particularly underemphasized given consistent epidemiologic data that heart disease and its complications are both the most likely cause of death among persons with diabetes (Brownson et al., 1993) and responsible for the bulk of excess healthcare, hospital, and pharmacologic costs associated with diabetes (Glauber & Brown, 1994).

The current emphasis on accountability in health care and the increasing emphasis on demand reduction (Sobel, 1995), and cost-containment demands that our interventions be cost-effective or cost-beneficial (Kaplan & Davis, 1986). Logically, behavioral and psychosocial procedures should be held to the same, rather than more stringent, standards as medico-pharmacological interventions. We currently find that our interventions are often subject to even higher standards, given that psychological services are often viewed as "add-ons" rather than an integral part of healthcare delivery.

Finally, following our "Levels of Influence Pyramid" (Figure 18.1), we feel that special priority should be placed on research that addresses Levels 3–6: healthcare systems, worksite/school, neighborhood/community, and cultural/policy/media factors related to diabetes care, given that the preponderance of psychosocial research has focused on the influences at the top two levels of the pyramid. In particular, studies of the integration of interventions across levels, and ways of assessing and changing behavior at these larger social levels, are needed.

REFERENCES

American Diabetes Association. (1995). *Mission statement.* Alexandria, VA: Author.

American Diabetes Association. (1995). Standards of Medical Care for Patients with Diabetes Mellitus. *Diabetes Care, 18*, 8–15.

American Diabetes Association. (1996). Nutrition recommendations and principles for people with diabetes mellitus. *Diabetes Care, Suppl. 19*, S16–S19.

American Diabetes Association Task Force to Revise the National Standards. (1995). National standards for diabetes self-management education programs. *Diabetes Care, 18*, 141–143.

Anderson, B. J. (1996). Involving family members in diabetes treatment. In B. J. Anderson & R. R. Rubin (Eds.), *Practical psychology for diabetes clinicians* (pp. 43–50). Alexandria,VA: American Diabetes Association.

Anderson, B. J., & Rubin, R. R. (1996). *Practical psychology for diabetes clinicians: How to deal with the key behavioral issues faced by patients and health care teams.* Alexandria, VA: American Diabetes Association.

Anderson, L. A. (1990). Health-care communication and selected psychosocial correlates of adherence in diabetes management. *Diabetes Care, 13*, 66–76.

Anderson, L. A., & Sharpe, P. A. (1991). Improving patient and provider communication: A synthesis and review of communication interventions. *Patient Education and Counseling, 17*, 99–134.

Anderson, R. M., Barr, P. A., Edwards, G. J., Funnell, M. M., Fitzgerald, J. T., & Wisdom, K. (1996). Using focus groups to identify psychosocial issues of urban black individuals with diabetes. *The Diabetes Educator, 22*, 28–33.

Anderson, R. M., Fitzgerald, J. T., Funnell, M. M., Barr, P. A., Stepien, C. J., Hiss, R. G., & Armbruster, B. A. (1994). Evaluation of an activated patient diabetes education newsletter. *The Diabetes Educator, 20*, 29–34.

Anderson, R. M., & Funnell, M. M. (1990). The role of the physician in patient education. *Practical Diabetology*, 10–12.

Anderson, R. M., Funnell, M. M., Butler, P. M., Arnold, M. S., Fitzgerald, J. T., & Feste, C. C. (1995). Patient empowerment: Results of a randomized controlled trial. *Diabetes Care, 18*, 943–949.

Ary, D. V., Toobert, D., Wilson, W., & Glasgow, R. (1986). Patient perspective on factors contributing to nonadherence to diabetes regimen. *Diabetes Care, 9*, 168–172.

Bond, G. G., Aiken, L. S., & Somerville, S. C. (1992). The health belief model and adolescents with insulin-dependent diabetes mellitus. *Health Psychology, 11*, 190–198.

Brown, S. A. (1990). Studies of educational interventions and outcomes in diabetic adults: A meta-analysis revisited. *Patient Education and Counseling, 16*, 189–215.

Brownson, R. C., Remington, P. L., & Davis, J. R. (1993). *Chronic disease epidemiology and control.* Baltimore, MD: Port City Press.

Clark, C. M., Jr., & Vinicor, F. (1996). Introduction: Risks and benefits of intensive management in NIDDM. *Annals of Internal Medicine, 124*, 81–85.

Clark, N. M., Becker, M. H., Lorig, K., Rakowski, W., & Anderson, L. (1991). Self-management of chronic disease by older adults: A review and questions for research. *Journal of Aging and Health, 3*, 3–27.

Clement, S. (1995). Diabetes self-management education. *Diabetes Care, 18*, 1204–1214.

Cohen, M. Z., Tripp-Reimer, T., Smith, C., Sorofman, B., & Lively, S. (1994). Explanatory models of diabetes: Patient-practitioner variation. *Social Science and Medicine, 38*, 59–66.

Cohen, S. J. (1983). Potential barriers to diabetes care. *Diabetes Care, 6*, 499–500.

Coonrod, B. A., Betschart, J., & Harris, M. I. (1994). Frequency and determinants of diabetes patient education among adults in the U.S. population. *Diabetes Care, 17*, 852–858.

Cox, D., Gonder-Frederick, L., Polonsky, W., Schlundt, D., Julian, D., & Clarke, W. (1995). A multi-center evaluation of blood glucose awareness training - II. *Diabetes Care, 18*, 523–528.

Cox, D. J., & Gonder-Frederick, L. (1992). Major developments in behavioral diabetes research. *Journal of Consulting and Clinical Psychology, 60*, 628–638.

Cox, D. J., Gonder-Frederick, L., & Clarke, W. L. (1996). Helping patients reduce severe hypoglycemia. In B. J. Anderson & R. R. Rubin (Eds.), *Practical psychology for diabetes clinicians* (pp. 93–104). Alexandria, VA: American Diabetes Association.

Cox, D. J., Gonder-Frederick, L., Julian, D. M., & Clarke, W. (1994). Long-term follow-up evaluation of blood glucose awareness training. *Diabetes Care, 17*, 1–5.

Cox, D. J., Gonder-Frederick, L., Lee, J. H., Julian, D. M., Carter, W. R., & Clarke, W. L. (1989). Effects and correlates of blood glucose awareness training among patients with IDDM. *Diabetes Care, 12*, 313–318.

Davis, R. M. (1995). Tobacco policy research comes of age. *Tobacco Control, 4*, 6–9.

Davis, W. K., Hess, G. E., & Hiss, R. G. (1988). Psychosocial correlates of survival in diabetes. *Diabetes Care, 11*, 538–545.

DCCT Research Group. (1993). The effect of intensive treatment of diabetes on the development and progression of long-term complications in insulin-dependent diabetes mellitus. *New England Journal of Medicine, 329*, 977–986.

Diabetes Guidelines Advisory Group (1996). *Continuous quality improvement guidelines: Diabetes mellitus*. Oregon Health Division, Portland, OR.

Dunn, S. M. (1990). Rethinking the models and modes of diabetes education. *Patient Education and Counseling, 16*, 281–286.

Eakin, E. G., & Glasgow, R. E. (1996). The physician's role in diabetes self-management: Helping patients to help themselves. *The Endocrinologist, 6*, 1–10.

Etzwiler, D. D. (1994). Diabetes translation: A blueprint for the future. *Diabetes Care, 17*, 1–4.

Ewart, C. (1991). Social action theory for a public health psychology. *American Psychologist, 46*, 931–946.

Fiore, M. C. (1991). The new vital sign. Assessing and documenting smoking status (commentary). *Journal of the American Medical Association, 266*, 3183–3184.

Fisher, E. B., Jr., Arfken, C. L., Heins, J., Houston, C., Jeffe, D., & Sykes, R. (1996). Acceptance of diabetes in adults. In D. S. Gochman (Ed.), *Handbook of health behavior research* (pp. 189–212). New York: Plenum.

Fisher, E. B., Jr., Lorenz, R. A., Heins, J. M., Marrero, D. G., Hiss, R. G., McNabb, W. L., & Wylie-Rosett, J. (1994). *Metabolic control matters: Nationwide translation of the Diabetes Control and Complications Trial: Analysis and recommendations*. Manuscript submitted for publication.

Fisher, E. B., Jr., Ziff, S. L., & Haire-Joshu, D. (1996). Smoking cessation in diabetes. In B. J. Anderson & R. R. Rubin (Eds.), *Practical psychology for diabetes clinicians* (pp. 121–132). Alexandria, VA: American Diabetes Association.

Glanz, K., Lankenau, B., Foerster, S., Temple, S., Mullis, R., & Schmid, T. (1995). Environtmental and policy approaches to cardiovascular disease prevention through nutrition: Opportunities for state and local action. *Health Education Quarterly, 22*, 512–527.

Glanz, K., & Rimer, B. K. (1995). *Theory at a glance: A guide for health promotion practice*. Bethesda, MD: National Cancer Institute.

Glasgow, R. E. (1995). A practical model of diabetes management and education. *Diabetes Care, 18*, 117–126.

Glasgow, R. E. (1996). Are research and policy advocacy two separate worlds? *Diabetes Care, 19*, 1165–1166.

Glasgow, R. E., & Anderson, B. J. (1995). Future directions for research on pediatric chronic disease management: Lessons from diabetes. *Journal of Pediatric Psychology, 20*, 389–402.

Glasgow, R. E., & Eakin, E. G. (1996). Dealing with complexity: The case of diabetes self-management. In B. J. Anderson & R. R. Rubin (Eds.), *Practical psychology for diabetes clinicians* (pp. 53–62). Alexandria, VA: American Diabetes Association.

Glasgow, R. E., McCaul, K. D., & Schafer, L. C. (1986). Barriers to regimen adherence among persons with insulin-dependent diabetes. *Journal of Behavioral Medicine, 9*, 65–77.

Glasgow, R. E., McCaul, K. D., & Schafer, L. C. (1987). Self-care behaviors and glycemic control in Type I diabetes. *Journal of Chronic Diseases, 40*, 399–412.

Glasgow, R. E., & Osteen, V. L. (1992). Evaluating diabetes education: Are we measuring the most important outcomes? *Diabetes Care, 15*, 1423–1432.

Glasgow, R. E., Toobert, D. J., & Hampson, S. E. (1996). Effects of a brief office-based intervention to facilitate diabetes dietary self-management. *Diabetes Care, 19*, 835–842.

Glasgow, R. E., Toobert, D. J., Hampson, S. E., Brown, J. E., Lewinsohn, P. M., & Donnelly, J. (1992). Improving self-care among older patients with Type II diabetes: The "Sixty Something . . ." study. *Patient Education and Counseling, 19*, 61–74.

Glasgow, R. E., Toobert, D. J., Hampson, S. E., & Noell, J. W. (1995). A brief office-based intervention to facilitate diabetes self-management. *Health Education Research: Theory & Practice, 10*, 467–478.

Glasgow, R. E., Wagner, E., Kaplan, R. M., Vinicor, F., Smith, L., & Norman, J. (1996). *If diabetes is a public health problem, why not treat it as one? A population-based approach to diabetes care.* Manuscript submitted for publication.

Glauber, H., & Brown, J. (1994). Impact of cardiovascular disease on health care utilization in a defined diabetic population. *Journal of Clinical Epidemiology, 47*, 1133–1142.

Golin, C. E., DiMatteo, M. R., & Gelberg, L. (1996). The role of patient involvement in the doctor visit: Implications for adherence to diabetes care. *Diabetes Care*, 19, 1153–1164.

Green, L. W., & Kreuter, M. W. (1991). *Health promotion planning: An education and environmental approach*. Mountain View, CA: Mayfield.

Greenfield, S., Kaplan, S. H., Ware, J. E., Yano, E. M., & Frank, H. (1988). Patients' participation in medical care: Effects on blood sugar control and quality of life in diabetes. *Journal of General Internal Medicine, 3*, 448–457.

Greenlick, M. R. (1992). Educating physicians for population-based clinical practice. *Journal of the American Medical Association, 267*, 1645–1648.

Haire-Joshu, D. (1991). Smoking, cessation, and the diabetes health care team. *The Diabetes Educator, 17*, 54–64.

Hampson, S. E., Glasgow, R. E., & Foster, L. (1995). Personal models of diabetes among older adults: Relation to self-management and other variables. *The Diabetes Educator, 21*, 300–307.

Harris, M. I., Eastman, R. C., & Siebert, C. (1994). The DCCT and medical care for diabetes in the U.S. *Diabetes Care, 17*, 761–764.

Irvine, A. A., Saunders, J. T., Blank, M. B., & Carter, W. R. (1990). Validation of scale measuring environmental barriers to diabetes-regimen adherence. *Diabetes Care, 13*, 705–711.

Johnson, S. B. (1993). Compliance and control in insulin-dependent diabetes: Does behavior really make a difference? In N. A. Krasnegor, L. Epstein, S. B. Johnson, & S. J. Yaffe (Eds.), *Developmental aspects of health compliance behavior* (pp. 275–297). Hillsdale, NJ: Lawrence Erlbaum.

Johnson, S. B. (1994). Health behavior and health status: Concepts, methods and applications. *Journal of Pediatric Psychology, 19*, 129–141.

Kaplan, R. M. (1990). Behavior as the central outcome in health care. *American Psychologist, 45*, 1211–1220.

Kaplan, R. M., & Davis, W. K. (1986). Evaluating the costs and benefits of outpatient diabetes education and nutrition counseling. *Diabetes Care, 9*, 81–86.

Kaplan, S. H., Greenfield, S. W., & Ware, J. E. (1989). Assessing the effects of physician-patient interactions on the outcomes of chronic disease. *Medical Care, 27*, 5110–5127.

King, A. C., Jeffery, R. W., Fridinger, F., Dusenbury, L., Provence, S., Hedlund, S. A., & Spangler, K. (1995). Environmental and policy approaches to cardiovascular disease prevention through physical activity: Issues and opportunities. *Health Education Quarterly, 22*, 499–511.

Kingery, P. M., & Glasgow, R. E. (1989). Self-efficacy and outcome expectations in the self-regulation of non-insulin dependent diabetes mellitus. *Health Education, 20*, 13–19.

Kirkman, M. S., Weinberger, M., Landsman, P. B., Samsa, G. P., Shortliffe, E. A., Simel, D. L., & Feussner, J. R. (1994). A telephone-delivered intervention for patients with NIDDM. *Diabetes Care, 17*, 840–846.

Lasker, R. D. (1993). The Diabetes Control and Complications Trial: Implications for policy and practice. *New England Journal of Medicine, 329*, 1035–1036.

Litzelman, D. K., Slemenda, C. W., Langefeld, C. D., Hays, L. M., Welch, M. A., Bild, D. E., Ford, E. S., & Vinicor, F. (1993). Reduction of lower extremity clinical abnormalities in patients with non-insulin-dependent diabetes mellitus: A randomized, controlled trial. *Annals of Internal Medicine, 119*, 36–41.

Lorenz, R. A., Bubb, J., Davis, D., Jacobson, A., Jannasch, K., Kramer, J., Lipps, J., & Schlundt, D. (1996). Changing behavior: Practical lessons from the Diabetes Control and Complications Trial. *Diabetes Care, 19*, 648–652.

Lorig, K. R., Mazonson, P. D., & Holman, H. R. (1993). Evidence suggesting that health education for self-management in patients with chronic arthritis has sustained health benefits while reducing health care costs. *Arthritis and Rheumatism, 36*, 439–446.

Lustman, P. J., Griffith, L. S., & Clouse, R. E. (1996). Recognizing and managing depression in patients with diabetes. In B. J. Anderson & R. R. Rubin (Eds.), *Practical psychology for diabetes clinicians* (pp. 143–154). Alexandria, VA: American Diabetes Association.

Marrero, D. G. (1994). Current effectiveness of diabetes health care in the U.S. *Diabetes Reviews, 2*, 292–309.

Mazze, R. S. (1994). A systems approach to diabetes care. *Diabetes Care, 17*, 5–11.

McCulloch, D. K., Glasgow, R. E., Hampson, S. E., & Wagner, E. (1994). A systematic approach to diabetes management in the post-DCCT era. *Diabetes Care, 17*, 765–769.

National Institutes of Health. (1995). *Diabetes in America.* (NIH Publication No.

95–1468). Bethesda, MD: National Institute of Diabetes and Digestive and Kidney Diseases.

Orme, C. M., & Binik, Y. M. (1989). Consistency of adherence across regimen demands. *Health Psychology, 8*, 27–43.

Padgett, D., Mumford, E., Hynes, M., & Carter, R. (1988). Meta-analysis of the effects of educational and psychosocial interventions on management of diabetes mellitus. *Journal of Clinical Epidemiology, 41*, 1007–1030.

Padgett, D. L., Nord, W. R., Heins, J. M., & Arfken, C. L. (1996). Managing diabetes in the workplace: Critical factors. *Diabetes Spectrum, 9*, 13–20.

Peyrot, M., & Rubin, R. R. (1994). Living with diabetes: The patient-centered perspective. *Diabetes Spectrum, 7*, 205–206.

Rubin, R. R., & Peyrot, M. (1992). Psychosocial problems and interventions in diabetes. *Diabetes Care, 15*, 1640–1657.

Rubin, R. R., & Peyrot, M. (1994). Implications of the DCCT: Looking beyond tight control. *Diabetes Care, 17*, 235–236.

Ruggiero, L., & Prochaska, J. O. (1993). Introduction: Readiness for change: Application of the transtheoretical model to diabetes. *Diabetes Spectrum, 6*, 22–24.

Sallis, J. F., & Owen, N. (1996). Ecological models. In K. Glanz, F. M. Lewis, & B. K. Rimer (Eds.), *Health behavior and health education: Theory, research and practice* (pp. 403–424). San Francisco, CA: Jossey-Bass.

Schlundt, D. G., Pichert, J. W., Gregory, B., & Davis, D. (1996). Eating and diabetes: A patient-centered approach. In B. J. Anderson & R. R. Rubin (Eds.), *Practical psychology for diabetes clinicians* (pp. 63–72). Alexandria, VA: American Diabetes Association.

Schlundt, D. G., Rea, M. R., Kline, S. S., & Pichert, J. W. (1994). Situational obstacles to dietary adherence for adults with diabetes. *Journal of the American Dietetic Association, 94*, 874–876.

Slavin, R. E. (1986). Best-evidence synthesis: An alternative approach to traditional and meta-analytic reviews. *Educational Research, 15*, 5–11.

Sobel, D. (1995). Rethinking medicine: Improving health outcomes with cost-effective psychosocial interventions. *Psychosomatic Medicine, 57*, 234–244.

Stauber, J., & Rampton, S. (1995). *Toxic sludge is good for you! Lies, damn lies and the public relations industry*. Monroe, ME: Common Courage Press.

Stokols, D. (1996). Translating social ecological theory into guidelines for community health promotion. *American Journal of Health Promotion, 10*, 282–298.

Toobert, D. J., & Glasgow, R. E. (1991). Problem-solving and diabetes self-care. *Journal of Behavioral Medicine, 14*, 71–86.

U.S. Department of Health and Human Services. (1992). 1992 national survey of worksite health promotion activities: Summary. *American Journal of Health Promotion, 7*, 452–464.

U.S. Preventive Services Task Force. (1996). *Guide to clinical preventive services* (2nd ed.). Baltimore, MD: Williams & Wilkins.

Vinicor, F. (1994). Is diabetes a public-health disorder? *Diabetes Care, 17*, 22–27.

Vogt, T. M. (1993). Paradigms and prevention. *American Journal of Public Health, 83*, 795–796.

Von Korff, M., Gruman, J., Schaefer, J., Curry, S. J., & Wagner, E. H. (1997).

Collaborative management of chronic illness. *Annals of Behavioral Medicine, 127*, 1097–1102.

Wasson, J., Gaudette, C., Whaley, F., Sauvigne, A., Baribeau, P., & Welch, H. G. (1992). Telephone care as a substitute for routine clinic follow-up. *Journal of the American Medical Association, 267*, 1788–1793.

Wing, R. R. (1996). Improving weight loss and maintenance in patients with diabetes. In B. J. Anderson & R. R. Rubin (Eds.), *Practical psychology for diabetes clinicians* (pp. 113–120). Alexandria, VA: American Diabetes Association.

Wing, R. R., & Anglin, K. (1996). Effectiveness of a behavioral weight control program for blacks and whites with NIDDM. *Diabetes Care, 19*, 409–413.

Wing, R. R., Epstein, L. H., Nowalk, M. P., & Lamparski, D. M. (1986). Behavioral self-regulation in the treatment of patients with diabetes mellitus. *Psychological Bulletin, 99*, 78–89.

Wing, R. R., Epstein, L. H., Paternostro-Bayles, M., Kriska, A., Nowalk, M. P., & Gooding, W. (1988). Exercise in a behavioural weight control programme for obese patients with type II (non-insulin-dependent) diabetes. *Diabetologia, 31*, 902–909.

Wysocki, T., Hough, B. S., Ward, K. M., & Green, L. B. (1992). Diabetes mellitus in the transition to adulthood: Adjustment, self-care and health status. *Journal of Developmental and Behavioral Pediatrics, 13*, 194–201.

19

Adherence Issues Among Cancer Patients

Amy H. Peterman and David F. Cella

Treatment adherence research among cancer patients is in its infancy compared to that among patients with other chronic illnesses (e.g., DiMatteo, Sherbourne, et al., 1993; Kravitz et al., 1993) or the general population (Janz & Becker, 1984). A large portion of the existing literature with cancer patients is focused simply on documenting rates of adherence to treatment. Significantly less attention has been paid to variables associated with adherence or to interventions designed to improve adherence. One potential reason for the relative lack of attention to adherence in this population is the widely held assumption that patients facing a possibly terminal illness like cancer will adhere without question to whatever recommendations are made (Lewis, Linet, & Abeloff, 1983; Tebbi, 1993). That is, health professionals have assumed that patients will adhere if the likely alternative is death. However, comparisons of adherence rates among diseases varying in severity do not confirm this assumption (DiMatteo, Hays, & Sherbourne, 1992; Kaplan & Simon, 1990).

This chapter reviews the literature on adherence among people who have been diagnosed with cancer. Adherence to cancer-prevention efforts among the general population is not addressed here, as this topic is well-covered elsewhere in this book. The term "adherence" is used in this chapter to refer to "the degree to which a patient 'voluntarily' follows the regimen recommended by a provider" (Barofsky, 1984, p. 43). The implication is that patients are active participants in their medical care. However, the majority of the literature reviewed for this paper used the term "compliance" with treatment and recommended care. This is, in part, reflective of the fact that most of the literature on this subject appears in medical journals, where the term "compliance" is more common. It may also reflect the fact that cancer treatment has traditionally been viewed as something, like intravenous (IV) chemotherapy, to be administered to a passive patient. The active (participatory) component implied by the term "adherence" has traditionally not been recognized. However, cancer treatment requires a great deal of commitment and energy on the part of the patient, and "adherence" seems to better capture this process.

The chapter is organized as follows: First, the significance of adherence to treatment success is discussed. Next, measurement issues are addressed. Third, investigations that have estimated adherence rates for different treatment-related behaviors are reviewed in an effort to establish the magnitude of the problem of adherence. Fourth, research investigating various determinants of adherence, special issues among children/adolescents with cancer, and interventions to improve adherence are examined. The chapter concludes with a discussion of future directions for research.

RELATIONSHIP OF ADHERENCE TO TREATMENT OUTCOMES: WHY STUDY ADHERENCE?

The bottom-line significance of adherence is assumed to be an impact on the eventual success of treatment and ultimately the physical health and survival of the patient. One frequently cited investigation documented that treatment success was significantly lower among patients who received less than 85% of their planned dosages of adjuvant chemotherapy (Bonadonna & Valagussa, 1981). Although adherence was not evaluated in this study, the findings of this and similar dose-intensity studies have been generalized to support a role for adherence in treatment outcome (Y. N. Lee, 1983). That is, if nonadherence contributes to a patient receiving a lesser amount of treatment, then the nonadherence may lead to a poorer treatment outcome.

However, while some treatments have shown a clear dose-response relationship with survival, there are numerous reports of treatment inefficacy as well (e.g., Carey et al., 1979; Feld, Rubinstein, Thomas, and the Lung Cancer Study Group, 1993; Fisher et al., 1990; Makela et al., 1993). In addition, other investigations have failed to show a survival advantage to treatment acceptance and follow-up recommendations. For example, in a retrospective study comparing patients who accepted and refused treatment, there was no significant survival advantage for accepting treatment for several different types of cancer (Huchcroft & Snodgrass, 1993). In an investigation of follow-up visits after breast cancer treatment, no differences were found in time to recurrence or overall survival for patients receiving more vs. less intensive follow-up (Liberati, & the GIVIO Investigators, 1995).

Additionally, it is quite difficult to judge the significance of nonadherence, as there are multiple factors affecting outcome, only one of which is adherence. Frequently, the current state of scientific knowledge does not allow an accurate assessment of the impact of treatment. Adjuvant chemotherapy, for example, is given in the absence of any visible evidence of disease. As such, there is no way to reliably monitor the success of treatment, unless the treatment fails and there is a recurrence. Additionally, it is very difficult to specify what a particular patient must do to ensure a response from a treatment: dosage requirements are made on the basis of group data, and thus any particular individual may need more or less treatment for the cure or control of disease (Barofsky, 1984). Thus, while adherence is likely to play an important role, it is but one of many factors affecting treatment outcomes.

Methods for Measuring Adherence

There are three general categories of measurement available for assessing adherence (Hays & DiMatteo, 1987). These include self-reports, collateral reports, and objective measures. Each of these has particular advantages and disadvantages as applied to the wide variety of treatment-related behaviors required of cancer patients.

That self-reported treatment adherence is frequently inaccurate has been well-documented within a general medical population (Cannell, Oksenberg, & Converse, 1977). The few investigations that attempted to validate the self-report of cancer patients by comparison with objective measures have shown equivocal results. A comparison of self-report data and adherence rates obtained from blood levels of a drug treatment suggested that adherence rates derived from blood levels were half that of self-reported adherence rates (Levine et al., 1987). However, two measures of smoking cessation, cotinine levels and self-reports, among head and neck cancer patients were in agreement 89.6% of the time (Gritz et al., 1993). One hundred percent agreement between self-report and serum drug levels was reported in a study of children and adolescents (Tebbi et al., 1986).

It is, therefore, possible that patients can be relatively accurate reporters of their own behavior. Nonetheless, the variability in these concordance rates suggests that it is necessary to approach self-reports with some skepticism, and to consider the context of the treatment. Sources of inaccuracy in self-report by other medical populations are multiple, including fear of embarrassment or rejection by the healthcare provider, desire for support and approval, and misunderstandings about treatment recommendations (Hays

& DiMatteo, 1987). In addition, self-report does not allow for an assessment of unintentional nonadherence, due to forgetfulness or neglect: by definition, people can't self-report about nonadherence of which they are unaware. Although these variables have not been investigated with cancer patients, there is no reason to expect that they would not also operate in this population.

Collateral reports of adherence can be obtained from family, friends, and healthcare providers. These sources of collateral information have apparently been little used in the cancer population. In apparently the only study to utilize this kind of data, Dolgin, Katz, Doctors, and Siegel (1986) asked physicians to rate their adolescent cancer patients' treatment adherence and estimate the threat that nonadherence posed to treatment outcome. However, they did not obtain self-reports of adherence, so it was not possible to judge the accuracy of the physicians' report. Often, physicians' estimates of patients' adherence have been found to be quite inaccurate (Caron & Roth, 1968, 1971; Davis, 1966).

Chart reviews have been used extensively as one source of objective information on cancer patient adherence to appointments for IV chemotherapy and follow-ups (e.g., Berger, Braverman, Sohn, & Morrow, 1988; Moul, Paulson & Walther, 1990). Pill counts, electronic bottles, and urine or blood levels of medication in the patient's body also provide objective measures of treatment adherence, particularly cancer patients' adherence to oral chemotherapy and supportive medications. For example, the presence of 17-ketogenic steroids in urine has been shown to be a reliable indicator of adherence to oral prednisone in pediatric cancer patients (Smith, Rosen, Trueworthy, & Lowman, 1979).

Other investigators have also utilized blood-serum levels of drugs and their metabolites to measure adherence (Lebovits et al.,1990; Richardson et al., 1987). Differing adherence rates have been found depending on whether the blood level of the parent drug or the metabolite was used. For example, Richardson et al. found that 77% of patients were nonadherent to allopurinol as measured by the detection of the drug itself in the blood, but that only 43.3% of patients would be classified as nonadherent based on detection of oxipurinol, a metabolite of allopurinol. These authors suggest that such different levels might indicate poor or inconsistent medication ingestion. This interpretation has not been tested empirically, and other authors have questioned the value of this method due to individual variability in drug distribution and metabolism (C. R. Lee, Nicholson, Souhami, & Deshmukh, 1992).

Another alternative for measuring adherence to oral medication is the use of an electronic pill bottle that can record the times of day that the bottle is opened. This method is a particularly powerful objective measurement tool because it picks up both intentional and unintentional sources of nonadherence. Lee et al. (1992) reported the use of such a container with patients receiving oral chemotherapy. They documented almost perfect adherence with the regimen by comparing the number of bottle openings with the number of times expected if adherence was perfect. In addition, they were able to reveal the pattern of pill-taking by noting discrepancies between the time the bottle was opened and the time it was supposed to be opened. Pill bottles were opened the correct number of times on 80.9% of days.

Given the "fallibility" of individual methods, Hays and DiMatteo (1987) advocated the use of a multi-trait, multi-method approach to the assessment of treatment adherence. Thus, patients might be defined as nonadherent if their self-report, the report of their physician or their spouse, or serum drug levels indicated nonadherence to the recommended treatment.

ADHERENCE RATES

The range of behaviors requested of cancer patients is wide. Patients are asked initially to accept treatment recommendations, then can be required to attend multiple appointments for treatment and check-ups, to take oral and IV medications, to make lifestyle changes, and, finally, to attend frequent follow-up visits after treatment completion. These various behaviors all carry implications for likelihood of adherence or degree of difficulty of adherence. Therefore, it is difficult to classify a particular patient simply as adherent or not adherent. The situation is more complex when considering the adherence behaviors of groups of patients, to whom quite different sets of behaviors or treatments have been recommended to maximize the likelihood of a positive treatment outcome. Thus, it is important to consider the literature on adherence among cancer patients by types of behaviors studied.

After a cancer diagnosis, patients are given treatment recommendations which may involve surgery, chemotherapy, radiation therapy, and other possible medications or behavioral changes. The initial choice point for the patient is whether to even receive these recommendations. Following this decision, the required choice is whether to agree to initiate the recommended treatment(s).

In the few extant empirical reports of outright treatment refusal, relatively low rates have been found. In a retrospective study of women with breast cancer, Taylor, Lichtman & Wood (1984) found that 2 of 78 (2.5%) respondents stated that they had rejected chemotherapy without trying it at all and an additional 6 women (7.7%) stated that they had initially refused chemotherapy before eventually agreeing. Moul et al. (1990) determined that 5% of testicular cancer patients refused chemotherapy, 0.5% refused surgical treatment and no patients refused radiation therapy when offered it. In patients suffering a relapse during or after chemotherapy treatment for the highly aggressive germ-cell tumors, 9% of the 55 patients refused further chemotherapy (Josefsen, Ous, Hoie, Stenwig, & Fossa, 1993). However, at least 2 of these patients subsequently opted for radiation or surgical treatment.

Given patients' initial agreement to a recommended cancer-treatment course, adherence to the ensuing recommendations can then be evaluated. Much chemotherapy treatment is still administered intravenously within a medical setting. A primary source of information about adherence rates is reports of the results of clinical trials and other particular treatment protocols, which usually report the rates in brief terms without much accompanying information. Adherence rates in clinical trials/treatment protocols vary widely.

Some protocols report extremely low nonadherence. For example, no one was nonadherent to an early protocol offering adjuvant chemotherapy to breast cancer patients (Carey et al., 1979). Other reports document nonadherence rates around 2–8% (Blay et al., 1995; Brown et al., 1994; Makela et al., 1993; Moertel et al., 1990; Ryder, Rizzi, Metivier, Karani, & Williams, 1996). In their evaluation of 1548 breast cancer patients who received a total of 20,765 courses of adjuvant chemotherapy, Glass et al. (1981) found that nonadherence to chemotherapy for reasons other than treatment toxicity ranged from 2.5% to 6.9%, depending on the protocol. These are strikingly low rates, particularly when one considers that the very rationale of adjuvant therapy implies that the vast majority of patients receiving it do not need it (i.e., they are already cured without the therapy, or the cancer will recur despite the therapy).

Investigations of adherence to chemotherapy for late stage cancers have reported significantly higher nonadherence rates. For example, Feld et al. (1993; Feld, Rubinstein, & Thomas, 1994) reported on a trial of adjuvant chemotherapy for operable non-small cell lung cancer. Only 80% of patients enrolled in the trial actually received their first treatment dose, 66% of patients received at least two of the four planned courses of treatment, and only 54% of patients completed all four courses. Others have similarly documented nonadherence rates ranging from 10–15% (Buccheri & Ferrigno, 1994; Jehn, 1994; Verdonck et al., 1992) to 20–25% (Berger et al., 1988; Schumacher et al., 1994) to greater than 30% (Y. N. Lee, 1983; Rivkin et al., 1993). The reason for the disparity in adherence across these trials is not readily apparent.

Adherence rates gleaned from reports of clinical trials and treatment protocols are specific to the particular treatment under investigation. Thus, it is possible, even likely, that some patients reported as nonadherent to a particular treatment in the above reports actually followed through with a different treatment that was preferable to them for some reason. For example, Zanetta et al. (1993) reported that 1 of 24 patients refused to continue the chemotherapy treatment being investigated for locally advanced cervical cancer; however, the report indicates that this patient did agree to radiation therapy. Chevallier et al. (1993) reported a similar situation in which 7 of 31 patients refused surgical treatment for inflammatory breast cancer, but agreed to receive radiation therapy instead. However, poor adherence to chemotherapy has been shown to be predictive of poor adherence to subsequent radiotherapy (Jacobs et al., 1994), suggesting that patients who are nonadherent to one treatment will be more likely to be nonadherent to another.

Reports such as these raise two important points. First, the context of patients' nonadherence must be specified (i.e., nonadherent to a particular treatment, or to treatment overall). The causes and potential implications of nonadherence to different treatment recommendations may vary significantly. Second, the majority of cancer patients are not treated within the context of clinical trials (Friedman & Cain, 1990). Only a small proportion are eligible for participation (approximately 25%; Gotay, 1991) and only a percentage of those eligible agree to participate (an average of 40%; Gotay, 1991). There is some suggestion that participants in clinical trials may be significantly different from other cancer patients (Gotay, 1991). Thus, it is difficult to know whether the adherence rates found in clinical trials are generalizable or even applicable to the larger population of cancer patients.

However, one study that surveyed 78 women after their treatment for breast cancer, without regard for the treatment received, documented a moderate rate of nonadherence (Taylor et al., 1984); 7.7% initially refused chemotherapy before eventually agreeing to it, and 2.5% of patients reported being intermittently nonadherent during their treatment. Thus, approximately 10% of this general population of breast cancer patients were not adherent to chemotherapy at some point in their treatment. This figure may underestimate nonadherence. The response rate for the study was only 49%, and it seems likely that those who were nonadherent to treatment might also have refused to participate in the study.

Oral chemotherapies are used as adjuncts to IV chemotherapy for a number of cancers. In addition, oral medications are often used for supportive care to decrease the incidence of side effects from IV therapy so that patients can tolerate more aggressive treatments. Such self-administration of pills in adults (special issues of children and adolescents are discussed below) has been associated with lower adherence than IV chemotherapies.

For example, Richardson et al. (1987) evaluated adherence to allupurinol, a supportive medication taken daily to prevent uric acid nephropathy from chemotherapy, and prednisone, taken 5 consecutive days each month as an antineoplastic drug. Nonadherence rates for patients who did not receive an intervention designed to increase adherence (discussed below) ranged from 43.3% to 77% for allopurinol, depending on the blood metabolite analyzed.

Self-reports of adherence suggested patients were nonadherent approximately 52% of the time. Nonadherence to prednisone administration ranged from 24.8% to 31.2%, again depending on the metabolite analyzed. Lebovits et al. (1990) found similar nonadherence rates with orally administered Cytoxan or prednisone, 37% and 38% respectively.

Adherence to appointments during the period of active cancer treatment or evaluation has also been examined. Garrett, Ashford, and Savage (1986) conducted a prospective examination of clinic attendance among 100 cancer patients receiving chemotherapy, hormone therapy, or supportive/palliative care. Eighty-nine percent of all scheduled visits were kept; 53% of patients kept all of their appointments, and 69% of patients kept 80% or more of their appointments. Glass et al. (1981) and Berger et al. (1988) documented that patients kept over 90% of their scheduled appointments during treatment.

Rates of adherence to behavioral recommendations made during treatment have also been investigated. These recommendations are thought to improve the effectiveness of treatment or decrease the likelihood of relapse. For example, breast cancer patients are advised to continue performing breast self-exams (BSE) in hope of catching any local recurrence early. Taylor, Lichtman, Wood, Bluming, et al. (1984) found that 43% of their sample of breast cancer patients practiced breast self-exam (BSE) at least monthly.

Several investigations into adherence to a low-fat diet have also been reported: it has been suggested that low fat diets might decrease the risk of breast cancer (Goodwin & Boyd, 1987). Adherence rates in such intervention studies are relatively low. Boyar et al. (1988) documented 74% completion of their 6-month study: Holm, Nordevang, Ikkala, Hallstrom and Callmer (1990) reported that 52% of breast cancer patients completed their 2-year trial.

Finally, cancer patients are typically followed closely during the period immediately after treatment, with frequency of follow-ups decreasing with time. While the utility of follow-ups for detecting recurrence has been questioned (e.g., Ormiston, Timoney, & Qureshi, 1985; Tomlin & Donegan, 1987; Winchester et al., 1979), they are standard practice (Tomiak & Piccart, 1993). However, such check-ups can be associated with a high degree of anxiety that may influence adherence.

As with other types of treatment-related behaviors, adherence to follow-up visits varies widely. Seventy-seven percent to 93% of testicular cancer patients kept all of their scheduled follow-up appointments. The actual percentage varied depending upon the type of previous treatment received (Young, Bultz, Russell, & Trew, 1991). Using a different type of follow-up measure, 84% of colon cancer patients who had been treated with surgery adhered to a fairly intensive follow-up procedure, including 3 haemoccult tests, a clinical examination, and sigmoidoscopy every 3 months (Crowson, Jewkes, Acheson, & Fielding, 1991). Only 22% of breast cancer patients studied by Tomlin and Donegan (1987) completed all recommended follow-up visits for 5 years or more. However, 100% of a medically indigent population with breast cancer completed 5 years of follow-up after treatment (Smith et al., 1995). Finally, 80% of patients diagnosed with colon cancer returned for at least one follow-up colonoscopy after treatment, although this percentage later dropped, then rose over the 7-year period of the investigation (Eckardt, Fuchs, Kanzler, Remmele, & Stienen, 1988).

In summary, rates of adherence to IV chemotherapy, oral chemotherapy and supportive medications, treatment appointments, behavioral changes, and follow-up visits vary widely. In many cases, nonadherence rates are quite low. However, for some behaviors, such as adherence to oral medication or follow-up visits, there can be nonadherence rates comparable to those found in the general medical population. Nonadherence may therefore be as significant a problem among cancer patients as it is among patients with other chronic illness or general medical conditions, where nonadherence rates have ranged from 15–93% (Kaplan & Simon, 1990). This challenges the widely held notion that people will always be adherent to treatment for life-threatening illness. It also affirms the necessity of investigating sources of nonadherence and potential interventions to improve adherence.

PREDICTORS OF ADHERENCE

One of the primary explanations advanced for nonadherence to cancer treatments has been their toxic side effects (Hoagland, Morrow, Bennett, & Carnrike, 1983; Y. N. Lee, 1983). Lee, for example, found that 65% of the breast cancer patients who did not receive at least 85% of their planned treatment did so due to treatment toxicity; however, the remaining 35% did not adhere due to non-drug related reasons such as family problems, out-of-town trips, depression, or other medical procedures unrelated to breast cancer. Other investigations have also documented that one of the major reasons patients are removed from specific treatments is toxicity (Glass et al., 1981).

However, removal from treatment is not nonadherence. In published reports, it is often not possible to determine whether a treatment was discontinued because a patient requested it due to subjective toxicity (nonadherence), because of objective toxicity such as bone marrow suppression (treatment discontinuation), or due to other life- or health-threatening reasons. There is wide variability in the proportion of patients reported to have discontinued treatment due to side effects. For example, Glass et al. (1981) stated that, of the 1% of patients who refused to complete their treatment, there was no indication that the reason was toxicity. However, Feld et al.

(1994) reported that chemotherapy-induced nausea was the major reason for poor compliance (<60%) in their trial and stated that the side effects were particularly poorly tolerated by patients who were aware they had no evidence of disease after tumor resection. Similarly, Jehn (1994) stated that the 14% of patients who refused a second round of treatment intended for maintenance or consolidation of treatment did so because they did not feel the additional treatment was necessary after having reached a complete response from the initial treatment. Patients who refused further treatment did not differ from those who continued with treatment on any pretreatment characteristics, including age, comorbidity, or factors predictive of likely poor long-term outcome.

Richardson, Marks and Levine (1988) investigated the relationship of the nature, frequency, intensity, and difficulty of side effects to adherence to oral chemotherapy and appointments for IV chemotherapy. The experience and frequency of side effects such as hair loss, nausea, loss of appetite, and pain, were not associated with any aspect of adherence. However, for those who did report particular side effects, both difficulty dealing with the side effect and the extent to which the side effect interfered with normal daily activities were negatively associated with adherence to clinic appointments. None of the side-effect variables were related to self-report or biochemical detection of oral chemotherapy medications. It was proposed that patients associated the IV chemotherapy they received at their clinic appointments with the side effects they found most difficult. Thus, side effects appeared to have a specific effect on compliance with the treatment apparently causing them, but not a more general effect on overall compliance. The authors suggest that better management of side effects and education about how to continue with normal activities despite side effects may improve adherence. Others have made similar suggestions (Fallowfield, 1992; Love, Leventhal, Easterling, & Nerenz, 1989).

Several treatment variables have been associated with adherence. Treatment length was related to poorer adherence, with fewer patients continuing with longer treatments (Berger et al., 1988; Rivkin et al., 1993; Schumacher et al., 1994). The anticipation of longer treatment may be enough, in some cases, to decrease adherence. Rivkin et al. (1993) found that patients assigned to a 2-year treatment were less likely to complete even 6 months of treatment than were those assigned to a 1-year treatment arm. More complex treatment regimens are also associated with poorer adherence (Richardson et al., 1987). Additionally, type of treatment received may be related to adherence to follow-up visits (Young et al., 1991). Patients with testicular cancer who were treated with surgery only attended fewer of their scheduled follow-ups than patients who received both surgery and chemotherapy.

The relationship of demographic variables to adherence has also been explored. Younger age has been related to lower likelihood of treatment refusal after a new cancer diagnosis (Huchcroft & Snodgrass, 1993), greater likelihood of smoking cessation after treatment for head and neck cancer (Gritz et al., 1993), greater tendency to practice breast self-examinations after breast cancer (Taylor et al., 1984) and better appointment attendance (Berger et al., 1988). However, others have found no age differences in likelihood of treatment refusal (Moul et al., 1990) or treatment completion (Berger et al., 1988; Jehn, 1994).

Socioeconomic status also has an indeterminate relationship with adherence. Some investigations suggest that lower-income patients are less adherent (Lebovits et al., 1990), while others document excellent adherence in samples gleaned from hospitals serving the medically indigent (Berger et al., 1988). Gender is typically not associated with adherence (Levine et al., 1987), although men were more likely to have refused treatment in one study (Huchcroft & Snodgrass, 1993). Other demographic variables, such as marital status, ethnicity, country of birth, and primary language, to the extent they have been studied, appear to be unrelated to cancer treatment adherence (Berger et al., 1988; Lebovits et al., 1990).

Disease-specific variables are also inconsistently related to treatment adherence. Disease severity (Levine et al., 1987) and comorbidity (Jehn, 1994) were unrelated to adherence to treatment. However, patients with a poorer prognosis were found to be more likely to refuse or discontinue treatment (Huchcroft & Snodgrass, 1993; Rivkin et al., 1993).

Sophisticated models of adherence predictors have been developed and tested in other populations with chronic diseases (DiMatteo, Sherbourne, et al., 1993; Janz & Becker, 1984; de Weerdt, Visser, Kok, & van der Veen, 1990). However, very few variables that have been shown to be important in other samples have been investigated with cancer patients, and the level of generalizability is unknown. In apparently the only adherence work in oncology with a theoretical basis, DiMatteo, Hays, et al. (1993) developed a scale to measure variables potentially related to adherence, the Adherence Determinants Questionnaire (ADQ), using several populations of cancer patients and healthy persons at some risk for cancer. Variables associated with patients' intentions to adhere to treatment included the perceived utility of recommendations and perceived susceptibility to cancer. The presence of supports and absence of barriers to adherence were the most consistent predictors of adherence. Previous levels of general medical adherence and intentions to adhere were also important predictors.

ADHERENCE AMONG CHILDREN AND ADOLESCENTS WITH CANCER

The adherence of children and adolescents with cancer deserves separate attention for several reasons. First, nonadherence rates in this population have been strikingly high. One of the earliest investigations utilizing an objective measure of adherence was conducted with children and adolescents taking oral chemotherapy (Smith et al., 1979). Nonadherence was 33% over all ages and 59% among adolescents. Subsequent research has confirmed that adherence is a significant problem for this population, with other estimates for medication nonadherence ranging from 19% to 52% (Dolgin et al., 1986; Festa, Tamaroff, Chasalow, & Lanzkowsky, 1992; Manne, Jacobsen, Gorfinkle, Gerstein & Redd, 1993; Tebbi et al., 1986). However, the rate of nonadherence to appointment-keeping appears to be significantly lower (1–10%; Manne et al., 1993).

A second reason for examining adherence in the younger age group separately is that, with significant improvements in treatment, cancer therapy for children is often given with curative, rather than palliative, intent (Festa et al., 1992; Tebbi & Koren, 1983). Thus, adherence appears to take on a heightened significance. Third, it has been proposed that adherence among young people must be considered within the context of their psychosocial development (Kellerman & Katz, 1977). Hence, attention has been focused on psychological and developmental explanations for nonadherence among children.

In general, demographic and disease-related variables, other than age, are not predictive of adherence among young people. Thus, gender and ethnicity (Manne et al., 1993; Tamaroff, Festa, Adesman, & Walco, 1992) have not been found to affect adherence. The presence of more siblings was related to poorer adherence in one study (Tebbi et al., 1986). Higher SES was linked to better adherence to appointments in another study (Manne et al., 1993), but not to treatment adherence in that study or in others (Tebbi et al., 1986). Treatment complications, side effects, disease stage or severity, complexity of medical regimen, and cancer type have not been shown to significantly affect adherence (Manne et al., 1993; Tamaroff et al., 1992; Tebbi et al., 1986). The presence of side effects and of visible physical consequences of treatment were related to physicians' estimates of treatment adherence among their adolescent patients; patients' beliefs were not studied (Dolgin et al., 1986).

Several studies have investigated the effects of parenting style and parent-child relationships on adherence to cancer treatments. Tebbi et al. (1986; Tebbi, Richards, Cummings, Zevon, & Mallon, 1988) found that better agreement between parent and child on issues such as who is responsible for medication administration, how to take medication, and effectiveness of medication was linked to better adherence. This study also documented high levels of disagreement, even for variables such as number and severity of side effects, suggesting that the lack of parent-child communication often found with adolescents (e.g., Fogelman, 1976) extends to healthcare issues also. A parenting style characterized by less sensitivity to the child, a more restrictive attitude, and less nurturance has been associated with more problems with appointment-keeping and symptom-reporting behaviors (Manne et al., 1993), but only among children with better physical functioning. Better parental supervision was unrelated to adherence in another investigation (Festa et al., 1992).

Some psychological and cognitive variables appear to be related to adherence. Adolescent and young adult patients found to be more adherent to oral medication also had a better understanding of the causality and prognosis of their illness, were less likely to use denial to cope with illness, and were less likely to be reassured by the absence of symptoms as an indicator of good health (Festa et al., 1992). In a study of 23 adolescents receiving follow-up care after remission from cancer, better cooperation with follow-up, as rated by nurses, was associated with a more positive self-image, an external locus of control focused on Powerful Others, and a belief that cancer is a powerful disease (Jamison, Lewis, & Burish, 1986). Fear of recurrence was not associated with better cooperation.

Psychological variables may also play a role in outright treatment refusal among adolescents (Blotcky, Cohen, Conatser, & Klopovich, 1985). Ten adolescents who refused cancer treatment for approximately 6 months were compared with 10 who consented to treatment. After matching on demographic and disease variables, refusers were found to have lower state anxiety and subjective distress, but higher trait anxiety, religiosity, and an external locus of control. The authors interpret the results of this study as suggesting that perhaps the refusers' external locus of control and high religiosity lead them to feel their medical situation was outside the realm of anybody's control, thus justifying their refusal. This is in contrast to the results of the study discussed above (Jamison et al., 1986), in which patients with an external locus of control focused on a Powerful Other were more adherent; a higher score on that subscale suggests a belief that putting things into the hands of a powerful other (e.g., a doctor) will be beneficial.

Finally, this study also interviewed 9 of the 10 refusers to determine their reasons for refusing treatment. In order of importance, the reasons were fear of how they would look, fear of friends' reactions, side effects of treatment, and painful medical procedures. All 9 refusers also believed that their disease was not changing or was getting better during their treatment refusal, and that their chances of a cure were good or excellent. Reasons for this high level of possible denial were not given.

Overall, it appears that the high rates of nonadherence among children and adolescents may be explained by a combination of variables. A realistic attitude toward the disease and treatment, good parent-child communication, and a good understanding of medication use and potential effectiveness appear to increase adherence. The findings of these studies suggest that better adherence might be promoted through facilitation of communication between parents and children regarding the disease and its treatment. Future research should continue to explore the role that complex developmental factors and family patterns play in treatment adherence in younger patients.

INTERVENTIONS TO IMPROVE ADHERENCE AMONG CANCER PATIENTS

Very few interventions to improve adherence have been conducted in this population and equivocal results have been found in the few studies reported to date. Perhaps this is the result of inadequate knowledge of the predictors of adherence, as discussed above, making it difficult to determine an appropriate focus for an intervention. Nonetheless, because nonadherence rates are relatively high and the costs of nonadherence potentially so great, interventions to improve adherence are particularly important. Therefore, the three investigations that have been conducted to date will be described in some detail below.

The relative effectiveness of three intervention packages for improving adherence to oral medications and clinic appointments for patients with hematologic malignancies was evaluated by Richardson and colleagues (Levine et al., 1987; Richardson et al., 1987). The interventions contained various combinations of three components: education about the disease and its treatment, shaping procedures for pill-taking, and a home visit by a nurse. Patients received either education and a home visit, education and shaping, or all three components. All three intervention packages significantly improved adherence to allopurinol, the oral supportive medication taken in conjunction with IV chemotherapy, and clinic appointments relative to a control group. The three interventions did not differ from each other. Adherence to prednisone, taken for a 5-day period once a month, did not differ between the control and any of the three intervention groups. Because the effectiveness of the three intervention groups did not differ, it was not possible to determine which component or components were responsible for improving adherence.

The impact of an interactive educational intervention on adherence to prescribed pain medication was evaluated in 230 cancer patients (Rimer et al., 1987). The intervention was designed to educate patients about the pain control regimen, to explain the rationale for compliance, to counter concerns about medication tolerance and addiction, and to assist the patient in implementing the regimen. Patients who received the intervention were more likely to take their medicine correctly, and were less likely to stop taking their medication when they felt better. Intervention patients were not less likely to forget to take their medication. The intervention was successful in countering patients' concerns about addiction and tolerance.

Gritz et al. (1991, 1993) evaluated the effectiveness of a smoking-cessation intervention for newly diagnosed head and neck cancer patients who had smoked cigarettes within the past year. The intervention, composed of educational materials, self-help guides, and social support materials for family members, was delivered by patients' usual oncology providers early in their treatment and was followed by six monthly booster sessions during their follow-up visits. The control group received standardized "usual care" advice about the risks of smoking and advice on quitting. Rates of smoking cessation were quite high and did not differ significantly between the intervention and control groups. The authors attribute this to greater readiness to change smoking behavior among control subjects, as measured at baseline.

Finally, traditional cognitive-behavioral interventions designed to reduce side effects have also been considered to be important in improving adherence (e.g., Fallowfield, 1992). Thus, relaxation training and systematic desensitization, which can help to decrease nausea/vomiting, are predicted to increase adherence. However, this has apparently not been tested empirically.

CONCLUSIONS AND FUTURE RESEARCH DIRECTIONS

Contrary to early medical opinion, a significant body of literature documents that nonadherence to cancer treatment and associated recommendations is a serious problem. Although some studies report extremely low nonadherence rates, the average among cancer patients appears to be approximately 25%–35%. That one-fourth to one-third of cancer patients do not adhere to some portion of their treatment may have significant effects on individual treatment outcome and the evaluation of treatment outcomes across groups of patients, such as in clinical trials. Further refinement of the measurement of adherence will contribute to a better understanding of the extent of the problem.

Future research should also be directed toward understanding the multiple factors that may predict adherence in this population of patients who are facing a life-threatening illness. The limited research conducted to date suggests that demographic and disease-related variables are poor predictors of adherence. Investigation of the relationship of adherence to psychosocial variables, such as coping styles and social support, physician characteristics, and physician-patient communications, might be profitable. Another potentially fruitful area of investigation is further specification of the relationship between treatment, side effects, interference with daily functioning, and adherence (e.g., the degree to which treatment affects quality of life might be explored as a predictor of adherence). Finally, it will be necessary for future research to evaluate multivariate models of the relationship between a number of predictive variables and adherence, as it appears that a full understanding of adherence to cancer therapy will require concurrent attention to multiple contributing factors.

REFERENCES

Barofsky, I. (1984). Therapeutic compliance and the cancer patient. *Health Education Quarterly, 10*, 43–56.

Berger, D., Braverman, A., Sohn, C.K., & Morrow, M. (1988). Patient compliance with aggressive multimodal therapy for locally advanced breast cancer. *Cancer, 61*, 1453–1456.

Blay, J. Y., Bouhour, D., Carrie, C., Bouffet, E., Brunat-Mentigny, M., Philip, T., & Biron, P. (1995). The C5R protocol: A regimen of high-dose chemotherapy and radiotherapy in primary cerebral Non-Hodgkin's lymphoma of patients with no known cause of immunosuppression. *Blood, 86*, 2922–2929.

Blotcky, A. D., Cohen, D. G., Conatser, C., & Klopovich, P. (1985). Psychosocial characteristics of adolescents who refuse cancer treatment. *Journal of Consulting and Clinical Psychology, 53*, 729–731.

Bonadonna, G., & Valagussa, P. (1981). Dose-response effect of adjuvant chemotherapy in breast cancer. *New England Journal of Medicine, 304*, 10–15.

Boyar, A. P., Rose, D. P., Loughridge, J. R., Engle, A., Palgi, A., Laakso, K., Kinne, D., & Wynder, E. L. (1988). Response to a diet low in total fat in women with postmenopausal breast cancer: A pilot study. *Nutrition and Cancer, 11*, 93–99.

Brown, E. R., Nichols, C. R., Turns, M., Williams, S. D., Loehrer, P. J., Roth, B. J., Lazarus, H. M., & Einhorn, L. H. (1994). Early salvage therapy for germ cell cancer using high dose chemotherapy with autologous bone marrow support. *Cancer, 73*, 1716–1720.

Buccheri, G., & Ferrigno, D. (1994). A randomised trial of MACC chemotherapy with or without lonidamine in advanced non-small cell lung cancer. *European Journal of Cancer, 30A*, 1424–1431.

Cannell, C. F., Oksenberg, L., & Converse, J. M. (Eds.). (1977). *Experiments in interviewing techniques: Field experiments in health reporting, 1971–1977*. Ann Arbor, MI: Survey Research Center, Institute for Social Research.

Carey, R. W., Sohier, W. D., Kaufman, S., Weitzman, S. A., Kelley, R. M., Lew, R. A., & Halpern, E. (1979). 5-drug adjuvant chemotherapy for breast cancer. *Cancer, 44*, 35–41.

Caron, H. S., & Roth, H. P. (1968). Patients' cooperation with a medical regimen. *Journal of the American Medical Association, 203*, 922–926.

Caron, H. S., & Roth, H. P. (1971). Objective assessment of cooperation with an ulcer diet: Relation to antacid intake and to assigned physician. *American Journal of Medical Science, 261*, 61–66.

Chevallier, B., Bastit, P., Graic, Y., Menard, J. F., Dauce, J. P., Julien, J. P., Clavier, B., Kunlin, A., & D'Anjou, J. (1993). The Centre H. Becquerel studies in inflammatory non metastatic breast cancer. Combined modality approach in 178 patients. *British Journal of Cancer, 67*, 594–601.

Crowson, M. C., Jewkes, A. J., Acheson, N., & Fielding, J. (1991). Haemoccult testing as an indicator of recurrent colorectal cancer: A 5-year prospective study. *European Journal of Surgical Oncology, 17*, 281–284.

Davis, M. S. (1966). Variations in patients' compliance with doctors' orders: Analysis of congruence between survey responses and results of empirical investigations. *Journal of Medical Education, 41*, 1037–1048.

de Weerdt, I., Visser, A. P., Kok, G., & van der Veen, E. A. (1990). Determinants of active self-care behaviour of insulin-treated patients with diabetes: Implications for diabetes education. *Social Science and Medicine, 30*, 605–615.

DiMatteo, M. R., Hays, R. D., Gritz, E. R., Bastani, R., Crane, L., Elashoff, R., Ganz, P., Heber, D., McCarthy, W., & Marcus, A. (1993). Patient adherence to cancer control regimens: Scale development and initial validation. *Psychological Assessment, 5*, 102–112.

DiMatteo, M. R., Hays, R. D., & Sherbourne, C. D. (1992). Adherence to cancer regimens: Implications for treating the older patient. *Oncology, 6(2 Suppl)*, 50–57.

DiMatteo, M. R., Sherbourne, C. D., Hays, R. D., Ordway, L., Kravitz, R. L., McGlynn, E. A., Kaplan, S., & Rogers, W. H. (1993). Physicians' characteristics influence patients' adherence to medical treatment: Results from the Medical Outcomes Study. *Health Psychology, 12*, 93–102.

Dolgin, M. J., Katz, E. R., Doctors, S. R., & Siegel, S. E. (1986). Caregivers' perceptions of medical compliance in adolescents with cancer. *Journal of Adolescent Health Care, 7*, 22–27.

Eckardt, V. F., Fuchs, M., Kanzler, G., Remmele, W., & Stienen, U. (1988). Follow-up of patients with colonic polyps containing severe atypia and invasive carcinoma. *Cancer, 61*, 2552–2557.

Fallowfield, L. J. (1992). Behavioural interventions and psychological aspects of care during chemotherapy. *European Journal of Cancer, 28A (Suppl 1)*, S39–S41.

Feld, R., Rubinstein, L., & Thomas, P. A. (1994). Adjuvant chemotherapy with cyclophosphamide, doxorubicin, and cisplatin in patients with completely resected Stage I non-small cell lung cancer. *Chest, 106(6 Sup,)*, 307S–309S.

Feld, R., Rubinstein, L., Thomas, P.A., and the Lung Cancer Study Group. (1993). Adjuvant chemotherapy with cyclophosphamide, doxorubicin, and cisplatin in patients with completely resected Stage I non-small-cell lung cancer. *Journal of the National Cancer Institute, 85*, 299–306.

Festa, R. S., Tamaroff, M. H., Chasalow, F., & Lanzkowsky, P. (1992). Therapeutic adherence to oral medication regimens by adolescents with cancer: I. Laboratory assessments. *Journal of Pediatrics, 120*, 807–811.

Fisher, B., Brown, A., Wolmark, N., Fisher, E. R., Redmond, C., Wickerham, L., Margolese, R., Dimitrov, N., Pilch, Y., Glass, A., Sutherland, C., & Foster, R. (1990). Evaluation of the worth of corynebacterium parvum in conjunction with chemotherapy as adjuvant treatment for primary breast cancer. *Cancer, 66*, 220–227.

Fogelman, K. (1976). *Britain's sixteen-year-olds*. London: National Children's Bureau.

Friedman, M. A., & Cain, D. F. (1990). National Cancer Institute sponsored cooperative clinical trials. *Cancer, 65*, 2376–2382.

Garrett, T. J., Ashford, A., & Savage, D. G. (1986). Oncology clinic attendance at an inner city hospital. *Cancer, 58*, 793–795.

Glass, A., Wieand, H. S., Fisher, V., Redmond, C., Lerner, H., Wolter, J., Shibata, H., Plotkin, D., Foster, R., Margolese, R., Wolmark, N., and Other NSABP Investigators. (1981). Acute toxicity during adjuvant chemotherapy for breast cancer: The National Surgical Adjuvant Breast and Bowel Project (NSABP) experience from 1717 patients receiving single and multiple agents. *Cancer Treatment Reports, 65*, 363–376.

Goodwin, P. J., & Boyd, N. F. (1987). Critical appraisal of the evidence that dietary fat intake is related to breast cancer risk in humans. *Journal of the National Cancer Institute, 79*, 473–485.

Gotay, C. C. (1991). Accrual to cancer clinical trials: Directions from the research literature. *Social Science Medicine, 33*, 569–577.

Gritz, E. R., Carr, C. R., Rapkin, D., Abemayor, E., Chang, L. J. C., Won, W. K., Belin, T. R., Calcaterra, T., Robbins, K. T., Chonkich, G., Beumer, J., & Ward, P. H. (1993). Predictors of long-term smoking cessation in head and neck cancer patients. *Cancer Epidemiology, Biomarkers & Prevention, 2*, 261–270.

Gritz, E. R., Carr, C. R., Rapkin, D. A., Chang, C., Beumer, J., & Ward, P. H. (1991). A smoking cessation intervention for head and neck cancer patients: Trial design, patient accrual, and characteristics. *Cancer Epidemiology, Biomarkers, & Prevention, 1*, 67–73.

Hays, R. D., & DiMatteo, M. R. (1987). Key issues and suggestions for patient compliance assessment: Sources of information, focus of measures, and nature of response options. *The Journal of Compliance In Health Care, 2*, 37–53.

Hoagland, C., Morrow, G. R., Bennett, J. M., Carnrike, C. L., Jr. (1983). Oncologists' views of cancer patient noncompliance. *American Journal of Clinical Oncology, 6*, 239–244.

Holm, L. E., Nordevang, E., Ikkala, E., Hallstrom, L., & Callmer, E. (1990). Dietary intervention as adjuvant therapy in breast cancer patients: A feasibility study. *Breast Cancer Research and Treatment, 16*, 103–109.

Huchcroft, S. A., & Snodgrass, T. (1993). Cancer patients who refuse treatment. *Cancer Causes and Control, 4*, 179–185.

Jacob, J. R., Casiano, R. R., Schuller, D. E., Pajak, T. F., Laramore, G. E., & Al-Sarraf, M. (1994). Chemotherapy as a predictor of compliance. *Journal of Surgical Oncology, 55*, 143–148.

Jamison, R. N., Lewis, S., & Burish, T. G. (1986). Cooperation with treatment in adolescent cancer patients. *Journal of Adolescent Health Care, 7*, 162–167.

Janz, N. K., & Becker, M. H. (1984). The health belief model: A decade later. *Health Education Quarterly, 11*, 1–47.

Jehn, U. (1994). Long-term outcome of postremission chemotherapy for adults with acute myeloid leukemia using different dose-intensities. *Leukemia and Lymphoma, 15*, 99–112.

Josefson, D., Ous, S., Hoie, J., Stenwig, A. E., & Fossa, S. D. (1993). Salvage treatment in male patients with germ cell tumours. *British Journal of Cancer, 67*, 568–572.

Kaplan, R. M., & Simon, H. J. (1990). Compliance in medical care: Reconsideration of self-predictions. *Annals of Behavioral Medicine, 12*, 66–71.

Kellerman, J., & Katz, E. R. (1977). Adolescents with cancer: Theoretical, clinical and research issues. *Journal of Pediatric Psychology, 2*, 127–131.

Kravitz, R. L., Hays, R. D., Sherbourne, C. D., DiMatteo, M. R., Rogers, W. H., Ordway, L., & Greenfield, S. (1993). Recall of recommendations and adherence to advice among patients with chronic medical conditions. *Archives of Internal Medicine, 153*, 1869–1878.

Lebovits, A. H., Strain, J. J., Schleifer, S. J., Tanaka, J. S., Bhardwaj, S., & Messe, M. R. (1990). Patient noncompliance with self-administered chemotherapy. *Cancer, 65*, 17–22.

Lee, C. R., Nicholson, P. W., Souhami, R. L., & Deshmukh, A. A. (1992). Patient compliance with oral chemotherapy as assessed by a novel electronic technique. *Journal of Clinical Oncology, 10*, 1007–1013.

Lee, Y. N. (1983). Adjuvant chemotherapy (CMF) for breast carcinoma. *American Journal of Clinical Oncology, 6*, 25–30.

Levine, A. M., Richardson, J. L., Marks, G., Chan, K., Graham, J., Selser, J. N., Kishbaugh, C., Shelton, D. R., & Johnson, C. A. (1987). Compliance with oral drug therapy in patients with hematologic malignancy. *Journal of Clinical Oncology, 5*, 1469–1476.

Lewis, C., Linet, M. S., & Abeloff, M. D. (1983). Compliance with cancer therapy by patients and physicians. *American Journal of Medicine, 74*, 673–678.

Liberati, A., & the GIVIO Investigators. (1995). The GIVIO trial on the impact of follow-up care on survival and quality of life in breast cancer patients. *Annals of Oncology, 6(Suppl 2)*, S41–S46.

Love, R., Leventhal, H., Easterling, D., & Nerenz, D. R.(1989). Side-effects and emotional distress during cancer chemotherapy. *Cancer, 63*, 604–612.

Makela, J., Tikkakoski, T., Leinonen, A., Siniluoto, T., Karttunen, A., & Kairaluoma, M. I. (1993). Superselective intra-arterial chemotherapy with Mitomycin C in hepatic neoplasms. *European Journal of Surgical Oncology, 19*, 348–354.

Manne, S. L., Jacobsen, P. B., Gorfinkle, K., Gerstein, F., & Redd, W. H. (1993). Treatment adherence difficulties among children with cancer: The role of parenting style. *Journal of Pediatric Psychology, 18*, 47–62.

Moertel, C. G., Fleming, T. R., MacDonald, J. S., Haller, D. G., Laurie, J. A., Goodman, P. J., Ungerleider, J. S., Emerson, W. A., Tormey D. C., Glick, J. H., Veeder, M. H., & Mailliard, J. A. (1990). Levamisole and fluorouracil for adjuvant therapy of resected colon carcinoma. *New England Journal of Medicine, 322*, 352–358.

Moul, J. W., Paulson, D. F., & Walther, P. J. (1990). Refusal of cancer therapy in testicular cancer: Recognizing and preventing a significant problem. *World Journal of Urology, 8*, 58–62.

Ormiston, M. C., Timoney, A. G., & Qureshi, A. R. (1985). Is follow up of patients after surgery for breast cancer worthwhile? *Journal of the Royal Society of Medicine, 78*, 920–921.

Richardson, J. L., Marks, G., Johnson, C. A., Graham, J. W., Chan, K. K., Selser, J. N., Kishbaugh, C., Barranday, Y., & Levine, A. M. (1987). Path model of multidimensional compliance with cancer therapy. *Health Psychology, 6*, 183–207.

Richardson, J. L., Marks, G., & Levine, A. (1988). The influence of symptoms of disease and side effects of treatment on compliance with cancer therapy. *Journal of Clinical Oncology, 6*, 1746–1752.

Rimer, B., Levy, M. H.., Keintz, M. K., Fox, L., Engstrom, P. F., & MacElwee, N. (1987). Enhancing cancer pain control regimens through patient education. *Patient Education and Counseling, 10*, 267–277.

Rivkin, S. E., Green, S., Metch, B., Jewell, W. R., Costanzi, J. J., Altman, S. J., Minton, J. P., O'Bryan, R. M., & Osborne, C. K. (1993). One versus 2 years of CMFVP adjuvant chemotherapy in axillary node-positive and estrogen receptor-negative patients: A Southwest Oncology Group Study. *Journal of Clinical Oncology, 11*, 1710–1716.

Ryder, S. D., Rizzi, P. M., Metivier, E., Karani, J., & Williams, R. (1996). Chemoembolisation with lipiodol and doxorubicin: Applicability in British patients with hepatocellular carcinoma. *Gut, 38*, 125–128.

Schumacher, M., Bastert, G., Bojar, H., Hubner, K., Olschewski, M., Sauerbrei, W., Schmoor, C., Beyerle, C., Neumann, R. L. A., & Rauschecker, H. F. for the German Breast Cancer Study Group. (1994). Randomized 2 × 2 trial evaluating hormonal treatment and the duration of chemotherapy in node-positive breast cancer patients. *Journal of Clinical Oncology, 12*, 2086–2093.

Smith, R. G., Landry, J. C., Hughes, L. L., Moore, M. R., Lynn, M. J., Davis, L. W., Styblo, T., Crocker, I. R., & Wood, W. D. (1995). Conservative treatment of early-stage breast cancer in a medically indigent population. *Journal of the National Medical Association, 87*, 500–504.

Smith, S. D., Rosen, D., Trueworthy, R. C., & Lowman, J. T. (1979). A reliable method for evaluating drug compliance in children with cancer. *Cancer, 43*, 169–173.

Tamaroff, M. H., Festa, R. S., Adesman, A. R., & Walco, G. A. (1992). Therapeutic adherence to oral medication regimens by adolescents with cancer. II. Clinical and psychologic correlates. *Journal of Pediatrics, 120*, 812–817.

Taylor, S. E., Lichtman, R. R., & Wood, J. V. (1984). Compliance with chemotherapy among breast cancer patients. *Health Psychology, 3*, 553–562.

Taylor, S. E., Lichtman, R. R., Wood, J. V., Bluming, A. Z., Dosik, G. M., & Leibowitz, R. L. (1984). Breast self-examinations among diagnosed breast cancer patients. *Cancer, 54*, 2528–2532.

Tebbi, C. K. (1993). Treatment compliance in childhood and adolescence. *Cancer, 71*, 3441–3449.

Tebbi, C. K., Cummings, K. M., Zevon, J. M. A., Smith, L., Richards, M., & Mallon, J. (1986). Compliance of pediatric and adolescent cancer patients. *Cancer, 58*, 1179–1184.

Tebbi, C. K., & Koren, B. G. (1983). A specialized unit for adolescent oncology patients: Is it worth it? *Journal of Medicine, 14*, 161–184.

Tebbi, C. K., Richards, M. E., Cummings, K. M., Zevon, M. A., & Mallon, J. C. (1988). The role of parent-adolescent concordance in compliance with cancer chemotherapy. *Adolescence, 13*, 599–611.

Tomiak, E., & Piccart, M. (1993). Routine follow-up of patients after primary therapy for early breast cancer: Changing concepts and challenges for the future. *Annals of Oncology, 4*, 199–204.

Tomlin, R., & Donegan, W. L. (1987). Screening for recurrent breast cancer: Its effectiveness and prognostic value. *Journal of Clinical Oncology, 5*, 62–67.

Verdonck, L. F., Dekker, A. W., de Gast, G. C., van Kempen, M. L., Lokhorst, H. M., & Nieuwenhuis, H. K. (1992). Salvage therapy with ProMACE-MOPP followed by intensive chemoradiotherapy and autologous bone marrow transplantation for patients with Non-Hodgkin's lymphoma who failed to respond to first-line CHOP. *Journal of Clinical Oncology, 10*, 1949–1954.

Winchester, D. P., Sener, S. F., Khandekar, J. D., Oviedo, M. A., Cunningham, M. P., Caprini, J. A., Burkett, F. E., & Scanlon, E. F. (1979). Symptomatology as an indicator of recurrent or metastatic breast cancer. *Cancer, 43*, 956–960.

Young, B. J., Bultz, B. D., Russell, J. A., & Trew, M. S. (1991). Compliance with follow-up of patients treated for non-seminomatous testicular cancer. *British Journal of Cancer, 64*, 606.

Zanetta, G., Landoni, F., Colombo, A., Pellegrino, A., Maneo, A., & Leventis, C. (1993). Three-year results after neoadjuvant chemotherapy, radical surgery, and radiotherapy in locally advanced cervical carcinoma. *Obstetrics and Gynecology, 82*, 447–450.

SECTION VI
Adherence Issues in Clinical Trials

Eleanor B. Schron, Editor

The adherence of study participants is a critical component in the conduct of clinical trials. Indeed, the integrity of the results of a trial can be undermined if participants are not able to follow through with protocol requirements. If the effect of a treatment is to be evaluated, such as the efficacy of a drug, the drug has to be taken. Well-designed and well-managed trials do not automatically guarantee optimal adherence from participants. Attention to adherence throughout all phases of a clinical trial, as well as within the context of the clinical practice setting, is important.

The following chapters address different aspects of adherence unique to the conduct of clinical trials as well as the clinical practice setting. Because of the importance of adherence to the outcome of a trial, it is very tempting to consider enrolling into a study only those individuals who will most likely be adherent. This raises a question about whether such selection is possible and, if it is, whether or not such preselection could have any untoward consequences. In Chapter 20, "Prerandomization Compliance Screening: A Statistician's View," Davis shows how the statistical power of a trial can be increased by excluding those who will not follow a treatment regimen. He then examines the tradeoff between increased study power and loss of generalizability of study results.

Addressing the question of whether or not early detection of poor adherence is possible, Dunbar and colleagues review the literature on adherence for evidence relating personal behaviors and characteristics such as psychological, motivational, and somatic factors to adherence outcomes. In Chapter 21, "Predictors of Patient Adherence," they present evidence from a number of studies that suggest that initial adherence to treatment predicts longer-term adherence. The finding that the initial adherence performance of participants was strongly associated with their long-term adherence efforts is worthy of note. It suggests that researchers and clinicians early on should preferentially allocate time and resources for the management of the initial adherence problems that people encounter as they attempt to adopt a new regimen, rather than emphasize remedial effects during the course of treatment.

20

Prerandomization Compliance Screening: A Statistician's View

C. E. Davis

In the conduct of clinical trials, the "intent-to-treat" rule is used as a standard data analysis procedure. The intent-to-treat rule states that the data from a participant entered into a clinical trial should be analyzed with the group to which he or she was assigned, regardless of whether the intended treatment was applied. For example, in a clinical trial of medicine versus surgery in the treatment of severe coronary disease, patients assigned to medical treatment who subsequently have surgery would be treated as through they were only treated by medical means. This rule is used in order to ensure that the comparison of the two (or more) treatment groups is unbiased. If the more severely ill patients among those assigned to medical treatment were to have surgery, counting subsequent deaths among these patients as attributable to surgical treatment would make the medically treated group appear to fare better than it actually did.

The use of the intent-to-treat rule in data analysis leads to another similar issue related to patient adherence to the behavior regimen assigned within a particular treatment. For example, if participants assigned to a diet or drug therapy do not adhere to the regimen, their data will be analyzed as though they had followed the prescription. This concept has led to the proposal that prospective participants in a clinical trial should be excluded if they are unable or unwilling to follow the procedures that will be used in the trial. Such issues as reporting to the clinic as requested or keeping a dietary record may be used as possible tests to see if the potential participant is likely to cooperate during the trial. An additional possibility is to ask the participant to take medication, usually placebo, single-masked, to determine capability to adhere to the required medication schedule. The participant, if unable to follow the prescribed behavioral pattern well, is not entered into the full study. In this brief presentation, I review some of the pros and cons of this latter procedure, and briefly describe the interim results of an NIH-sponsored trial that used the method.

SHOULD A PRERANDOMIZATION ADHERENCE SCREEN BE USED?

The major reason for using a prerandomization adherence screen is to protect the statistical power of the clinical trial. Suppose we are to conduct a clinical trial using a response variable that is normally distributed with means $\mu 1$ (control group) and $\mu 2$ (treated group), and common variance δ^2. If the proportion of participants in the treated group who do not adhere to the assigned regimen is p, it follows that the expected treatment difference is $(1 - p)(\mu 1 - \mu 2)$, rather than $\mu 1 - \mu 2$. With perfect adherence, the sample size for significance level a and power 1-b is

$$2n = \delta 2\ (z_\alpha + z_\beta)^2/(\mu_1 - \mu_2)^2$$

However, with the proportion of participants in the treated group not adhering equal to p, the sample size is:

$$2n = \delta 2(z_\alpha + z\beta)^2/(\mu_1 - \mu_2)^2\ (1 - p)^2$$

Thus the size of the study is increased by a factor of $(1 - p)^{-2}$. The following table gives values for the increase in sample size for a given level of adherence.

Increase in Sample Size for Adherence *p*

p	*k*
.01	1.02
.05	1.11
.10	1.23
.20	1.56
.50	4.00

To use the table, one can compute the sample size, assuming all participants adhere, and then multiply that sample size by k (a constant) to account for poor adherence. For example, if we computed an estimated sample size of 100 for a trial, then assuming that 10% of the participants would not adhere to the treatment implies that we should have a sample of $100 \times 1.23 = 123$ participants; that is, a 10% poor adherence proportion leads to a need for 23% more participants in order to maintain the same statistical power.

In the above sample computation, we assume that poor adherence to placebo will not effect the study. Of course, if participants who are assigned to the placebo group begin to receive the active treatment, the power will be further diminished. Clearly, the cost of poor adherence is great, and thus we should try our best to minimize poor adherence. This has led to the proposal for a prerandomization adherence screen (run-in).

This proposal is based on the assumption that those participants identified as poor adherers in the prerandomization screen will be the same as those who would subsequently be poor adherers in the main study. There is some evidence to support this idea from observational data. In Chapter 21 of this volume, Dunbar et al. presents data from the LRC-CPPT indicating that participants who took their medication regularly during the early portion of the study tended to take their medication regularly throughout the study. While this observation supports the idea that we should be able to predict persons who will be poor adherers, Davis, Applegate, Gordon, Curtis, & McCormick (1995) found that a placebo run-in did not substantially affect the amount of cholesterol change in a study of lipid-lowering in older persons. Trivedi and Rush (1994) also found no appreciable effect of a placebo run-in in a meta analysis of 101 studies of antidepressant drugs. The assumption that a placebo run-in is a cost-effective way to increase adherence should be studied further by replication of these two studies.

The major criticism of the prerandomization adherence screen is that the removal of a subset of potential participants restricts the generalizability of the results. If we ask the question "Does drug A reduce mortality in patients with disease X?", we are asking what will happen if we apply drug A to the entire population of patients with disease X. However, if we remove from consideration those patients who do not follow instructions during the prerandomization phase, we are answering the question "Does drug A reduce mortality in patients with disease X who behave as we request?" This criticism will be valid in some settings and not in others.

For example, if I want to design a trial to answer the question "Will the introduction of a low-fat diet reduce the incidence of coronary disease in the population?" it would not be proper to have a prerandomization adherence screen, since the question is clearly asking what will happen in the entire population. However, if we design a trial to answer the question, "Will a low-fat diet reduce the *risk* of coronary disease?", we may choose to eliminate from the study those persons who do not pass a prerandomization screen, since the question concerns whether the diet has any effect at all on coronary disease. In demonstration and prevention research where the acceptability of an intervention may play a role, we should rarely use prerandomization screening, but in research designed primarily to look at the efficacy of treatment, such a screen may be warranted. Clearly, we should think carefully about these issues before making such a decision.

There are, of course, logistical problems associated with a prerandomization screen, particularly in double-masked studies. If a participant takes a placebo for a few days and then at randomization is given the active treatment, the side effects or symptomatic relief may lead them to conclude that they are on the active treatment and thus threaten the masking. The degree to which this might effect the validity of the study will no doubt be dependent on the type of treatment and its side effects. Nonetheless, the possibility of damaging the study through breaking the blind should be considered before one embarks on a run-in.

Two other potential problems associated with a run-in period should be noted. First, to the extent that nonadherers are misidentified, the gain in statistical power may be reduced. Second, the addition of a run-in period will almost certainly make recruitment more difficult.

PRERANDOMIZATION SCREENING IN SOLVD

The National Heart, Lung, and Blood Institute sponsored a clinical trial in patients with low ejection fractions (reduced emptying of the ventricular chamber associated with normal beating of the heart), the Studies of Left Ventricular Dysfunction (SOLVD). In this study, potential participants with ejection fractions less than or equal to 35 were randomly assigned to an angiotensin-converting enzyme inhibitor (enalapril) or a placebo. The endpoint of interest was total mortality, and follow-up was for a minimum of 2 years (SOLVD, 1990).

In this study there were two types of prerandomization screenings. Since it has been reported that in a small number of persons the first exposure to enalapril may lead to severe hypotension, it was decided to give each potential participant a small test dose of the active drug, so that participants in whom the drug was contraindicated could be excluded. Thus, at the first clinic visit, each patient was put on a 2.5 mg bid (2 times per day) dose of the active drug for a period of from 2 to 7 days. Although the intent of this "test dosing" was to protect the safety of the participants, it was decided to exclude participants who took less than 75% of the prescribed medication during this period. A participant judged to be eligible following this "test dosing" was then prescribed 2 weeks of placebo. Participants who did not take at least 80% of the medication during this 2-week period were excluded from the trial.

TABLE 20.1 Participants Excluded from SOLVD, March, 1987—Preliminary Data

			Excluded			
Visit	Included	Percentage	Poor Adherence	Percentage	Other	Percentage
Test dose	1390	97.0	30	2.1	13	0.1
Placebo dose	1230	96.2	26	2.0	22	1.7

Note. The data in Table 20.1 were presented at a SOLVD Steering Committee meeting in March, 1987.

SOLVD began recruitment in July 1986 and as of the data (March, 1987) presented here, 1342 participants had been entered toward a goal of 7100. Table 20.1 gives a summary of the results of the prerandomization screening to date. Clearly, a small proportion (approximately 4%) of the potential participants are being excluded for lack of adherence. Nevertheless, if we use the rough rule outlined above, correcting for a 4% reduction in adherence, we would need 8.5% more participants to make up for this loss in power. Thus, although the percentage of potential participants excluded is small, the potential gain in the power of the study is not negligible. It is interesting to consider the question of the effect of the prerandomization adherence screen on the generalizability of the study. Table 20.2 compares some of the characteristics of the participants excluded for poor adherence with those of the participants who were not excluded.

In Table 20.2, it is noticeable that characteristics that seem to be associated with poor adherence are older age, female sex, non-White race, more severe disease (as noted by the New York Heart Association (NYHA) classification but not by ejection fraction), and taking vasodilators. This latter characteristic is probably not a surprise, since it seems well-recognized that the more behaviors we ask of a person, the less likely they are to be able to carry out all of them. It appears from these data that SOLVD is slightly changing the characteristics of its sample by requiring adherence to be good during the prerandomization phase. The effects of this on the generalizability of the study are debatable.

SUMMARY

The exclusion of potential participants who will not follow a treatment regimen possibly increases the statistical power of the clinical trial. However,

TABLE 20.2 Characteristics of Participants Excluded in SOLVD Compared to Those Not Excluded, March, 1987—Preliminary Data

	Not Excluded		Excluded Poor Adherence	
Characteristic	E dose[a]	P dose[b]	E dose[a]	P dose[b]
Mean age (yrs.)	59	59	63	61
Percentage male	85	86	73	77
Percentage white	82	83	73	62
Percent NYHA > 2	24	23	50	35
Taking vasodilators (%)	29	27	36	36
Mean EF (%)	25	26	23	25

[a]enalapril; [b]placebo

Note: The data in Table 20.2 were presented at a SOLVD Steering Committee meeting in March, 1987.

this increase in power may be purchased by reducing the generalizability of the results of the study, possibly interfering with the double-masking and possibly making recruitment more difficult. Thus, one should consider the relative merits of these issues in deciding whether or not to have a prerandomization adherence screen in any particular study.

REFERENCES

Davis, C. E., Applegate, W. B., Gordon, D. J., Curtis, R. C., & McCormick, M. (1995). An empirical evaluation of the placebo run-in. *Controlled Clinical Trials, 16*, 41–50.

The SOLVD Investigators. (1990). Studies of left ventricular dysfunction (SOLVD)—rationale, design and methods: Two trials that evaluate the effect of enalapril in patients with reduced ejection fraction. *American Journal of Cardiology, 66*, 315–322.

Trivedi, M. H., & Rush, H. (1994). Does a placebo run-in or a placebo treatment cell affect the efficacy of antidepressant medications? *Neuro–psychopharmacology, 11*, 33–43.

21

Predictors of Patient Adherence: Patient Characteristics

Jacqueline M. Dunbar-Jacob, Elizabeth A. Schlenk, Lora E. Burke, and Judith T. Matthews

With nonadherence rates ranging from 20% to 80% in practice and research settings, considerable healthcare resources are utilized in either remediating nonadherence or in treating the consequences of inadequately treated disease or risk factors. In the clinical research arena, further resources may be expended in the recruitment and management of additional subjects to compensate for the loss of power due to dropouts or poor adherers. Resources might be better utilized at the outset of treatment or subject recruitment if those individuals likely to have difficulty adhering could be identified. And, indeed, investigations have been undertaken directed toward the prediction of adherence.

A number of studies have examined factors under the control of the provider that are likely to lead to nonadherence, such as prescription of multiple and/or complex regimens, lack of consistency in care providers, care provider behavior toward patients, adequacy of instructions, and convenience. Other sets of predictors are those that are more specific to the person than to the regimen, provider, or clinical setting. It is this latter set of factors that is addressed in this review. That is, what characteristics of the

This paper was supported in part by the National Institute of Health, National Institute of Nursing Research (5 P30 NR03924-02).

individual are likely to influence subsequent adherence to a healthcare regimen? A number of areas have been examined, including (a) psychological characteristics, (b) cognitive-motivational factors, (c) behavior itself, and (d) somatic and cognitive factors.

PSYCHOLOGICAL CHARACTERISTICS AS PREDICTORS OF ADHERENCE

Overall, the literature shows little support for personality traits as predictors of patient adherence. On the other hand, certain psychological states may influence adherence, although the data are not clear. For example, depression has been found to be associated with adherence in some studies (Blumenthal, Williams, Wallace, Williams, & Needles, 1982; Heiby, Onorato, & Sato, 1985; Nelson, Stason, Neutra, Solomon, & McArdle, 1978; O'Leary, Rohsenow, & Chaney, 1979) but not in others (Graveley & Oseasohn, 1991; Welsh, Labbé, & Delaney, 1991). Differences may be attributable to the patient populations being studied. However, within exercise both Welsh et al. (1991) and Heiby et al. (1985) studied exercise adherence in healthy populations with opposing results. Similarly, Graveley and Oseasohn (1991) and Nelson et al. (1978) studied medication adherence in persons with chronic disorders and found opposing results. In contrast, feelings of euphoria after training runs have predicted completion of a marathon (Heiby et al., 1985) and optimism has been associated with adherence to medical follow-up recommendations following detection of a suspicious skin lesion (Friedman, Webb, Bruce, Weinberg, & Cooper, 1995).

Anxiety has also been associated with adherence in some, but not all, studies. High anxiety has been associated with poor medication adherence among patients with hypertension (Nelson et al., 1978) and overuse of medications among patients with asthma (Mawhinney et al., 1993) whereas lower anxiety predicted greater exercise behavior among older adults (Emery, Hauck, & Blumenthal, 1992). In contrast, anxiety did not predict adherence to prenatal class attendance among primagravidas (Michie, Marteau, & Kidd, 1990) nor did it predict exercise adherence among healthy women (Welsh et al., 1991). Michie et al. (1990) did find that avoidant coping predicted attendance, suggesting that how individuals cope with anxiety may be the more powerful predictor. Interestingly, avoidant coping also predicted adherence in the Medical Outcomes Study (Sherbourne, Hays, Ordway, DiMatteo, & Kravitz, 1992).

Other psychological state characteristics have been examined as well, although in few studies. For example, ambiguity to antiepileptic medication was higher among nonadherers whereas unpredictability regarding their disease was higher among adherers (DiLorio, Faherty, & Manteuffel, 1991).

The authors speculated that individuals high in ambiguity regarding their disease might be more prone to experiment with their medication, whereas individuals who believed that the disease was unpredictable might be more prone to take regular steps to prevent a seizure.

Hostility has also been examined in the context of adherence. Lee et al. (1992) reported that patients with hypertension who scored higher in hostility, assessed by the Hostility Scale of the Brief Symptom Inventory, reported skipping more doses of medication than those lower in hostility, although they did not report any greater difficulty in remembering to take medication. Asthma patients with greater reports of anger and irritation about their disease were more likely to attend an asthma education program (Yoon, McKenzie, Miles, & Bauman, 1991). Hostility has also been identified as a component of Type A behavior. Type A behavior as well as Type H, "hard-driving," measured by the Jenkins Activity Survey, were also examined in relation to adherence to exercise. Both were related to attendance in an exercise program designed for healthy women (Welsh et al., 1991). Self-motivation has also been considered as a possible patient characteristic which might influence adherence. Indeed, Welsh et al. (1991) reported that self-motivation was not associated with exercise program attendance, but was associated with exercise frequency.

The Medical Outcomes Study reported that emotional distress over one's health also predicted adherence (DiMatteo et al., 1993). In the Lipid Research Clinics Coronary Primary Prevention Trial[1] (CPPT), psychological distress more broadly conceived was found to relate to adherence prospectively. Psychological distress, which included the self-reported presence or history of tranquilizer use, excessive fatigue, difficulty sleeping, moodiness, and irritability, as well as depression, was assessed during prerandomization screening. A multiple regression analysis showed statistical significance ($p < .001$) between tranquilizer use and excessive fatigue and reduced adherence at year 1. Further, these two factors and difficulty sleeping were associated with reduced adherence over 7 years. However, such a small proportion of the variance was accounted for ($r = .012$, $r = .022$ respectively) that one could

[1] The Lipid Research Clinics-Coronary Primary Prevention Trial (LRC-CPPT) was a multicenter, randomized, double-blind, controlled clinical trial testing the cholesterol hypothesis among healthy, hyperlipidemic males aged 35 to 59 at entry. Participants were on a cholesterol-lowering medication or placebo dispensed in packets for at least 7 years. All volunteers completed a medical history and examination during the screening phase of the recruitment effort, prior to randomization into the study. Three months after this assessment was completed, the clinic visits for the 7 to 10 volunteers were randomized to either active medication or placebo and followed bimonthly. Adherence was assessed at each clinic visit by means of an unobtrusive packet count. The predicted behavior was adherence over the first year of the trial and over 7 years of the trial.

conclude that psychological distress did not predict adherence (Dunbar & Knoke, 1986). The pattern of the relationship between psychological distress and adherence, however, was toward lower adherence given the presence of psychological distress during the prerandomization period or ever in the past (see Table 21.1).

The question arises as to why psychological states might predict adherence. A study examining a cognitive-behavioral model of adherence to health-related exercise by Heiby and colleagues (1985) suggests that depression and anxiety may be components of motivation. In a factor analysis, these investigators found that trait anxiety, depression, self-reinforcement, and self-motivation loaded on the same factor such that low trait anxiety and low depression scores were associated with high self-reinforcement and high self-motivation. It may be speculated that the pessimistic and self-deprecating cognitions typically found in depression contribute to lowered self-reinforcement and self-motivation. This would be an interesting avenue for further exploration.

COGNITIVE-MOTIVATIONAL PREDICTORS OF ADHERENCE

Beliefs and other cognitions have also been examined as potential predictors of patient adherence. It is in this area that much of the research on the characteristics of the patient as an influence on adherence has taken place. The principal models include health beliefs, intentions, self-efficacy, and stages of change.

Most commonly cited is the Health Belief Model, a cognitive-motivational model described by Rosenstock (1966) and refined by Becker and others (e.g., Becker, Drachman, & Kirscht, 1974; Janz & Becker, 1984; Rosenstock, 1974). The model essentially states that recommended health actions will be taken if an individual believes:

1. that he himself is susceptible to the illness;
2. the consequences of the illness or of noncompliance are serious;
3. the recommended action is beneficial or efficacious in reducing risk or severity; and
4. the barriers or costs of action do not exceed the benefits.

In addition to these beliefs, general health motivation is, at times, included in the model. General health motivation consists of both positive factors, for example, engagement in healthy behaviors, as well as negative factors, for example, worry or concern over health.

Most investigations of the utility of the Health Belief Model have been concurrent or retrospective studies. Behavior of interest and health beliefs

TABLE 21.1 History of Tranquilizer Use and Medication Adherence at Year 1 and Over 7 Years in the LRC-CPPT: Cumulative Adherence as Measured at Two-Time Intervals in a Study

Tranquilizer Use	Medication Adherence	
	1 Year	7 Years
Never used	81%	66%
Used in past	77%	59%
Used during screening	71%	48%

were assessed at the same time. These studies have shown modest relationships between beliefs and behavior.

Twenty-four prospective studies have been reported in the literature that have undertaken an examination of the influence of health beliefs on subsequent behavior. Two of these studies will not be included in this discussion, due to methodologic limitations. Both investigations evaluated interventions designed to change health beliefs through educational procedures and measured postintervention adherence (Inui, Yourtee, & Williamson, 1976) and contraceptive practices of adolescents (Eisen, Zellman, & McAlister, 1985). The postintervention assessment was carried out on a group of patients largely different from those assessed pretreatment in the Inui et al. study. Further, the inclusion of an intervention targeted to the modification of health beliefs confounded the utility of initial beliefs as predictors of adherence in the absence of a control group in the Eisen et al. study. Thus, 22 prospective prediction studies remain.

The types of behaviors and the period between assessment of health beliefs and subsequent adherence varied among these 22 prospective prediction studies. For example, these studies variously examined healthcare utilization (6), participation in screening programs (6), medication adherence (5), smoking cessation (3), modification of activity (2), stress management (2), dietary adherence (2), acquisition of immunizations (1), self-report of drinking and driving (1), weight loss (1), and breast self-examination practices (1). The period between assessment of health beliefs and subsequent behavior ranged from 1 week (screening attendance) to 8 years (smoking cessation). Susceptibility, severity, benefits, and health motivation were typically assessed. In general, barriers were not examined in these studies.

Fourteen of the prospective studies examined perceived susceptibility to disease. Variations were found in the populations and the health behaviors that were associated with this patient characteristic. Perceived susceptibility was associated with medical care utilization among medical facility populations

(Berkanovic, Telesky, & Reeder, 1981) and HMO populations (Leavitt, 1979), but not in a population-based random sample (Berkanovic et al. 1981). Perceived susceptibility predicted well-child visits but not illness or accident visits in a pediatric clinic (Becker, Nathanson, Drachman, & Kirscht, 1977). Further, it predicted medication adherence and appointment-keeping for children with otitis media (Becker et al., 1974) and children's weight loss in an obesity program (Becker, Maiman, Kirscht, Haefner, & Drachman, 1977). Perceived susceptibility did not predict adolescents' compliance with dental appointments (West, DuRant, & Pendergrast, 1993), follow-up appointment-keeping in adults and children with otitis media (Jones, Jones, & Katz, 1989), or medical follow-up for suspicious lesions in a skin cancer detection program (Friedman et al., 1995). It did not predict adherence to antihypertensive medications (Taylor, 1979) or participation in fecal occult blood testing (Myers et al., 1994; Sandler, DeVellis, Blalock, & Holland, 1989) among adults. Lastly, perceived susceptibility predicted participation in a breast-screening program (Calnan, 1984; Calnan & Moss, 1984), but not the actual practice of breast self-examination (Calnan & Moss, 1984) and mammography utilization in a population-based community sample (Bastani, Marcus, Maxwell, Das, & Yan, 1994). Even when perceived susceptibility was successful as a predictive variable, power was low with gamma coefficients[2] ranging from .3 to .5 and correlation coefficients ranging from .01 to -.03.

Personal susceptibility was examined in the LRC-CPPT program in a somewhat different manner (Dunbar & Knoke, 1986). In this case, personal susceptibility was dichotomously operationalized as the presence or absence of known risk factors for cardiovascular disease during the screening period. This type of definition is similar to that utilized by Croog and Richards (1977) in assessing health beliefs and smoking cessation; that is, symptoms or risk factors are seen as associated with a threat to individual susceptibility. Croog and Richards (1977) used such indicators as occurrences of chest pain, heart palpitations, breathlessness, and other symptoms as well as rehospitalization, use of physician services, and disability days. In the LRC-CPPT the risk factors included:

---

[2] Gamma is an index of rank-order association. In the special case of the 2×2 table, gamma is a function of the odds ratio. A simple way to test its significance is to compute and test the contingency chi-square value. Numerically gamma is larger than the corresponding phi coefficient, which is equal to the Pearson Product Moment Correlation between 0–1 indicator variables. In the case of the 2×2 table, for crude test purposes, or for comparing it with results stated as correlations, dividing the gamma by two is not too misleading for gammas up to .60. A computational formula can be found in the SPSS Statistical Algorithms manual, and a more detailed discussion in Goodman and Kruskal (1954). (R. Ulrich, (1986) personal communication.)

1. systolic blood pressure greater than 104 mmHg and/or diastolic blood pressure above 90 mmHg;
2. greater than 120% of ideal weight using the 1979 Metropolitan Life tables;
3. current smoker;
4. lack of exercise;
5. over age 47;
6. previously advised by a physician to follow a cholesterol-lowering diet; and
7. a family history, in a first-degree relative, of cardiovascular disease or stroke.

These particular risk factors were all those that were in the subject's awareness.

Family history of cardiovascular disease, age, and smoking were statistically significant predictors of adherence both during the first year of the trial and over the 7-year duration of the study; however, the proportion of variance accounted for was low. The multiple regression equation yielded an R^2 of .024 (p = .0001) for year 1 and an R^2 of .039 (p = .001) over the seven years of the trial. However, with the exception of smoking, the trend across all of the risk factors was for higher susceptibility to be associated with higher adherence.

The results of these studies suggest that the utility of perceived susceptibility as a predictor of adherence may vary with the timing of assessment, the population sampled, and the health behavior of interest. Susceptibility appears to be associated with attendance at screening or prevention visits, as well as with mothers' adherence to pediatric regimens and childhood weight loss, at least when assessed after diagnosis is made. It does not appear to be predictive of health practice or medication adherence when assessment is prior to diagnosis, at least for adult populations. While some interesting and consistent trends were noted in an adult clinical trial population with the above definition for susceptibility, the proportion of variance accounted for by this patient characteristic had little, if any, predictive power.

Perceived severity is the second component of the Health Belief Model. It has been shown to predict well-child and illness visits in a well-child clinic population (Becker, Nathanson, et al. 1977) weight loss among obese children (Becker, Maiman, et al. 1977), and treatment adherence among children with otitis media (Becker et al., 1974). Perceived severity has also been associated with appointment-keeping among children and adults with otitis media (Jones et al., 1989) and participation in colorectal cancer screening in a HMO population (Myers et al., 1994). The gamma coefficients range from 16 for well-child visits to .5 for weight loss. The proportion of variance accounted for is again low. Perceived severity did not, however, predict visits in an adult HMO (Leavitt, 1979) or in an adult community sample (Berkanovic et al. 1981), nor did it predict dental follow-up for adolescents (West et al., 1993) or medication adherence in chronically ill adults (Lorenc & Branthwaite, 1993). It is interesting to note that mothers' management of children's healthcare appears to be the population where severity is most likely to influence subsequent behavior. An examination of the interaction of populations and health behavior with beliefs about severity of the illness or its consequences and the effects on health behavior would be of interest.

Perceived benefits or efficacy of health behaviors as a modifier of disease, a third component in the Health Belief Model, were found to be predictive of screening attendance, but had little predictive power (Calnan, 1984; King, 1984). Modest correlations (*r* .25 and .27, respectively) also were found with adolescent self-report of driving while drinking (Beck, 1981) and of mothers' adherence to medication regimen for children with otitis media (Becker et al., 1977). Further, a positive relationship has been demonstrated between perceived benefits and medication adherence in myocardial infarction (MI) patients (Miller, Wikoff, McMahon, Garrett, & Ringel, 1988) and colorectal cancer (Myers et al., 1994) and mammography screening (Bastani et al., 1994) in a HMO population and a population-based community sample, respectively. However, perceived benefits did not predict follow-up appointment-keeping in adults and children with otitis media (Jones et al., 1989) and medication adherence among adults with chronic conditions (Lorenc & Branthwaite, 1993). It is interesting that little attention has been given to this factor in the prospective prediction studies, particularly in light of the recent work in the area of efficacy and health behavior.

Examination of perceived barriers to health behavior has also yielded mixed findings in the few studies located that have considered this fourth component of the Health Belief Model. Perceived barriers have been predictive of medication adherence in adults with chronic conditions (Lorenc & Branthwaite, 1993) and mammography utilization in community-based women (Bastani et al., 1994). In contrast, perceived barriers were not associated with adolescents' appointment-keeping for dental follow-up (West et al., 1993).

With the exception of studies examining mothers' management of children's health regimens, there appears to be some inconsistency in the findings regarding the ability of health beliefs to predict subsequent behavior. Less favorable findings appear when adult health practices are examined, for example, studies on breast self-examination practices and adherence to antihypertensive drug regimens, than when screening practices are examined. The predictive ability of health beliefs may vary between populations, as noted in the examination of studies of perceived severity and medical care utilization. The number of studies in each of the abovementioned areas is small, but those that have been undertaken suggest than an important direction in the study of health beliefs is an examination of the interaction of specific beliefs with types of health behaviors prescribed, as well as with the population of patients and the setting in which patients are seen.

A complicating factor in evaluating the effect of health beliefs on adherence is the time at which the assessment of health beliefs was undertaken in relation to diagnosis. Health beliefs may be modified with experience with a particular regimen (Beck, 1981; Taylor, 1979). In the single study that assessed health beliefs prior to diagnosis and again 6 months and 12 months after diagnosis and initiation of treatment, prediagnostic beliefs did not predict subsequent adherence (Taylor, 1979). After 6 months of exposure to antihypertensive treatment, beliefs both corresponded to current adherence and offered some prediction of adherence at 12 months. It would appear from this study that the ability of health beliefs to predict behavior is related to whether or not individuals have experienced the behavior and adjusted their beliefs accordingly. This is consistent with much of the attitude/behavior research.

A number of studies found other cognitive-motivational factors to be more predictive than health beliefs. Seven of the 22 studies reported that behavioral intentions were the most powerful predictor of behavior (Beck, 1981; Calnan, 1984; Calnan & Moss, 1984; Cummings, Jette, Brock, & Haefner, 1976; King, 1982, 1984; Myers et al., 1994). These findings are consistent with the cognitive-motivational model posed by Fishbein (1975), which postulated a major role of intention and social influence in predicting subsequent behavior. In contrast, no association was demonstrated between intentions during hospitalization and adherence with activity, stress management, and medication and diet prescriptions 2 years later in post-MI patients (Miller, Wikoff, Garrett, McMahon, & Smith, 1990). Interestingly, four of these studies found associations between selected health beliefs and intentions. Perceived severity was related to intentions, as was perceived efficacy (Cummings et al., 1976; King, 1982, 1984). Consistent with the Preventive Health Model, an integrated framework derived from the Health Belief Model, the Theory of Reasoned Action, and Social Learning Theory, perceived salience and coherence of a preventive action—that is, the extent to which it is perceived to be effective, convenient, personally beneficial, and supported by significant others—was also found to be related to intentions (Myers et al., 1994) The nature of these studies did not lend themselves to an examination of the direction of influence. However, a path model developed by Cummings et al. (1976) suggests that perceived severity effects perceived efficacy. This in turn effects behavioral intention both directly and in conjunction with other variables, such as past experience and social influence. The findings of these studies suggest an interesting avenue for further exploration, that is, the role of behavioral intentions in predicting adherence and the influence, if any, of health beliefs on those intentions.

Following yet a third cognitive-motivational model, Bandura (1977) has postulated in his Self-Efficacy Theory of behavior that individuals will engage in or persist with a behavior to the extent that they believe themselves capable of carrying out that behavior (efficacy expectancy) and to the extent that they believe the behavior will lead to a desired outcome (outcome expectancy). Conversely, "people avoid activities that they believe exceed their coping capabilities" (p. 123) as well as those in which "they expect their efforts to produce no results" (p. 140) (Bandura, 1982). Moreover, these expectations tend to be specific to the behavior in question, rather than general expectations of competence or outcomes (Grusec, 1992; Kaplan, Atkins, & Reinsch, 1984). Interestingly, this specificity was also a finding in the Health Belief area (Becker, Nathanson, et al., 1977b).

A line of investigation examining the role of efficacy in modifying risk behaviors and promoting healthy lifestyles has provided evidence that self-efficacy can serve as a predictor of future performance (Condiotte and Lichtenstein, 1981; Ewart, Taylor, Reese, & DeBusk, 1983; Ewart et al., 1986; Gormley, Carrieri-Kohlman, Douglas, & Stulbarg, 1993; Gortner & Jenkins, 1990; McCann, Follette, Driver, Brief, & Knopp, 1988). Recent research across behavior domains and disease regimens suggests that the self-efficacy model has utility in explaining why individuals adopt or sustain health behaviors, for example, adherence to preventive screening recommendations (Friedman et al., 1995; Myers et al., 1994), and adherence to chronic disease regimens (Kavanagh, Gooley, & Wilson, 1993; McAuley, 1993; McCaul, Glasgow, & Schafer, 1987; Taal, Rasker, Seydel, & Wiegman, 1993).

Bandura (1982) proposes that behavioral skills training and practice alter self-efficacy on the precept that authentic mastery experiences are the best mechanism for providing efficacy information. This has been demonstrated in the research on self-efficacy. For example, Kaplan et al. (1984) reported that patients with chronic obstructive pulmonary disease who were given training in compliance with a walking prescription significantly increased their exercise in contrast to a control group of patients who were only given the exercise prescription and attention. They found that efficacy expectations regarding walking mediated the gains in exercise. Expectations regarding gains in behaviors other than walking changed as a function of their similarity to walking. Similar findings were reported in a study of the effects of exercise testing on physical activity patterns among men post-myocardial infarction (Ewart et al., 1983). In a study of dietary therapy for hyperlipidemia, McCann and colleagues (1995) demonstrated changes in self-efficacy, which were related to the extent of change in eating patterns and reductions in serum lipid levels, following four weekly sessions with a dietitian. Further, self-efficacy was found to be a factor in the adoption of new behaviors in a study of self-management among children with asthma (Evans, 1987), and was a strong predictor of regimen adherence among adolescents with insulin dependent diabetes (McCaul et al., 1987).

Few investigators have examined outcome expectancy alone, or in conjunction with self-efficacy. A few prospective studies have focused on the prediction of adherence to treatment regimens. McCaul and colleagues (1987) found both efficacy and outcome expectancies to be the strongest predictors of adherence for both the concurrent and prospective analyses in their study of IDDM patients. These findings held up among both adults and adolescents and across the three regimens of diabetes management: glucose monitoring and insulin administration, diet, and exercise. Efficacy and outcome expectancies were examined as determinants of adherence to exercise (Desharnais, Bouillon, & Godin, 1986), medication-taking for rheumatoid arthritis (Dunbar-Jacob et al., 1993), and a cholesterol-lowering diet (Burke, Dunbar-Jacob, Sereika, & Rohay, 1996). Dunbar-Jacob and colleagues (1993) found outcome expectancy to be related to self-reported medication-taking, but not to unobtrusive monitoring of medication-taking. At least one study had noted that self-efficacy is a stronger predictor of adherence than outcome expectancy. Desharnais et al. (1986) reported that at the outset of an exercise program participants who became dropouts displayed lower efficacy expectancy pertaining to attendance, while expressing higher outcome expectancy.

A fourth cognitive-motivational model, the Transtheoretical Model of Stages of Change (DiClemente et al., 1991; Prochaska & DiClemente, 1983; Prochaska, DiClemente, & Norcross, 1992) addresses self-initiated and professionally assisted change. According to this theory, individuals move through five stages as they attempt to modify behavior: precontemplation, contemplation, preparation, action, and maintenance. Rather than postulating a linear progression through these stages, the theory proposes that most people recycle through them, suggesting adherence might take a varying course over time. The theory addresses the processes of change, using a decisional balance model. Research has supported the validity of the stages-of-change model (Kristeller, Rossi, Ockene, Goldberg, & Prochaska, 1992; Prochaska, Norcross, Fowler, Follick, & Abrams, 1992). While the theory is promising in predicting who might adhere at a given point in time, empirical reports to date tend to address clinical outcomes rather than adherence to treatment regimens.

Cognitive-motivational models, therefore, have contributions to make to the understanding of patient adherence to a health care regimen. Each proposes a slightly different schema for the understanding of the relationship between motivational cognitions and subsequent behavior. In most cases, the proportion of the variance in adherence behavior accounted for is low. Further, studies in the health belief area suggest that the effect of beliefs on behavior may vary as a function of the population and setting studied, as well as a function of the time at which assessment of beliefs is undertaken. Intentions and self-efficacy seem particularly promising as predictors of adherence. Aspects of health beliefs also appear to be promising in predicting mothers' adherence behaviors and more general screening behaviors. They may also have a mediational role with intentions. Both self-efficacy and health beliefs appear to be influenced by experience, suggesting that studies need to assess these dimensions prior to the onset of the regimen of interest, if interest is in initial adherence. This is not to diminish the role of altered cognitions of this sort as predictors of longer-term adherence, once experience has been gained with the regimen. As self-efficacy and health beliefs appear to change in the direction of the behavior change, however, one wonders if behavior itself would be predictive of future adherence.

HEALTH BEHAVIORS AS PREDICTORS OF SUBSEQUENT ADHERENCE

Health behavior as a predictor of subsequent adherence can be examined along two dimensions. The first is whether adherence to a specific behavior predicts adherence to that same behavior in the future. The second is whether adherence to a specific behavior or set of behaviors predicts adherence to another health behavior in the future.

It can be hypothesized that if individuals adhere to a health care regimen at one time they are likely to do so at a later time. Indeed, such a hypothesis is supported in the few studies that have examined the effect of adherence to a specific regimen on subsequent adherence to the same regimen. This has been particularly evident with screening behaviors for cancer. Past practice with breast self-examination (BSE) has been shown to be the best predictor of BSE after a BSE class (Calnan & Moss, 1984); past mammography has been shown to be the best predictor of participation in mammography screening (Bastani et al., 1994); and the best predictor of follow-up on suspicious skin lesions following a skin cancer screening program was frequency of skin self-examination (Friedman et al., 1995). Interestingly, Myers (1994) found that while past colorectal screening was predictive of screening in univariate analyses, in regression analysis, past screening predicted intentions only, and not actual screening, although intentions and screening behaviors were correlated. Dental health behaviors are included in the area of preventive practice. Past dental appointments have been shown to be predictive of these behaviors when examined in an adolescent population (West et al., 1993). Thus, there is mounting evidence that, at least with regard to screening and preventive practices, past engagement is a significant predictor of subsequent behavior.

Support for the value of past adherence as a predictor of subsequent adherence to treatment regimens has been found in several studies. In the Lipid Research Clinics Coronary Primary Prevention Trial (CPPT), a 10-year study of the cholesterol hypothesis, adherence to the study medication during the first month postrandomization accounted for 34.5% of the variance in adherence in the first year (Dunbar & Knoke, 1986). The addition of the next three most significant individual patient predictors of adherence (age, smoking status, and psychological distress) in a multiple regression equation raised the R^2 to .36 (p=.001). The same set of factors predicted adherence over the 7 years of the study with an R^2 of .24 (p=.001). Initial adherence continued to make the major contribution. Since that time, three other studies have also suggested that initial adherence to treatment predicts longer-term adherence. First-month adherence to tuberculosis preventive therapy was the strongest predictor of adherence at 6 months (Dubanoski, 1988) while adherence to nasal continuous positive airway pressure (CPAP) adherence in the first month predicted usage at 3 months among patients with sleep apnea (Kribbs et al., 1993). The Medical Outcomes Study also reported that baseline adherence was associated with adherence 2 years later (Di Matteo et al., 1993). While not measuring adherence directly, it has also been noted that weight loss in the initial phase of treatment predicts weight loss at the end of treatment (Wadden et al., 1992). The ability of initial adherence to predict subsequent adherence over a 3-month to 7-year duration suggests a certain stability to adherence within a specific regimen based upon a pattern established early. This growing body of evidence for the ability of early behavior to predict subsequent behavior suggests interesting and valuable directions for the continued study of adherence to health regimens, both in efforts to understand as well as to promote adherence.

Health behaviors other than early adherence performance to an intervention do not predict adherence to a specific regimen. For example, while prior experience with otitis media predicted mothers' adherence to follow-up appointments for otitis media care, it did not predict adherence to appointments for other reasons (Becker et al., 1974). In the LRC-CPPT study, visit attendance during the first month postrandomization was associated with subsequent medication adherence in the first year and over the 7 years of the study. However, the substitution of initial-visit adherence for initial-medication adherence in a multiple regression equation lowered substantially the proportion of variance accounted for in subsequent medication adherence (R^2 = .095 contrasted with R^2 = .36). Thus, a related but not identical health behavior reduced the ability to predict future adherence.

Other behaviors were examined among the LRC-CPPT participants to determine the predictive ability of health-oriented behaviors on subsequent adherence to the medication regimen. During screening the participants were interviewed regarding their current and past practices with regard to smoking, exercise, weight, alcohol intake, and multivitamin use. Univariate analyses showed no statistically significant association over 1 year or over 7 years for regularity of exercise, relative weight, alcohol consumption, or multivitamin usage. While smoking status during screening did predict medication adherence over 1 year and over 7 years, the proportion of variance accounted for was very small, 1.2% the first year and 2% over the 7 years. Smokers had lower adherence than nonsmokers.

These studies suggest that behavior can predict behavior. The more similar the initial behavior is to the behavior to be predicted, the greater the ability to predict. However, there does not appear to be a set of behaviors characterizing an individual that would allow prediction of adherence to a specific health regimen; that is, there is not an individual who is health-oriented, as defined by the practice of a set of healthy behaviors, and whose adherence could be predicted on the basis of that practice alone. However, the studies suggest that a history of adherence to a specific regimen would predict subsequent adherence to that regimen. Further study of the ability of behavior to predict subsequent adherence would be of interest and would be most useful in the selection of subjects for clinical research efforts where maximal adherence to protocol regimen is desired.

SOMATIC AND COGNITIVE FACTORS AS PREDICTORS OF ADHERENCE

Eleven studies have examined the aversive effects, as well as the relief of symptoms due to treatment, as predictors of adherence. For example, physical discomforts during running does predict dropping out of a marathon training program (Heiby et al., 1985). Indeed, the amount of running done by the dropouts was a function of the number of injuries experienced. Other researchers similarly reported that adverse side effects, especially the number, nature, and perceived intensity, were inversely related to adherence in adolescents receiving iron supplements (Cromer, Steinberg, Gardner, Thornton, & Shannon, 1989) and in women prescribed ethinylestradiol (Kruse, Eggert-Kruse, Rampmaier, Runnebaum, & Weber, 1993).

Adherence to self-management procedures for adults with diabetes, hypertension, and cardiopulmonary disease were related to fewer symptoms (Kravitz et al., 1993; Nagy & Wolfe, 1984). Other researchers found that less shortness of breath predicted metered-dose inhaler adherence in patients with chronic obstructive pulmonary disease (COPD) (Rand, Nides, Cowles, Wise, & Connett, 1995). In contrast, more severe dyspnea predicted adherence to nebulizer therapy among patients with COPD (Turner, Wright, Mendella, & Anthonisen, 1995). Two randomized clinical trials found that symptoms were not predictive of adherence (Jones et al., 1989; Yoon et al., 1991). Asthma severity did not differ between attenders and nonattenders of an asthma education program after discharge from the hospital (Yoon et al., 1991). Duration and intensity of otitis media symptoms did not predict follow-up appointment keeping in adults and children presenting to an emergency department (Jones et al., 1989). Thus, patients with fewer symptoms were more likely to adhere to self-management regimens. However, severity of respiratory symptoms as well as duration and intensity of otitis media symptoms were less consistently predictive of adherence.

Given, Given, and Coyle (1985) noted further that patients with hypertension participating in an intervention study who perceived themselves to have more severe symptoms were more likely to drop out. This investigation suggests that beliefs about symptoms may be important predictors of nonadherence. This notion is further supported by Meyer, Leventhal, and Guttman (1985) in a study of hypertensive patients' models of their illness. These investigators noted that a majority of patients believed they could monitor their own blood pressure changes through physiological symptoms. Indeed, 71% of new patients, 92% of continuing patients, and 94% of returning patients reported such an ability. Those patients who believed treatment relieved their symptoms reported adhering to treatment. Thus, the notion of somatic factors predicting subsequent adherence may be confounded by the patient's perception of those symptoms and by the inclusion of somatic factors in their model of a disease and its treatment.

Four prospective studies examined the ability of cognitive factors to predict adherence with mixed results. Graveley and Oseasohn (1991) reported that cognitive impairment was not a predictor of medication adherence among elderly male veterans. Other researchers found that visual and verbal memory were correlated with medication adherence among elderly outpatients (Isaac & Tamblyn, 1993). Faster psychomotor speed in sedentary, elderly, cognitively intact subjects predicted exercise behavior at 1-year follow-up in a randomized clinical trial (Emery et al., 1992). A randomized clinical trial conducted with elderly adults demonstrated that the group receiving both cognitive aids (an organizational chart and medication organizer) had fewer drug omission errors than the other groups (Park, Morrell, Frieske, & Kincaid, 1992). Thus, more research is needed on the effect of cognitive factors on adherence behavior as well as devices to promote adherence among elderly, cognitively impaired persons.

SUMMARY

A variety of factors specific to the patient have been reviewed that predict subsequent patient adherence. Included in these factors are psychological characteristics, particularly psychological distress; cognitive-motivational factors drawn from theories regarding health beliefs, intentions and behavior, self-efficacy, and stages of change; and health behaviors and somatic and cognitive factors. Whereas each of these areas has something to contribute to the prediction of patient adherence to a healthcare regimen, the predictive power tends to be modest at best for any single factor. The most promising of these seem to be self-efficacy, intentions, and adherence behavior itself. Not to be lost, however, is the role of psychological distress, perceived vulnerability or susceptibility to illness or its consequences, and the experience or perceived experience of somatic complaints. Many questions still arise in the area of prediction of patient adherence. How do beliefs interact with populations, healthcare settings, and the type of behavior to influence adherence? Also, how do these multiple factors interact, if at all, to lead to adherence or nonadherence? Further, how do each of these factors independently act to influence adherence, if at all? Whereas more is becoming known about patient factors predictive of adherence, the relatively modest associations suggest that there is still much to be learned.

REFERENCES

Bandura, A. (1977). Self-efficacy: Toward a unifying theory of behavioral change. *Psychological Review, 84*, 191–215.

Bandura, A. (1982). Self-efficacy mechanism in human agency. *American Psychologist, 37*, 122–147.

Bastani, R., Marcus, A. C., Maxwell, A. E., Das, I. P., & Yan, K. X. (1994). Evaluation of an intervention to increase mammography screening in Los Angeles. *Preventive Medicine, 23*, 83–90.

Beck, K. H. (1981). Driving while under the influence of alcohol: Relationship to attitudes and beliefs in a college population. *American Journal of Drug and Alcohol Abuse, 8*, 377–386.

Becker, M. H., Drachman, R. H., & Kirscht, J. P. (1974). A new approach to explaining sick-role behavior in low-income populations. *American Journal of Public Health, 64*, 205–216.

Becker, M. H., Maiman, L. A., Kirscht, J. P., Haefner, D. P., & Drachman, R. H. (1977). The health belief model and prediction of dietary compliance: A field experiment. *Journal of Health and Social Behavior, 18*, 348–366.

Becker, M. H., Nathanson, C. A., Drachman, R. H., & Kirscht, J. P. (1977). Mothers' health beliefs and children's clinic visits: A prospective study. *Journal of Community Health, 3*, 125–135.

Berkanovic, E., Telesky, C., & Reeder, S. (1981). Structural and social psychological factors in the decision to seek medical care for symptoms. *Medical Care, 19*, 693–709.

Blumenthal, J. A., Williams, R. S., Wallace, A. G., Williams, R. B., & Needles, T. L. (1982). Physiological and psychological variables predict compliance to prescribed exercise therapy in patients recovering from myocardial infarction. *Psychosomatic Medicine, 44*, 519–527.

Burke, L. E., Dunbar-Jacob, J., Sereika, S., & Rohay, J. (1996). Outcome expectations vs. self-efficacy as predictive of dietary adherence in cardiac rehabilitation patients (Abstract). Paper presented at the 4th International Congress of Behavioral Medicine. *Annals of Behavioral Medicine, 18*(Suppl), S088.

Calnan, M. (1984). The health belief model and participation in programmes for the early detection of breast cancer: A comparative analysis. *Social Science and Medicine, 19*, 823–830.

Calnan, M. W., & Moss, S. (1984). The health belief model and compliance with education given at a class in breast self-examination. *Journal of Health and Social Behavior, 25*, 198–210.

Condiotte, M.. M., & Lichtenstein, E. (1981). Self-efficacy and relapse in smoking cessation programs. *Journal of Consulting and Clinical Psychology, 49*, 648–658.

Cromer, B. A., Steinberg, K., Gardner, L., Thornton, D., & Shannon, B. (1989). Psychosocial determinants of compliance in adolescents with iron deficiency. *American Journal of Diseases in Children, 143*, 55–58.

Croog, S. H., & Richards, N. P. (1977). Health beliefs and smoking patterns in heart patients and their wives: A longitudinal study. *American Journal of Public Health, 67*, 921–930.

Cummings, K. M., Jette, A. M., Brock, B. M., & Haefner, D. P (1976). Psychosocial determinants of immunization behavior in a swine influenza campaign. *Medical Care, 17*, 639–649.

Desharnais, R., Bouillon, J., & Godin, G. (1986). Self-efficacy and outcome expectations as determinants of exercise adherence. *Psychological Reports, 59*, 1155–1159.

DiClemente, C. C., Prochaska, J. O., Fairhurst, S. K., Velicer, W. F., Velasquez, M. M., & Rossi, J. S. (1991). The process of smoking cessation: An analysis of precontemplation, contemplation, and preparation of stages of change. *Journal of Consulting and Clinical Psychology, 58*, 295–304.

DiLorio, C., Faherty, B., & Manteuffel, B. (1991). Cognitive-perceptual factors associated with antiepileptic medication compliance. *Research in Nursing and Health, 14*, 329–338.

DiMatteo, M. R., Sherbourne, C. D., Hays, R. D., Ordway, L., Kravitz, R. L., McGlynn, E. A., Kaplan, S., & Rogers, W. H. (1993). Physicians' characteristics influence patients' adherence to medical treatment: Results from the Medical Outcomes Study. *Health Psychology, 12*, 93–102.

Dubanoski, J. P. (1988). Preventive health behavior: A model of adherence prediction. *Dissertation Abstracts International, 48*(10-B), 3152.

Dunbar, J., & Knoke, J. (1986, March). *Prediction of medication adherence at one year and seven years: Behavioral and psychological factors*. Paper presented at the Society for Clinical Trials Annual Conference, Montreal, Canada.

Dunbar-Jacob, J., Sereika, S., Burke, L. E., Kwoh, C. K., McCall, M., Locke, C., Holmes, J., Bondi, K., Canty, T., & Starz, T. (1993). Perceived treatment efficacy: Assessment in rheumatoid arthritis(Abstract). Paper presented at the 14th annual Scientific Sessions, Society of Behavioral Medicine. *Annals of Behavioral Medicine, 15*(Suppl), S147.

Eisen, M., Zellman, G. L., & McAlister, A. L. (1985). A health belief model approach to adolescents' fertility control: Some pilot program findings. *Health Education Quarterly, 12*, 185–210.

Emery, C. F., Hauck, E. R., & Blumenthal, J. A. (1992). Exercise adherence or maintenance among older adults: 1-year follow-up study. *Psychology and Aging, 7*, 466–470.

Evans, D. (1987, April). *School-based health education for children with asthma.* Paper presented at the NHLBI National Working Conference on the Adoption and Maintenance of Behaviors for Optimal Health, Bethesda, MD.

Ewart, C. K., Stewart, K. J., Gillilan, R. E., Kelemen, M. H., Valenti, S. A., Manley, J. D., & Kelemen, M.D. (1986). Usefulness of self-efficacy in predicting overexertion during programmed exercise in coronary artery disease. *American Journal of Cardiology, 57*, 557–561.

Ewart, C. K., Taylor, C B., Reese, L., & DeBusk, R. F. (1983). Effects of early post myocardial infarction exercise testing on self-perception and subsequent physical activity. *The American Journal of Cardiology, 51*, 1076–1080.

Fishbein, M. (1975). *Belief, attitude, intention, and behavior.* Reading, MA: Addison-Wesley.

Friedman, L. C., Webb, J. A., Bruce, S., Weinberg, A. D., & Cooper, H. P. (1995). Skin cancer prevention and early detection intentions and behavior. *American Journal of Preventive Medicine, 11*, 59–65.

Given, C. W., Given, B A., & Coyle, B. W. (1985). Prediction of patient attrition from experimental behavioral interventions. *Nursing Research, 34*, 293–298.

Goodman, L. A., & Kruskal, W. H. (1954). Measures of association for cross classifications. *Journal of the American Statistical Association, 49*, 732–764.

Gormley, J. M., Carrieri-Kohlman, V., Douglas, M. K., & Stulbarg, M. S. (1993). Treadmill self-efficacy and walking performance in patients with COPD. *Journal of Cardiopulmonary Rehabilitation, 13*, 424–431.

Gortner, S. R., & Jenkins, L. S. (1990). Self-efficacy and activity level following cardiac surgery. *Journal of Advanced Nursing, 15*, 1132–1138.

Graveley, E. A., & Oseasohn, C. S. (1991). Multiple drug regimens: Medication compliance among veterans 65 years and older. *Research in Nursing and Health, 14*, 51–58.

Grusec, J. E. (1992) Social learning theory and developmental psychology; The legacies of Robert Sears and Albert Bandura. *Developmental Psychology, 28*, 776–786.

Heiby, E. M., Onorato, V. A., & Sato, R. A. (1985, August) *A cognitive-behavioral model of adherence to health-related exercise.* Poster session presented at the American Psychological Association 93rd Annual Convention, Los Angeles, CA.

Inui, T. S., Yourtee, E. L., & Williamson, J. W. (1976). Improved outcomes in hypertension after physician tutorials: A controlled trial. *Annals of Internal Medicine, 84*, 646–651.

Isaac, L. M., & Tamblyn, R. M. (1993). Compliance and cognitive function: A methodological approach to measuring unintentional errors in medication compliance in the elderly. McGill-Calgary Drug Research Team. *The Gerontologist, 33*, 772–781.

Janz, N. K., & Becker, M. H. (1984). The Health Belief Model: A decade later. *Health Education Quarterly 11*, 1–47.

Jones, S. L., Jones, P. K., & Katz, J. (1989). A nursing intervention to increase compliance in otitis media patients. *Applied Nursing Research, 29*, 68–73.

Kaplan, R. M., Atkins, D. J., & Reinsch, S. (1984). Specific efficacy expectations mediate exercise compliance in patients with COPD. *Health Psychology, 3*, 233–242.

Kavanagh, D. J., Gooley, S., & Wilson, P. H. (1993). Prediction of adherence and control in diabetes. *Journal of Behavioral Medicine, 6*, 509–522.

King, J. B. (1982). The impact of patients' perceptions of high blood pressure on attendance at screening: An extension of the health belief model. *Social Science and Medicine, 16*, 1079–1091.

King, J. B. (1984). Illness attributions and the health belief model. *Health Education Quarterly, 10*, 287–312.

Kravitz, R. L., Hays, R. D., Sherbourne, C. D., DiMatteo, M. R., Rogers, W. H., Ordway, L., & Greenfield, S. (1993). Recall of recommendations and adherence to advice among patients with chronic medical conditions. *Archives of Internal Medicine, 153*, 1869–1878.

Kribbs, N. B., Pack, A. I., Kline, L. R., Smith, P. L., Schwartz, A. R., Schubert, N. M., Redline, S., Henry, J. N., Getsy, J. E., & Dinges, D. F. (1993). Objective measurement of patterns of nasal CPAP use by patients with obstructive sleep apnea. *American Review of Respiratory Disorders, 147*, 887–895.

Kristeller, J. L., Rossi, J. S., Ockene, J. K., Goldberg, R., & Prochaska, J. O. (1992). Processes of change in smoking cessation: A cross-validation study in cardiac patients. *Journal of Substance Abuse, 4*, 263–276.

Kruse, W., Eggert-Kruse, W., Rampmaier, J., Runnebaum, B., & Weber, E. (1993). Compliance and adverse drug reactions: A prospective study with ethinylestradiol using continuous compliance monitoring. *Clinical Investigator, 71*, 483–487.

Leavitt, F. (1979). The health belief model and utilization of ambulatory care services. *Social Science and Medicine, 13A*, 105–112.

Lee, D., De Leon, C. F. M., Jenkins, C. D., Croog, S. H., Levine, S., & Sudilovsky, A. (1992). Relation of hostility to medication adherence, symptom complaints, and blood pressure reduction in a clinical field trial of antihypertensive medication. *Journal of Psychosomatic Research, 36*, 181–190.

Lorenc, L., & Branthwaite, A. (1993). Are older adults less compliant with prescribed medication than younger adults? *British Journal of Clinical Psychology, 32*, 485–492.

Mawhinney, H., Spector, S. L., Heitjan, D., Kinsman, R. A., Dirks, J. F., & Pines, I. (1993). As-needed medication use in asthma usage patterns and patient characteristics. *Journal of Asthma, 30*, 61–71.

McAuley, E. (1993). Self-efficacy and the maintenance of exercise in older adults. *Journal of Behavioral Medicine, 16*, 103–113.

McCann, B. S., Bovbjerg, V. E., Brief, D. J., Turner, C., Follette, W. C., Fitzpatrick, V., Dowdy, A. Retzlaff, B., Walden, C. E., & Knopp, R. H. (1995). *Annals of Behavioral Medicine, 17*, 221–226.

McCann, B. S., Follette, W. C., Driver, J. L., Brief, D. J., & Knopp, R. H. (1988, August). *Self-efficacy and adherence in the dietary treatment of hyperlipidemia.* Paper presented at the 96th Annual Convention of the American Psychological Association, Atlanta, GA.

McCaul, K. D., Glasgow, R. E., & Schafer, L. C. (1987). Diabetes regimen behaviors: Predicting adherence. *Medical Care, 25*, 868–881.

Meyer, D., Leventhal, H., & Gutmann, M. (1985). Common sense models of illness: The example of hypertension. *Health Psychology, 4*, 115–135.

Michie, S., Marteau, T. M., & Kidd, J. (1990). Cognitive predictors of attendance at antenatal classes. *British Journal of Clinical Psychology, 29*, 193–199.

Miller, P., Wikoff, R., Garrett, M. J., McMahon, M., & Smith, T. (1990). Regimen compliance two years after myocardial infarction. *Nursing Research, 39*, 333–336.

Miller, P., Wikoff, R., McMahon, M., Garrett, M. J., & Ringel, K. (1988). Influence of a nursing intervention on regimen adherence and societal adjustments post-myocardial infarction. *Nursing Research, 37*, 297–302.

Myers, R. E., Ross, E., Jepson, C., Wolf, T., Balshem, A., Millner, L., & Leventhal, H. (1994). Modeling adherence to colorectal cancer screening. *Preventive Medicine, 23*, 142–151.

Nagy, V T., & Wolfe, G. R. (1984). Cognitive predictors of compliance in chronic disease patients. *Medical Care, 22*, 912–921.

Nelson, E. C., Stason, W. B., Neutra, R. R., Solomon, H. S., & McArdle, P. J. (1978). Impact of patient perceptions on compliance with treatment for hypertension. *Medical Care, 16*,893–906.

O'Leary, M. R., Rohsenow, D. J., & Chaney, E. F. (1979). The use of multivariate personality strategies in predicting attrition from alcoholism treatment. *Journal of Clinical Psychiatry, 40*, 190–193.

Park, D. C., Morrell, R. W., Frieske, D., & Kincaid, D. (1992). Medication adherence behaviors in older adults: Effects of external cognitive supports. *Psychology and Aging, 7*, 252–256.

Prochaska, J. O., & DiClemente, C. C. (1983). Stages and processes of self-change in smoking: Toward an integrative model of change. *Journal of Consulting and Clinical Psychology, 5*, 390–395.

Prochaska, J. O., DiClemente, C. C., & Norcross, J. C. (1992). In search of how people change. *American Psychologist, 47*, 1102–1114.

Prochaska, J. O., Norcross, J. C., Fowler, J. L., Follick, M. J., & Abrams, D. B. (1992). Attendance and outcome in a worksite weight control program: Processes and stages of change as process and predictor variables. *Addictive Behaviors, 17*, 35–45.

Rand, C. S., Nides, M., Cowles, M. K., Wise, R. A., & Connett, J. (1995). Long-term metered-dose inhaler adherence in a clinical trial. Lung Health Study Research Group. *American Journal of Respiratory and Critical Care Medicine, 152*, 580–588.

Rosenstock, I. M. (1966). Why people use health services. *Milbank Memorial Fund Quarterly, 44*, 94–127.

Rosenstock, I. M. (1974). The historical origins of the health belief model. *Health Education Monographs, 2*, 328–335.

Sandler, R. S., DeVellis, B. M., Blalock, S. J., & Holland, K. L. (1989). Participation of high-risk subjects in colon cancer screening. *Cancer, 63*, 2211–2215.

Sherbourne, C. D., Hays, R. D., Ordway, L., DiMatteo, M. R., & Kravitz, R. L. (1992). Antecedents of adherence to medical recommendations: Results from the

Medical Outcomes Study. *Journal of Behavioral Medicine, 15*, 447–468.

Taal, E., Rasker, J. J., Seydel, E. R., & Wiegman, O. (1993). Health status, adherence with health recommendations, self-efficacy and social support in patients with rheumatoid arthritis. *Patient Education and Counseling, 20*, 63–76.

Taylor, D. W. (1979). A test of the health belief model in hypertension. In R. B. Haynes, D. W. Taylor, & D. L. Sackett (Eds.), Compliance in health care (pp. 103–109). Baltimore: Johns Hopkins University Press.

Turner, J., Wright, E., Mendella, L., & Anthonisen, N. (1995). Predictors of patient adherence to long-term home nebulizer therapy for COPD. IPPB Study Group. *Chest, 108*, 394–400.

Wadden, T. A., Foster, G. D., Wang, J., Pierson, R. N., Yang, M. U., Moreland, K., Stunkard, A. J., & VanItallie, T. B. (1992). Clinical correlates of short- and long-term weight loss. *American Journal of Clinical Nutrition, 56*, 271S–274S.

Welsh, M. C., Labbé, E. E., & Delaney, D. (1991). Cognitive strategies and personality variables in adherence to exercise. *Psychological Reports, 68*, 1327–1335.

West, K. P., DuRant, R. H., & Pendergrast, R. (1993). An experimental test of adolescents' compliance with dental appointments. *Journal of Adolescent Medicine, 14*, 384–389.

Yoon, R., McKenzie, D. K., Miles, D. A., & Bauman, A. (1991). Characteristics of attenders and non-attenders at an asthma education programme. *Thorax, 46*, 886–890.

SECTION VII
Lifestyle Change and Adherence: The Broader Context

Sally A. Shumaker, Editor

As discussed throughout this book, obstacles to adherence may arise from a number of factors, including the complexity of a particular regimen; behavioral or biological disincentives to changing behaviors; poor communication between individuals and their health providers; public policies and social contexts that reinforce negative health behaviors; and the complex needs of specific populations. Furthermore, there is a persistent inadequacy in theoretical models to help investigators frame questions and to assist them in understanding adherence and behavior change. Also, defining, measuring, and interpreting information about adherence continues to be a formidable challenge for both researchers and health providers. In spite of these problems, however, there is an implicit assumption throughout this book that better adherence is almost always worth pursuing and will result in better health outcomes for most individuals. Thus, our focus has been on identifying and pursuing methods to enhance adherence and the adoption and maintenance of healthy behaviors.

In this final section of this book, the authors step back from the assumption that adherence is primae facie good and should be relentlessly pursued by both consumers and healthcare providers. These authors consider the possibly unintended consequences of "good" adherence, who in society is ultimately responsible for health behavior changes, and the underlying ethical issues inherent in the contracts been health providers and their patients. The authors in this section discuss adherence within a broader social context and challenge health providers and researchers to look more carefully at the implications of adherence to health behavior interventions for the individual and society.

In Chapter 22, Czajkowski, Chesney, and Smith discuss the potential consequences of adherence in experimental studies which include placebo and treatment groups. These authors consider how various factors, including one's belief in the efficacy of treatment, can produce treatmentlike effects in the placebo condition. Further, this "placebo effect" is strengthened by adherence. These authors suggest that as long as the placebo effect is treated as a nuisance variable rather than as a real phenomenon worthy of study in its own right, differences in adherence between treatment and placebo groups may lead to incorrect interpretations of data. Further, health providers may be underutilizing the strength of personal commitment embodied in the placebo effect to improve health. Czajkowski, Chesney, and Smith describe several models to explain the placebo effect and discuss its implications for clinical research and for assumptions regarding treatment efficacy.

In Chapter 23, Ribsl and Humphreys consider a basic philosophical issue that is at the core of adherence and health behavior: whether health is primarily a personal responsibility or a societal obligation. Contrasting the extreme views of a paternalistic society in which health prescriptions are pursued at the risk of personal freedom, versus "rugged individualism" in which all health decisions are individually determined with disregard for the larger social context or societal good, these authors develop an alternative model. In this model collaboration is pursued between individuals' behaviors as mediated by structures in the community, and the health promotion professionals. Ribsl and Humphrey carefully examine the philosophical context underlying the extreme views of paternalism versus individualism and from this develop the collaborative model with mediating structures, with several examples provided to elucidate the model.

We end the book with a consideration of the ethics that underlie recommended behavior changes. In Chapter 24, Faden highlights the key moral issues relevant to the question of adherence to lifestyle changes. She discusses the differences implied in normative and applied ethics when considering adherence in three very different contractual relationships: the clinician and the patient, the researcher and the subject, and the government and its citizenry.

Adherence and the Placebo Effect

Susan M. Czajkowski,
Margaret A. Chesney, and
Ashley W. Smith

Traditionally, adherence has been viewed as a critical element in the success of a treatment or health regimen, for without it patients may not receive the full benefit of treatment. Given the importance of adherence to treatment success, other chapters in this volume focus on factors that predict or influence adherence to a specific treatment and on strategies for increasing adherence. In contrast, in this chapter we consider adherence from another perspective: the potential effects of adherence on treatment effectiveness and health outcomes. We propose that, in addition to its role in maximizing the active, specific effects of the treatment, adherence may also increase treatment effectiveness by activating nonspecific or placebo effects that influence treatment success. Thus, the mere act of adhering to a treatment regimen may in itself produce positive health outcomes, regardless of the actual efficacy of the intervention, due to a placebo effect.

We begin with a brief review of studies documenting an association between adherence to treatment and health outcomes. We then outline a hypothetical model of the role adherence may play in enhancing the nonspecific, or placebo, effects of an intervention and thus in affecting treatment outcome. A brief overview of placebo effects is presented, including a discussion of possible mechanisms through which placebos exert their influence. Applying the model, we then suggest an explanation for why adherence to a treatment may enhance a placebo response, and finally, discuss implications of the model for both clinical applications and research.

THE RELATIONSHIP OF ADHERENCE TO TREATMENT OUTCOME

A number of studies have now documented an association between adherence, to either active treatment or placebo, and health outcomes. Good adherence to either treatment or placebo has been associated with benefit, and poor adherence with negative effects, in studies of treatments for myocardial infarction (MI) (The Coronary Drug Project Research Group, 1980; Horwitz et al., 1990; Verter & Friedman, 1984); cancer (Dolin et al., 1982; Pizzo et al., 1983) and schizophrenia (Pledger, 1992).

In one of the earliest studies to document this effect, the Coronary Drug Project (CDP) (Coronary Drug Project Research Group, 1980), male patients who had experienced a myocardial infarction within 3 months of study entry were randomly assigned to either a condition in which they received clofibrate or to a placebo control group. The results showed no significant difference in 5-year mortality between the two groups: for the 1103 men treated with clofibrate, 5-year mortality was 20%; for the 2789 men given placebo, it was 20.9%.

Further analyses performed to determine whether adherence to clofibrate influenced 5-year mortality showed that good adherers (defined as patients who took 80% or more of the drug during the 5-year follow-up period) had a significantly lower 5-year mortality (15%) than did poor adherers (24.6%; see Table 22.1). However, this was true for those receiving the placebo as well; good adherers to placebo had significantly lower mortality than poor adherers to placebo (15.1% for good adherers versus 28.2% for poor adherers). Furthermore, this effect held even when multivariate statistical methods were used to adjust for baseline differences between the two groups on 40 variables that were related to 5-year mortality (e.g., indices of disease severity, use of hypertensive medication).

In the CDP, flaws in the way adherence was measured may account for the relationship found between adherence and mortality. In this study, adherence was determined by physician estimates of the number of pills taken by patients each day. These estimates were based not only on the number of pills returned by patients at their clinic visits, but also on physician's interviews in which patients were questioned about problems with the medication, including side effects, that may have affected adherence to the regimen. Because of the subjective nature of the latter measure of adherence, assessments of patients' adherence may have been influenced by physicians' assessments of the health of individual patients. Thus, the

TABLE 22.1 Influence of Adherence on Five-Year Mortality Rates in the Coronary Drug Project

	Treatment group	
Adherence	Clofibrate	Placebo
Good adherers (< 80% adherence)	15.0% (15.7)*	15.1% (16.4)
Poor adherers (> 80% adherence)	24.6% (22.5)	28.2% (25.8)

*The figures in parentheses are adjusted for 40 baseline characteristics.

Note. From The Coronary Drug Project Research Group. "Influence of adherence to treatment and response of cholesterol on mortality in the Coronary Drug Project." *The New England Journal of Medicine, 8*, 1039. Copyright the Massachusetts Medical Society.

healthier patients may have been classified as highly adherent, and their lower mortality rate may have simply reflected this bias in classification to the high-adherence "condition."

However, similar results have been found in other studies using more objective measures of adherence. For example, in the Aspirin Myocardial Infarction Study (AMIS), in which adherence was assessed using three different measures (pill count, urine salicylate, and platelet aggregation), lower mortality rates were found for good adherers to the aspirin treatment (6.1%) and to placebo (5.1%) relative to poor adhererers to either aspirin (21.9%) or placebo (22%). An analysis of the relationship of adherence to mortality in the Beta-Blocker Heart Attack Trial (BHAT) also found good adherers to have better health outcomes than poor adherers: patients who demonstrated poor adherence, whether assigned to treatment or placebo, were two and one-half to three times as likely to die within one year of follow-up than patients with good adherence (Horwitz et al., 1990). Other studies demonstrating this effect include trials of antibiotic prophylaxis to reduce fever or infection in cancer patients (Dolin et al., 1982; Pizzo et al., 1983) and a trial of chlorpromazine versus placebo in schizophrenic patients (Pledger, 1992).

These results have most often been used to demonstrate the problems associated with analyzing clinical trial data using subgroups based on patient responses, such as adherence, since individuals who demonstrate good adherence may differ from poor adherers on any number of variables that may also cause differences in mortality (Coronary Drug Project Research Group, 1980; Friedman, Furberg, & DeMets, 1996). Perhaps the healthier patients in these studies were better able to tolerate the medication and so adhered better to it, while the sicker patients were less able to tolerate the medication and so discontinued using it. Alternatively, the poor adherers in studies such as the CDP may have been individuals who abused drugs or alcohol and who were therefore negligent about taking their medication. If these individuals were also less healthy than adherers, as would be expected, their survival rates over the 5-year follow-up period would be lower than those in the "high-adherence" group. In this case, both adherence and mortality would result from a third, unmeasured variable—e.g., alcohol/drug abuse—and would actually be unrelated to each other when that variable was controlled.

At least two of the studies cited above used multivariate analyses to control for sociodemographic, psychosocial, and health-related factors that might account for the adherence-mortality relationship in an attempt to determine the variable or variables that underlie the adherence-mortality relationships found (Coronary Drug Project Research Group, 1980; Horwitz et al., 1990). Adjustment for these variables, including various indices of disease severity, psychosocial factors such as stress, and unhealthy behaviors such as smoking, did not weaken the adherence-mortality association. Nevertheless, it is possibile that some key explanatory variable was not measured and therefore not able to be used in the adjusted analyses. For example, Kellet (1990) suggests that depression, which has been independently associated with mortality in coronary artery disease and myocardial infarction patients (Ahern et al., 1990; Carney et al., 1988; Frasure-Smith, Lesperance, & Talajic, 1993) and with adherence to cardiac risk factor modification and cardiac rehabilitation (Blumenthal, Williams, Wallace, Williams, & Needles, 1982; Guiry, Conroy, Hickey, & Mulcahy, 1987), may have contributed to both low levels of adherence and higher mortality in the heart-disease treatment trials (AMIS, CDP and BHAT).

Apart from their value in justifying intent-to-treat approaches to data analysis in clinical trials, some have argued that these findings reflect an interesting phenomenon in its own right—that there is something related to adherence, or characteristic of individuals who demonstrate good adherence, that is associated with positive health outcomes (Epstein, 1984; Horwitz & Horwitz, 1993). Epstein (1984) raises the possibility that patient expectancies of the efficacy of treatment may play a role in the relationship between adherence and health outcomes found in these studies. Horwitz and colleagues (Horwitz et al., 1990; Horwitz & Horwitz, 1993) suggest that adherence may be a marker for a variety of psychological, social, and behavioral variables that affect the outcomes of treatment (e.g., a patient's ability to control aspects of life that affect disease progression), and recommend further research using more extensive and refined measures of psychosocial and behavioral factors.

In this chapter we extend these arguments, and explore the possibility that the very act of adherence itself, and/or characteristics of individuals who demonstrate good adherence, may affect health outcomes by activating the nonspecific or placebo effects of an intervention. In the next section, we propose a hypothetical model that demonstrates the ways in which adherence might influence treatment outcome via nonspecific effects.

MODEL: THE NONSPECIFIC EFFECTS OF ADHERENCE

The model (see Figure 22.1) proposed here is one in which adherence to an intervention is seen as enhancing not only the effects of active treatment components, but also the effects of nonspecific components of that intervention as well. The model suggests that adherence enhances the following nonspecific components that can influence intervention outcomes: (1) patient and provider expectancies of the intervention's success, and (2) the social support available to the patient from the provider and others in the patient's environment.

In several chapters in this volume, expectancies and social support have been described as predictors of adherence. The model presented here suggests that these factors may also be "effects" of adherence. Adherence influences the expectancy of treatment success to the extent that patients who follow an intervention develop the expectation that they will experience positive health outcomes. Conversely, patients who do not adhere should have a diminished expectancy of positive outcomes from the intervention. Patient adherence also impacts provider expectancies regarding the outcome of the intervention. For example, a physician is more likely to expect lower serum cholesterol levels in a patient who is adhering to a prescribed low-fat diet than in a patient who continues to eat a high-fat diet. Patient adherence may also influence the amount of social support extended to patients by providers and others in the patient's social network, since adhering to a prescribed medical regimen is likely to be rewarded by positive responses from family, friends, and caretakers.

As portrayed in the model, the relationship between adherence and the nonspecific components of treatment is a reciprocal one. Expectancies and social support are affected by adherence and, in turn, influence subsequent adherence. For example, the patient who adheres to the low-fat diet, and meets with a physician who expresses a positive expectancy for lower cholesterol levels and praises the patient for adhering, is more likely to continue adhering to the prescribed diet.

In the model, expectancy and social support are considered not only in terms of their relationship to adherence, but in terms of their roles as nonspecific factors influencing treatment outcomes. This aspect of the model is based on evidence that these two variables are important in influencing

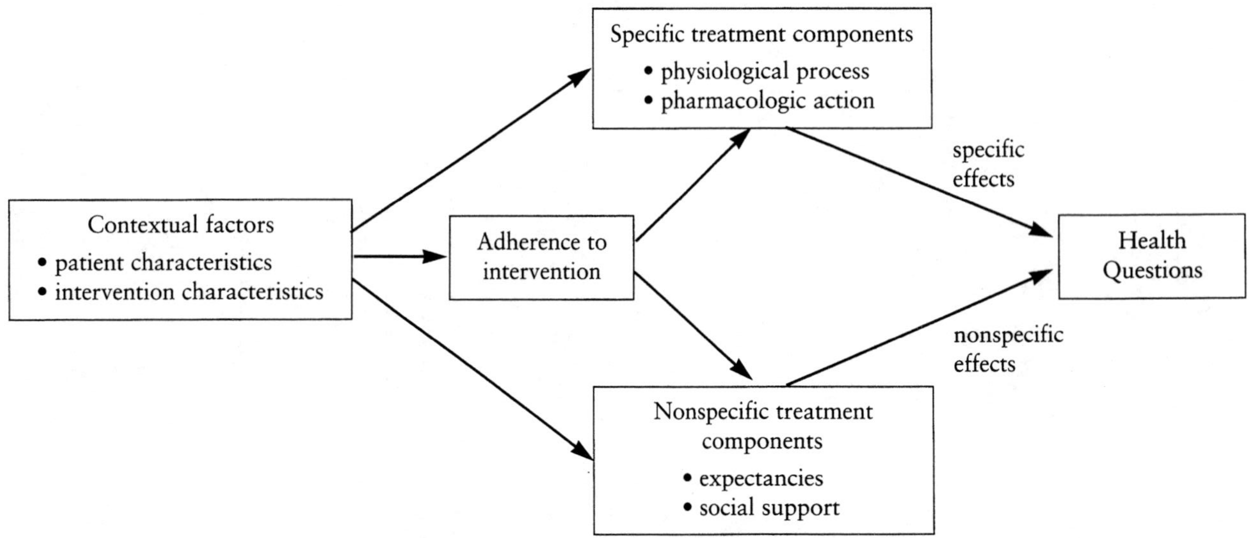

Figure 22.1 The effects of adherence on health outcomes.

health outcomes (Agras, Horne, & Taylor, 1982; Berkman, Leo-Summers, & Horwitz, 1992; Hovell et al., 1986; Williams et al., 1992). Thus, the perspective added by this model is that the expectancies and social support fostered by adherence may have an effect on health that is independent of any active treatment the patient may receive.

Finally, the literature indicates that nonspecific effects are influenced by some of the same factors known to influence adherence. These factors include patient characteristics (e.g., attitudes toward the provider, self-efficacy, and positive expectancies) and intervention characteristics (e.g., therapeutic setting, provider characteristics, treatment cost, and method of treatment delivery). Figure 22.1 shows these characteristics as having effects on adherence and on nonspecific treatment components; in addition, patient characteristics can directly influence specific treatment effects (e.g., due to individual differences in sensitivity to the therapeutic agent).

OVERVIEW OF THE PLACEBO EFFECT

Shapiro and Shapiro (1984, p. 372) define a placebo as

> any therapy or component of therapy that is deliberately used for its nonspecific, psychological, or psychophysiological effect, or that is used for its presumed specific effect but is without specific activity for the condition being treated.

A placebo effect is defined as "the psychological or psychophysiological effect produced by placebos" (Shapiro & Shapiro, 1984, p. 372). This definition implies that active treatments may have placebo components and that the effects of specific therapies (i.e., nonplacebos) are often due to both placebo and nonplacebo effects (Shapiro & Shapiro, 1984).

Historically, the term "placebo" has referred to inactive pills or tablets given to control subjects in drug trials. Over time, however, the term "placebo effect" has come to refer to a variety of nonspecific effects on health outcomes that are integrally related to the delivery and monitoring of treatment but that are not attributable to the specific therapeutic agent under study. In this chapter, the terms "placebo" and "nonspecific" will be used interchangeably.

The nonspecific effects of treatments are well documented in the literature on medical and behavioral interventions. Placebo effects have been studied in medical conditions as diverse as pain (Peck & Coleman, 1991); ulcerative colitis (Meyers & Janowitz, 1989) and irritable bowel syndrome (Dobrilla, Imbimbo, Piazzi, & Benzi, 1990); and congestive heart failure (Archer & Leier, 1992; Packer, 1990). Beecher (1955), in his classic review of placebo responses in patients suffering a wide variety of illnesses, found that in 35% of patients (averaged across the studies), symptoms were "satisfactorily relieved" by the placebo.

Recently, placebo effects have received increased attention in clinical trials that have found greater than expected improvements in the health of participants in placebo control groups. In the area of hypertension control, for instance, a number of studies, including the Multiple Risk Factor Intervention Trial (Multiple Risk Factor Intervention Trial Research Group, 1982), the Hypertension Detection and Follow-up Program (Hypertension Detection and Follow-up Program Cooperative Group, 1979), and the Australian National Blood Pressure Study (Management Committee, 1980) have found reductions in blood pressure greater than would be expected due to regression toward the mean alone for usualcare or placebo control groups. Similar results have been reported for several other studies that compared the effects of behavioral treatments for hypertension (e.g., relaxation training, biofeedback, cognitive restructuring) with the effects of placebo treatment (e.g., flexibility training) or blood pressure monitoring alone (Agras et al., 1987; Chesney et al., 1987; Jacob et al., 1986; Ward et al., 1987). The results of these studies have stimulated inquiry into possible explanations for the significant improvements or changes found for control groups, and have focused attention on the impact of nonspecific and behavioral factors on control groups in clinical trial research (Kramer & Shapiro, 1984).

It is important to note that in the clinical trials mentioned above, as well as in other studies, nonspecific effects have been demonstrated to involve not only improvements in subjective symptoms, but also objectively measured cardiovascular risk factor and end-organ changes as well (Gould, Davies, Mann, Altman, & Raftery, 1981). Indeed, the physiological effects of placebos are acknowledged as being very powerful. Placebos can induce addiction and have been reported to be more effective than, or even to reverse the effects of, some pharmacologic agents (Shapiro & Shapiro, 1984). In addition, the range of physiological processes that have been shown to exhibit placebo effects are very broad and include inhibited gastric acid secretion, reduced adrenocortical activity, and decreased serum lipoproteins (Bush, 1974).

MECHANISMS OF THE PLACEBO EFFECT

The recognition that nonspecific treatment components may influence health outcomes raises questions regarding the mechanisms underlying these effects. Placebos are thought to exert their effects through both psychological and biological mechanisms (Wilkins, 1985).

Psychological Mechanisms

Models that focus on the psychological mechanisms underlying the placebo effect fall into two categories: (1) learning-theory models, which explain placebo effects as classical conditioning phenomena; and (2) cognitively oriented models, which emphasize the role of mental processes, such as expectancy.

Learning-Theory Models

Models based on a learning theory approach focus on the placebo effect as a conditioned response. According to this explanation, the complex of stimuli surrounding the administration of a drug (e.g., taking a pill) become conditioned stimuli because of their repeated association with drug administration and relief from suffering during the person's developmental history (Wickramasekera, 1985). For example, a patient who derives pain relief from aspirin may eventually respond in a similar fashion to medications with similar characteristics (e.g., small, white pills). Support for the learning-theory model involves mostly animal research, which has confirmed the conditioning of physiologic and pharmacologic responses as an important element in placebo phenomena (Ader, 1985). This model is useful in explaining placebo effects associated with the administration of drugs; however, it is less applicable to situations involving nonpharmacologic treatments, such as behavioral or lifestyle interventions.

Cognitive Models

Currently, the most widely accepted cognitively based explanation for the placebo effect is that it is based on people's expectations of therapeutic benefit or success. The expectancy model of placebo effects is similar to an early cognitively based hypothesis that postulated a relationship between individuals' responses to placebo and their suggestibility. However, although it is commonly believed that individuals who score high on measures of suggestibility are more prone to the placebo response, no consistent relationship has been found between this response and either suggestibility or hypnotizability (Evans, 1985).

Another early cognitive model of placebo effects involved anxiety reduction, resulting from an individual's belief in the pain-reducing effects of a treatment. According to this model, placebo effects are attributable to decreased perceptions of pain and distress associated with anxiety reduction. This hypothesis was supported by studies showing that for chronically anxious individuals, feelings of reduced anxiety following placebo ingestion lead to a significant increase in pain tolerance (Evans, 1985). While the anxiety-reduction hypothesis addresses the effects of placebos on pain, it does not generalize easily to the many other physiological processes affected by placebos.

More recently, studies have shown that individuals' expectations regarding the effects of a drug or treatment influence their responses to placebo treatments. For example, study participants who received a caffeine placebo and were led to expect improved performance on a psychomotor task showed improved performance relative to participants who received the caffeine placebo and were told they could expect impairment (Fillmore, Mulvihill, & Vogel-Sprott, 1994). Similarly, the belief that alcohol has been consumed and expectations about the effects of alcohol have been shown to influence a variety of responses to consumption of nonalcoholic beverages, including pain reduction (Cutter, Maloof, Kurtz, & Jones, 1976) and alcohol craving (Ludwig, Wikler, & Stark, 1974). Study participants given placebos that were described as analgesics have also reported less pain than no-treatment controls (Gelfand, Ullman, & Krasner, 1963; Liberman, 1964), and the content of placebo instructions has been found to be a powerful influence on study participants' responses to dental pain (Gryll & Katahn, 1978). Other studies have demonstrated changes in physiological responses such as blood pressure and pulse rate based on participants' expectancies about the effects of the placebo being administered (Kirsch & Weixel, 1988). M. Ross & Olson (1981), in an examination of double-blind drug outcome studies, conclude that participants' expectancies are key determinants of placebo responses, and that participants provided placebos will respond in ways that are congruent with expected symptoms or physical responses.

Studies in clinical settings have also shown that responses to treatment are mediated by patient expectancies generated within the therapeutic relationship. In one study, students who expected a relaxation procedure to produce an immediate lowering of blood pressure had significantly lower systolic blood pressures immediately following the procedure than did a group of participants who were led to believe that the relaxation training would produce a delayed effect (Agras et al., 1982). In contrast, Wadden (1984) found no differences in blood pressure reduction between participants assigned to a cognitive-therapy condition, which involved a positive expectancy of blood pressure change, and those assigned to relaxation therapy. Results from several other studies, however, suggest that the effects of relaxation therapy may be primarily due to nonspecific factors, such as positive expectancy or social support (Brauer, Horlick, Nelson, Farquhar, & Agras, 1979; Luborsky et al., 1982).

Evidence suggests that the placebo effect is influenced not only by patient expectancies but by doctor or experimenter expectations. For example, when the physician believes a powerful drug is being used in a double-blind study, the placebo effect is stronger than if he or she believes the medication is less effective (Evans,1985). Thus, the physician's belief about a drug's efficacy may be communicated to the patient, and appears to mediate treatment effectiveness.

An individual's expectations about treatment success may be influenced by a variety of factors. For example, the social support received from family, friends, and health providers may enhance patients' beliefs or expectations about the efficacy of therapy. When a spouse is supportive of the patient receiving a specific form of therapy, the patient may come to believe such therapy will be beneficial. The effect of social support from members of a patient's network can be especially powerful when those others are seen as credible sources of information and when the patient has a great deal of faith in them. Plotkin (1985) emphasizes the impact of the patients' faith in the therapist as an important condition for behavioral change to occur in therapy.

The powerful influence of social support on health outcomes, including morbidity and mortality, is now well-documented (Berkman et al., 1992; Williams et al., 1992). Given these effects, one might expect that supportive interactions with health care personnel might influence response to treatment. One study demonstrated a positive effect for personalized care, operationalized as greater personal attention and warmth shown to the patient, on blood-pressure reduction in hypertensive patients (Hovell et al., 1986). In this study, patients receiving personalized care differed significantly in the magnitude of their blood-pressure reductions from those receiving usual care. Several other studies have documented similar effects for personalized versus usual care, although the mechanisms for such effects remain unknown (Dunbar, Marshall, & Hovell, 1979; Finnerty, Mattie, & Finnerty, 1973). Hovell et al. (1986) speculate that personalized care may evoke a generalized relaxation response, and suggest that future research is needed to determine the mechanisms underlying the effects of social support on blood pressure reduction.

Biological Models

There have been few attempts to investigate the ways in which psychological processes, such as expectancy, translate into the physiological changes observed in placebo phenomena. Levine, Gordon, and Fields (1978) hypothesize that placebo effects are based on biochemical processes that produce psychological and somatic changes. According to their model, placebo expectancies activate the endorphin system, which reduces pain. Evidence supporting this model includes several studies showing that with dental postoperative pain, naloxone (an opiate antagonist that blocks the release of endorphins) counteracts placebo-induced analgesia (Levine, Gordon, & Fields, 1978, 1979). Further research is needed on the biological bases of the placebo effect, using both pain and nonpain paradigms, since the existing literature in this area has been criticized for methodological problems and failure to replicate (Gracely, Wolshee, Deeter, & Dubner, 1982; Grevert & Goldstein, 1977, 1978; Mihic & Binkert, 1978).

ADHERENCE AND THE PLACEBO EFFECT

Returning to the thesis outlined earlier that adherence may activate or enhance placebo effects, how might adherence influence these effects? There are two leading explanations: (1) that adherence per se activates nonspecific components of treatment; or (2) certain characteristics of individuals who adhere to a treatment enhance the nonspecific components of treatment.

With the first explanation, given the hypothesis discussed in the previous section that expectancies of therapeutic benefit or success activate placebo effects, then any factor in a therapeutic situation that enhances such expectancies would indirectly influence placebo effects as well. Adherence to treatment may be one such factor, since adherence is integrally related to patient expectancies in a therapeutic situation.

Patient adherence to treatment is influenced by the expectation that the treatment will produce the desired effect (e.g., lower cholesterol, reduce weight). For example, individuals will be more likely to adhere to a low-calorie diet if they believe that doing so will be effective in producing weight loss *and* if they see themselves as capable of adhering to the diet. Bandura (1977) refers to the former belief as an outcome expectancy (the belief that a given behavior will lead to a particular outcome) and the latter as an efficacy expectation (the belief that one is capable of implementing the required behavior). According to Bandura (1977), success in a therapeutic situation is based on the acquisition of expectancies of increased personal effectiveness, or efficacy expectancies. High-efficacy expectancies are related to perseverance of effort at a task (e.g., adherence) and thus to maintenance of therapeutic improvement.

Thus, expectations about treatment effectiveness and one's ability to comply to a treatment are important determinants of actual adherence to treatment. However, as noted earlier, the relationship is reciprocal, since expectancies of success can also be a consequence of complying with treatment: the more one adheres to the treatment regimen, the more likely one is to expect treatment success. By complying with treatment, the patient enhances the expectation that the treatment will work. Adherence may also affect patients' generalized feelings of well-being and increase expectations that they can control other aspects of their lives, such as health-related behaviors (Epstein, 1984), ultimately leading to changes in these behaviors (e.g., quitting smoking, adhering to other medications, and adopting healthy dietary and exercise regimens). Expectancies of change and improvement are therefore important as both antecedents and consequences of adherence.

If this is true, then efforts to increase adherence (especially by enhancing expectancies of treatment success) may increase treatment effectiveness not only because they maximize the extent to which the patient receives active treatment, but also because these adherence-induced expectancies activate placebo responses to treatment. In the same way, social support may influence patients' beliefs or expectations about the efficacy of treatment and thus influence nonspecific treatment responses.

The second explanation of how adherence influences placebo effects—that there are certain characteristics of adherers that activate nonspecific components of treatment—may also be based on an expectancy effect. For example, if adherers are more likely to have an enhanced sense of control over events in their lives, and therefore more likely to believe that they can affect their health positively by complying to treatment, then treatment effectiveness may be due primarily to the greater expectancies for treatment success held by these individuals, rather than to the treatment itself. Other characteristics that differentiate adherers from nonadherers (e.g., "hardiness" or greater resiliency under stress; optimism) may also be important determinants of treatment success to the extent that they influence patient expectancies regarding treatment outcomes.

More adherent individuals may also be more likely to engage in a variety of health-related behaviors, such as adopting healthier diets and exercise regimens and avoiding stressors, than nonadherers. Adoption of these behaviors, which may increase expectations of better health, may also contribute to better medical outcomes in these individuals. Finally, Horwitz & Horwitz (1993) suggest that in individuals with chronic disease, adherence may reflect better adaptation to the stress of illness and an enhanced capability to respond to such stress. This enhanced adaptive response may itself generate both positive health-related behaviors and increased expectancies for treatment success, both of which may result in improvements in health.

IMPLICATIONS AND RESEARCH DIRECTIONS

There has been no research to date that adequately tests the model proposed in this chapter concerning the role that adherence may play in enhancing nonspecific treatment effects. This may be partly due to the lack of attention paid to nonspecific treatment components in health research. Although placebo effects are acknowledged as being of sufficient importance to necessitate the inclusion of placebo controls in most studies of medical or behavioral interventions, biomedical researchers have not made use of the placebo condition as an opportunity to examine and better understand the nonspecific effects of treatment. Placebos have traditionally been viewed as nuisance variables to be controlled for, or have been used to produce blinding (masking) of treatment groups, unrelated to expectations of nonspecific effects. They are rarely if ever viewed as important for study in their own right or as important adjuncts to active treatment (Evans, 1985).

This is in contrast to the emphasis on nonspecific factors in psychotherapy outcome studies (Frank, 1971; Garfield, 1980, 1982; Smith, Glass, & Miller, 1980; Stone, Imber, & Frank, 1966). In this literature, psychotherapy researchers have identified a number of nonspecific factors, or "common ingredients," as being important contributors to positive therapy outcomes, regardless of the particular mode of therapy used (Garfield,1982). The nonspecific factor thought to be most central to therapeutic outcome is the patient's expectation of benefit (Frank, 1961, 1983; Garfield, 1982; Goldstein, 1962), which has also been implicated as an important mechanism underlying placebo effects.

The model presented in this chapter suggests that adherence to treatment may affect health outcomes by enhancing or activating nonspecific effects of treatment (e.g., expectancies, social support). This has important implications for clinical trials and other research studies involving interventions, since there are several situations in which such adherence-induced placebo effects could lead to inaccurate conclusions about treatment efficacy.

While placebo control conditions are commonly used in studies involving the evaluation of drug therapies, studies evaluating other types of interventions (especially behavioral or lifestyle interventions) often do not use placebo conditions or use inadequate placebo controls. This is due to the difficulty in designing a placebo control condition when the treatment is behavioral in nature. When the treatment is pharmacological, it is possible to manufacture a pill that is identical in every respect (e.g., in appearance) to the pharmacological agent being used. But it is often difficult to devise a placebo for a behavioral treatment that is identical to the treatment itself in every way except that it has no active component (Buck & Donner, 1982). Clearly, given the possibility that adherence to an intervention may affect the evaluation of a treatment's effectiveness, the design of placebo conditions for all studies involving patient adherence to some intervention—whether behavioral or pharmacological in nature—should be given serious consideration.

Problems may arise even when adequate placebo controls are used if adherence rates differ between the treatment and control groups. One reason for different adherence rates that could influence patient expectancies regarding treatment success (and therefore affect treatment effectiveness via those expectancies) is that some patients receiving treatment who are particularly sensitive to physiological cues and sensations might interpret the presence or absence of such sensations as indicating whether or not they are receiving the active treatment (Wilkins, 1985). Because patients in the active treatment group would be more likely to become "unblinded" in this way, and therefore more likely to adhere to treatment and to expect a successful outcome, it would be difficult to pull apart the actual treatment effect from an expectancy-induced effect. In this case, a more positive outcome for the treatment group could be inaccurately attributed to treatment efficacy when it was actually due to increased expectations of treatment success. This suggests that adherence rates between the treatment and placebo conditions should always be assessed to rule out the possibility that adherence-induced placebo effects are responsible for any effects found.

The model presented in this chapter has implications not only for the internal validity of studies that involve adherence to interventions, but also for the generalizabiliy of such studies. For example, one disadvantage of prerandomization screening (also known as the "run-in" phase of a clinical trial) is that by screening out nonadherers, any effects found for a particular treatment can only be generalized to those individuals who are likely to adhere to a treatment regimen. Since these individuals may have certain psychosocial characteristics that affect their adherence behavior (e.g., high self-efficacy) and that may also affect treatment success, the finding of a treatment effect would be applicable only to a narrow subgroup of patients —those who adhere to treatment. More studies are needed of the characteristics of nonadherers, and the ways in which they are similar to or differ from good adherers, to determine whether the results of studies using "run-ins" can be generalized to those individuals who are typically less adherent.

Future research should attempt to: (1) determine whether adherence-induced expectancies do in fact activate placebo effects; and (2) identify and evaluate aspects of the act of adherence or characteristics of those that comply that may enhance placebo effects. Furthermore, clinical trials and other studies that evaluate the effects of interventions should use designs that allow researchers to partial out or control for these effects. Rosenthal (1985) and S. Ross & Buckalew (1985) suggest experimental designs that can be used to better understand how nonspecific effects may impact on evaluations of treatment effectiveness.

A method that may help clarify whether or not patient expectancies are mediating the effects of adherence on mortality and morbidity is a causal modeling approach that tests the effect of adherence on health outcomes directly and indirectly (via expectancy as a mediating variable). Aspects of the model presented in this chapter can also be tested experimentally. Examples of this approach include laboratory studies in which participants' expectations about the effects of a particular treatment are manipulated (see Agras et al., 1982; Fillmore et al., 1994; Kirsch & Weixel, 1988). A classic design in this regard is the balanced placebo design proposed by Marlatt & Rohsenow (1980), which allows independent evaluation of drug effects, expectancy effects, and their interaction. Design of studies to include a placebo and nonplacebo control group may also clarify expectancy effects.

An implication of the research presented here is that treatment effects in placebo-controlled trials may be conservative, since nonspecific benefits occur in both groups which would add to a treatment's benefit in clinical practice. Recently, some behavioral and biomedical researchers have called for increased attempts to understand and harness the power of the placebo effect to benefit patients in clinical practice settings (Benson & Friedman, 1996; Chaput de Saintonge & Herxheimer, 1994; Connelly, 1991). Clearly, more attention should be focused on the role of nonspecific factors in health-related research, similar to the prominent role given to such factors in psychotherapy outcome research (Garfield, 1982). Perhaps certain components of healthcare interventions, such as enhanced expectations of benefit or the perceived social support available from the healthcare provider, are "common ingredients" that enhance health-related outcomes, regardless of the treatment or disease process involved. Future research should focus on identifying such common ingredients and using them to increase the effectiveness of health-related interventions.

REFERENCES

Ader, R. (1985). Conditioned immunopharmacological effects in animals: Implications for a conditioning model of pharmacotherapy. In I. L. White, B. Tursky, & G. E. Schwartz (Eds.) *Placebo: Theory, research and mechanisms* (pp. 306–331). New York: Guilford Press.

Agras, W. S., Horne, M., & Taylor, C. B. (1982). Expectation and blood pressure-lowering effects of relaxation. *Psychosomatic Medicine, 44*, 389–395.

Agras, W. S., Taylor, C. B., Kraemer, H. C., Southam, M. A., & Schneider, O. A. (1987). Relaxation training for essential hypertension at the worksite: II. The poorly controlled hypertensive. *Psychosomatic Medicine, 49*, 264–273.

Ahern, D. K., Gorkin, L., Anderson, J. L., Tierney, C., Hallstrom, A., Ewart, C., Capone, R. J., Schron, E., Kornfeld, D., & Herd, J. A. (1990). Biobehavioral variables and mortality or cardiac arrest in the Cardiac Arrhythmia Pilot Study (CAPS). *American Journal of Cardiology, 66*, 59–62.

Archer, T. P., & Leier, C. V. (1992). Placebo treatment in congestive heart failure. *Cardiology, 81*, 125–133.

Bandura, A. (1977). Self-efficacy: Toward a unifying theory of behavior change. *Psychological Review, 84*, 191–215.

Beecher, H. K. (1955). The powerful placebo. *Journal of the American Medical Association, 159*, 1602–1606.

Benson, H., & Friedman, R. (1996). Harnessing the power of the placebo effect and renaming it "remembered wellness." *Annual Review of Medicine, 47*, 193–199.

Berkman, L. F., Leo-Summers, L., & Horwitz, R. I. (1992). Emotional support and survival after myocardial infarction. *Annals of Internal Medicine, 117*, 1003–1009.

Blumenthal, J. A., Williams, R. S., Wallace, A. G., Williams, R. B., & Needles, T. L. (1982). Physiological and psychological variables predict compliance to prescribed exercise therapy in patients recovering from myocardial infarction. *Psychosomatic Medicine, 44*, 519–527.

Brauer, A. P., Horlick, L., Nelson, E., Farquhar, J. W., & Agras, W. S. (1979). Relaxation therapy for essential hypertension. *Journal of Behavioral Medicine, 2*, 21–29.

Buck, C., & Donner, A. (1982). The design of controlled experiments in the evaluation of non-therapeutic interventions. *Journal of Chronic Diseases, 35*, 531–538.

Bush, P. J. (1974). The placebo effect. *Journal of the American Pharmaceutical Association, NS14*, 671–672.

Carney, R. M., Rich, M. W., Freedland, K. E., Saini, J., teVelde, A., Simeone, C., & Clark, K. (1988). Major depressive disorder predicts cardiac events in patients with coronary artery disease. *Psychosomatic Medicine, 50*, 627–633.

Chaput de Saintonge, D. M., & Herxheimer, A. (1994). Harnessing placebo effects in health care. *The Lancet, 344*, 995–998.

Chesney, M. A., Black, G. W., Swan, G. E., & Ward, M. M. (1987). Relaxation training for essential hypertension at the worksite: 1. The untreated mild hypertensive. *Psychosomatic Medicine, 49*, 250–263.

Connelly, R. J. (1991). Nursing responsibility for the placebo effect. *The Journal of Medicine and Philosophy, 16*, 325–341.

Coronary Drug Project Research Group. (1980). Influence of adherence to treatment and response of cholesterol on mortality in the Coronary Drug Project. *New England Journal of Medicine, 18*, 1038–1041.

Cutter, H. S., Maloof, B., Kurtz, N. R., & Jones, W. C. (1976). "Feeling no pain:" Differential responses to pain by alcoholics and non-alcoholics before and after drinking. *Journal of Studies on Alcohol, 37*, 273–277.

Dobrilla, G., Imbimbo, B. P., Piazzi, L., & Benzi, G. (1990). Long-term treatment of irritable bowel syndrome with cimetropium bromide: A double-blind placebo controlled clinical trial. *Gut, 31*, 355–358.

Dolin, R., Reichman, R. C., Madore, H. P., Maynard, R., Linton, P. N., & Webber-Jones, J. (1982). A controlled trial of amantadine and rimantadine in the prophylaxis of influenza A infection. *New England Journal of Medicine, 307*, 580–583.

Dunbar, J., Marshall, G., & Hovell, M. (1979). Behavioral interventions in compliance. In R. B. Haynes, D. W. Taylor, & D. L. Sackett (Eds.), *Compliance with therapeutic and preventive regimens*, (pp. 174–190). Baltimore, MD: Johns Hopkins University Press.

Epstein, L. (1984). The direct effects of compliance on health outcome. *Health Psychology, 3*, 385–393.

Evans, F. J. (1985). Expectancy, therapeutic instructions and the placebo response. In L. White, B. Tursky, & G. E. Schwartz (Eds.), *Placebo: Theory, research and mechanisms* (pp. 215–278). New York: Guilford.

Fillmore, M. T., Mulvihill, L. E., & Vogel-Sprott, M. (1994). The expected drug and its expected effect interact to determine placebo responses to alcohol and caffeine. *Psychopharmacology, 115*, 383–388.

Finnerty, F. A., Jr., Mattie, E. C., & Finnery, E. A., III. (1973). Hypertension in the inner city: I. Analysis of clinic dropouts. *Circulation, 47*, 73–75.

Frank, J. D. (1961). *Persuasion and healing: A comparative study of psychotherapy*. Baltimore, MD: Johns Hopkins University Press.

Frank, J. D. (1971). Therapeutic factors in psychotherapy. *American Journal of Psychotherapy, 25*, 350–361.

Frank, J. D. (1983). The placebo is psychotherapy. *Behavioral and Brain Sciences, 6*, 291–292.

Frasure-Smith, N., Lesperance, F., & Talajic, M. (1993). Depression following myocardial infarction: Impact on 6-month survival. *Journal of the American Medical Association, 270*, 1819–1825.

Friedman, L., Furberg, C., & DeMets, D. (1996). *Fundamentals of clinical trials*. St. Louis, MO: Mosby-Year Book.

Garfield, S. L. (1980). *Psychotherapy: An eclectic approach*. New York: Wiley.

Garfield, S. L. (1982). Eclecticism and integration in psychotherapy. *Behavior Therapy, 13*, 610–623.

Gelfand, S., Ullman, L. P. & Krasner, L. (1963). The placebo response: An experimental approach. *Journal of Nervous and Mental Disorders, 136*, 379–387.

Goldstein, A. P. (1962). *Therapist-patient expectancies in psychotherapy*. New York Macmillan.

Gould, B. A., Davies, A. B., Mann, S., Altman, D. G., & Raftery, E. B. (1981) Does placebo lower blood pressure? *Lancet, ii*, 1377–1381.

Gracely, R. H., Wolshee, P. J., Deeter, W. R., & Dubner, R. (1982). Natural and placebo alter postsurgical pain by independent mechanisms. *Society for Neuroservice Abstracts, 8*, 264.

Grevert, P., & Goldstein, A. (1977). Effects of naloxone on experimentally produced ischemic pain and on mood in human subjects. *Proceedings of the National Academy of Sciences USA, 74*, 1291–1294.

Grevert, P., & Goldstein, A. (1978). Endorphins: Naloxone fails to alter experimental pain or mood in humans. *Science, 199*, 1093–1095.

Gryll, S. L., & Katahn, M. (1978). Situational factors contributing to the placebo effect. *Psychopharmacology, 57*, 253–261.

Guiry, E., Conroy, R. M., Hickey, N., & Mulcahy, R. (1987). Psychological response to an acute coronary event and its effect on subsequent rehabilitation and lifestyle change. *Clinical Cardiology, 10*, 256–260.

Horwitz, R. I., & Horwitz, S. M. (1993). Adherence to treatment and health outcomes. *Archives of Internal Medicine, 153*, 1863–1868.

Horwitz, R. I., Viscoli, C. M., Berkman, L., Donaldson, R. M., Horwitz, S. M., Murray, C. J., Ransohoff, D. F., & Sindelar, J. (1990). Treatment adherence and risk of death after a myocardial infarction. *Lancet, 336*, 542–545.

Hovell, M. E., Black, D. R., Mewborn, C. R., Geary, D., Agras, W. S., Kamachi, K., Kirk, R., Walton, C., & Dawson, S. (1986). Personalized versus usual care of previously uncontrolled hypertensive patients: An exploratory analysis. *Preventive Medicine, 15*, 673–684.

Hypertension Detection and Follow-up Program Cooperative Group. (1979). Five year findings of the Hypertension Detection and Follow-up Program: I. Reduction in mortality of persons with high blood pressure, including mild hypertension. *Journal of the American Medical Association, 242*, 2562–2571.

Jacob, R. G., Shapiro, A. P., Reeves, R. A., Johnsen, A. M., McDonald, R. H., & Cobum, P. C. (1986). Relaxation therapy for hypertension: Comparison of effects with concomitant placebo, diuretic and beta blocker. *Archives of Internal Medicine, 146*, 2335–2340.

Kellet, J. M. (1990). Compliance and clinical trials in heart disease. *The Lancet, 336*, 1003.

Kirsch, I., & Weixel, L. J. (1988). Double-blind versus deceptive administration of a placebo. *Behavioral Neuroscience, 102*, 319–323.

Kramer, M. S., & Shapiro, S. H. (1984). Scientific challenges in the application of randomized trials. *Journal of the American Medical Association, 252*, 2739–2745.

Levine, J. D., Gordon, N. C., & Fields, H. L. (1978). The mechanism of placebo analgesia. *Lancet, 2*, 654–657.

Levine, J. D., Gordon, N. C., & Fields, H. L. (1979). Naloxone dose dependently produces analgesia and hyperalgesia in postoperative pain. *Nature, 278*, 740–741.

Levine, J. D., Gordon, N. C., Jones, R. T., & Fields, H. L. (1978). The narcotic antagonist naloxone enhances clinical pain. *Nature, 272*, 826–827.

Liberman, R. (1964). An experimental study of the placebo phenomenon under three different situations of pain. *Journal of Psychiatric Research, 2*, 233–246.

Luborsky, L., Crits-Christoph, P., Brady, J. P., Kron, R. E., Weiss, T., Cohen, M., & Levy, L. (1982). Behavioral versus pharmacological treatments for essential hypertension–A needed comparison. *Psychosomatic Medicine, 44*, 203–213.

Ludwig, A. M., Wikler, A., & Stark, L. H. (1974). The first drink: Psychological aspects of craving. *Archives of General Psychiatry, 30*, 539–547.

Management Committee. (1980). The Australian therapeutic trial in mild hypertension. *Lancet*, 1261–1267.

Marlatt, G. A., & Rohsenow, D. J. (1980). Cognitive processes in alcohol use: Expectancy and the balanced placebo design. In N. K. Mello (Ed.), *Advances in substance abuse: Behavioral and biological research* (pp. 159–199). Greenwich, CT: JAI.

Meyers, S., & Janowitz, H. D. (1989). The "natural history" of ulcerative colitis: an analysis of the placebo response. *Journal of Clinical Gastroenterology, 11*, 33–37.

Mihic, D., & Binkert, E. (1978). Is placebo analgesia mediated by endorphine? Paper presented at the Second World Congress on Pain, Montreal, Quebec August.

Multiple Risk Factor Intervention Trial Research Group. (1982). Multiple Risk Factor Intervention Trial: Risk factor changes and mortality results. *Journal of the American Medical Association, 248*, 1465–1477.

Packer, M. (1990). The placebo effect in heart failure. *American Heart Journal, 120*, 1579–1582.

Peck, C., & Coleman, G. (1991). Implications of placebo therapy for clinical research and practice in pain management. *Theoretical Medicine, 12*, 247–270.

Pizzo, P. A., Robichaud, K. J., Edwards, B. K., Schumaker, C., Kramer, B. S., & Johnson, A. (1983). Oral antibiotic prophylaxis in patients with cancer: A double-blind randomized placebo-controlled trial. *Journal of Pediatrics,102*, 125–133.

Pledger, G. W. (1992). Basic statistics: Importance of adherence. *Journal of Clinical Research in Pharmacoepidemiology, 6*, 77–81.

Plotkin, E. B. (1985). A psychological approach to placebo: The role of faith in therapy and treatment. In L. White, B. Tursky, & G. E. Schwartz (Eds.), *Placebo: Theory, research and mechanisms* (pp. 237–254). New York: Guilford.

Rosenthal, R. (1985). Designing, analyzing, interpreting and summarizing placebo studies. In L. White, B. Tursky, & G. E. Schwartz (Eds.), *Placebo: Theory, research and mechanisms* (pp. 110–136). New York: Guilford.

Ross, M., & Olson, J. M. (1981). An expectancy-attribution model of the effects of placebos. *Psychological Review, 88*, 408–437.

Ross, S., & Buckalew, L. W. (1985). Placebo agentry: Assessment of drug and placebo effects. In L. White, B. Tursky, & G. E. Schwartz (Eds.), *Placebo: Theory, research and mechanisms* (pp. 67–82). New York: Guilford.

Shapiro, A. K., & Shapiro, E. (1984). Patient-provider relationships and the placebo effect. In J. D. Matarazzo, S. M. Weiss, J. A Herd, N. E. Miller, & S. M. Weiss (Eds.), *Behavioral health: A handbook of health enhancement and disease prevention* (pp. 371–383). New York: Wiley.

Smith, M. L., Glass, E. V., & Miller, T. (1980). *The benefits of psychotherapy.* Baltimore, MD: Johns Hopkins University Press.

Stone, A. R., Imber, S. D., & Frank, J. D. (1966). The role of non-specific factors in short-term psychotherapy. *Australian Journal of Psychology, 18*, 210–217.

Verter, J., & Friedman, L. (1984). Adherence measures in the Aspirin Myocardial Infarction Study (AMIS). *Controlled Clinical Trials, 5*, 306.

Wadden, T. (1984). Relaxation therapy for essential hypenension: Specific or non-specific effects? *Journal of Psychosomatic Research, 28*, 53–61.

Ward, M. M., Swan, G. E., & Chesney, M. A. (1987). Arousal reduction treatments for mild hypertension: A meta-analysis of recent studies. In S. Julius (Ed.), *Handbook of hypertension. Volume 10. Behavioral factors in hypertension* (pp. 285–302). New York: Elsevier.

Wickramasekera, L. (1985). A conditioned response model of the placebo effect: Predictions from the model. In L. White, B. Tursky, & G. E. Schwartz (Eds.), *Placebo: Theory, research and mechanisms* (pp. 255–287). New York: Guilford.

Wilkins, W. (1985). Placebo controls and concepts in chemotherapy and psychotherapy research. In L. White, B. Tursky, & G. E. Schwartz (Eds.), *Placebo: Theory, research and mechanisms* (pp. 83–109). New York: Guilford.

Williams, R. B, Barefoot, J. C., Califf, R. M., Haney, T. L., Saunders, W. B., Pryor, D. B., Hlattky, M. A., Siegler, I. C. & Mark, D. B. (1992). *Journal of the American Medical Association, 267*, 520–524.

23

Collaboration Between Professionals and Mediating Structures in the Community: Toward a "Third Way" in Health Promotion

Kurt M. Ribisl and Keith Humphreys

Many of the chapters in this volume address how professionals can encourage adherence to their health promotion and medical recommendations. Like all health promotion issues, adherence occurs in a philosophical context and is defined as a problem because of a corresponding set of assumptions about how professionals and citizens should interact. The purpose of this chapter is to illuminate the philosophical context in which adherence and other health promotion issues are debated. Particularly, this chapter discusses the philosophical issue of whether health is primarily a personal responsibility or a societal obligation (Beauchamp, 1980, 1987; Charlton, 1993; Kilwein, 1989; Rosenstock, 1990; Wikler, 1987). One extreme viewpoint on this issue is health-promotion paternalism, in which the behavioral

We thank Todd Rogers, C. Barr Taylor, and the members of the VA/Stanford Writing Seminar for helpful comments on these ideas. Preparation of this manuscript was supported by Public Health Service Grant No. F32 CA 69731 from the National Cancer Institute (Kurt M. Ribisl) and the Veterans Affairs Mental Health Strategic Health Group (Keith Humphreys).

prescriptions of health experts should be adhered to even if this involves sacrifices in the freedom of citizens to eat, drink, smoke, and live as they wish (e.g., Terris, 1980). The contrasting extreme is "rugged individualism" (e.g., Ardell, 1977; Kass, 1975) in which health is viewed as a direct consequence of personal lifestyle decisions that should be made freely, rather than in adherence to outside expert opinion. Both of these ends of a philosophical continuum have generally been rejected, leaving most health-promotion professionals looking for a "third way" that transcends the limitations of each extreme. In this paper, we offer one proposal for a third way: Collaboration between health promotion professionals and mediating structures in the community.

PHILOSOPHICAL CONTEXT

We begin our discussion with two extreme views on responsibility for health, which we label "rugged individualism" and "paternalism." Although neither view is particularly compelling in its pure form, some analysis of each is warranted because each has positive elements that could be integrated into a "third way" of health promotion. Rugged individualism is a quintessentially American ideal (Bellah, Madsen, Sullivan, Swidler, & Tipton, 1985) in which each citizen is given maximal personal freedom and expected to accept the consequences of how that freedom is used. In the area of health, extreme rugged individualism implies that diet, exercise, smoking, drinking and other health habits should not be subjected to outside intervention (e.g., mandatory motorcycle helmet laws, steep tax increases on alcohol). Further, society's responsibility to help unhealthy people is minimized by attributing poor health to individual decisions and individual failings (e.g., lack of willpower). Thus, reliance on purely self-directed behavior change reflects a ruggedly individualistic approach.

Paternalism is the philosophical counterpoint to rugged individualism. In its extreme form, paternalism holds that experts have a moral responsibility to identify and solve health problems because individuals and communities lack the experience or ability to effect change. Extensive interventions by professionals and policymakers into individuals' lives without their input is justified in the name of the health of society as a whole, which is considered a widely agreed-upon public good. The proper role of citizens in this framework is simply to adhere to the policies and advice of health professionals. This framework generally views unhealthy people as victims of circumstances who should not be blamed for their problems.

There is little point in arguing the extreme views of rugged individualism and paternalism; both are "straw men." However, both philosophies contain some compelling elements that merit inclusion in a "third way" of thinking about health promotion. Here, we restrict our focus to a comparison of the philosophies in four areas: (1) Sharing of control between professionals and the community; (2) Respect for diversity in health decisions; (3) Social compassion, and (4) Utilization of scientific knowledge. We focus on these areas because they seem important criteria of evaluation for health-promotion efforts, and because they illuminate how the two philosophies' strengths and weaknesses mirror each other.

STRENGTHS OF RUGGED INDIVIDUALISM

Sharing of Control of Health Promotion

Rugged individualists insist that those in need of altering their health behavior should have a large measure of control over what behaviors are deemed problematic and how they are addressed. Rugged individualism's insistence on democratic control of health serves an important function, because even well-meaning interventions by health professionals into others' lives can result in unintended negative consequences (Biglan, 1995). For example, Becker (1986) has noted that several health-promotion recommendations made by experts (e.g., ideal weight, proper cholesterol intake, moderate alcohol consumption) have later been withdrawn or altered because they proved either of no benefit or harmful. Hence, the skepticism embodied in the rugged individualist's philosophy against toward blindly following "expert" advice is warranted.

Additionally, keeping some control for health in the hands of those desiring behavior change is beneficial, because it can enhance the sense of efficacy that leads to positive health changes (Bandura, 1986). Both the perception and experience of personal control increase individuals' abilities to change their behaviors (Kanfer & Scheft, 1988). Thus, if the public believes in a rugged individualistic philosophy of health promotion, they may have more faith in their ability, and hence more success, at implementing health-behavior changes in their own lives. Lastly, if experts design and completely control a health intervention, as might happen under an extremely paternalistic philosophy, the intervention and its effects typically fade from view shortly after the professional moves on to a new problem (Green & Kreuter, 1991).

Allowing for Diversity in Health Decisions

Rugged individualism respects diverse views of the importance (or unimportance) of health, what constitutes good health, and how good health can be achieved and promoted. Rugged individualism places great stock in the freedom of ordinary citizens, and, perhaps most importantly, is the freedom to be different from others. In contrast, paternalist health-promotion efforts can disregard diversity by imposing solutions for health on a society that force some of the population to trade off other aspects of life that are more important to them (Charlton, 1993; Fuchs, 1974). That is, rugged individualists recognize that for some people, the utilities or benefits associated with unhealthy pleasures override the utilities associated with health. A pluralistic democracy allows for diverse value systems, including one in which individuals can decide that they prefer marbled steak, a bottle of merlot, and an imported cigar over the possibility of reduced cardiovascular morbidity.

STRENGTHS OF PATERNALISM

Social Compassion

Evaluating health-promotion efforts regarding social compassion involves asking questions like: "How harsh is this approach on people who have trouble changing?"; "Does this intervention have a prosocial orientation?"; and "Does this intervention reach out to people who are experiencing difficulty?" Health paternalism stands up well under such criteria.

Paternalistic health-promotion efforts are usually intended to reduce health disparities between different segments of society, which is desirable from many perspectives on social justice (Beauchamp, 1980). For example, the paternalistic intervention mentioned by Terris (1980) of outlawing saturated fats in baked goods would provide comparable health benefits to all consumers of baked goods. In contrast, voluntary individually focused health recommendations (e.g., diet guidelines) tend to be most beneficial for well-educated, literate, and already healthy people, and thus may distribute health benefits unequally.

Paternalism is also socially compassionate because it recognizes the limits of individual control and the power of environmental influences on health-related behaviors (Brownell, Marlatt, Lichtenstein, & Wilson, 1986). Because they recognize that unhealthy people are often victims of circumstance, paternalists are less likely than rugged individualists to misdirect health-behavior change efforts at the individual level when the problem is more heavily influenced by environmental factors (e.g., social pressure, poverty, or seductive advertising).

Lastly, health-behavior change may be easier to achieve, more prosocial in orientation, and simply more fun if it is not solely an individual activity. A society full of rugged individuals doing solitary push-ups in their private exercise rooms seems a dubious goal.

Use of Scientific Knowledge

Professionals have developed a powerful scientific base in health psychology and public health that can guide the health behavior change process. Another strength of paternalistic health-promotion efforts is that they are usually informed by that knowledge base, because paternalistic programs are typically implemented by experts who have some scientific grounding in health issues. In contrast, rugged individualism leaves individuals to seek out their own health information. This can lead individuals to engage in health behaviors whose effectiveness or ineffectiveness is hard to see at an individual level, but could be clearly demonstrated in a scientific study of a representative sample (e.g., attempting to follow a diet published in a supermarket tabloid).

SUMMARY

To summarize the strengths and weaknesses of each philosophy, rugged individualism serves to promote shared control of health promotion and respect for diversity, but can be a socially harsh and uninformed approach to health. In contrast, paternalistic approaches tend to be guided by social concern and scientific knowledge, but can deprive individuals of control of their lives and force a "one-size-fits-all" approach that does not respect diversity. An ideal "third way" would avoid the liabilities of each philosophical extreme and would combine the strengths of the two philosophies by maximizing participant control, allowing for diversity in health decisions, being socially compassionate, and using scientific knowledge to full advantage. We now turn to how health promotion initiatives can measure up to this formidable challenge.

COLLABORATING WITH MEDIATING STRUCTURES

Mediating structures are organizations and institutions that stand between individuals' private lives and the larger institutions of public life (Berger & Neuhaus, 1977). Examples of mediating structures are churches, families, voluntary associations, and neighborhoods. Mediating structures can be contrasted with larger, more impersonal institutions, such as the government, capitalist enterprise, and bureaucracies such as the school system, which are often alienating to ordinary people not only because of their size, but because they are perceived to be controlled by powerful and nonresponsive others (Berger & Neuhaus, 1977).

Several writers (Eng & Hatch, 1991; McLeroy, Bibeau, Steckler & Glanz,

1988; Robertson & Minkler, 1994; Steckler et al., 1995) have acknowledged the potential role of mediating structures in promoting health. Our focus here is to urge health-promotion practitioners and researchers to view mediating structures not merely as convenient intervention sites, but as entities worthy of collaboration. Similarly, Eng and Hatch (1991) noted that African American churches are more than just handy recruiting centers for people with health problems; within the church there exists a social support system that can be readily linked with the professional service delivery system, and these linkages can shift the dynamics from a provider-client mode to more of a group-collaborator mode.

Collaboration with mediating structures by health-promotion professionals has the potential to combine the strengths of the two philosophies described above, and to minimize their drawbacks. Because mediating structures involve collective activity that is entirely or primarily voluntary, they increase the freedom and power of their members. This makes it more likely that health-promotion efforts conducted in collaboration with the community will leave some control in the hands of the community. Also, because the mediating structure has its own "center of gravity," consultation and advice by a professional will less easily turn into a controlling relationship. Generally, there is less potential for outside coercion or exploitation and greater potential for sustainability when community members and institutions are actively involved in shaping interventions (Altman, 1995; Green & Kreuter, 1991; Stokols, 1992).

Diversity in health decisions can be easily achieved through collaboration with mediating structures. Unlike paternalistic interventions, that take a "one-size-fits-all" approach to health promotion, the same community may produce multiple mediating structures that attack a given health problem in different ways. For example, one community with a high incidence of HIV infection may have a community coalition of gay activists who advocate for better medications and health care, a group of ministers who reinvigorate the standards of monogamy and premarital abstinence with their parishioners, and a group of former heroin-dependent people who start a storefront peer-counseling and needle-exchange program.

Collaboration with mediating structures also offers some of the benefits associated with paternalism, such as a prosocial orientation. By definition, creation of a mediating structure overrides the concept of harsh, rugged individualism. That is, mediating structures involve social activity in the context of which health and better living generally can be humanely promoted. Further, because mediating structures involve many individuals, knowledge can be disseminated and applied more efficiently than in one-on-one encounters with individuals who have health-behavior problems.

Collaboration with mediating structures has the potential to improve health-promotion practice by serving as a conduit between individual- and population-based approaches to health promotion. In the last two decades, there has been greater awareness of the need for ensuring community involvement in defining and solving health problems (Flynn, Ray, & Rider, 1994; Green & McAlister, 1994). Prior to this time, many health-promotion efforts were focused on either individual behavior (health psychology) or on larger population-based (public health) strategies (Roberts, 1989; Winett, King, & Altman, 1989). Dissatisfaction with these disparate micro- and macro-level approaches has spurred several theorists to propose multi-level ecological models that seek to bridge the gap between the health psychology and public health models (Abrams, Elder, Carleton, Lasater, & Artz, 1986; Kersell & Milsum, 1985; McLeroy et al., 1988; Roberts, 1989; Stokols, 1992; Winett et al., 1989). Although these theoretical developments have provided a more comprehensive and unified conceptualization of health promotion, progress still needs to be made in the implementation of integrated multi-level (e.g., individual, social, policy) intervention strategies. For instance, evaluations from recent multi-level intervention strategies have thus far produced only modest results (COMMIT Research Group, 1995; Glasgow, Terborg, Hollis, Severson, & Boles, 1995; Glasgow et al., 1994), though as our understanding of multi-level interventions becomes more sophisticated, their impact could be greater. Just as early health-promotion theory had gaps between individual- and system-level approaches, health-promotion intervention practice has gaps that may be filled partially by greater collaboration with mediating structures.

Green and Raeburn (1990) argued persuasively that the new focus of attention for health promotion should be engaging the community in a more participatory way, with a focus on enabling community groups or mediating structures. Certainly, it is not new to rely on mediating structures such as voluntary health associations or grassroots coalitions to ameliorate health problems; nevertheless, we suggest there are several types of mediating structures that deserve greater attention (e.g., mutual help groups, the Internet) or could be collaborated with more closely (e.g., churches). Further, mediating structures are more commonly used as convenient intervention settings than as active collaborators in the health-promotion process. We now turn to a discussion of promising programs for improving health in collaboration with four types of mediating structures: mutual help organizations, the Internet, community coalitions, and religious organizations. Although this is only a partial account of the many mediating structures in our society, it provides practical illustrations of the value of collaborating with them in health promotion efforts.

Mutual Help Groups

Mutual help groups (also known as self-help groups) are peer-led, voluntary associations of people who share some status that results in difficulties that the group tries to address. A large proportion of mutual help groups focus on health-related issues, such as smoking, alcoholism, obesity, diabetes, sexually transmitted diseases, multiple sclerosis, and depression, to name just a few (for a comprehensive listing, see White & Madara, 1995). Approximately 10 million Americans participated in mutual help groups in the past year (Kessler, Mickelson, & Zhao, 1997), indicating that these organizations have become a significant mediating structure in American society. Although health professionals have helped create or otherwise assisted some mutual help organizations, ultimate control of these organizations lies with their members.

Both narrative reviews (e.g., Humphreys & Rappaport, 1994; Kurtz, 1990; Kyrouz and Humphreys, 1996; Lieberman, 1986) and meta-analyses (e.g., Emrick, Tonigan, Montgomery, & Little, 1993) of the literature on mutual help groups have concluded that they generally have favorable effects on participants. This conclusion applies both to health status per se (e.g., weight loss among obese people, reduced drinking by alcoholic individuals) and other areas (e.g., life satisfaction, enhanced friendship networks, reduced stigma).

Given their goal of improving individual and community health, one might expect that public health researchers and health psychologists would show great interest in mutual help organizations. Although some health professionals refer patients to self-help groups, as yet health promotion professionals have generally shown little interest in the self-help group movement. Inspection of the citation lists of the major reviews of the mutual-help literature reveals numerous reports in journals within community, counseling, and developmental psychology; gerontology; psychiatry; social work; sociology, and substance abuse, but scarcely an article in leading health journals such as the *American Journal of Public Health, Health Education Quarterly*, or *Health Psychology*. Also, popular health promotion texts (Breckon, Harvey, & Lancaster, 1994; Green & Kreuter, 1991) have little, if any, discussion of the potential roles for mutual help groups. Taylor and Stunkard's (1993) recent assertion that in the area of weight control, the full potential of lay-led mutual help groups may not have been realized in the United States applies equally well to a variety of other health problems.

One instructive exception to this general pattern was recently reported by Simmons (1992), who was one of a group of health-promotion workers in the Coventry Diabetes Study who facilitated a successful collaboration with a mutual help group. The project was conducted in England in a community with a large population of people who had immigrated from South Asia. The staff of the Coventry Diabetic Study conducted a house-to-house survey of residents to ascertain the prevalence of diabetes. They used the survey interviews as an opportunity to distribute information on diabetes and to solicit interest in a self-help group. Members of the study then met with local diabetic Asian immigrants who were interested in founding a mutual help group.

The research team, in conjunction with diabetic community members, publicized the group and also occasionally provided guest speakers on diabetes to the group. The meetings of the mutual help group were run entirely by local diabetic residents. The language spoken during meetings was Punjabi, except when Gujerati residents were present, in which case Hindi was spoken. Attendance varied from 15–50 diabetic residents and their families. At the meetings, members provided each other with mutual support, social contact, and occasional cultural and recreational activities (e.g., celebration of the festival of Diwali). Information about diabetes was also provided, and health professionals were sometimes invited to discuss diet, foot care, eye care, and the like.

The research team also supported the mutual help group by conducting a longitudinal evaluation of its effects. Over a 12-month period, individuals who attended the group showed increases in their knowledge about diabetes and decreases in their high-glycated hemoglobin. A comparison group of diabetic nonattenders showed no such changes.

Perhaps most importantly, after relying on the research team in its early stages, the group became increasingly independent. Two years after its inception, it became completely independent of the Coventry Diabetes Study, and had been running for 4 years at the time of Simmons's article in 1992. Instead of fading away when the professionals moved on, this self-help group was still being run entirely by residents after the study had ended. The study team successfully avoided the ruggedly individualistic extreme of not helping the group get started at all, and the paternalistic extreme of trying to control it themselves. The net result of their collaboration is that the community has created a mediating structure that continues to serve as a cost-free, accessible resource for residents. Such "seeding" of new groups represents an exciting opportunity for future health-promotion efforts.

The advantages to collaborating with mutual help groups on health-promotion projects are potentially great. First, these groups encourage people to help each other with health problems, thus setting a powerful norm that serves as a counterweight to the American cultural prescription of rugged individualism in dealing with health problems. Second, because mutual help groups expect members to give as well as receive help, everyone being helped by the group has the opportunity to help others and also influence how the group operates. Third, they foster diversity, instead of a one-size-fits-all approach to health promotion such as what occurs in paternalistic health promotion policies. For example, alcoholic individuals can choose from mutual help groups that emphasize abstinence (e.g., Alcoholics Anonymous) or moderate drinking (e.g., Moderation Management); that are for men and women (e.g., Smart Recovery), or women only (e.g., Women for Sobriety); and groups that have an atheistic and rational philosophy (e.g., Rational Recovery) or groups that are steeped in fundamentalist Christian thought (e.g., Alcoholics for Christ).

The Electronic Community on the Internet

The Internet can be viewed as a form of community and as a mediating structure. In the book, *The Virtual Community*, Rheingold (1994) described many facets of community on the WELL or Whole Earth 'Lectronic Link. Rheingold believes that a virtual community forms when enough people have maintained continued discourse "with sufficient feeling, to form webs of personal relationships in cyberspace" (p.5). Many components of the Internet have already been used to promote health or link people interested in health promotion (e.g., Glowniak, 1995; Harris, 1995; Rheingold, 1994). The Internet and the other "new media" offer many advantages over more traditional sources of health information such as magazines, booklets, newspapers, and videos. The Internet excels at allowing educational materials to be customized along a number of dimensions such as the individual's preferred learning style, literacy level, existing level of knowledge, and motivation, among others (Dede & Fontana, 1995; Gustafson, Bosworth, Chewning, & Hawkins, 1987; Vickery, 1995). Thus, these technologies can avoid paternalism by allowing for sufficient local customization and promoting active learner involvement in the educational process.

Another advantage of the Internet is that content can be presented in very interesting and motivating formats. The multimedia and hypertext capabilities of the World Wide Web can generate more user interest than the noninteractive written materials commonly used by health educators. At the same time, the Internet overcomes the alienation inherent in rugged individualism by linking people across different states, nations, and cultures. Furthermore, the democratic spirit of rugged individualism is maintained, because consumers can readily access health and medical information from an array of diverse sources at a time and place they choose. Thus, the Internet features many of the best aspects of mediating structures: it is mostly run by lay people; its offerings reflect a very broad array of interests; and it has excellent potential for sustainability.

In some ways, the virtual environment is no substitute for face-to-face human interaction, but in many ways this is a benefit because of the flexibility and anonymity it affords. "Hi-touch" is not always better than hi-tech. Vickery (1995) noted that one of the greatest challenges facing the computerized technologies is attempting to meet people's needs for "emotional and social support in dealing with major health problems and decisions" (p. 57). Interestingly, Vickery noted that this has usually been one of the strengths of mutual help groups, leading him to advocate for the integration of new media technologies with mutual help. Forming mutual help groups online provides the best of both worlds; with online mutual help groups, responses to problems or concerns can be thoughtfully prepared offline and then posted, giving them the feel of a slow motion mutual help group (Madara, 1995). Online groups also overcome many of the barriers to traditional groups, such as lack of an existing group to attend, rarity of the condition, lack of transportation, and demanding 24-hour caregiver responsibilities (Madara, 1995). Although in some cases individuals find comfort on the Internet from helping professionals, overwhelmingly most of the support and assistance appears to come from fellow participants.

Community Coalitions

Community coalitions, which are also called partnerships, can have many different forms. In general, they are "an organization of individuals representing diverse organizations, factions or constituencies who agree to work together in order to achieve a common goal" (Feighery & Rogers, 1990, p. 1). Coalitions have many functions, such as broadening the mission of member organizations, developing wider support for issues, developing financial and human resources, and strengthening local organizations and institutions to respond better to the needs and aspirations of their constituents (Chavis, 1995). In general, there are three types of coalitions: grassroots coalitions that seek to pressure political decisionmakers to act; professional coalitions that strive to increase their power and influence; and community-based coalitions that are composed of both grassroots and professional members (Feighery & Rogers, 1990).

If the number of times coalitions are mentioned in published journal articles and community health texts is an appropriate indicator of interest, then community coalitions appear to be very popular health-promotion vehicles. Several recent reports (Butterfoss, Goodman & Wandersman, 1993; Kumpfer, Turner, Hopkins & Librett, 1993) attest to the interest and potential for community coalitions to be excellent vehicles to achieve health goals and to promote community input and empowerment. These different forms of coalitions are mediating structures in the truest sense. They represent the community (often disenfranchised groups) and they subvert the problems of paternalism by relying on grassroots experiences and local control. Furthermore, because they usually help unify a broad segment of the population, they also avoid many of the pitfalls of rugged individualism.

One successful coalition grappled with the issue of gay rights in Oregon, where a proposed ballot measure (Measure 13) restricting gay rights sparked considerable community debate. More interesting than the fact that the measure failed was the innovative process of community unification and coalition-building that resulted in the midst of this divisive political issue. Because communities are not homogenous, many health issues can generate friction from opposing community groups (Robertson & Minkler, 1994), which can derail any possible health gains unless health promoters can help find common ground.

In Oregon, factions representing religious and conservative groups clashed with more liberal factions promoting gay rights. To bridge what seemed to be irreconcilable differences, a group called "A New Community Meeting" was created by community organizers. Basically, participants agreed that they would disagree on some of the issues, but still met behind closed doors in mediated sessions. Eventually, the group produced a 12-page document on their agreements! Although the process did not generate complete consensus on the issue, an editorial in Eugene's Register-Guard ("Common ground exists," 1994) commented that it produced many agreements and successfully "lowered the temperature of the debate." This process, developed by dispute resolution specialists, is notable for fostering community unity in the face of an acrimonious debate. This is an important lesson for those in community health promotion: it is feasible to find common ground on seemingly intractable issues, and collaboration means acknowledging disparate community voices, especially viewpoints starkly different from our own.

A case study of a mental-health coalition provides an intimate portrayal of the aspirations, struggles, and victories of one coalition in Canada (Nelson, 1994). A private citizen whose son was a mental-health consumer initiated the group in close collaboration with a local researcher. Their first step was to conduct a needs assessment, which they presented at a community forum. The needs assessment results revealed that many consumers lacked social support and experienced significant housing problems. A broad-based coalition was formed consisting of mental health and community service providers, parents, families, friends, and consumers. This group established an organizational structure and mutually agreed that their primary goal would be to increase housing and aftercare support programs for consumers through advocacy and community education. Details about coalition activities spanning 6 years were well-documented by Nelson (1994). These activities ultimately led to many of the desired outcomes. For instance, the number of supportive housing options for consumers rose over 300% from the baseline period, and community mental health funding increased by more than 400%, which far exceeded funding increases for other health programs in that period. In summary, because the fruitful collaboration between the researcher and the community groups contributed to many of the successes of this group, this example serves as a good role model for the process of health professionals collaborating with mediating structures like coalitions.

Religious Organizations

Another key mediating structure in our society is provided by churches and religious organizations. Virtually all Americans (96%) report believing in God or a universal spirit, and 88% say that religion is important in their lives (Gallup Organization, 1995). Religious involvement or religiosity is a robust predictor of not developing alcohol and drug problems (Gorsuch, 1988), has been related to better recovery from surgery (Pressman, Lyons, Larson, & Strain, 1990) and even reduced probability of death following cardiac surgery (Oxman, Freeman, & Manheimer, 1995). Churches have also been a constant, stable source of inspiration and fellowship for many ethnic and racial populations: "Schools open, schools close, factories come in, and factories leave, but the church door is always open. Ministers, pastors, priests, elders, bishops, and other church leaders work 24 hours a day, 7 days a week" (Tuggle, 1995, p. 635). Religious settings have had a long history of caring for the body as well as the soul, and therefore make great companions for health promotion activities. Many are already involved in health-related activities; about two-thirds of Northern Black churches reported sponsoring a community outreach program, focusing on topics such as human sexuality, AIDS education, pregnancy and drug abuse prevention, and domestic violence (Thomas, Quinn, Billingsley & Caldwell, 1994).

More recently, health-promotion professionals have sought greater collaborative relationships with religious organizations, even though religious groups have a long history of promoting member health on their own. This synergy, which draws on the strengths of each party, has excellent potential for improving health and closing the existing gaps in health status, especially for racial and ethnic populations (Carter Center and The Park Ridge Center, 1990). Early interventions with religious organizations were usually limited to using them as a convenient recruiting sites for professionally delivered interventions, such as screenings for blood pressure or diabetes, and for cardiovascular risk reduction (e.g., National Heart, Lung, and Blood Institute, 1989). Later, church members were enlisted to deliver or assist with intervention delivery, usually as trained lay health advisors (DePue, Wells, Lasater, & Carleton, 1990).

Most recently, religious organizations have entered into partnerships or coalitions with health organizations. For example, there is the Heart, Body, and Soul program, which a broad-based collaborative effort of CURE (Clergy United for the Renewal of East Baltimore), The Johns Hopkins University, a health department, community groups, and various local churches (Levine et al., 1992). A unique aspect of this project is the collaborative spirit of the endeavor. The project was designed to be community-based, community-owned, community-directed, and developed in conjunction with the expertise within an academic medical center. The organizational structure of the project also reflects the equal standing within the partnership of The Johns Hopkins School of Medicine and the CURE group. The goal of the project is to reduce morbidity and mortality and improve the health status of the African American population in East Baltimore. These goals were realized according to evaluation data that showed participants having significant increases in the rate of controlled hypertension, which led to decreased hospitalization and mortality due to uncontrolled hypertension (Levine et al., 1992).

Unfortunately, religious organizations have had mixed experiences with researchers. In the area of mental health promotion, Rappaport (1981) commented that despite the fact that most Americans are formal members of religious organizations and that these settings play many important roles in their lives, these settings have been routinely ignored by mental health professionals, or "conceptualized as if they were second-rate mental health agencies in need of psychological consultation, rather than as places for us to learn from" (p. 20). For this and other reasons, religious groups have been suspicious and reluctant to participate in activities with parties raising the health-promotion banner. The newer, more collaborative approaches to engaging religious organizations, however, serve as counteragents to the paternalistic approaches of the past.

Eng and Hatch (1991) encouraged researchers to modify their frame of reference when collaborating so that they are able to recognize, learn from, and draw upon the expertise that is indigenous to the religious setting. Others suggest that actively incorporating aspects of religious culture into intervention demonstrates sensitivity to religious and cultural customs. For example, the religious concept of "witnessing" by church members was employed to increase breast self-exam and mammography usage among African American women (Erwin, Spatz, & Turturro, 1992). Women with breast cancer testified to others (witnessed) about discovering the breast lump, the treatment process, and their own philosophy about survival. Another example of cultural tailoring is the use of *promotoras*, peer health workers, within the Companeros en la Salud (Partners in Health Project) (Castro et al., 1995). There is some evidence to suggest that religious and cultural tailoring may enhance the effectiveness of interventions. For instance, a multimodal culturally relevant and spiritually based approach to smoking cessation was more effective than standard self-help approaches, both of which were distributed at churches serving urban African American populations (Voorhees et al., 1996).

Religious settings are diverse and have different traditions of health and healing that need to be considered during collaboration (Carter Center and The Park Ridge Center, 1990; Thomas et al., 1994). Furthermore, individual religious organizations will desire differing levels of collaboration with health promotion programs; therefore, matching desired involvement and commitment is essential (Lasater, Carleton, & Wells, 1991). Finally, the sustainability of the intervention can be maximized by careful planning to ensure that the resulting product is truly community-owned and controlled (Altman, 1995; Lasater et al., 1991; Levine et al., 1992). Greater collaboration with religious organizations, like collaboration with other mediating structures, usually involves greater sharing of responsibility for development and implementation. Interestingly, greater involvement by health professionals in one church program did not offer advantages over lower involvement; churches with the lowest professional involvement conducted more health screenings of their members than churches with greater professional involvement (DePue et al., 1990; Lasater, Wells, Carleton & Elder, 1986).

CONCLUSIONS

Like others who have argued that it is unproductive to debate whether the focus of health promotion should be primarily ruggedly individualistic (i.e., micro) or paternalistic (i.e., macro) (Green & Raeburn, 1990; Robertson & Minkler, 1994; Yeo, 1993), the goal should be to strike a proper balance between these extremes. One way to maximize the strengths of these contrasting philosophies is to focus on collaboration with mediating structures in the community. According to the World Health Organization, health promotion has the potential to be a potent strategy for synthesizing the personal choice associated with rugged individualism and the social responsibility associated with paternalism (Working Group on the Concept and Principles of Health Promotion, 1986). Health researchers, clinicians, program managers, and health psychologists can increase their effectiveness by focusing more energy on collaboration with mediating structures such as mutual help groups, the Internet, community coalitions, and religious settings.

We have briefly mentioned strategies and tactics for achieving collaborative relationships. In the program evaluation literature, advocates have outlined innovative approaches to ensuring collaborative relationships (Guba & Lincoln, 1989; Patton, 1982). Similarly, community psychologists (Rappaport, 1990; Serrano-Garcia, 1990) provide detailed approaches that strongly encourage researchers to involve community members and groups in all stages of community research, including the very beginning stages. Collectively, these approaches indicate a "doing with" orientation instead of a "doing to" or "doing for" approach, which Altman (1995) argues will lead to greater sustainability of programs and their effects. As Altman concedes, a collaborative or partnership model to community research may not be more effective than other approaches, but it is very likely to be more sustainable. Furthermore, these collaborative approaches can succeed in maximizing community control, allowing for substantial diversity in health decisions, being socially compassionate, and utilizing scientific knowledge. Labonte's (1994) advice on terms of authentic partnership is instructive and can help prevent the field from merely substituting the "tyranny of the community" for the "tyranny of the professional" (Robertson & Minkler, 1994).

This does not imply that mediating structures are always beneficent. Mediating structures can be wrong as easily as health professionals, leading Minkler (1994) to recommend "Honor thy community—but do not make it holy" (p. 528). Yet collaborating with mediating structures offers many important potential benefits, such as shared control between professionals and those they aim to serve, respect for diversity, prolonged program sustainability, and application of expert knowledge with coercive expert control.

REFERENCES

Abrams, D. B., Elder, J. P., Carleton, R. A., Lasater, T. M., & Artz, L. M. (1986). Social learning principles for organizational health promotion: An integrated approach. In M. F. Cataldo & T. J. Coates (Eds.), *Health and industry: A behavioral medicine perspective* (pp. 28–51). New York: John Wiley & Sons.

Altman, D. G. (1995). Sustaining interventions in community systems: On the relationship between researchers and communities. *Heath Psychology, 14*, 526–536.

Ardell, D. B. (1977). *High level wellness: An alternative to doctors, drugs and disease*. Emmaus, PA: Rodale.

Bandura, A. (1986). *Social foundations of thought and action: a social cognitive theory*. Englewood Cliffs, NJ: Prentice-Hall.

Beauchamp, D. (1987). Life-style, public health and paternalism. In S. Doxiadis (Ed.), *Ethical dilemmas in health promotion* (pp. 69–81). New York: John Wiley & Sons.

Beauchamp, D. E. (1980). Public health and individual liberty. *Annual Review of Public Health, 1*, 121–136.

Becker, M. H. (1986). The tyranny of health promotion. *Annals of Internal Medicine, 14*, 15–25.

Bellah, R. N., Madsen, R., Sullivan, W. M., Swidler, A., & Tipton, S. M. (1985). *Habits of the heart: Individualism and commitment in American life*. New York: Harper & Row.

Berger, P. L., & Neuhaus, R. J. (1977). *To empower people: the role of mediating structures in public policy*. Washington, DC: American Enterprise Institute for Public Policy Research.

Biglan, A. (1995). Ethical principles for changing cultural practices. *Changing cultural practices: A contextualist framework for intervention research* (pp. 179–204). Reno, NV: Context.

Breckon, D. J., Harvey, J. R., & Lancaster, R. B. (1994). *Community health education: Settings, roles, and skills for the 21st Century*. Gaithersburg, MD: Aspen.

Brownell, K. D., Marlatt, G. A., Lichtenstein, E., & Wilson, G. T. (1986). Understanding and preventing relapse. *American Psychologist, 41*, 765–782.

Butterfoss, F. D., Goodman, R. M., & Wandersman, A. (1993). Community coalitions for prevention and health promotion. *Health Education Research, 8*, 315–330.

Carter Center, The, and The Park Ridge Center. (1990). *Healthy People 2000: A role for America's religious communities*. Chicago: Author.

Castro, F. G., Elder, J., Coe, K., Tafoya-Barraza, H. M., Moratto, S., Campbell, N., & Talavera, G. (1995). Mobilizing churches for health promotion in Latino communities: Companeros en la Salud. *Journal of the National Cancer Institute Monographs, 18*, 127–135.

Charlton, B. G. (1993). Public versus personal health [Editorial]. *Public Health, 107*, 397–399.

Chavis, D. M. (1995). Building community capacity to prevent violence through coalitions and partnerships. *Journal of Health Care for the Poor and Underserved, 6*, 234–245.

COMMIT Research Group. (1995). Community Intervention Trial for Smoking Cessation (COMMIT): II. Changes in adult cigarette smoking prevalence. *American Journal of Public Health, 85*, 193–200.

Common ground exists. (1994, June 17). *The Register-Guard*, p. 18A.

Dede, C., & Fontana, L. (1995). Transforming health education via new media. In L. M. Harris (Ed.), *Health and the new media: Technologies transforming personal and public health* (pp. 163–183). Mahway, NJ: Erlbaum.

DePue, J. D., Wells, B. L., Lasater, T. M., & Carleton, R. A. (1990). Volunteers as providers of heart health program in churches: A report on implementation. *American Journal of Health Promotion, 4*, 361–366.

Emrick, C. D., Tonigan, J. S., Montgomery, H., & Little, L. (1993). Alcoholics Anonymous: What is currently known? In B. S. McCrady & W. R. Miller (Eds.), *Research on Alcoholics Anonymous: Opportunities and alternatives* (pp. 41–76). New Brunswick, NJ: Rutgers Center of Alcohol Studies.

Eng, E., & Hatch, J. W. (1991). Networking between agencies and Black churches: The lay health advisor model. *Prevention in Human Services, Vol 10*, 123–146.

Erwin, D. O., Spatz, T. S., & Turturro, C. L. (1992). Development of an African-American role model intervention to increase breast self-examination and mammography. *Journal of Cancer Education, 7*, 311–319.

Feighery, E., & Rogers, T. (1990). *Building and maintaining effective coalitions*. Palo Alto, CA: Stanford Health Promotion Resource Center.

Flynn, B. C., Ray, D. W., & Rider, M. S. (1994). Empowering communities: Action research through Healthy Cities. *Health Education Quarterly, 21*, 395–405.

Fuchs, V. R. (1974). *Who shall live? Health, economics, and social choice*. New York: Basic Books.

Gallup Organization, The. (1995). The Gallup Organization Religion Poll newsletter archive [on-line] : Available: http:\\www.gallup.com\newsletter\feb95\index.html.

Glasgow, R. E., Terborg, J. R., Hollis, J. F., Severson, H. H., & Boles, S. M. (1995). Take Heart: Results from the initial phase of a work-site wellness program. *American Journal of Public Health, 85*, 209–216.

Glasgow, R. E., Terborg, J. R., Hollis, J. F. et al. (1994). Modifying the dietary and tobacco use patterns in the worksite. The Take Heart Project. *Health Education*

Quarterly, 21, 69–82.

Glowniak, J. V. (1995). Medical resources on the Internet [see comments]. *Annals of Internal Medicine, 123*, 123–31.

Gorsuch, R. L. (1988). Psychology of religion. *Annual Review of Psychology, 39*, 201–221.

Green, L. W., & Kreuter, M. W. (1991). *Health promotion planning: An educational and environmental approach* (2nd ed.). Mountain View, CA: Mayfield.

Green, L. W., & McAlister, A. L. (1994). Macro-intervention to support health behavior: Some theoretical perspectives and practical reflections. *Health Education Quarterly, 11*, 322–339.

Green, L. W., & Raeburn, J. (1990). Contemporary developments in health promotion: Definitions and challenges. In N. Bracht (Ed.), *Health promotion at the community level* (pp. 29–44). Newbury Park, CA: Sage.

Guba, E. G., & Lincoln, Y. S. (1989). *Fourth generation evaluation.* Newbury Park, CA: Sage.

Gustafson, D. H., Bosworth, K., Chewning, B., & Hawkins, R. P. (1987). Computer-based health promotion: Combining technological advances with problem-solving techniques to effect successful health behavior changes. *Annual Review of Public Health, 8*, 387–415.

Harris, L. M. (1995). *Health and the new media: Technologies transforming personal and public health.* Mahway, NJ: Erlbaum.

Humphreys, K., & Rappaport, J. (1994). Researching self-help/mutual aid groups and organizations: Many roads, one journey. *Applied and Preventive Psychology, 3*, 217–231.

Kanfer, F. H., & Scheft, B. K. (1988). *Guiding the process of therapeutic change.* Champaign, IL: Research Press.

Kass, L. (1975). Regarding the end of medicine and the pursuit of health. *Public Interest, 40*, 11–42.

Kersell, M. W., & Milsum, J. H. (1985). A systems model of health behavior change. *Behavioral Science, 30*, 119–126.

Kessler, R. C., Mickelson, K. D., Zhao, S. (1997). Patterns and correlates of self-help group membership in the United States. *Social Policy, 27*, 27–46.

Kilwein, J. H. (1989). No pain, no gain: A puritan legacy [editorial]. *Health Education Quarterly, 16*, 9–12.

Kumpfer, K. L., Turner, C., Hopkins, R., & Librett, J. (1993). Leadership and team effectiveness in community coalitions for the prevention of alcohol and other drug abuse. *Health Education Research, 8*, 359–374.

Kurtz, L. F. (1990). The Self-Help Movement: Review of the past decade of research. *Social Work with Groups, 13*, 101–115.

Kyrouz, E. M., & Humphreys, K. (1996). Do psychiatrically disabled people benefit from participation in self-help/mutual aid organizations?: A research review. *Community Psychologist, 29*, 21–25.

Labonte, R. (1994). Health promotion and empowerment: Reflections on professional practice. *Health Education Quarterly, 21*, 253–268.

Lasater, T. M., Carleton, R. A., & Wells, B. L. (1991). Religious organizations and large-scale health related lifestyle change programs. *Journal of Heath Education, 22*, 233–239.

Lasater, T. M., Wells, B. L., Carleton, R. A., & Elder, J. P. (1986). The role of churches in disease prevention studies. *Public Health Reports, 101*, 125–131.

Levine, D. M., Becker, D. M., Bone, L. R., Stillman, F. A., Tuggle, M. B., Prentice, M., Carter, J., & Filippeli, J. (1992). A partnership with minority populations: A community model of effectiveness research. *Ethnicity & Disease, 2*, 296–305.

Lieberman, M. (1986). Self-Help groups and psychiatry. *Annual Review of Psychiatry, 5*, 744–760.

Madara, E. J. (1995, May). *Online self-help: National and world-wide networks.* Paper presented at the "The computer as a patient's assistant" Conference, Boston, MA.

McLeroy, K. R., Bibeau, D., Steckler, A., & Glanz, K. (1988). An ecological perspective on health promotion programs. *Health Education Quarterly, 15*, 351–377.

Minkler, M. (1994). Ten commitments for community health education. *Health Education Research, 9*, 527–534.

National Heart, Lung, and Blood Institute. (1989). *Churches as an avenue to high blood pressure control* (89–2725). Rockville, MD: Author.

Nelson, G. (1994). The development of a mental health coalition: a case study. *American Journal of Community Psychology, 22*, 229–255.

Oxman, T. E., Freeman, D. H., Jr., & Manheimer, E. D. (1995). Lack of social participation or religious strength and comfort as risk factors for death after cardiac surgery in the elderly. *Psychosomatic Medicine, 57*, 5–15.

Patton, M. Q. (1982). Collaborative evaluation practice with groups. In *Practical evaluation* (pp. 55–98). Beverly Hills, CA: Sage.

Pressman, P., Lyons, J. S., Larson, D. B., & Strain, J. J. (1990). Religious belief, depression, and ambulation status in elderly women with broken hips. *American Journal of Psychiatry, 147*, 758–760.

Rappaport, J. (1981). In praise of paradox: A social policy of empowerment over prevention. *American Journal of Community Psychology, 9*, 1–25.

Rappaport, J. (1990). Research methods and the empowerment social agenda. In P. Tolan, C. Keys, F. Chertok, & L. Jason (Eds.), *Researching community psychology: Issues of theory and methods* (pp. 51–63). Washington DC: American Psychological Association.

Rheingold, H. (1994). *The virtual community: Homesteading on the electronic frontier*. New York: HarperCollins.

Roberts, M. C. (1989). Public health and health psychology: Two cats of Kilkenny. *Professional Psychology: Research and Practice, 18*, 145–149.

Robertson, A., & Minkler, M. (1994). New health promotion movement: A critical examination. *Health Education Quarterly, 21*, 295–312.

Rosenstock, I. M. (1990). Personal responsibility and public policy in health promotion. In S. A. Shumaker, E. B. Schron, & J. K. Ockene (Eds.), *The handbook of health behavior change* (pp. 424–437). New York: Springer Publishing Company.

Serrano-Garcia, I. (1990). Implementing research: Putting our values to work. In P. Tolan, C. Keys, F. Chertok, & L. Jason (Eds.), *Researching community psychology: Issues of theory and methods* (pp. 171–182). Washington, DC: American Psychological Association.

Shinn, M. (1987). Expanding community psychology's domain. *American Journal of Community Psychology, 15*, 555–574.

Simmons, D. (1992). Diabetes self help facilitated by local diabetes research: The Coventry Asian Diabetes Support Group. *Diabetic Medicine, 9*, 866–869.

Steckler, A., Allegrante, J. P., Altman, D., Brown, R., Burdine, J. N., Goodman, R. M., & Jorgensen, C. (1995). Health education intervention strategies: Recommendations for future research. *Health Education Quarterly, 22*, 307–328.

Stokols, D. (1992). Establishing and maintaining healthy environments: Toward a social ecology of health promotion. *American Psychologist, 47*, 6–22.

Taylor, C. B., & Stunkard, A. J. (1993). Public health approaches to weight control. In A. J. Stunkard & T. A. Wadden (Eds.), *Obesity: theory and therapy* (pp. 335–353). New York: Raven.

Terris, M. (1980). Epidemiology as a guide to health policy. *Annual Review of Public Health, 1*, 323–344.

Thomas, S. B., Quinn, S. C., Billingsley, A., & Caldwell, C. H. (1994). The characteristics of northern Black churches with community health outreach programs. *American Journal of Public Health, 84*, 575–579.

Tuggle, M. B. (1995). New insights and challenges about churches as intervention sites to reach the African-American community with health information. *Journal of the National Medical Association, 87 (Supplement)*, 635–637.

Vickery, D. M. (1995). Demand management, self-care, and the New Media. In L. M. Harris (Ed.), *Health and the new media: Technologies transforming personal and public health*. Mahway, NJ: Lawrence Erlbaum.

Voorhees, C. C., Stillman, F. A., Swank, R. T., Heagerty, P. J., Levine, D. M., & Becker, D. M. (1996). Heart, Body, and Soul: Impact of church-based smoking cessation interventions on readiness to quit. *Preventive Medicine, 25*, 277–285.

White, B. J., & Madara, E. J. (1995). *The self-help sourcebook (5th ed.)*. Denville, NJ: American Self-Help Clearinghouse.

Wikler, D. (1987). Who should be blamed for being sick? *Health Education Quarterly, 14*, 11–25.

Winett, R. A., King, A. C., & Altman, D. A. (1989). *Health psychology and public health: An integrative approach*. New York: Pergamon Press.

Working Group on the Concept and Principles of Health Promotion. (1986). A discussion document on the concept and principles of health promotion. *Health Promotion, 1*, 73–76.

Yeo, M. (1993). Toward an ethic of empowerment for health promotion. *Health Promotion International, 8*, 225–235.

24

Ethical Issues in Lifestyle Change and Adherence

Ruth R. Faden

In this chapter I examine issues in lifestyle change and adherence from the perspective of normative ethics. Central to frameworks of ethical analysis in normative ethics is the notion that moral deliberation and justification ordinarily rest on principles, rules, and rights, understood as abstract action guides. These action guides, the choice and analysis of which are inherently controversial, together with questions of their relationship with one another and their relationship to a theory of virtues, constitute the heart of modern ethical theory.

Structures of principles and rules, rights, and virtues can be used to analyze questions of morality, in particular concrete situations and arenas of social life. Often such analysis is referred to as "applied ethics." Numerous areas of applied ethics have been identified, such as business ethics and journalism ethics.

Three areas of applied ethics of particular relevance to the themes of this volume are the ethics of the healing professions, research ethics, and ethics and public policy. For our purposes, these fields can be understood as the ethics of the professional-patient relationship, the ethics of the researcher-subject relationship, and the ethics of the government-citizenry relationship, respectively.

This chapter is reprinted from the first edition of this book.

In this chapter I highlight the origins and characteristics of some of the key moral issues related to life-style and adherence in each of these areas: clinician-patient, researcher-subject, and government-citizenry. Relevant principles and rules emerge as each area is discussed.

Before proceeding, however, one caveat is in order having to do with the difficulty of treating together questions of adherence in a clinical context and questions of life-style for the general public. The ethical issues raised by adherence with prescribed medical regimens for the clinically ill can be substantively different from the issues raised in relation to adoption of recommendations of the Surgeon General or the American Heart Association regarding healthy lifestyles. While it is beyond the scope of this chapter to take these differences systematically into account, the sections that follow vary in the extent to which they focus on adherence versus general life-style issues.

THE CLINICIAN-PATIENT RELATIONSHIP

Most of the chapters in this volume have focused specifically on adherence and life-style issues in health care services and the clinical encounter. In Freidman's chapter (Chapter 4), reference is made to how different models of the physician-patient relationship affect issues of adherence. Medical ethics also operate with models of the doctor-patient relationship. One such approach argues that the doctor-patient relationship in particular, and all health professional-patient relationships generally, are dominated by two competing models of moral responsibility—the beneficence model and the autonomy model (Beauchamp & McCullough, 1985).

Under the beneficence model, the *primary* obligation of clinicians is to seek the best balance of good over harm for their patients. Goods and harms are understood in strictly medical terms, such that the chief goods are health, the prevention or elimination of disease and injury, relief from pain and suffering, the amelioration of disabilities, and the prolongation of life. The principal harms at issue are death, disease, disability, pain, and suffering.

By contrast, under the autonomy model the values and beliefs of the patient become the primary moral consideration. If the patient's values conflict with the values of medicine, the clinician's primary moral obligation is to respect and facilitate the patient's preferences.

Both models speak to important moral truths about the professional-patient relationship. However, occasionally the requirements of these models can come into conflict. A central moral task is fixing the limits of each of these two models, in light of the demands of the other, in particular contexts.

The perspective of the beneficence model provides strong moral support for adherence interventions in clinical settings. Under this model, clinicians have a moral obligation, an affirmative duty, to take actions that will preserve the health of their patients and prevent them from disease and injury. Thus, insofar as clinicians are not taking seriously their obligations to secure the adherence of their patients to medically indicated regimens, clinicians are morally blameworthy. This moral obligation has been given legal force in a California case in which a physician was held liable for not adequately informing his patient of the risks of failing to have a Pap test (*Truman v. Thomas*, 1980).

There are, of course, limits under the beneficence model to the clinician's obligation to be proactive in securing patient adherence. It is a fundamental maxim of ethics that "ought implies can." Insofar as it is not possible for clinicians to implement adherence interventions or otherwise secure adherence, they have no obligation to do so. Whether or not it is possible for physicians to secure adherence raises a host of issues discussed in earlier chapters, including the amount of time and the kinds of skills needed to be successful in promoting adherence in clinical contexts.

A related point is the relative moral priority of competing clinical duties in a context of limited resources. When the amount of time and dollars to be spent on clinical encounters is limited, what priority is to be placed on activities that cure disease, as compared with those that allay suffering, prevent deterioration, or promote health? Although clinicians may have a prima facie obligation to seek adherence to medical regimens and lifestyle recommendations, these obligations may necessarily be less weighty than other duties competing for the clinician's attention.

In contrast to the beneficence model, the autonomy model does not provide clinicians with a direct moral warrant for securing adherence to medical recommendations. Under the autonomy model, if the patient's values do not include improving his or her health prospects by altering lifestyle or adhering to medications, then the clinician is obligated to respect that value preference.

This is not to say, however, that the autonomy model releases clinicians from any obligation in relation to adherence and lifestyle. At minimum, respect for the patient's autonomy requires the clinician to ascertain the basis for the patient's position and, in particular, to establish whether the patient's rejection of the clinician's recommendation is based on an adequate understanding of what is at stake. As Andrew Baum pointed out earlier in this volume (Commentary, Section 1), one cannot assume that naive theories of disease conform to medical theories of disease and thus that lay persons and clinicians will necessarily share an understanding of the importance of certain recommended behaviors in preventing or curing disease.

What if the clinician ascertains that the patient has a correct understanding of what is at stake in refusing to adhere to medical recommendations and still wishes to ignore them? In my view, the clinician's beneficence-based obligations require the clinician to attempt to persuade the patient to change his or her position. I have argued elsewhere that persuasive interventions, properly constrained, do not violate obligations to respect patient autonomy (Faden & Beauchamp, 1986). However, if, after reasonable attempts at persuasion, the patient's values remain fixed, these must be respected.

The ascendance of the autonomy model in thinking about the ethics of the physician-patient relationship has been reflected in the adherence literature. What was once referred to as the problem of "compliance with doctor's orders" has become the problem of "adherence to the recommendations of professionals." Even this second adherence formulation is not wholly satisfactory. In line with the autonomy model, a more desirable formulation would entail something like the following: "assisting individuals to make informed and reflective choices about whether to adopt or reject professional recommendations."

Contrasting the beneficence model of professional-patient relationships with the autonomy model helps highlight the central moral issues raised by adherence and lifestyle interventions in clinical settings. However, in isolation this approach draws too stark a contrast between competing moral principles and fails to capture much of the textual richness of the clinician-patient relation. An alternative approach in moral theory, frequently referred to as the care perspective, draws attention to issues of responsiveness and compassion in the moral life, including the need to respond to that which is unique and particular about the other in a moral relationship (Areen, 1988; Hanen & Nielsen, 1987). The care perspective reminds us to refrain from being formulaic in our approach to moral issues. In clinical encounters, each patient brings a unique history and life experience. From the care perspective, assisting "individuals to make informed and reflective choices" about medical regimens or lifestyle changes requires compassionate attention to the needs of the patient as a unique individual.

In providing such assistance, professionals should recognize that there exist genuine epistemic challenges to the validity of medical knowledge and thus to the force of medical opinion and recommendation. Earlier I made reference to the recognition that naive theories of disease are not always isomorphic with medical theories and thus that patients may be basing their decisions to reject medical recommendations on false beliefs and incomplete understanding. It is also the case, however, that naive theories of disease are not always so naive. That is, patients' beliefs about the etiology and treatment of disease can be more correct than the opposing beliefs of medical experts. As Rosenstock notes in Chapter 23, the medical community has a notable history of being wrong in its predictions and recommendations regarding both health risks and protective behaviors. Patients of the past who refused to increase their consumption of eggs and who refused to take swine flue shots were all at the time considered to be "noncompliers" who held "false beliefs" by contemporary medical standards. To a significant extent, this sort of disagreement between patient and physician is an epistemic problem about the nature of medical knowledge and its evidentiary base, in a context of ever-evolving scientific theories of disease and illness. At stake is whether physicians can offer anything stronger than medical opinions, a far cry from the tradition of the "doctor's order."

THE RESEARCHER-SUBJECT RELATIONSHIP

The ethics of the researcher-subject relationship has a different tradition and a different social imperative from that of the physician-patient relationship. In the clinical context, ethics is guided, at least in part, by the assumption that both clinician and patient share the goal of seeking to improve the patient's welfare. By contrast, in research the primary goal is not to benefit the subject but to produce generalizable, "scientific" knowledge. Because the welfare of the subject is not central to the research enterprise, there is no beneficence model in research ethics corresponding to that in clinical ethics. As a result, obligations to respect the autonomy of research subjects are generally difficult to validly override, even by appeal to arguments grounded in beneficence or conceptions of the public good.

The implications of this understanding of the ethics of the researcher-subject relationship for adherence issues in research are straightforward. In general, it is not morally permissible for researchers to overlook their obligations to seek valid informed consent from their subjects and respect potential subjects' decisions to refuse to participate or to drop out of studies, even when honoring these obligations threatens or compromises the scientific integrity of their research. When tensions arise between respecting the refusals of subjects and promoting the cooperation of subjects, the interventions of researchers should be restricted to persuasion and to inducements that do not substantially undermine the voluntariness of the subjects' decisions.

THE GOVERNMENT-CITIZENRY RELATIONSHIP

That government has both the obligation and the right to protect the public health is clear. What is less clear is the scope of this government obligation. What kinds of threats to health are covered under this government obligation? What means should the government use to control these threats?

The answers to these questions turn on a complex of principles and values, including, most prominently, respect for autonomy, justice, public welfare, and utility. How the demands of these principles are to be balanced or blended depends critically on one's theory of the state, in our case, on one's theory of the liberal state in a democratic society.

In Chapter 23, Dr. Rosenstock suggests that I and other writers on this subject have been internally inconsistent in our position on government-sponsored health campaigns. I have expressed concerns about autonomy issues in health education efforts while calling for restrictive government regulatory action (Faden, 1987). However, Rosenstock's criticism is a misreading of my analysis. There is no inconsistency involved; rather, there is an application of the principles to different cases, cases that differ in the extent to which the different principles come into play.

Strong state action is most clearly morally demanded when the health of innocent parties is placed at risk by the actions of others and there is a feasible way to remove the risk through regulation or environmental control. Classic examples here include asbestos and lead exposures in the workplace or the home, unsafe appliances, and carcinogenic food additives.

State action is demanded in such cases by a complex of principles including justice and utility. It should be noted that these cases do not raise relevant autonomy issues. That is, there is no substantive conflict between the demands of justice and obligations to respect autonomy. To be facetious, one rarely asserts a liberty right to be exposed to lead or asbestos.

Note also that the lead and asbestos cases are classic examples of what has been referred to in the literature as victim-blaming situations. Health education interventions to promote the wearing of respiratory protective gear among workers in inadequately ventilated plants or to promote more vigilant behavior among tenants in lead-contaminated apartments are indeed morally suspect, and in many circumstances morally unconscionable.

The moral issues are somewhat more complicated when we move to cases where there are plausibly some autonomy interests at issue, but the autonomy interests do not involve weighty liberty values. The classic example here is the seat belt and air bag controversy.

Those outside the automobile industry opposed to compulsory seat belt legislation claim, among other things, a liberty right to drive unharnessed. Those opposed to mandatory air bags claim, among other things, a liberty right to decide whether they wish to pay the additional costs of air bag installation, which will be passed on to consumers.

The position one takes in relation to this controversy depends to a significant extent on the value one places on these particular liberty interests, in comparison to values placed on the other principles. Whether media campaigns or other forms of behavioral interventions as alternatives to regulation are morally preferable or morally questionable turns on a complex balancing of these competing values and principles.

Not all health issues entail strong arguments for coercive state action—either because the autonomy interests outweigh any other consideration, or because effective technological or regulatory solutions do not exist or are by themselves insufficient. Here, interventions directed at individuals are particularly fitting. I have in mind such health issues as oral hygiene, breast self-exam, safer sexual practices, and exercise.

In many of these instances, where the autonomy interests are strong it is important to evaluate behavioral interventions in terms of their effect on autonomous choice. There is not, however, always consensus about which health issues entail strong autonomy interests, at least in part because of fundamental disagreements about the causal determinants of behavior. Nevertheless, at least for some people, many of the classic lifestyle issues of diet and exercise fall into this area. More paradigmatically, reproductive behaviors—abortion in the instance of fetuses who would be disabled, contraceptive use, and so on—are recognized by many to entail strong autonomy interests such that any intervention, behavioral or otherwise, must be carefully scrutinized for its impact on autonomous choice.

The discussion thus far has focused on ethics, to the exclusion of politics. However, any evaluation of the ethics of government lifestyle and adherence interventions must recognize that there are instances in which regulatory or environmental intervention is morally preferable but politically impossible, at least at the moment. How government officials and researchers ought to proceed under such circumstances is difficult to stipulate in the abstract. Consider, for example, Altman's discussion about smoking behavior and advertising in Chapter 13. Under such circumstances, there will certainly be situations in which interventions directed at individuals are morally permissible as the only available strategy for dealing with a health problem.

SUMMARY

This chapter focuses on traditional issues of justice and autonomy as they relate to adherence and lifestyle issues. One variant of the justice and autonomy themes not discussed is the morality of promoting healthier lifestyles in a context in which millions of Americans are denied access to basic health services. Any thorough examination of the ethics of lifestyle change and adherence must address not only whether the characteristics of specific interventions conform with obligations to respect autonomy, but also whether the resources needed to mount these interventions have been justly allocated.

A thorough examination of the ethics of lifestyle change and adherence must also address how our ethics affect our evaluation designs. To the extent that we claim that our objective is merely to encourage people to make informed voluntary decisions regarding their health, then should not our primary evaluation criterion be the quality of the choice made by those to which our interventions are aimed, rather than the choices themselves? If this is true, then our evaluation criterion is not how many subjects stayed in the trial, but how well they understood what was involved in participating in the trial, regardless of whether they consented or refused, stayed in or dropped out. The issue becomes not how many hypertensives took their medications according to directions, but how many made an informed reflective decision about whether they wanted to take the medication as recommended. Whether we are willing to have our evaluations conform with our ethics remains a challenge for the field.

REFERENCES

Areen, J. (1988). A need for caring. *Michigan Law Review, 86*, 967–1082.

Beauchamp, T. L., & McCullough, L. B. (1984). *Medical ethics*. Englewood Cliffs, NJ: Prentice-Hall.

Faden, R. R. (1987). Ethical issues in government sponsored public health campaigns. *Health Education Quarterly*, 14 (1), 27–37.

Faden, R. R., & Beauchamp, T. L. (1986). *A history and theory of informed consent*. New York: Oxford University Press.

Hanen, M., & Nielsen, K. (Eds.). (1987). Science, morality and feminist theory. *Canadian Journal of Philosophy, 13* (Supplement).

Truman v. Thomas, 165 Cal. Rptr. 308, 611 P.2d 902 (Cal. 1980).

Index

('i' indicates an illustration; 'n' indicates a note; 't' indicates a table)